Update on Non-Alcoholic Steatohepatitis

Editor

ZOBAIR M. YOUNOSSI

CLINICS IN LIVER DISEASE

www.liver.theclinics.com

Consulting Editor
NORMAN GITLIN

May 2023 • Volume 27 • Number 2

ELSEVIER

1600 John F. Kennedy Boulevard • Suite 1800 • Philadelphia, Pennsylvania, 19103-2899

http://www.theclinics.com

CLINICS IN LIVER DISEASE Volume 27, Number 2
May 2023 ISSN 1089-3261, ISBN-13: 978-0-323-96056-4

Editor: Kerry Holland
Developmental Editor: Ann Gielou M. Posedio

Clinics in Liver Disease (ISSN 1089-3261) is published quarterly by Elsevier Inc., 360 Park Avenue South, New York, NY 10010-1710. Months of issue are February, May, August, and November. Business and Editorial Offices: 1600 John F. Kennedy Blvd., Ste. 1800, Philadelphia, PA 19103-2899. Customer Service Office: 3251 Riverport Lane, Maryland Heights, MO 63043. Periodicals postage paid at New York, NY and additional mailing offices. Subscription prices are $339.00 per year (U.S. individuals), $100.00 per year (U.S. student/resident), $674.00 per year (U.S. institutions), $434.00 per year (international individuals), $200.00 per year (international student/resident), $837.00 per year (international instituitions), $393.00 per year (Canadian individuals), $100.00 per year (Canadian student/resident), and $837.00 per year (Canadian institutions). Foreign air speed delivery is included in all *Clinics* subscription prices. All prices are subject to change without notice. **POSTMASTER:** Send address changes to *Clinics in Liver Disease*, Elsevier Health Sciences Division, Subscription Customer Service, 3251 Riverport Lane, Maryland Heights, MO 63043. **Customer Service: Telephone: 1-800-654-2452 (U.S. and Canada); 314-447-8871 (outside U.S. and Canada). Fax: 314-447-8029. E-mail: journalscustomerservice-usa@elsevier.com (for print support); journalsonlinesupport-usa@elsevier.com (for online support).**

Reprints. For copies of 100 or more of articles in this publication, please contact the Commercial Reprints Department, Elsevier Inc., 360 Park Avenue South, New York, NY 10010-1710. Tel.: 212-633-3874; Fax: 212-633-3820; E-mail: reprints@elsevier.com.

Clinics in Liver Disease is covered in *MEDLINE/PubMed (Index Medicus)*, Science Citation Index Expanded, Journal Citation Reports/Science Edition, and Current Contents/Clinical Medicine.

Contributors

CONSULTING EDITOR

NORMAN GITLIN, MD, FRCP (LONDON), FRCPE (EDINBURGH), FAASLD, FACP, FACG
Head of Hepatology, Southern California Liver Centers, San Clemente, California, USA

EDITOR

ZOBAIR M. YOUNOSSI, MD, MPH
Betty and Guy Beatty Center for Integrated Research, Professor and Chairman, Department of Medicine, Center for Liver Diseases, Inova Fairfax Medical Campus, Inova Medicine, Liver and Obesity Research Program, Inova Health System, President, Inova Medicine Services, Claude Moore Health Education and Research Building, Falls Church, Virginia, USA

AUTHORS

MANAL F. ABDELMALEK, MD, MPH
Professor of Medicine, Director of Hepatobiliary Diseases, Division of Gastroenterology and Hepatology, Department of Medicine, Mayo Clinic, Rochester, Minnesota, USA

SALEH A. ALQAHTANI
Associate Professor of Medicine, Division of Gastroenterology and Hepatology, Johns Hopkins University, Baltimore, Maryland, USA; Professor of Medicine, Liver Transplant Center, King Faisal Specialist Hospital and Research Center, Riyadh, Saudi Arabia

KHALID ALSWAT, MD
Department of Medicine, Liver Disease Research Centre, College of Medicine, King Saud University, Riyadh, Saudi Arabia

JUAN PABLO ARAB, MD
Departamento de Gastroenterologia, Escuela de Medicina, Pontificia Universidad Catolica de Chile, Santiago, Chile; Division of Gastroenterology, Department of Medicine, Schulich School of Medicine, Western University and London Health Sciences Centre, Alimentiv, London, Ontario, Canada

MARÍA TERESA ARIAS-LOSTE, MD, PhD
Gastroenterology and Hepatology Department, Marqués de Valdecilla University Hospital, Clinical and Translational Digestive Research Group, IDIVAL, Santander, Spain

ANGELO ARMANDI, MD
Department of Medical Sciences, University of Turin, Torino, Italy

MARCO ARRESE, MD
Departamento de Gastroenterologia, Escuela de Medicina, Pontificia Universidad Catolica de Chile, Centro de Envejecimiento y Regeneración (CARE), Facultad de Ciencias Biológicas, Pontificia Universidad Católica de Chile, Santiago, Chile

RAMON BATALLER, PhD, MD
Division of Gastroenterology, Hepatology and Nutrition, Center for Liver Diseases, University of Pittsburgh Medical Center, Pittsburgh, Pennsylvania, USA

SARA BATTISTELLA, MD
Gastroenterology, Multivisceral Transplant Unit, Department of Surgery, Oncology and Gastroenterology, Padua University Hospital, Padua, Italy

DEBORA BIZZARO, BS, PhD
Gastroenterology, Multivisceral Transplant Unit, Department of Surgery, Oncology and Gastroenterology, Padua University Hospital, Padua, Italy

FERNANDO BRIL, MD
Division of Endocrinology, Diabetes and Metabolism, The University of Alabama at Birmingham, Birmingham, Alabama, USA

ELISABETTA BUGIANESI, MD, PhD
Department of Medical Sciences, University of Turin, Torino, Italy

PATRIZIA BURRA, MD, PhD
Professor, Gastroenterology, Head, Multivisceral Transplant Unit, Department of Surgery, Oncology and Gastroenterology, Padua University Hospital, Padua, Italy

JOSÉ LUIS CALLEJA, PhD, MD
Department of Gastroenterology and Hepatology, Puerta de Hierro University Hospital, Puerta de Hierro Health Research Institute (IDIPHIM), CIBERehd, Universidad Autonoma de Madrid, Majadahonda, Spain

MARLEN IVON CASTELLANOS-FERNANDEZ, MD
Institute of Gastroenterology, University of Medical Sciences of Havana, Havana, Panamericana, La Habana, Cuba

LAURENT CASTERA, MD
Université de Paris, UMR1149 (CRI), INSERM, Paris, France; Service d'Hépatologie, Assistance Publique-Hôpitaux de Paris (AP-HP), Hôpital Beaujon, Clichy, France

GRACIELA CASTRO-NARRO, MD, MSc
Department of Gastroenterology, National Institute of Medical Sciences and Nutrition Salvador Zubirán, Mexico City, Mexico

WAH-KHEONG CHAN
Professor, Gastroenterology and Hepatology Unit, Department of Medicine, Faculty of Medicine, University of Malaya, Kuala Lumpur, Malaysia

HUNZA CHAUDHRY, MD
University of California, San Francisco, Fresno, California, USA

JAVIER CRESPO, PhD, MD
Gastroenterology and Hepatology Department, Clinical and Translational Research in Digestive Diseases, Valdecilla Research Institute (IDIVAL), Marqués de Valdecilla

University Hospital, IDIVAL, Santander, Spains de Valdecilla University Hospital, Santander, Spain

KENNETH CUSI, PhD, MD
Division of Endocrinology, Diabetes and Metabolism, Department of Medicine, University of Florida, Gainesville, Florida, USA

ARKA DE, MD, DM
Department of Hepatology, Post Graduate Institute of Medical Education and Research, Chandigarh, India

JOHN F. DILLON, MD
Division of Molecular and Clinical Medicine, University of Dundee, Ninewells Hospital and Medical School, Dundee, United Kingdom

WINSTON DUNN, MD
Division of Gastroenterology and Hepatology, Department of Medicine, University of Kansas Medical Center, Kansas City, Kansas, USA

AJAY DUSEJA, MD, DM, FAMS, FAASLD, FACG, FSGEI, FISG, FINASL, Master-ISG
Professor and Head, Department of Hepatology, Post Graduate Institute of Medical Education and Research, Chandigarh, India

ERIC DYBBRO, MD
Division of Gastroenterology, Hepatology, and Nutrition, Children's Hospital Los Angeles, Los Angeles, California, USA

KATHERINE ELIZABETH EBERLY, MD
Inova Medicine, Inova Health System, Department of Medicine, Center for Liver Diseases, Inova Fairfax Medical Campus, Falls Church, Virginia, USA

MOHAMED EL-KASSAS, MD
Endemic Medicine Department, Faculty of Medicine, Helwan University, Cairo, Egypt

JIAN-GAO FAN, MD, PhD
Professor of Medicine, Department of Gastroenterology, Xinhua Hospital Affiliated to the Shanghai Jiao Tong University School of Medicine, Shanghai Key Lab of Pediatric Gastroenterology and Nutrition, Shanghai, China

SVEN FRANCQUE, MD, PhD
Professor, Department of Gastroenterology and Hepatology, Antwerp University Hospital, Laboratory of Experimental Medicine and Paediatrics (LEMP), Faculty of Medicine and Health Sciences, University of Antwerp, InflaMed Centre of Excellence, University of Antwerp, Translational Sciences in Inflammation and Immunology, University of Antwerp, Antwerp, Belgium; European Reference Network on Hepatological Diseases (ERN RARE-LIVER), Antwerp University Hospital, Edegem, Belgium

JACOB GEORGE, MD
Storr Liver Centre, The Westmead Institute for Medical Research, Westmead Hospital and University of Sydney, New South Wales, Australia

LYNN H. GERBER, MD
Department of Medicine, Betty and Guy Beatty Center for Integrated Research, Director for Research, Medicine Service Line, Inova Health System, Center for Liver Disease, Inova Fairfax Hospital, Falls Church, Virginia, USA

GIACOMO GERMANI, MD, PhD
Gastroenterology, Multivisceral Transplant Unit, Department of Surgery, Oncology and Gastroenterology, Padua University Hospital, Padua, Italy

PEGAH GOLABI, MD
Betty and Guy Beatty Center for Integrated Research, Department of Medicine, Center for Liver Disease, Inova Fairfax Medical Campus, Inova Medicine, Inova Health System, Falls Church, Virginia, USA

ZACHARY D. GOODMAN, MD, PhD
Center of Liver Diseases, Inova Fairfax Hospital, Falls Church, Virginia, USA

SAEED HAMID, MD
Department of Medicine, Aga Khan University, Karachi, Pakistan

LINDA HENRY, PhD
Department of Medicine, Center for Liver Diseases, Inova Fairfax Medical Campus, Betty and Guy Beatty Center for Integrated Research, Inova Health System, Inova Medicine, Liver and Obesity Research Program, Falls Church, Virginia, USA; Center for Outcomes Research in Liver Diseases, Washington, DC, USA

MARYAM K. IBRAHIM, MD
Department of Medicine, Massachusetts General Hospital, Harvard Medical School, Boston, Massachusetts, USA

PAULA IRUZUBIETA, PhD, MD
Gastroenterology and Hepatology Department, Clinical and Translational Research in Digestive Diseases, Valdecilla Research Institute (IDIVAL), Marqués de Valdecilla University Hospital, IDIVAL, Santander, Spains de Valdecilla University Hospital, Santander, Spain

VASILY ISAKOV, MD, PhD
Chief, Department of Gastroenterology and Hepatology, Federal Research Center for Nutrition and Biotechnology, Moscow, Russia

CAROLINA JIMÉNEZ-GONZÁLEZ, MSc
Gastroenterology and Hepatology Department, Marqués de Valdecilla University Hospital, Clinical and Translational Digestive Research Group, IDIVAL, Santander, Spain

TAKUMI KAWAGUCHI, MD, PhD
Professor, Department of Medicine, Division of Gastroenterology, Kurume University, School of Medicine, Kurume, Japan

ROHIT KOHLI, MBBS, MS
Division of Gastroenterology, Hepatology, and Nutrition, Children's Hospital Los Angeles, Los Angeles, California, USA

CHRISTOPHER J. KOPKA, JD
Independent Researcher, Salida, Colorado, USA

KRIS V. KOWDLEY, MD, FACP, FACG, FAASLD, AGAF
Liver Institute Northwest, Seattle, Washington, USA; Elson S. Floyd College of Medicine, Washington State University, Spokane, Washington, USA

AMEETA KUMAR, MD
Inova Medicine, Inova Health System, Department of Medicine, Center for Liver Diseases, Inova Fairfax Medical Campus, Falls Church, Virginia, USA

JEFFREY V. LAZARUS, PhD
Barcelona Institute for Global Health (ISGlobal), Hospital Clínic, Faculty of Medicine and Health Sciences, University of Barcelona, Barcelona, Spain; CUNY Graduate School of Public Health and Health Policy (CUNY SPH), New York, New York, USA

SIMON LEIGH, PhD
Organization for the Review of Care and Health Applications, Daresbury, United Kingdom; Institute of Digital Healthcare, University of Warwick, Coventry, United Kingdom

ROHIT LOOMBA, MD
Division of Gastroenterology and Hepatology, Department of Medicine, NAFLD Research Center, University of California San Diego, La Jolla, California, USA

NAHUM MÉNDEZ-SÁNCHEZ, MD, MSc, PhD, FAASLD, FACG, AGAF
Professor, Faculty of Medicine, National Autonomous University of Mexico, Coyoacán, Mexico City, Mexico; Liver Research Unit, Medica Sur Clinic and Foundation, Mexico City, Mexico

MARÍA LUZ MARTÍNEZ-CHANTAR, PhD
Liver Disease Laboratory, Center for Cooperative Research in Biosciences (CIC BioGUNE), Basque Research and Technology Alliance (BRTA), Centro de Investigación Biomedica en Red de Enfermedades Hepáticas y Digestivas (CIBERehd), Derio, Bizkaia, Spain

MIGUEL MATEO, MD
Pharmacy Organisation and Inspection, Government of Cantabria, Santander, Spain

MAZEN NOUREDDIN, MD, MHSc
Sherrie and Alan Conover Center for Liver Disease and Transplantation, Houston Methodist Hospital, Houston Research Institute and Houston Liver Institute, Houston, Texas, USA

JANUS ONG, MD
College of Medicine, University of the Philippines, Manila, Philippines

ANTONIO PÉREZ, PhD, MD
Endocrinology and Nutrition Department, Santa Creu i Sant Pau Hospital, Universitat Autónoma de Barcelona, IIB-Sant Pau and Centro de Investigación Biomedica en Red de Diabetes y Enfermedades Metabólicas Asociadas (CIBERDEM), Barcelona, Spain

SHREYA C. PAL, MD
Faculty of Medicine, National Autonomous University of Mexico, Coyoacán, Mexico City, Mexico; Liver Research Unit, Medica Sur Clinic and Foundation, Mexico City, Mexico

QIN PAN, MD
Research Scientist, Research Center, Zhoupu Hospital Affiliated to the Shanghai University of Medicine and Health Sciences, Department of Gastroenterology, Xinhua Hospital Affiliated to the Shanghai Jiao Tong University School of Medicine, Shanghai, China

FRANCESCO PAOLO RUSSO, MD, PhD
Professor, Gastroenterology, Multivisceral Transplant Unit, Department of Surgery, Oncology and Gastroenterology, Padua University Hospital, Padua, Italy

VLAD RATZIU, MD, PhD
Professor, Sorbonne Université, Institute of Cardiometabolism and Nutrition, Assistance Publique-Hôpitaux De Paris, Hôpital Pitié-Salpêtrière, INSERM UMRS 1138 CRC, Paris, France

LISA RICE-DUEK, MBA
Health Information Management Systems Society (HIMSS), Berlin, Germany

MARY E. RINELLA, MD, FAASLD
University of Chicago Pritzker School of Medicine, Director of the Metabolic and Fatty Liver Program, University of Chicago Hospitals, Department of Medicine, University of Chicago, Chicago, Illinois, USA

MANUEL ROMERO-GÓMEZ, PhD, MD
UCM Digestive Diseases and CIBERehd, Virgen Del Rocío University Hospital, Institute of Biomedicine of Seville, University of Seville, Seville, Spain

ALVARO SANTOS-LASO, PhD
Gastroenterology and Hepatology Department, Marqués de Valdecilla University Hospital, Clinical and Translational Digestive Research Group, IDIVAL, Santander, Spain

ARUN SANYAL, MD
Division of Gastroenterology, Hepatology and Nutrition, School of Medicine Internal Medicine, Virginia Commonwealth University Richmond, Virginia, USA

JÖRN M. SCHATTENBERG, PhD, MD
Metabolic Liver Research Program, Faculty of Social Welfare and Health Sciences, Department of Medicine, University Medical Centre Mainz, Mainz, Germany

DIPAM SHAH, MD
Inova Medicine, Inova Health System, Department of Medicine, Center for Liver Diseases, Inova Fairfax Medical Campus, Falls Church, Virginia, USA

SARAH SHALABY, MD
Gastroenterology, Multivisceral Transplant Unit, Department of Surgery, Oncology and Gastroenterology, Padua University Hospital, Padua, Italy

TRACEY G. SIMON, MD
Harvard Medical School, Division of Gastroenterology and Hepatology, Clinical and Translational Epidemiology Unit (CTEU), Massachusetts General Hospital, Boston, Massachusetts, USA

ASHWANI K. SINGAL, MD, MS, FACG, FAASLD, AGAF
Professor of Medicine, University of South Dakota Sanford School of Medicine, Avera Medical Group Liver Disease and Transplant Institute, Transplant Hepatologist, Avera McKennan University Hospital, Chief, Clinical Research Affairs Avera Transplant Institute, Veterans Affairs Medical Center, Sioux Falls, South Dakota, USA

AALAM SOHAL, MD
Liver Institute Northwest, Seattle, Washington, USA

MARIA STEPANOVA, PhD
Department of Medicine, Center for Liver Diseases, Inova Fairfax Medical Campus, Betty and Guy Beatty Center for Integrated Research, Inova Health System, Falls Church, Virginia, USA; Center for Outcomes Research in Liver Diseases, Washington, DC, USA

HIROKAZU TAKAHASHI, MD, PhD
Professor, Department of Laboratory Medicine, Liver Center, Saga University Hospital, Saga, Japan

JUAN TURNES, MD
Department of Gastroenterology and Hepatology, Complejo Hospitalario Universitario Pontevedra & IIS Galicia Sur, Pontevedra, Spain

MARCELA VILLOTA-RIVAS, MGH
Barcelona Institute for Global Health (ISGlobal), Hospital Clínic, University of Barcelona, Barcelona, Spain

MIRIAM B. VOS, MD, MSPH
Division of Gastroenterology, Hepatology, and Nutrition, Emory School of Medicine, Children's Healthcare of Atlanta, Atlanta, Georgia, USA

ROBERT WONG, MD, MS
Division of Gastroenterology and Hepatology, Stanford University School of Medicine, Gastroenterology Section, Veterans Affairs Palo Alto Healthcare System, Palo Alto, California, USA

VINCENT WONG, MD
Department of Medicine and Therapeutics, Medical Data Analytics Center, The Chinese University of Hong Kong, State Key Laboratory of Digestive Disease, Institute of Digestive Disease, The Chinese University of Hong Kong, Hong Kong, SAR

AARON YEOH, MD
Division of Gastroenterology and Hepatology, Stanford University School of Medicine, Palo Alto, California, USA

YUSUF YILMAZ, MD
Professor of Medicine, Department of Gastroenterology, School of Medicine, Recep Tayyip Erdoğan University, Rize, Turkey; Liver Research Unit, Institute of Gastroenterology, Marmara University, İstanbul, Turkey

ZOBAIR M. YOUNOSSI, MD, MPH
Betty and Guy Beatty Center for Integrated Research, Professor and Chairman, Department of Medicine, Center for Liver Diseases, Inova Fairfax Medical Campus, Inova Medicine, Liver and Obesity Research Program, Inova Health System, President, Inova Medicine Services, Claude Moore Health Education and Research Building, Falls Church, Virginia, USA

MING-LUNG YU
Professor, School of Medicine, College of Medicine, National Sun Yat-Sen University, Hepatitis Research Center, College of Medicine, Kaohsiung Medical University, Hepatobiliary Section, Department of Internal Medicine, Hepatitis Center, Kaohsiung Medical University Hospital, Division of Hepato-Gastroenterology, Department of Internal Medicine, Kaohsiung Chang Gung Memorial Hospital, Kaohsiung, Taiwan

ALBERTO ZANETTO, MD, PhD
Gastroenterology, Multivisceral Transplant Unit, Department of Surgery, Oncology and Gastroenterology, Padua University Hospital, Padua, Italy

SHIRA ZELBER-SAGI, RD, PhD
University of Haifa, School of Public Health, Mount Carmel, Haifa, Israel; Department of Gastroenterology, Tel-Aviv Medical Centre, Tel-Aviv, Israel

HIROKAZU TAKAHASHI, MD, PhD
Professor, Department of Laboratory Medicine, Liver Center, Saga University Hospital, Saga, Japan

JUAN TURNES, MD
Department of Gastroenterology and Hepatology, Complejo Hospitalario Universitario de Pontevedra & IIS Galicia Sur, Pontevedra, Spain

MARCELA VILLOTA-RIVAS, MSPH
Barcelona Institute for Global Health (ISGlobal), Hospital Clínic, University of Barcelona, Barcelona, Spain

MIRIAM B. VOS, MD, MSPH
Division of Gastroenterology, Hepatology, and Nutrition, Emory School of Medicine, Children's Healthcare of Atlanta, Atlanta, Georgia, USA

ROBERT WONG, MD, MS
Division of Gastroenterology and Hepatology, Stanford University School of Medicine, Gastroenterology Section, Veterans Affairs Palo Alto Healthcare System, Palo Alto, California, USA

VINCENT WONG, MD
Department of Medicine and Therapeutics, Medical Data Analytics Centre, The Chinese University of Hong Kong, State Key Laboratory of Digestive Disease, Institute of Digestive Disease, The Chinese University of Hong Kong, Hong Kong, SAR

AARON YEOH, MD
Division of Gastroenterology and Hepatology, Stanford University School of Medicine, Stanford, California, USA

YUSUF YILMAZ, MD
Professor of Medicine, Department of Gastroenterology, School of Medicine, Recep Tayyip Erdoğan University, Rize, Turkey; Liver Research Unit, Institute of Gastroenterology, Marmara University, İstanbul, Turkey

ZOBAIR M. YOUNOSSI, MD, MPH
[illegible]

MING-LUNG YU
Professor, School of Medicine, College of Medicine, National Sun Yat-Sen University, Hepatitis Research Center, College of Medicine, Kaohsiung Medical University, Hepatobiliary Section, Department of Internal Medicine, Hepatitis Center, Kaohsiung Medical University Hospital, Division of Hepato-Gastroenterology, Department of Internal Medicine, Kaohsiung Chang Gung Memorial Hospital, Kaohsiung, Taiwan

ALBERTO ZANETTO, MD, PhD
Gastroenterology, Multivisceral Transplant Unit, Department of Surgery, Oncology and Gastroenterology, Padua University Hospital, Padua, Italy

SHIRA ZELBER-SAGI, RD, PhD
University of Haifa, School of Public Health, Mount Carmel, Haifa, Israel; Department of Gastroenterology, Tel-Aviv Medical Center, Tel Aviv, Israel

Contents

Preface **xix**

Zobair M. Younossi

Nonalcoholic Fatty Liver Disease: Disease Burden and Disease Awareness **173**

Pegah Golabi, Vasily Isakov, and Zobair M. Younossi

Nonalcoholic fatty liver disease (NAFLD) has become the most common chronic liver disease worldwide and has been implying an unprecedented burden to health care systems. The prevalence of NAFLD has exceeded 30% in developed countries. Considering the asymptomatic nature of undiagnosed NAFLD, high suspicion and noninvasive diagnosis have utmost importance especially in primary care level. At this point, patient and provider awareness should be optimal for early diagnosis and risk stratification for patients at risk of progression.

Metabolic Syndrome and Its Association with Nonalcoholic Steatohepatitis **187**

Fernando Bril, Arun Sanyal, and Kenneth Cusi

The relationship between insulin resistance, metabolic syndrome (MetS), and nonalcoholic fatty liver disease (NAFLD) is complicated. Although insulin resistance is almost universal in people with NAFLD and MetS, NAFLD may be present without features of MetS and vice versa. While NAFLD has a strong correlation with cardiometabolic risk factors, these are not intrinsic components of this condition. Taken together, our knowledge gaps call for caution regarding the common assertion that NAFLD is the hepatic manifestation of the MetS, and for defining NAFLD in broad terms as a "metabolic dysfunction" based on a diverse and poorly understood constellation of cardiometabolic features.

Hepatic Outcomes of Nonalcoholic Fatty Liver Disease Including Cirrhosis and Hepatocellular Carcinoma **211**

Saleh A. Alqahtani, Wah-Kheong Chan, and Ming-Lung Yu

Nonalcoholic fatty liver disease (NAFLD) is the most common chronic liver disease worldwide and represents a significant cause of cirrhosis and hepatocellular carcinoma (HCC). Almost 20% of patients with NAFLD and advanced fibrosis develop cirrhosis, of which 20% can progress to decompensated liver stage. Although patients with cirrhosis or fibrosis continue to have a high risk for HCC progression, growing evidence shows that NAFLD-HCC can develop even in the absence of cirrhosis. Current evidence characterizes NAFLD-HCC primarily as a condition with late presentation, lower response to curative therapy, and poor prognosis.

Changings and Challenges in Liver Transplantation for Nonalcoholic Fatty Liver Disease/Steatohepatitis 225

Sarah Shalaby, Sara Battistella, Alberto Zanetto, Debora Bizzaro, Giacomo Germani, Francesco Paolo Russo, and Patrizia Burra

Liver transplantation for nonalcoholic fatty liver disease/steatohepatitis (NAFLD/NASH) is increasing rapidly worldwide. Compared with alcohol and viral-related liver disease, NAFLD/NASH is more frequently associated with a systemic metabolic syndrome, which significantly affects other organs, requiring multidisciplinary management, in all phases of liver transplant.

Extrahepatic Outcomes of Nonalcoholic Fatty Liver Disease: Cardiovascular Diseases 239

Angelo Armandi and Elisabetta Bugianesi

Patients with nonalcoholic fatty liver disease (NAFLD) are at high risk of cardiovascular disease, including carotid atherosclerosis, coronary artery disease, heart failure, and arrhythmias. The risk is partially due to shared risk factors, but it may vary according to liver injury. A fatty liver may induce an atherogenic profile, the local necro-inflammatory changes of nonalcoholic steatohepatitis may enhance systemic metabolic inflammation, and fibrogenesis can run parallel in the liver and in the myocardium and precedes heart failure. The detrimental impact of a Western diet combines with polymorphisms in genes associated with atherogenic dyslipidemia. Shared clinical/diagnostic algorithms are needed to manage the cardiovascular risk in NAFLD.

Extrahepatic Outcomes of Nonalcoholic Fatty Liver Disease: Nonhepatocellular Cancers 251

Maryam K. Ibrahim, Tracey G. Simon, and Mary E. Rinella

Nonalcoholic fatty liver disease (NAFLD) encompasses the entire spectrum of fatty liver disease in individuals without significant alcohol consumption, including isolated steatosis, steatohepatitis, and cirrhosis. The overall global prevalence of NAFLD is estimated to be 30%, and the associated clinical and economic burden will continue to increase. NAFLD is a multisystemic disease with established links to cardiovascular disease, type 2 diabetes, metabolic syndrome, chronic kidney disease, polycystic ovarian syndrome, and intra- and extrahepatic malignancies. In this article the authors review the potential mechanisms and current evidence for the association between NAFLD and extrahepatic cancers and the resultant impact on clinical outcomes.

Update on Nonalcoholic Steatohepatitis: Sarcopenia and Nonalcoholic Fatty Liver Disease 275

Takumi Kawaguchi, Hirokazu Takahashi, and Lynn H. Gerber

Dual diagnoses of sarcopenia and nonalcoholic fatty liver disease (NAFLD) increase the risk of all cause mortality and severe liver disease, regardless of nationality. General agreement about diagnostic criteria for sarcopenia includes loss of skeletal muscle mass, weakness, and reduced physical performance. Histopathology demonstrates loss of type 2 muscle fibers, more than type 1 fibers and myosteatosis, a risk factor for severe liver disease. Low skeletal mass and NAFLD are inversely related; the mechanism is through decreased insulin signaling and insulin resistance, critical for metabolic homeostasis. Weight loss, exercise, and increased protein intake have been effective in reducing NAFLD and sarcopenia.

Nonalcoholic Fatty Liver Disease in Asia, Africa, and Middle East Region 287

Janus Ong, Khalid Alswat, Saeed Hamid, and Mohamed El-Kassas

Non-alcoholic fatty liver disease (NAFLD) is one of the most common causes of chronic liver disease worldwide. The global prevalence of the disease varies according to the geographical region. Despite having distinct models for the western patterns of NAFLD, Africa, Asia, and the Middle East regions exhibited varying prevalence rates of NAFLD. The disease burden is anticipated to significantly increase in these areas. Furthermore, with an increase in NAFLD risk factors in these regions, the disease burden is expected to rise even more. Policies at the regional and international levels are required to address such growing burden of NAFLD consequences.

Nonalcoholic Fatty Liver Disease in Latin America and Australia 301

Marlen Ivon Castellanos-Fernandez, Shreya C. Pal, Marco Arrese, Juan Pablo Arab, Jacob George, and Nahum Méndez-Sánchez

The epidemiologic and demographical features of nonalcoholic fatty liver disease (NAFLD) vary significantly across countries and continents. In this review, we analyze current data regarding prevalence of NAFLD in Latin America and Caribbean and Australia and review some peculiarities found in these regions. We stress the need of greater awareness of NAFLD and the development of cost-effective risk stratification strategies and clinical care pathways of the disease. Finally, we highlight the need of effective public health policies to control the main risk factors for NAFLD.

Pathogenetic Pathways in Nonalcoholic Fatty Liver Disease: An Incomplete Jigsaw Puzzle 317

Qin Pan, Jian-Gao Fan, and Yusuf Yilmaz

Nonalcoholic fatty liver disease (NAFLD)—a condition of excess fat accumulation in hepatocytes associated with metabolic dysfunction—has surpassed viral hepatitis to become the most prevalent chronic liver disease worldwide. As of now, only modestly effective pharmacological therapies for NAFLD exist. The uncomplete understanding of the pathophysiology underlying the heterogeneous disease spectrum known as NAFLD remains one of the major obstacles to the development of novel therapeutic approaches. This review compiles current knowledge on the principal signaling pathways and pathogenic mechanisms involved in NAFLD, which are analyzed in relation to its main pathological hallmarks (ie, hepatic steatosis, steatohepatitis, and liver fibrosis).

Genetic Markers Predisposing to Nonalcoholic Steatohepatitis 333

Aalam Sohal, Hunza Chaudhry, and Kris V. Kowdley

The growing prevalence of nonalcoholic fatty liver disease (NAFLD) has sparked interest in understanding genetics and epigenetics associated with the development and progression of the disease. A better understanding of the genetic factors related to progression will be beneficial in the risk stratification of patients. These genetic markers can also serve as potential therapeutic targets in the future. In this review, we focus on the genetic markers associated with the progression and severity of NAFLD.

for NASH is limited, current treatment options include life-style modification and the use of medications to treat metabolic comorbidities. This review addresses current approaches to the treatment of NAFLD/NASH, including the impact of diet, exercise, and available pharmacotherapies on the histologic features of liver injury.

The Role Bariatric Surgery and Endobariatric Therapies in Nonalcoholic Steatohepatitis **413**

Aaron Yeoh, Robert Wong, and Ashwani K. Singal

Nonalcoholic fatty liver disease (NAFLD) is the most common cause of chronic liver disease worldwide. Disease spectrum varies from steatosis, steatohepatitis, fibrosis, cirrhosis, and hepatocellular carcinoma. Currently, there are no approved medical therapies, and weight loss through lifestyle modifications remains a mainstay of therapy. Bariatric surgery is the most effective therapy for weight loss and has been shown to improve liver histology. Recently, endoscopic bariatric metabolic therapies have also emerged as effective treatments for patients with obesity and NAFLD. This review summarizes the role of bariatric surgery and endoscopic therapies in the management of patients with NAFLD.

Future Treatment Options and Regimens for Nonalcoholic Fatty Liver Disease **429**

Sven Francque and Vlad Ratziu

Recent progress in our understanding of the pathogenic mechanisms that drive progression of nonalcoholic steatohepatitis as well as lessons learned from several clinical trials that have been conducted over the past 15 years guide our current regulatory framework and trial design. Targeting the metabolic drivers should probably be the backbone of therapy in most of the patients, with some requiring more specific intrahepatic anti-inflammatory and antifibrotic actions to achieve success. New and innovative targets and approaches as well as combination therapies are currently explored, while awaiting a better understanding of disease heterogeneity that should allow for future individualized medicine.

Special Population: Lean Nonalcoholic Fatty Liver Disease **451**

Ajay Duseja, Arka De, and Vincent Wong

Nonalcoholic fatty liver disease (NAFLD) is strongly associated with obesity but around 10% to 20% of patients with NAFLD have normal body mass index, a condition referred to as lean or nonobese NAFLD. Although lean patients more often have milder liver disease, a proportion may nonetheless develop steatohepatitis and advanced liver fibrosis. Both genetic and environmental factors contribute to the development of NAFLD. Noninvasive tests have similarly good accuracy as initial assessments for lean NAFLD. Future studies should determine the most appropriate treatment in this special population.

Special Population: Pediatric Nonalcoholic Fatty Liver Disease **471**

Eric Dybbro, Miriam B. Vos, and Rohit Kohli

Pediatric nonalcoholic fatty liver disease represents the most common liver disease in children and has been shown to carry significant morbidity. Widespread heterogeneity of disease, as well as the limitation of indirect

screening modalities, has made true prevalence of disease difficult to estimate as well as hindered ability to identify optimal prognostic factors in the pediatric population. Current therapeutic options are limited in pediatric patients with current mainstay of therapy, lifestyle modifications, has proven to have a limited efficacy in current clinical application. Current research remains needed in improved screening modalities, prognosticating techniques, and therapeutic options in the pediatric population.

Economic Burden and Patient-Reported Outcomes of Nonalcoholic Fatty Liver Disease **483**

Maria Stepanova, Linda Henry, and Zobair M. Younossi

In addition to adverse clinical outcomes such as liver-related morbidity and mortality, nonalcoholic fatty liver disease (NAFLD) is associated with a substantial public health and economic burden and could also potentially impair health-related quality of life and other patient-reported outcomes. The disease also affects multiple aspects of patients' quality of life which are the most pronounced in physical health-related and fatigue domains as well as work productivity, and get more severe in patients with advanced liver disease or with non-hepatic comorbidities. The economic burden of NAFLD is substantial and is increasing, with the highest costs in those with advanced disease.

Physicians' Use of Digital Health Interventions in the Management of Nonalcoholic fatty liver disease **515**

Jeffrey V. Lazarus, Marcela Villota-Rivas, Carolina Jiménez-González, Alvaro Santos-Laso, Paula Iruzubieta, María Teresa Arias-Loste, Lisa Rice-Duek, Simon Leigh, Christopher J. Kopka, Juan Turnes, José Luis Calleja, and Javier Crespo

Globally, the use of digital health interventions (DHIs) is expanding, along with growing scientific evidence of their effectiveness. Given the high and increasing prevalence of noncommunicable liver disease, we surveyed 295 physicians across Spain about their knowledge, beliefs, attitudes, practices, and access with regard to DHIs for patient care and in particular for liver diseases, including nonalcoholic fatty liver disease and nonalcoholic steatohepatitis. Physicians reported high familiarity with DHIs, although most had not recommended them in patient care. Addressing concerns, including limited available time, evidence of effectiveness, education, training, and access may contribute to an increased uptake of these technologies.

Research Priorities for Precision Medicine in Nonalcoholic fatty liver disease **535**

Paula Iruzubieta, Ramon Bataller, María Teresa Arias-Loste, Marco Arrese, José Luis Calleja, Graciela Castro-Narro, Kenneth Cusi, John F. Dillon, María Luz Martínez-Chantar, Miguel Mateo, Antonio Pérez, Mary E. Rinella, Manuel Romero-Gómez, Jörn M. Schattenberg, Shira Zelber-Sagi, Javier Crespo, and Jeffrey V. Lazarus

NAFLD is a multisystem condition and the leading cause of chronic liver disease globally. There are no approved NAFLD-specific dugs. To advance in the prevention and treatment of NAFLD, there is a clear need

to better understand the pathophysiology and genetic and environmental risk factors, identify subphenotypes, and develop personalized and precision medicine. In this review, we discuss the main NAFLD research priorities, with a particular focus on socioeconomic factors, interindividual variations, limitations of current NAFLD clinical trials, multidisciplinary models of care, and novel approaches in the management of patients with NAFLD.

Update on Non-Alcoholic Steatohepatitis

CLINICS IN LIVER DISEASE

FORTHCOMING ISSUES

August 2023
Acute-on-Chronic Liver Failure
Nikolaos T. Pyrsopoulos, *Editor*

November 2023
Hepatitis B Virus and Hepatitis D Virus
Robert G. Gish, *Editor*

February 2024
Autoimmune Hepatitis Including PBC and PSC
David E. Bernstein, *Editor*

RECENT ISSUES

February 2023
Updates in Consultations in Liver Disease
Steven L. Flamm, *Editor*

November 2022
Primary Biliary Cholangitis
Binu V. John, *Editor*

August 2022
Pediatric Liver Disease
Philip Rosenthal, *Editor*

SERIES OF RELATED INTEREST

Gastroenterology Clinics of North America
https://www.gastro.theclinics.com

Preface

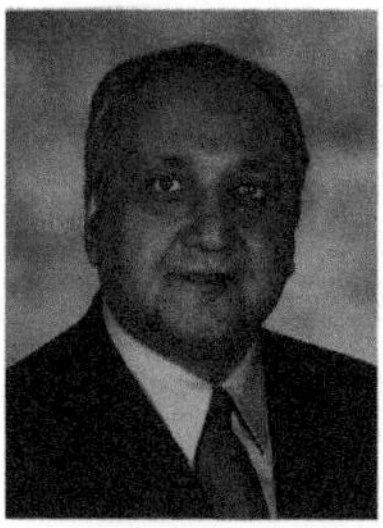

Zobair M. Younossi, MD, MPH
Editor

Epidemiologic data published in 2023 suggest that nonalcoholic fatty liver (NAFLD) and nonalcoholic steatohepatitis (NASH) affect around 30% and 5% of the world population and is on track to become the most common cause of cirrhosis and hepatocellular carcinoma (HCC), the most common cause for liver death, and the most common indication for liver transplantation. Driven by the global pandemic of obesity and type 2 diabetes, the global burden of NAFLD can be measured not only in clinical terms (liver mortality, cirrhosis, HCC) but also by its negative impact on patient-reported outcomes and the economic burden of the disease.

Over the last decades, many advances have been made to better understand the epidemiology and pathogenesis of NAFLD. In addition, a number of validated noninvasive tests have become available to be used in clinical practice. Although we are still hoping for risk stratification an approved drug regimen to treat NASH, there is a great potential to achieve this goal in the near future. Despite these gains, disease awareness remains low, and recognition of NAFLD as an important noncommunicable disease by the World Health Organization or similar other international bodies remains elusive.

In this issue of the *Clinics in Liver Disease*, leaders in the field of NAFLD/NASH provide cutting-edge information about different aspects of this important liver disease. The data presented in these articles should prove useful and practical to all stakeholders engaged in the filed of NAFLD/NASH.

Zobair M. Younossi, MD, MPH
President, Inova Medicine Services
Professor and Chairman
Department of Medicine
Inova Fairfax Medical Campus
3300 Gallows Road
Falls Church, VA 22042, USA

E-mail address:
Zobair.Younossi@inova.org

Clin Liver Dis 27 (2023) xix
https://doi.org/10.1016/j.cld.2023.02.001
1089-3261/23/© 2023 Published by Elsevier Inc.

Nonalcoholic Fatty Liver Disease: Disease Burden and Disease Awareness

Pegah Golabi, MD[a,b,c], Vasily Isakov, MD, PhD[d], Zobair M. Younossi, MD, MPH[a,b,c,e,*]

KEYWORDS

• Fatty liver • Epidemiology • Prevalence • Disease burden • Awareness

KEY POINTS

- The global prevalence of NAFLD has been increasing for the last two decades.
- South America, Middle East and Asia have the highest prevalence of NAFLD while some regions in Africa have reported the lowest prevalence.
- Among NAFLD, the proportion of patients with NASH is increasing as well, which will, in turn, increase the number of patients with advanced liver disease in the coming years.
- The disease awareness in both the patients and providers is suboptimal.Even though primary care settings could represent the first level of encounter for patients with undiagnosed NASH and provide an opportunity for risk stratification, very few programs are being implemented in clinical practice.
- Considering the worsening burden of NAFLD and related adverse outcomes, more needs to be done to increase disease awareness across different stakeholder groups.

INTRODUCTION

After four decades since the term nonalcoholic steatohepatitis (NASH) and nonalcoholic fatty liver disease (NAFLD), there is growing evidence to suggest that they are rapidly becoming the most common causes of liver disease across the world.[1]

[a] Betty and Guy Beatty Center for Integrated Research, Inova Health System, Falls Church, VA, USA; [b] Department of Medicine, Center for Liver Disease, Inova Fairfax Medical Campus, 3300 Gallows Road, Falls Church, VA 2202, USA; [c] Inova Medicine, Inova Health System, Falls Church, VA, USA; [d] Department of Gastroenterology & Hepatology, Federal Research Center for Nutrition and Biotechnology, 21 Kashirskoe Shosse, Moscow 115446, Russia; [e] Inova Medicine Services, Department of Medicine, Inova Fairfax Medical Campus, Betty and Guy Beatty Center for Integrated Research, Claude Moore Health Education and Research Building, 3300 Gallows Road, Falls Church, VA 22042, USA

* Corresponding author. Inova Medicine Services, Department of Medicine, Inova Fairfax Medical Campus, Betty and Guy Beatty Center for Integrated Research, Claude Moore Health Education and Research Building, 3300 Gallows Road, Falls Church, VA 22042.

E-mail address: zobair.younossi@inova.org

Clin Liver Dis 27 (2023) 173–186
https://doi.org/10.1016/j.cld.2023.01.001
1089-3261/23/

As the name implies, fatty infiltration of hepatocytes in the absence of secondary causes, including excessive alcohol consumption, is the cornerstone of NAFLD. It encompasses a spectrum of liver pathology, ranging from simple steatosis to NASH, which is regarded as the more progressive form of NAFLD.[2] It has been shown that some patients with NASH develop hepatic fibrosis leading to cirrhosis and hepatocellular carcinoma.[3–7]

NAFLD has become a highly prevalent, alarming health care providers and policy makers across the globe in the last decades. NAFLD prevalence has been increasing at an unprecedented rate, with an estimated global prevalence rate ranging between 24% and 38%.[1,4,8,9] It is also estimated that up to 20% of patients with NAFLD may have underlying NASH.[10] Understandably, those rates are even higher among patients with type 2 diabetes (T2DM), obesity, and especially those undergoing bariatric surgery (see chapter 16).[11] However, NAFLD prevalence is not uniform globally and demonstrates variations based on the population studied. Possible explanations for this heterogeneous prevalence rate include different rates of risk factors across different geographic regions, genetic factors, environmental factors, and cultural elements.[12]

Although NAFLD is a liver disease, it is regarded as a part of multisystemic diseases that include cardiovascular disease, extrahepatic cancers, sarcopenia, and other conditions associated with metabolic syndrome[13–15] (see chapters 2, 5-7). In fact, underlying insulin resistance seems to be the underpinning of NAFLD and other related comorbidities. It is also important to note that the presence of T2DM is an independent predictor of advanced fibrosis and mortality among NAFLD population.[16,17]

The progression of NASH seems to be nonlinear with patients following a slowly progressive course for a period of time, followed by periods of regression. Given the sheer number of patients with NAFLD and NASH, a large number of patients can present with advanced fibrosis, cirrhosis, hepatocellular carcinoma, and requirement for liver transplantation[18,19] (see chapter 3,4). In fact, after the introduction of effective treatment options for viral hepatitis in the last decade, NAFLD/NASH and alcoholic liver disease have become the main indications for liver transplantation in the United States[20,21] (see chapter 14). In addition to clinical consequences, NAFLD/NASH also causes significant economic burden as well as impairment with its patient-related outcomes. This comprehensive burden not only affects patients but also communities and the whole health care systems.

Even though NAFLD/NASH is highly prevalent and possesses an unquestionable burden to patients and health care systems (see chapter 20), treatment options are very limited (see chapter 15). In fact, lifestyle modification with diet and exercise has been cornerstone of treatment of NAFLD.[2] However, in practice, the proportion of patients who can achieve and sustain the recommended weight loss remains very small. In the last decade, there have been significant efforts to develop pharmacologic agents for the treatment of NASH and related fibrosis.[22,23] Multicenter and multinational trials are being carried out without a successfully approved pharmacologic regimen[24,25] (see chapter 17). Considering the high prevalence and progressive nature of NAFLD/NASH, it is important to identify patients who are at risk of progressive liver disease and adverse outcomes. In this context, risk stratification algorithms are being developed to identify NAFLD patients at risk for developing advanced fibrosis and cirrhosis and link these patients for specialty care such as gastroenterology and hepatology. In addition to limited treatment options, awareness about the disease is poor at primary care and other front-line provider settings. Programs to improve awareness, case finding, and linkage of those at risk will be of great importance.

In the following sections, the authors review the burden of NAFLD related to prevalence and mortality.

NONALCOHOLIC FATTY LIVER DISEASE BURDEN

As stated above, most recent reports suggest that the global prevalence of NAFLD is around 30% to 32% in the general population. More importantly, NASH prevalence has been increasing and is now estimated to be around 5.3% globally.[8–10,26] The highest prevalence rates have been reported from South America, Middle East, and Asia, whereas the lowest rates were seen in some parts of Africa.[27,28]

North America

In North America, the vast majority of data originate from the United States. Understandably, noninvasive methods, such as imaging or blood tests, were most recently used, rather than liver biopsy, which is still regarded as the gold standard for diagnosis. In the general US population, NAFLD prevalence has continued to worsen in the last decade. Even though a previous meta-analysis reported a prevalence rate of 24% in the general US population, the most recent meta-analysis suggests a pooled global prevalence rate of 31.2% from 1990-2019.[9,26] In fact, the prevalence for 2016-2019 was 38.2%.9 Nevertheless, NAFLD prevalence shows variations in different ethnic groups, and Hispanic Americans and Americans from European descent have higher NAFLD rates than African Americans.[29,30] Furthermore, even within a certain ethnic group, NAFLD prevalence shows variations based on the country of origin. It has previously been demonstrated that although NAFLD prevalence is 29% among Hispanic Americans, it is 33% among those of Mexican origin, 18% among those of Puerto Rican origin, and 16% among those of Dominican origin.[31] These rates suggest both potential genetic predisposition and environmental factors that may affect diet and activity habits. More studies are needed to better understand the ethnic differences among NAFLD patients in North America.

South America (see chapter 9)

Compared with the United States, NAFLD prevalence seems to be higher in South America, with an estimated prevalence rate of 44.4% in the general population.[9,32,33] In a multicenter study in Brazil among 1280 patients, the prevalence of NAFL, NASH, and fibrosis was 42%, 58%, and 27%, respectively.[34] Furthermore, NAFLD prevalence of 26.6% was reported among young males in Colombia, whereas the rate was 22% in Chile.[35,36] Finally, a cohort study among 2500 patients in Mexico showed a prevalence rate of 17.1%.[37] It is important to note that study design and modalities used to establish the diagnosis of NAFLD can explain some of the differences in the reported rates.

Similar to North America, the prevalence of NAFLD and NASH in these multiethnic populations is affected by different genetic factors such as single-nucleotide polymorphism of patatin-like phospholipase domain containing protein 3 (PNPLA3) as well as environmental factors affecting diet and activity.

Asia (see chapter 8)

NAFLD prevalence rates demonstrate a wide variation in Asian countries, likely due to different levels of economic development and dietary habits. Even within the same country, such as China, significant regional differences have been observed. In a recent meta-analysis, the prevalence of NAFLD was 33.9% in South Asia, 33.1% in Southeast Asia, 29.7% in East Asia, and 28% in Asia Pacific region.[9] Again, the method of diagnosis and study design could impact these reported prevalence rates. In this context, previous studies have shown that the prevalence of NAFLD according to proton magnetic resonance spectroscopy was 19.3% in nonobese patients and 60.5% in obese individuals from Hong Kong.[38] On the other hand, in Shanghai, NAFLD diagnosis based on ultrasound reported a prevalence rate of 38.2% among 7152 individuals.[39] Even though lower rates were also reported in some rural regions of China, dietary habits and lifestyle differences seem to be responsible for these differences. Similar to China, a significant difference in the NAFLD prevalence rates was observed between rural (9%) and urban (32%) areas of India.[40,41] In Japan and Korea, NAFLD prevalence rates were found to be comparable to North America, with 26% and 27%, respectively.[42,43]

Africa and Middle East (see chapter 9)

There have been very limited epidemiologic data from Africa, making it difficult to assess the prevalence of NAFLD reliably. Nevertheless, the prevalence of NAFLD in Africa seems to follow the prevalence of obesity and T2DM. Overall, the prevalence seems to be lower. In fact, NAFLD prevalence was reported to range from 1.2% to 4.5% in Nigeria. On the other hand, 50% to 69% of diabetics in Sudan and Nigeria seem to have NAFLD.[44–47]

In contrast, the rates of NAFLD in the North African countries are similar to those reported from the Middle East. In fact, the Middle East and North Africa region has one of the highest NAFLD prevalence rates and experiences a very high burden of disease.[27] Based on the most recent meta-analytic assessments, NAFLD prevalence in this region has reached 36.5%, which is higher than previously reported rates.[4,9] At the country level, population-based reports from Iran reported that NAFLD prevalence might be as high as 39%, with urban areas being affected more heavily than rural areas.[48,49] The scenario is even worse in the neighboring country, Turkey where a recent cross-sectional study among 15 centers with more than 113,000 participants reported the prevalence of ultrasound-based NAFLD of 48.3%.[50] These rates were higher among older individuals (>50 years of age, 65.6%) and males (65%). Again, lifestyle choices and dietary habits seem to play a role in NAFLD prevalence even within the same country. In this context, the NAFLD prevalence was lower in the Aegean region of Turkey (West), where the Mediterranean diet is common as compared with Central Anatolia (39.8% vs 57.1%) and a more carbohydrate and a red meat-rich diet is common. Furthermore, this study demonstrated 22% increase in NAFLD prevalence between 2007 to and 2010 (43.5%) and 2014 to 2016 (53.1%) years.[50]

Europe

Depending on the region, NAFLD prevalence ranges between 20% and 30% across Europe in the general population level.[9] Most of the reports diagnosed NAFLD based on ultrasound data in this region. Not surprisingly, if the focus is turned into "at-risk" populations, such as those with T2DM, NAFLD prevalence rates increase substantially. A multicenter, cross-sectional, population-based study in Spain, across 25 centers with more than 750 patients demonstrated an NAFLD prevalence of 25.8%, with NAFLD rates being higher among males (33.4%).[51] In Germany, a recent cross-sectional, population-based study among almost 15,000 participants reported a prevalence of 37.5%, but it needs to be noted that rather than ultrasound data, the authors defined NAFLD by fatty liver index.[52] The Dionysos nutrition study, albeit about two decades old, demonstrated an NAFLD prevalence of 25% in Northern Italy.[53] In this context, a multicentric study of the Italian Atherosclerotic Society reported that among patients with metabolic syndrome, NAFLD rates were as high as 78%.[54]

Similar rates were reported from the United Kingdom, France, Hungary, and Romania.[28,55]

The prevalence of NAFLD and NASH in Eastern European countries is difficult to estimate not only due to a few epidemiologic studies, but also because of in these countries there exists a unique combination of epidemiologic factors that favor the increase in prevalence of advanced liver diseases and its complications and liver-related mortality. Indeed, it is difficult to evaluate the real prevalence of NAFLD/NASH by screening the population with high consumption of alcohol, high prevalence of viral hepatitis and obesity.

The largest epidemiologic studies among Eastern European countries were performed in Russia, in which the prevalence of NAFLD/NASH was assessed in primary care physicians' patients who visited them for any reason. Abdominal ultrasound, blood tests, and physical examination were performed. Among 30,787 patients who were enrolled into the DIREG1 study in 2007, 24% of patients were found to have liver steatosis, in 3.3% with elevated ALT, and in 0.8% of the studied population liver cirrhosis was found.[56] Six years later, the study was repeated and among 50,145 patients enrolled 28.1% of patients demonstrated liver steatosis at abdominal ultrasonography (US), in 9.1% of patients with elevated alanine aminotransferase (ALT) and in 0.84% with cirrhosis.[57] However, there were serious drawbacks in both studies including the unclear method for assessment of alcohol consumption (as the widely accepted CAGE or Alcohol Use Disorders Identification Test (AUDIT) questionnaires were not used); poor standardization of US protocol (different equipment and operators); and age disproportion between two studies (33% younger than 40 in DIREG1 compared with only 10% in DIREG2). The prevalence of viral hepatitis markers was surprisingly low for the Russian population in the first study (1.8% for HBV and 1.4% for hepatitis B virus [HCV]), and it was not mentioned at all in the second one.

Recently, two population-based studies have been performed (Ural Eye and Medical Study and Ural Very Old Study), in which the prevalence and associated factors of NAFLD were evaluated in rural and urban regions in Bashkortostan, Russia, and included 5852 participants aged 40 + years and 1130 participants of 85 + years, respectively. Defining NAFLD by the absence of consuming alcohol on a regular basis and by abnormally high ALT and aspartate aminotransferase (AST) levels or by an AST/ALT ratio of greater than 1.0, they found that 789/1130 (69.8%; 95%CI 67.1, 72.3) individuals of 85+ years had NAFLD. In multivariable analysis, a higher NAFLD prevalence was associated with female sex (OR 2.24; 95%CI 1.66, 3.01; $P < .001$), higher serum concentrations of low-density lipoproteins (OR 1.34; 95%CI 1.17, 1.55; $P < .001$), lower prothrombin index (OR 0.98; 95%CI 0.96, 0.99; $P = .002$), and lower ankle-brachial index (OR 0.03; 95%CI 0.02, 0.29; $P = .003$).[58] However, in Ural Eye and Medical Study, the prevalence of NAFLD was 2341/5852 or 40.0% (95%CI 38.8, 41.3). In univariable analysis, a higher NAFLD prevalence was associated ($P \leq .10$) with older age, female sex, and non-Russian ethnicity.[58] The major drawback of both studies was the use of only ALT or ALT/AST ratio as the criteria for NAFLD, without exclusion of viral hepatitis, and other numerous reasons for ALT elevation. The absence of regular alcohol abuse was confirmed by questions about alcohol consumption (since when or when stopped, alcohol consumption-related wrongdoing); however, there is no information how it was validated or compared with widely accepted questionnaires or scales used for the evaluation of alcohol consumption.

Conclusions of all four studies should be accepted with caution, as the high alcohol consumption (7–10 L per capita/year) and HCV-infection (4.5–5 million of HCV-positive) are still the major causes of liver steatosis and hepatitis in the population.

However, in all mentioned studies, both factors may be underestimated due to methodological weakness of the study protocols.

Large multicenter observational study (PRELID 2) was performed in 100 medical centers to evaluate the prevalence of NAFLD among patients seeking general practitioners' and gastroenterologists' help in Ukraine. Concomitant pathology, metabolic syndrome, and its individual criteria in patients with confirmed and unconfirmed diagnosis of NAFLD were also evaluated. Among 5000 patients enrolled nonalcoholic steatosis was diagnosed in 3153 (62.72%), NASH—in 1517 (30.30%), and liver cirrhosis—in 44 (0.88%) patients.[59] However, only in 3571 (71.42%) cases, the diagnosis was confirmed, because doctors included in the study the patients with suspected NAFLD. In the presence of metabolic syndrome, the diagnosis of NAFLD was confirmed in 76.07% of cases, with a low level of high-density lipoproteins—in 71.25%, with hypertriglyceridemia—in 77.15%. The results of this study are difficult to extrapolate to the general population as it was performed in tertiary centers (gastroenterology departments), and it is not clear how alcohol consumption and other causes of liver steatosis were excluded in the studied population.

In other Eastern European countries, the prevalence of NAFLD or NASH has not been evaluated in large population-based studies; however, several single-center studies should be mentioned. In Belarus, 548 office workers were enrolled into the study for the assessment of NAFLD risk factors, and in 26% of them, liver steatosis was revealed by US, but in 5.2% presumed NASH was diagnosed by chronic ALT elevation and exclusion of other common reasons of liver inflammation including hepatotropic viruses, drugs, and alcohol consumption.[60] The combination of abdominal obesity, hypertension, and dyslipidemia was found in 90% of patients with liver steatosis and in half of patients with NASH, all other patients with NASH except one were diabetic. Abdominal obesity itself was associated only with 8% of patients with liver steatosis, and it was only a risk factor in one patient with NASH.

In Moldova, there were no specific studies evaluating the prevalence of NAFLD/NASH in the general population, but World health organization (WHO) regularly performed studies evaluating the risk factors for noncommunicable diseases in the frame of STEP survey,[61,62] the results of which can be interesting for defining probable level of prevalence of liver steatosis and NASH in the population. The combined results of reports published in 2013 and in 2020 demonstrate that the prevalence of overweight individuals in the population was 56% and it was increasing with age up to 79.8% in women of 45 to 59 years old, but obesity was found in 26.1% of men and in 45.7% of women of the same age group. More than 58% of middle-aged men and women have raised blood pressure, 19.7%—elevated blood glucose and 42.3%—raised blood cholesterol. Taking it all into account, it can be said that high prevalence of NAFLD/NASH in Moldova looks quite probable. However, the same reports showed that around 70% of men of all ages and 57% of women consume alcohol and at least 30% of men and 10% of women reported heavy episodes of drinking.[62] Viral hepatitis is still prevalent in Moldova,[63] and as a consequence, there is a substantial number of liver cirrhosis and more than 80% of all cases of HCC are related to hepatotropic viruses.[64]

FUTURE PROJECTIONS

Considering that about one third of the world's general population is affected by NAFLD and the epidemiologic trends in obesity, diabetes, and metabolic syndrome have been worsening, the burden of NAFLD and NASH is expected to worsen over the years, not only in developed countries but also in the developing countries. In this context, research has shifted toward predicting the future impact of these conditions; thus, different Markov models were developed to reliably anticipate the clinical, economic, and total health care burden of NAFLD and NASH in the coming decades. A study by Estes and colleagues used a dynamic model for assessing the future burden of NAFLD for the United States for the year 2030. It was reported that compared with 2015, by 2030, NAFLD population was projected to increase by 21%, NAFLD prevalence to increase by 10% and reach 33.5%, NASH population to increase by 63%, advanced fibrosis (F3/F4) to increase by 160%, compensated cirrhosis to increase by 163%, the number of decompensated cirrhosis to increase by 180%, hepatocellular carcinoma cases to increase by 146%, and liver transplant cases to increase by 59%.[65] However, future projections are not very different for European countries, as models demonstrate that the burden of NAFLD and NASH will continue to worsen. It is estimated that by 2030, the number of NAFLD cases will increase by 13.5% in Germany, and up to 20.2% in the United Kingdom, and NAFLD prevalence will reach 23.6% in France and to 29.5% in Italy.[65] These data as well as data from population-based databases suggest that the prevalence and burden of NAFLD are expected to worsen in the next decades. These alarming statistics require an effective and urgent public health strategy to deal with the pandemic of obesity and related NAFLD.

NONALCOHOLIC FATTY LIVER DISEASE AWARENESS

Despite the rising prevalence and burden of NAFLD/NASH, knowledge and awareness about the disease are still highly suboptimal and unsatisfactory. In this context, raising awareness among patients and health care providers, especially among those in the primary care setting, must become a priority. This increase in awareness must be coupled with programs and algorithms to identify NAFLD patients at highest risk of progression to adverse outcomes (see chapter 14). Unfortunately, the lack of awareness and delays in diagnosis is a major challenge with the majority of cirrhotic patients with NASH present in decompensated state and advanced hepatocellular carcinoma.[66,67] In the context of awareness, both patient and provider and patients and providers' perspectives must be considered.

Patient Knowledge and Awareness

From the patient's perspective, NAFLD can go undiagnosed for years, as symptoms are mild and unrecognized until more advanced stages of liver disease is reached. In many cases, NAFLD is suspected when abnormalities in liver enzyme levels are detected, or fatty infiltration of hepatic parenchyma is detected in ultrasound incidentally.[68–70] Despite this recognition, further assessment is ignored, and patients have a false sense of security that NAFLD is a "benign" disease. A recent study using NHANES database for 2011 to 2016 period demonstrated that only 5.1% of NAFLD patients were aware of having a liver disease; this rate was only 1.8% for non-Hispanic Blacks, and 8.4% for those with a college or higher degree, emphasizing the role of race and education in disease awareness.[68] Another multicenter, prospective cohort study in the United States reported similar findings. Almost 2800 patients with risk factors for coronary artery disease participated in the 25th year of the cohort study, filled out a survey and underwent non-contrast computed tomography of the abdomen.[69] The prevalence of computed tomography (CT)-diagnosed NAFLD was 23.9% in this study, and only 2.4% of the participants were aware of their liver condition. This study did not demonstrate any difference in education levels between NAFLD aware and unaware groups.[69] A recent study compared disease awareness between NAFLD and viral hepatitis and included more than 37,000 subjects.[71] This study demonstrated that even though the prevalence of

NAFLD was considerably higher than viral hepatitis, there were striking differences in disease awareness, as only 4.4% of patients with NAFLD were aware of their liver condition, as opposed to 42.4% of patients with HCV and 17.2% with hepatitis B virus (HBV).[71]

It is certain that NAFLD awareness should be increased in the population level and a study from Brazil may provide some insights in terms of possible ways to achieve this. Almost 2000 individuals participated in a recent population-based survey sponsored by the Brazilian Liver Institute and per the results, NAFLD ranked second as the mostly recognized cause of liver cancer, following alcohol.[72] It can be suggested that social media could play an important role in improving disease awareness.

Clinician Knowledge and Awareness

Besides patients', health care providers also have significant challenges related to NAFLD/NASH knowledge and awareness. Even though NAFLD has been growing at an unprecedented rate, it is estimated that 20% and possibly fewer cases of NAFLD have been diagnosed.[73] Even though routine screening for NAFLD is not recommended by the American Association for the Study of Liver Diseases, it is the primary care level that "at risk" population should be identified and linked to specialty care. In this context, the optimal knowledge and awareness efforts must target the primary care providers and endocrinologists who see the largest number of patients at risk with T2DM and obesity.[74–76]

To illustrate these challenges, a recent global survey of 2202 providers across 40 countries (primary care, endocrinologists, gastroenterologists, and hepatologists) suggested a significant knowledge gap, especially among the primary care physician (PCPs).[77] In terms of knowledge, expectedly, the proportion of correct answers was highest for hepatologists, followed by gastroenterologists, endocrinologists, and primary care providers. Even though 80% of endocrinologists and 66% of primary care doctors reported that they would screen patients for NAFLD if they had diabetes or dyslipidemia, 9.2% of primary care providers reported not screening for NAFLD at all. Interestingly, more than 50% of primary care providers were not familiar with NAFLD fibrosis score and were not aware that cardiovascular disease was the leading cause of mortality among NAFLD cohort.[77] Similar to other reports from different parts of the world, this finding emphasizes the importance of provider training.

Another study from Australia among 108 PCPs provides daunting results.[74] In fact, half of the participants thought NAFLD prevalence was less than 10% in the general population, a quarter of the participants thought liver enzyme levels were sensitive for detecting NAFLD, and 71% stated they were unlikely to refer a patient to hepatology unless liver enzymes were abnormal.[74]Finally, a study from France evaluated the awareness of diabetologists and general practitioners about chronic liver disease.[78] Among a total of 678 providers (500 general practitioners and 178 diabetologists), NAFLD was identified as the main cause of chronic liver disease (CLD) in 36% and as the second most common cause of CLD in another 36%. About 82% of general practitioners and 96% of diabetologists were correct in NAFLD prevalence trends. Interestingly, even though 74% of general practitioners reported being familiar with noninvasive tests, FIB4 was cited by only 15% of them.[78] Similarly, two-thirds of primary care clinicians in Australia were unsure whether FIB4 or enhanced liver fibrosis score could help identifying advanced fibrosis.[74]

These data raise a few questions at different provider settings. "What needs to happen for a simple noninvasive test to be performed at primary care level?" Considering the primary source of knowledge for NAFLD among primary care providers is the

Internet, the answer to this question should be providing online computer-based modules and regular webinars for updates.

Besides the patients' and providers' awareness of NAFLD, it is also worth mentioning the countries' preparedness for the growing global burden of NAFLD. Recent studies clearly demonstrate that no country has a national strategy for NAFLD and only 32 countries have national NAFLD guidelines.[79,80] It is certain that to control the worsening NAFLD burden, there is an urgent need for policy improvements across the globe.

SUMMARY

NAFLD prevalence is increasing all over the world due to rising rates of obesity and T2DM. Future projections estimate that the proportion of NASH and NAFLD will continue to increase, resulting in more patients with advanced stages of liver disease, a rise in hepatocellular cancer cases, and the demand for liver transplantation. In order to combat this daunting clinical and economic burden of NAFLD/NASH, effective programs to raise awareness and identify patients at risk must be undertaken. These efforts must be implemented as national and regional guidelines and policies and should be coupled with the development of new therapeutic regimens for progressive NASH.

CLINICS CARE POINTS

- Non-alcoholic fatty liver disease (NAFLD) is the most common cause of chronic liver disease that affects around 30% of the global population.
- NAFLD is a disease spectrum ranging from simple steatosis to non-alcoholic steatohepatitis (NASH), which can progress to cirrhosis, HCC.
- NAFLD and NASH are responsible for the rapidly growing clinical, patient reported outcomes (PROs) and economic burden around the world.
- NAFLD patients with type 2 diabetes (T2D) and other components of metabolic syndrome are especially at high risk for adverse outcomes and should be the main targets of risk stratification and management.
- Awareness of NAFLD is low across all countries There is an urgent need to take public health action to increase awareness of NAFLD.

POTENTIAL COMPETING INTERESTS

Dr Z.M. Younossi is a consultant to BMS, Gilead, AbbVie, Abbott, Novo Nordisk, Merk, Siemens, and Intercept. All other authors have no conflict of interest to disclose.

FUNDING

None.

REFERENCES

1. Henry L, Paik J, Younossi ZM. Review article: the epidemiologic burden of non-alcoholic fatty liver disease across the world. Aliment Pharmacol Ther 2022; 56(6):942–56.
2. Cusi K, Isaacs S, Barb D, et al. American association of clinical endocrinology clinical practice guideline for the diagnosis and management of nonalcoholic

fatty liver disease in primary care and endocrinology clinical settings: co-sponsored by the American association for the study of liver diseases (AASLD). Endocr Pract 2022;28:528–62.
3. Anstee QM, Targher G, Day CP. Progression of NAFLD to diabetes mellitus, cardiovascular disease or cirrhosis. Nat Rev Gastroenterol Hepatol 2013;10:330–44.
4. Sayiner M, Koenig A, Henry L, et al. Epidemiology of nonalcoholic fatty liver disease and nonalcoholic steatohepatitis in the United States and the rest of the world. Clin Liver Dis 2016;20:205–14.
5. Kabarra K, Golabi P, Younossi ZM. Nonalcoholic steatohepatitis: global impact and clinical consequences. Endocr Connect 2021;10(10):R240–7.
6. Younossi Z, Stepanova M, Sanyal AJ, et al. The conundrum of cryptogenic cirrhosis: adverse outcomes without treatment options. J Hepatol 2018;69:1365–70.
7. Gao E, Hercun J, Heller T, et al. Undiagnosed liver diseases. Transl Gastroenterol Hepatol 2021;6:28.
8. Riazi K, Azhari H, Charette JH, et al. The prevalence and incidence of NAFLD worldwide: a systematic review and meta-analysis. Lancet Gastroenterol Hepatol 2022;7(9):851–61.
9. Younossi Z, Golabi P, Paik J, et al. The global epidemiology of nonalcoholic fatty liver disease (NAFLD) and non-alcoholic steatohepatitis (NASH): a systematic review. Hepatology 3 (2023),10–97.
10. El-Kassas M, Cabezas J, Iruzubieta P, et al. Non-alcoholic fatty liver disease: current global burden. Semin Liver Dis 2022. https://doi.org/10.1055/a-1862-9088.
11. Soresi M, Cabibi D, Giglio RV, et al. The prevalence of NAFLD and fibrosis in bariatric surgery patients and the reliability of noninvasive diagnostic methods. Biomed Res Int 2020;2020:5023157.
12. Cotter TG, Rinella M. Nonalcoholic fatty liver disease 2020: the state of the disease. Gastroenterology 2020;158:1851–64.
13. Golabi P, Otgonsuren M, de Avila L, et al. Components of metabolic syndrome increase the risk of mortality in nonalcoholic fatty liver disease (NAFLD). Medicine 2018;97:e0214.
14. Lim S, Kim J-W, Targher G. Links between metabolic syndrome and metabolic dysfunction-associated fatty liver disease. Trends Endocrinol Metab 2021;32:500–14.
15. Jarvis H, Craig D, Barker R, et al. Metabolic risk factors and incident advanced liver disease in non-alcoholic fatty liver disease (NAFLD): a systematic review and meta-analysis of population-based observational studies. Plos Med 2020;17:e1003100.
16. Younossi ZM, Golabi P, de Avila L, et al. The global epidemiology of NAFLD and NASH in patients with type 2 diabetes: a systematic review and meta-analysis. J Hepatol 2019;71:793–801.
17. Powell EE, Wong VW-S, Rinella M. Non-alcoholic fatty liver disease. Lancet 2021;397:2212–24.
18. Cotter TG, Dong L, Holmen J, et al. Nonalcoholic fatty liver disease: impact on healthcare resource utilization, liver transplantation and mortality in a large, integrated healthcare system. J Gastroenterol 2020;55:722–30.
19. Lonardo A, Targher G. NAFLD in the 20's. From epidemiology to pathogenesis and management of nonalcoholic fatty liver disease. Curr Pharm Des 2020;26:991–2.

20. Paik JM, Golabi P, Younossi Y, et al. Changes in the global burden of chronic liver diseases from 2012 to 2017: the growing impact of nonalcoholic fatty liver disease. Hepatology 2020;72(5):1605–16.
21. Paik JM, Golabi P, Biswas R, et al. Nonalcoholic fatty liver disease and alcoholic liver disease are major drivers of liver mortality in the United States. Hepatol Commun 2020;4:890–903.
22. Younossi ZM, Loomba R, Rinella ME, et al. Current and future therapeutic regimens for nonalcoholic fatty liver disease and nonalcoholic steatohepatitis. Hepatology 2018;68:361–71.
23. Neuschwander-Tetri BA. Therapeutic landscape for NAFLD in 2020. Gastroenterology 2020;158:1984–98, e3.
24. Harrison SA, Goodman Z, Jabbar A, et al. A randomized, placebo-controlled trial of emricasan in patients with NASH and F1-F3 fibrosis. J Hepatol 2020;72:816–27.
25. Younossi ZM, Ratziu V, Loomba R, et al. Obeticholic acid for the treatment of nonalcoholic steatohepatitis: interim analysis from a multicentre, randomised, placebo-controlled phase 3 trial. Lancet 2019;394:2184–96.
26. Younossi ZM, Koenig AB, Abdelatif D, et al. Global epidemiology of nonalcoholic fatty liver disease-Meta-analytic assessment of prevalence, incidence, and outcomes. Hepatology 2016;64:73–84.
27. Golabi P, Paik JM, AlQahtani S, et al. The burden of nonalcoholic fatty liver disease in Asia, Middle East and North Africa: data from global burden of disease 2009-2019. J Hepatol 2021;75(4):795–809.
28. Younossi Z, Anstee QM, Marietti M, et al. Global burden of NAFLD and NASH: trends, predictions, risk factors and prevention. Nat Rev Gastroenterol Hepatol 2018;15:11–20.
29. Pan J-J, Fallon MB. Gender and racial differences in nonalcoholic fatty liver disease. World J Hepatol 2014;6:274–83.
30. Schneider ALC, Lazo M, Selvin E, et al. Racial differences in nonalcoholic fatty liver disease in the U.S. population. Obesity 2014;22:292–9.
31. Fleischman MW, Budoff M, Zeb I, et al. NAFLD prevalence differs among hispanic subgroups: the Multi-Ethnic Study of Atherosclerosis. World J Gastroenterol 2014;20:4987–93.
32. Younossi ZM. Non-alcoholic fatty liver disease-A global public health perspective. J Hepatol 2018;70(3):531–44.
33. López-Velázquez JA, Silva-Vidal KV, Ponciano-Rodríguez G, et al. The prevalence of nonalcoholic fatty liver disease in the Americas. Ann Hepatol 2014;13:166–78.
34. Cotrim P, Oliveira L. Nonalcoholic fatty liver disease in Brazil. Clinical and histological profile. Ann Hepatol 2011;10(1):33–7.
35. Perez M, Gonzáles L, Olarte R, et al. Nonalcoholic fatty liver disease is associated with insulin resistance in a young Hispanic population. Prev Med 2011;52:174–7.
36. Riquelme A, Arrese M, Soza A, et al. Non-alcoholic fatty liver disease and its association with obesity, insulin resistance and increased serum levels of C-reactive protein in Hispanics. Liver Int 2009;29:82–8.
37. Lizardi-Cervera J, Laparra DIB, Chávez-Tapia NC, et al. [Prevalence of NAFLD and metabolic syndrome in asymtomatic subjects]. Rev Gastroenterol Mex 2006;71:453–9.
38. Wei JL, Leung JC-F, Loong TC-W, et al. Prevalence and severity of nonalcoholic fatty liver disease in non-obese patients: a population study using proton-magnetic resonance spectroscopy. Am J Gastroenterol 2015;110:1306–14.

39. Hu X, Huang Y, Bao Z, et al. Prevalence and factors associated with nonalcoholic fatty liver disease in Shanghai work-units. BMC Gastroenterol 2012;12:123.
40. Das K, Das K, Mukherjee PS, et al. Nonobese population in a developing country has a high prevalence of nonalcoholic fatty liver and significant liver disease. Hepatology 2010;51:1593–602.
41. Amarapurkar D, Kamani P, Patel N, et al. Prevalence of non-alcoholic fatty liver disease: population based study. Ann Hepatol 2007;6:161–3.
42. Hamaguchi M, Kojima T, Takeda N, et al. The metabolic syndrome as a predictor of nonalcoholic fatty liver disease. Ann Intern Med 2005;143:722–8.
43. Jeong EH, Jun DW, Cho YK, et al. Regional prevalence of non-alcoholic fatty liver disease in Seoul and Gyeonggi-do, Korea. Clin Mol Hepatol 2013;19:266–72.
44. Olusanya TO, Lesi OA, Adeyomoye AA, et al. Nonalcoholic fatty liver disease in a Nigerian population with type II diabetes mellitus. Pan Afr Med J 2016;24:20.
45. Onyekwere CA, Ogbera AO, Balogun BO. Non-alcoholic fatty liver disease and the metabolic syndrome in an urban hospital serving an African community. Ann Hepatol 2011;10:119–24.
46. Almobarak AO, Barakat S, Suliman EA, et al. Prevalence of and predictive factors for nonalcoholic fatty liver disease in Sudanese individuals with type 2 diabetes: is metabolic syndrome the culprit? Arab J Gastroenterol 2015;16:54–8.
47. Afolabi BI, Ibitoye BO, Ikem RT, et al. The relationship between glycaemic control and non-alcoholic fatty liver disease in Nigerian type 2 diabetic patients. J Natl Med Assoc 2018;110:256–64.
48. Moghaddasifar I, Lankarani KB, Moosazadeh M, et al. Prevalence of non-alcoholic fatty liver disease and its related factors in Iran. Int J Organ Transpl Med 2016;7:149–60.
49. Etminani R, Manaf ZA, Shahar S, et al. Predictors of nonalcoholic fatty liver disease among middle-aged Iranians. Int J Prev Med 2020;11:113.
50. Değertekin B, Tozun N, Demir F, et al. The changing prevalence of non-alcoholic fatty liver disease (NAFLD) in Turkey in the last decade. Turk J Gastroenterol 2021;32:302–12.
51. Caballería L, Pera G, Auladell MA, et al. Prevalence and factors associated with the presence of nonalcoholic fatty liver disease in an adult population in Spain. Eur J Gastroenterol Hepatol 2010;22:24–32.
52. Huber Y, Schulz A, Schmidtmann I, et al. Prevalence and risk factors of advanced liver fibrosis in a population-based study in Germany. Hepatol Commun 2022;6:1457–66.
53. Foschi FG, Bedogni G, Domenicali M, et al. Prevalence of and risk factors for fatty liver in the general population of Northern Italy: the Bagnacavallo Study. BMC Gastroenterol 2018;18(1):177.
54. Soresi M, Noto D, Cefalù AB, et al. Nonalcoholic fatty liver and metabolic syndrome in Italy: results from a multicentric study of the Italian Arteriosclerosis society. Acta Diabetol 2013;50:241–9.
55. Younossi Z, Tacke F, Arrese M, et al. Global perspectives on non-alcoholic fatty liver disease and non-alcoholic steatohepatitis. Hepatology 2018;69(6):2672–82.
56. Drapkina O, Evsyutina Y, Ivashkin V. Prevalence of non-alcoholic fatty liver disease in the Russian federation: the open, multicenter, prospective study, DIREG 1. Am J Clin Med Res 2015;3:31–6.
57. Ivashkin V, Drapkina O, Maev I, et al. Prevalence of non-alcoholic fatty liver disease in out-patients of the Russian Federation: DIREG 2 study results. Russ J Gastroenterol Hepatol Coloproctol 2015;6:31–41 (In Russian).

58. Bikbov MM, Gilmanshin TR, Zainullin RM, et al. Prevalence of non-alcoholic fatty liver disease in the Russian ural Eye and medical study and the ural very old study. Sci Rep 2022;12:7842.
59. Stepanov YM. Results of the observational cross-over PRELID 2 study (2015–2016). Part 1. The prevalence of non-alcoholic fatty liver disease, the characteristics of concomitant pathology, metabolic syndrome and its individual criteria in patients seeking general pract. GASTRO 2019;53:26–33.
60. Silivonchik N, Goloborodko V, Lednik A, et al. Evaluation of risk factors and prevalence of non-alcoholic fatty liver disease. Fam Doctor 2012;1:17–20 (In Russian).
61. Prevalence of noncommunicable disease risk factors in the Republic of Moldova STEPS 2013. Copenhagen: WHO Regional office to Europe; 2014. p. 221.
62. Gender and noncommunicable diseases in Republic of Moldova. Analysis of STEPS data. WHO Regional Office for Europe. Copenhagen: World Health Organization; 2014. p. 44. Available at: https://apps.who.int/iris/handle/10665/337487. Accessed January 8, 2022.
63. Spinu C, Sajin O, Isac M, et al. Viral hepatitis B, C and D in the Republic of Moldova: achievements and problems. Public Health Economy Management Med 2019;82:352–63.
64. Turcanu A, Pitel E, Dumbrava V-T, et al. Profile of hepatocellular carcinoma in the Republic of Moldova: first-hand information on the presentation, distribution and etiologies. Rom J Intern Med 2019;57:37–46.
65. Estes C, Anstee QM, Arias-Loste MT, et al. Modeling NAFLD disease burden in China, France, Germany, Italy, Japan, Spain, United Kingdom, and United States for the period 2016–2030. J Hepatol 2018;69:896–904.
66. Goutté N, Sogni P, Bendersky N, et al. Geographical variations in incidence, management and survival of hepatocellular carcinoma in a Western country. J Hepatol 2017;66:537–44.
67. Dam Fialla A, Schaffalitzky de Muckadell OB, Touborg Lassen A. Incidence, etiology and mortality of cirrhosis: a population-based cohort study. Scand J Gastroenterol 2012;47:702–9.
68. Le MH, Yeo YH, Cheung R, et al. Ethnic influence on nonalcoholic fatty liver disease prevalence and lack of disease awareness in the United States, 2011-2016. J Intern Med 2020;287:711–22.
69. Cleveland ER, Ning H, Vos MB, et al. Low awareness of nonalcoholic fatty liver disease in a population-based cohort sample: the CARDIA study. J Gen Intern Med 2019;34:2772–8.
70. Ghevariya V, Sandar N, Patel K, et al. Knowing what's out there: awareness of non-alcoholic fatty liver disease. Front Med 2014;1:4.
71. Alqahtani SA, Paik JM, Biswas R, et al. Poor awareness of liver disease among adults with NAFLD in the United States. Hepatol Commun 2021;5(11):1833–47.
72. Bittencourt PL, Oliveira CP, Codes L, et al. Internet search engines and social media are improving awareness on nonalcoholic fatty liver disease in Brazil. J Hepatol 2022;77(4):1217–9.
73. Alexander M, Loomis AK, Fairburn-Beech J, et al. Real-world data reveal a diagnostic gap in non-alcoholic fatty liver disease. BMC Med 2018;16:130.
74. Patel PJ, Banh X, Horsfall LU, et al. Underappreciation of non-alcoholic fatty liver disease by primary care clinicians: limited awareness of surrogate markers of fibrosis. Intern Med J 2018;48:144–51.
75. Polanco-Briceno S, Glass D, Stuntz M, et al. Awareness of nonalcoholic steatohepatitis and associated practice patterns of primary care physicians and specialists. BMC Res Notes 2016;9:157.

76. Casler K, Trees K, Bosak K. Providing care for fatty liver disease patients: primary care nurse practitioners' knowledge, actions, and preparedness. Gastroenterol Nurs 2020;43:E184–9.
77. Younossi ZM, Ong JP, Takahashi H, et al. A global survey of physicians knowledge about nonalcoholic fatty liver disease. Clin Gastroenterol Hepatol 2022;20:e1456–68.
78. Canivet CM, Smati S, Lannes A, et al. Awareness of chronic liver diseases, a comparison between diabetologists and general practitioners. Clin Res Hepatol Gastroenterol 2022;46:101848.
79. Lazarus JV, Mark HE, Villota-Rivas M, et al. The global NAFLD policy review and preparedness index: are countries ready to address this silent public health challenge? J Hepatol 2022;76:771–80.
80. Lazarus JV, Ekstedt M, Marchesini G, et al. A cross-sectional study of the public health response to non-alcoholic fatty liver disease in Europe. J Hepatol 2020;72:14–24.

Metabolic Syndrome and Its Association with Nonalcoholic Steatohepatitis

Fernando Bril, MD[a,*], Arun Sanyal, MD[b], Kenneth Cusi, MD[c]

KEYWORDS

• Insulin resistance • Diabetes • Obesity • NASH • Treatment of type 2 diabetes

KEY POINTS

- The presence of insulin resistance is almost universal in patients with nonalcoholic fatty liver disease (NAFLD) and/or metabolic syndrome (MetS).
- Insulin resistance, and lipotoxicity, are systemic processes that can affect multiple organs, including the liver. Genetic and epigenetic factors determine which organs are affected, and thus defining the specific phenotype of the patient.
- Nonalcoholic fatty liver disease can exist in the absence of the cardiometabolic risk factors that define the metabolic syndrome.
- Targeting insulin resistance in clinical practice should be a major target, including interventions to achieve weight loss, and medications that are insulin sensitizers.

INTRODUCTION

The close relationship between the metabolic syndrome (MetS) and nonalcoholic fatty liver disease (NAFLD) is well described in the literature.[1,2] Indeed, due to this strong association, NAFLD has oftentimes been referred to as the hepatic expression of the MetS, and recently suggested that NAFLD should be renamed metabolic-associated (dysfunction) fatty liver disease (MAFLD).[3] Moreover, a recently proposed definition of MAFLD introduced the idea of using metabolic parameters to establish the presence of MAFLD, in a similar fashion that we currently determine the presence of the MetS in the clinic.[4] Many consider a name change premature[5] and the issue is being actively debated in the field as the true nature of this relationship is only incompletely understood. It is important to highlight that NAFLD and nonalcoholic

[a] Division of Endocrinology, Diabetes and Metabolism, University of Alabama at Birmingham, Birmingham, AL, USA; [b] Division of Gastroenterology, Hepatology and Nutrition, School of Medicine Internal Medicine, Virginia Commonwealth University; [c] Division of Endocrinology, Diabetes and Metabolism, University of Florida, Gainesville, FL, USA

* Corresponding author. Endocrinology, Diabetes and Metabolism, Department of Medicine, University of Alabama at Birmingham, 510 20th Street S, FOT 803, Birmingham, AL.
E-mail address: Fbril@uab.edu

Clin Liver Dis 27 (2023) 187–210
https://doi.org/10.1016/j.cld.2023.01.002

steatohepatitis (NASH) are much more than insulin resistance or some of its cardiometabolic risk factors. Although insulin resistance is an obvious common factor for NAFLD and MetS, not all patients with insulin resistance develop NAFLD or MetS. Indeed, some patients may develop one of these entities without any manifestation of the other one, or neither of them.

This review will aim to address some frequently overlooked questions. Are NAFLD and MetS just common final pathways of insulin resistance or is there an interaction between them? What determines which patients manifest one or the other? Should we consider them the same thing? Is NAFLD really the hepatic manifestation of MetS? Does the coexistence of NAFLD and MetS predispose patients to more severe liver disease? Can we identify and target insulin resistance in clinical practice to prevent or treat NAFLD? In this article, we aimed to answer the above questions by summarizing the available evidence.

INSULIN RESISTANCE: BASIC CONCEPTS

In simple terms, insulin resistance could be understood as the inability of insulin to exert its action on target tissues. However, the concept of insulin resistance is significantly more complicated, as it affects some specific metabolic pathways while leaving other pathways unaffected.[6] As a result of this, because one of the initial responses to insulin resistance is a compensatory hyperinsulinemia to maintain euglycemia, insulin-dependent pathways that are relatively unaffected by insulin resistance may actually be overactivated (ie, hepatic lipogenesis). Therefore, patients with insulin resistance have both up- and down-regulated insulin-dependent pathways.[7]

Insulin resistance is oftentimes considered by primary care providers as only a risk factor to develop hyperglycemia. However, independently of hyperglycemia, insulin resistance should be understood as a detrimental systemic entity, with multiple metabolic consequences. Indeed, even in the presence of severe insulin resistance, more often than not, hyperglycemia does not manifest at all (eg, in most patients with obesity without glucose intolerance or type 2 diabetes [T2D]), or is only a very late manifestation. Whether hyperglycemia develops will depend on the ability of pancreatic ß-cells to maintain an adequate compensatory hyperinsulinemia.[8]

Although a systemic condition, insulin resistance impacts each tissue differently, thus the variable phenotype seen across patients.[9] A combination of genetic, epigenetic, and environmental factors is likely responsible for the variable degree of insulin resistance affecting each tissue in a particular patient. It is also important to note that although in this article we frequently refer to elevated weight (overweight/obesity) and sedentarism as the main reasons for the development of insulin resistance, there are other contributors and etiologies of insulin resistance. In addition to genetic factors, other acquired factors that can promote insulin resistance are hyperglycemia, subclinical inflammation, pregnancy, and medications, such as highly active antiretroviral treatment (eg, protease inhibitors), glucocorticoids, nicotinic acid, and atypical antipsychotics (eg, olanzapine). It should be noted that many lean individuals are insulin-resistant and may develop NASH.[1,2,7] In the following sections, we will try to explain how insulin resistance affects different insulin-sensitive tissues and may contribute to the development of NAFLD and features of the MetS.

Insulin Resistance Across the Spectrum of Body Mass Index

In broad terms, insulin resistance is the result of the interplay between acquired and genetic defects.[10–12] Although the relative contribution of these factors is likely variable from patient to patient, pure genetic defects (ie, monogenic syndromes of insulin resistance) are rare,[11] and environmental factors seem to play a determinant role in most of the patients. However, even when exposed to similar environmental factors, patients manifest different degrees of insulin resistance, suggesting that genetic/epigenetic factors somehow modulate this response. Among acquired factors that promote insulin resistance, weight excess is likely the best recognized and characterized.[10]

Of note, adipose tissue excess does not affect insulin sensitivity equally in all patients. For example, in a study measuring insulin-stimulated glucose uptake by means of an insulin suppression test, changes in body mass index (BMI) only explained ~22% of the variability of insulin sensitivity.[13] Among 113 patients with BMIs between 19.5 and 29.9 kg/m^2, BMI was not associated with insulin resistance after adjustment for other variables, such as hepatic triglyceride content.[14] Among factors affecting the relationship between BMI and insulin sensitivity, ethnicity has been well recognized as a major factor in the literature.[15] Specifically, patients of Asian ethnicity seem to develop insulin resistance at lower BMI levels,[16] which has resulted in a lower threshold to define overweight and obesity in this ethnic group. This explains why lower cut-off points for BMI were also included for Asian patients in the definition of MetS. Even among Asian populations, there seem to be differences in how BMI affects insulin resistance when different subgroups (ie, Chinese, Malays, and Asian-Indians) are compared.[17]

Studies comparing the relationship between BMI and insulin resistance in African-American and non-Hispanic White ethnicities have been inconclusive. Although some studies have shown increased whole-body insulin resistance in African-American patients,[18] others showed no differences.[19] There is evidence that African-American patients have a distinctive pattern of lipid accumulation, which is significantly different than non-Hispanic White patients.[15] Specifically, they tend to accumulate less visceral and hepatic fat than BMI-matched non-Hispanic White counterparts,[20] which may result in lower hepatic insulin resistance (despite similar insulin resistance in other tissues).[19] An opposite situation has been observed in Hispanic patients, with higher visceral and hepatic fat accumulation, even after matching for insulin resistance.[21]

In addition to ethnicity and location of lipid accumulation, other factors that are likely to affect the relationship between BMI and insulin resistance are age, sex, physical activity, family history, and concomitant medications. In summary, the absence of a 'linear' relationship between BMI and insulin resistance supports the frequent clinical observation that the degree of obesity does not necessarily correlate with the severity of insulin resistance.[13] Moreover, this concept could have been anticipated given the existence of lean individuals with severe insulin resistance, as well as metabolically healthy patients with obesity.[22]

Insulin Resistance: A Systemic Problem Affecting Different Tissues

Although the concept of lipotoxicity was first introduced to explain the detrimental effects of increased FFA levels on β-cell function,[23] it is oftentimes used with a broader meaning to describe deleterious effects of FFAs on ectopic tissues such as skeletal muscle, liver, myocardium, and others, as described below.[24] We defer to recent in-depth reviews on the molecular mechanisms[6,7] to focus on the clinical aspects of insulin resistance relevant to the development of NAFLD/NASH. It is important to understand that lipotoxicity is a systemic entity simultaneously affecting most tissues. It is characterized by increased rates of adipose tissue lipolysis and of plasma FFA levels despite concomitant hyperinsulinemia, leading to ectopic fat accumulation with cellular dysfunction and even necrosis/apoptosis.[25] Owing to its high capacity for fat accumulation, the liver has frequently been identified as a key end-organ for cellular lipotoxicity. However, less is known about the consequences of lipotoxicity in other organs, such as kidneys, heart, and others.

Adipose tissue insulin resistance

Insulin resistance in the adipose tissue develops as a result of the interplay between genetic factors and adipocyte hypertrophy secondary to excess caloric intake.[26] Its most important clinical consequence is the inability of insulin to adequately inhibit hormone-sensitive lipase (HSL), which leads to an increased rate of triglyceride breakdown (ie, lipolysis) and the increased flow of free fatty acids (FFAs) from adipose tissue to ectopic tissues. It has been well-established that despite higher plasma insulin levels, in states of insulin resistance (whether individuals are lean or obese) plasma FFAs are inadequately within the "normal range" or even elevated.[25,27] In addition to excess lipolysis, a dysfunctional adipose tissue is also characterized by over secretion of pro-inflammatory cytokines (eg, tumor necrosis factor-α and interleukin-6, among others),[28] which may further contribute to the development of insulin resistance. Moreover, adiponectin is typically downregulated in dysfunctional adipocytes in insulin-resistant states, further contributing to ectopic fat accumulation and abnormal glucose and lipid metabolism.[28]

Skeletal muscle insulin resistance

In the fasting state (ie, low plasma insulin levels) skeletal muscle relies on FFA as an energy supply. In the post-prandial state, the increase of plasma insulin concentration results in increased glucose uptake, metabolism, and storage as glycogen, with a switch from fat to glucose as the main source of energy. This transition from fasting to fed states, with the consequent shift from FFA to glucose as an energy substrate is referred to as metabolic flexibility.[29] Metabolic inflexibility[30] is a key feature of insulin-resistant states such as obesity, NAFLD, and T2D. Skeletal muscle insulin resistance is characterized as a decrease in insulin-stimulated glucose uptake and metabolism and an inappropriate shift in energy source when transitioning from fasting to a postprandial state and vice versa.[31] Finally, it should be noted that in addition to adipose-tissue derived FFA oversupply/FFA flux, intramyocellular glucose metabolism defects include impaired mitochondrial fatty acid oxidation and accumulation of toxic lipid metabolites such as diacylglycerols and ceramides that impair insulin action and promote cellular inflammation.[32–34]

Hepatic insulin resistance

Fig. 1 summarizes how a dysfunctional adipose tissue, in combination with other factors, such as diet and hyperinsulinemia, contribute to triglyceride accumulation in the liver (ie, NAFLD) and the metabolic derangements that constitute the MetS. Briefly, increased FFA pool in the liver originates from three different sources: adipose tissue lipolysis (arrow 1), FFA spillover from chylomicrons, and *de novo* lipogenesis (DNL) from carbohydrates and other small molecules (arrow 2) [35,36] Of these, adipose tissue-derived FFAs are likely the most important source, contributing to over two-thirds of the hepatic FFA pool, emphasizing the key role of adipose tissue in this condition.[37] Although the relative contribution of DNL to the FFA pool is relatively small, several studies have suggested that this pathway exhibits the most significant increment in patients with NAFLD compared with those without NAFLD.[38,39] Glucose, fructose, and insulin are key promoters of increased DNL in patients with NAFLD.[40]

In response to FFA surplus, the liver responds by accumulating them as triglycerides (arrow 3). It is currently believed that triglyceride accumulation in the liver is not harmful for the liver *per se*.[37] Moreover, we can consider triglyceride accumulation as a defense

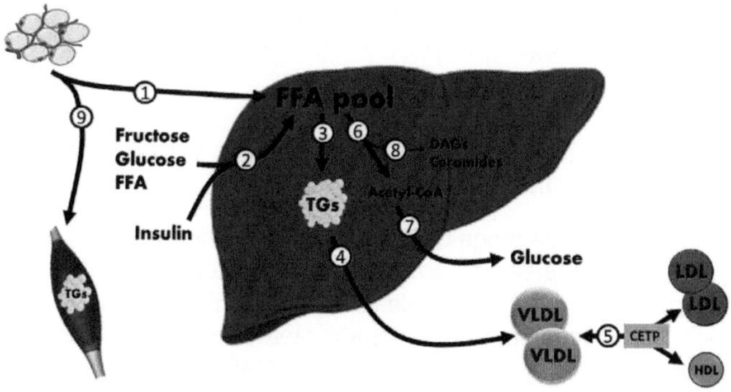

Fig. 1. Free fatty acid (FFA) sources and fate in NAFLD. FFA pool in the liver comes from adipose tissue lipolysis (*arrow 1*), FFA spillover from lipoproteins, and de novo lipogenesis (*arrow 2*). They can be stored as triglycerides (*arrow 3*) and secreted as part of VLDL molecules (*arrow 4*). Once in VLDL, triglycerides can be exchanged by cholesterol in HDL and LDL particles (*arrow 5*). FFAs in the liver can also be oxidized to obtain energy (*arrow 6*), and molecules generated in this process will later fuel gluconeogenesis (*arrow 7*). Incomplete oxidation of FFAs can lead to accumulation of pro-inflammatory intermediates, like diacylglycerols and ceramides (*arrow 8*). Of note, lipotoxicity is a systemic process and similar mechanisms occur in other tissues other than the liver (*arrow 9*).

mechanism to avoid more toxic FFAs from generating lipid intermediates (ie, DAGs, ceramides) or reactive oxygen species. However, this triglyceride accumulation promotes over secretion of triglyceride-rich very-low-density lipoprotein (VLDL) particles (arrow 4), which in turn contributes to the typical atherogenic dyslipidemia seen in insulin-resistant states (ie, high triglycerides, low high-density lipoprotein-cholesterol [HDL-C], small dense low-density lipoprotein-cholesterol [LDL-C]). In normal conditions, VLDL particles exchange TG and cholesterol with LDL and HDL particles, a process that is regulated by cholesterol ester transfer protein (CETP).[35] In patients with NAFLD, over secretion of large triglyceride-rich VLDL particles leads to a higher transfer of triglycerides to HDL and LDL particles (arrow 5). These triglycerides are metabolized as these particles circulate, ultimately leading to small HDL and LDL particles. Small HDL particles are cleared by the kidneys, which results in the typical low HDL-C levels in these patients. In addition, small and dense LDL particles are highly atherogenic, contributing to the high cardiovascular risk of these patients.

As also shown in **Fig. 1**, triglyceride accumulation and VLDL secretion are not the only potential fates of increased FFA in the liver.[37] When these mechanisms are unable to meet the demands of the FFA excess, FFAs end up undergoing increased β-oxidation (arrow 6). This leads to increased production of acetyl-CoA, which is an allosteric activator of pyruvate carboxylase, resulting in increased hepatic glucose production (ie, gluconeogenesis) (arrow 7). This increased hepatic glucose production, likely combined with the inability of skeletal muscle to appropriately uptake glucose and a lower insulin clearance, contributes to a compensatory hyperinsulinemia.[7] Although beneficial to maintain glucose levels at normal values, hyperinsulinemia also stimulates DNL further promoting hepatic steatosis.[41] Chronic hyperinsulinemia additionally promotes insulin resistance by downregulating insulin receptor signaling and defects in downstream signaling steps.[42] Finally, in addition to promoting high rates of hepatic gluconeogenesis, increased hepatic FFA oxidation also leads to incomplete lipid oxidation (arrow 8), with the generation of lipid intermediates (eg, ceramides and diacylglycerols) and reactive oxygen species (ROS) that promote hepatic insulin resistance and inflammation.[37] It should be noted that they may contribute to the progression of NAFLD, although the pathogenesis of NASH involves many other pathways beyond those linked with insulin resistance.

NONALCOHOLIC FATTY LIVER DISEASE AND METABOLIC SYNDROME: UNDERSTANDING THEIR COMPLEX RELATIONSHIP

NAFLD encompasses a wide range of liver conditions, which are characterized by the presence of hepatic steatosis in the absence of other secondary causes.[43,44] Hepatic steatosis is defined as liver fat accumulation ≥5% by histology or ≥5.56% by magnetic resonance-based techniques.[43] If hepatic steatosis coexists with lobular inflammation and hepatocyte ballooning it is considered NASH, which can in turn progress to liver fibrosis.[43,44] In the case of MetS, the situation is more complicated, as there are several definitions. In **Table 1** we have summarized the ones usually used in clinical practice. As can be observed, they are usually based on detecting central obesity and/or insulin resistance in combination with metabolic abnormalities (hypertension, dyslipidemia, and/or hyperglycemia). However, the most clinically widespread definition (ATP III) uses only the presence of three out of five metabolic traits to define MetS, irrespectively of the presence of obesity and/or insulin resistance (see **Table 1**).

Although NAFLD and MetS frequently coexist, this is not true in a significant number of patients. There are different scenarios, where we can clearly delineate the differences between NAFLD and MetS.

Nonalcoholic Fatty Liver Disease in the Absence of Metabolic Syndrome

Based on the IDF definition, the MetS is defined by the presence of increased waist circumference or obesity and at least 2 metabolic traits. However, it is possible that some patients with NAFLD can have insulin resistance without central obesity, and therefore could have NAFLD in the absence of MetS. As mentioned above, although central obesity is extremely common in patients with dysfunctional adipose tissue in NAFLD and MetS, there are other determinants of adipose tissue dysfunction. This is particularly true in patients of Asian ethnicity, who oftentimes present with insulin resistance in the absence of obesity as defined by their ethnicity cutoffs (although possibly the majority would have subtle increases in visceral adiposity).

NAFLD in patients that are lean has been increasingly recognized in the literature, and it is associated with similar metabolic and hepatic abnormalities as in people with overweight or obesity and NAFLD.[45] In a meta-analysis including a total of 10,530,308 patients, among all patients with NAFLD, 19.2% were lean.[46] Moreover, these patients showed a significant progression to more severe forms of liver disease, with 29.2% of patients with lean NAFLD having clinically significant fibrosis.[46] In different studies assessing complications and overall mortality, NAFLD in lean patients was associated with similar degrees of complications and mortality as NAFLD in obese patients.[47,48] It is likely that distinctive genetic/epigenetic factors may play a role in the development of NAFLD in lean patients. For example, lean patients with NAFLD have been found to have a stronger association with the pathogenic variant of PNPLA3.[49,50]

Unlike the IDF definition, the NCEP ATP definition does not require obesity for the diagnosis of MetS (see **Table 1**). Therefore, lean patients with NAFLD can still be considered as having MetS, if abnormal metabolic traits are found. In this setting, it is important to note that metabolic abnormalities, depending on genetic/epigenetic factors, can be a relatively late manifestation of insulin resistance. Therefore, in cases of mild NAFLD, it is possible that this entity can exist even in the absence of clinical evidence of MetS.

Table 1
Definitions of metabolic syndrome

	NCEP ATPIII (2005)	IDF (2005)	WHO (1998)	EGIR (1999)	AACE (2003)
Absolutely required	–	Waist circumference ≥94 cm (men) or ≥80 cm (women) Or BMI ≥ 30 kg/m^2	IFG, IGT, T2D or evidence of IR by euglycemic clamp	Insulin resistance or fasting hyperinsulinemia in nondiabetics	Any of: NAFLD, PCOS, acanthosis nigricans; FH of T2D, HTN, CVD; History of GD; Sedentary lifestyle; Age > 40; non-Caucasian ethnicity; or BMI >25.0 kg/m^2 (or WC ≥ 102 cm [men] or ≥88 cm [women]) in nondiabetics
Additional criteria	≥3 of the following:	≥2 of the following:	≥2 of the following:	≥2 of the following:	≥2 of the following:
	Waist circumference ≥102 cm (men) or ≥88 cm (women)	–	Waist-to-hip ratio >0.90 (men) or >0.85 (women), and/or BMI ≥ 30 kg/m^2	Waist circumference ≥94 cm (men) or ≥80 cm (women)	–
	TG ≥ 150 mg/dL or receiving treatment	TG ≥ 150 mg/dL or receiving treatment	TG ≥ 150 mg/dL and/or HDL-C <35 mg/dL (men) or <39 mg/dL (women), or receiving treatment	TG ≥ 177 mg/dL or HDL-C <39 mg/dL, or receiving treatment	TG ≥ 150 mg/dL or receiving treatment
	HDL-C <40 mg/dL (men) or <50 mg/dL (women), or receiving treatment	HDL-C <40 mg/dL (men) or <50 mg/dL (women), or receiving treatment			HDL-C <40 mg/dL (men) or <50 mg/dL (women), or receiving treatment
	SBP ≥130 mm Hg, DBP ≥85 mm Hg, or receiving treatment	SBP ≥130 mm Hg, DBP ≥85 mm Hg, or receiving treatment	SBP ≥140 mm Hg, DBP ≥90 mm Hg, or receiving treatment	SBP ≥140 mm Hg, DBP ≥90 mm Hg, or receiving treatment	SBP ≥130 mm Hg, DBP ≥85 mm Hg, or receiving treatment
	FPG ≥100 mg/dL or receiving treatment	FPG ≥100 mg/dL or receiving treatment	–	FPG ≥110 mg/dL, but not diabetes	FPG 110 to 125 mg/dL or 2-h OGTT glucose 140 to 199 mg/dL
	–	–	Microalbuminuria (UAER ≥20 μg/min or ACR ≥30 mg/g)	–	–

Metabolic Syndrome in the Absence of Nonalcoholic Fatty Liver Disease

It is well-known that the prevalence of NAFLD is higher in patients with T2D.[51] However, ~35% to 40% of patients with diabetes do not have NAFLD, despite an abnormal metabolic profile. The mechanisms protecting these patients from fat accumulation are not well understood, but may include an increased capacity of hepatic fat oxidation.[37,52] Another frequent example of patients with MetS without NAFLD are patients of African-American ethnicity. These patients show a lower prevalence of NAFLD when compared with Caucasian patients.[20,53] The underlying mechanisms of such a difference are not well understood. Lower rates of NAFLD result in overall lower triglyceride levels and higher HDL-C values as these depend on hepatic VLDL secretion as explained above. Paradoxically, even when having a lower risk for NAFLD, these patients show an increased risk of developing diabetes and hypertension. Therefore, although these patients can be diagnosed with MetS based on the presence of obesity, hyperglycemia, and hypertension, they oftentimes do not have concomitant NAFLD.

The scenarios presented above are just 2 examples of how NAFLD and MetS can exist independently of each other. Although it is common in clinical practice to observe most of these metabolic abnormalities clustered together, this is not always the case. As mentioned above, the development of overweight or obesity results in a dysfunctional adipose tissue and lipotoxicity. The mechanisms that determine which organs or tissues are specifically impacted by lipotoxicity in each individual (and thus their phenotypic manifestations), are not well-understood. In **Fig. 2**, we have represented how the effects of lipotoxicity in different tissues could result on different manifestations of the MetS. It is likely that the interaction of genetic, epigenetic, as well as other environmental factors, can determine which metabolic traits manifest in each individual patient. In addition, the adaptive capacity of each organ to deal with increased FFA flux and lipotoxicity may also determine whether metabolic abnormalities elicit. For

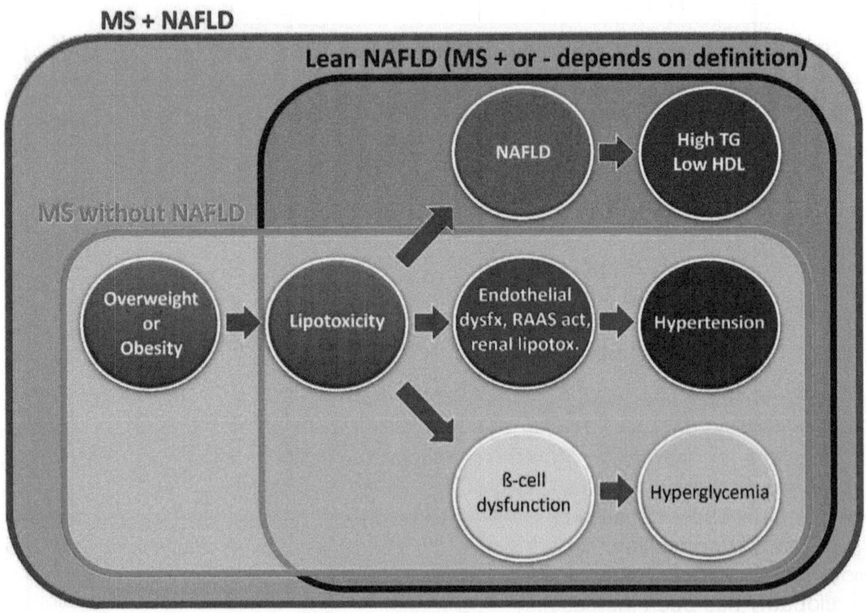

Fig. 2. Diagram showing that NAFLD and MetS can exist independently of each other.

example, patients with PNPLA3 polymorphism (I148 M rs738409) are at increased risk of developing NAFLD, but usually have lower plasma triglycerides and higher HDL-C.[54] These patients store more lipids in the liver (thus worse NAFLD), but as a consequence they secrete less VLDL (better lipid profile). Whether this SNP is associated with worse cardiovascular disease is still unknown. Among 4814 participants in the third National Health and Nutrition Examination Survey (NHANES 1991 to 1994), no increased cardiovascular mortality was noted in patients homozygous for PNPLA3 I148 M with NAFLD after a follow-up period of ~20 years.[55]

Does the Presence of Metabolic Syndrome Influence the Progression of Nonalcoholic Fatty Liver Disease?

Several guidelines recognize MetS as a risk factor for the progression of liver disease in NAFLD.[43,44,56] This is in part due to multiple observational studies showing an association between NASH and/or advanced liver fibrosis and the number of components of the MetS.[57,58] Many of these studies have performed multiple logistic analyses to isolate the effect of MetS on liver histology independently of other metabolic factors. However, the reality is that metabolic traits are usually clustered in patients with NAFLD, and it is practically impossible to isolate the effect of one from the others. Statistical analyses, even when complex, are unlikely to help us answering this question, as they can only adjust for known factors (ie, obesity, triglyceride levels, A1c, etc.), but not for other common factors that usually go unmeasured (ie, tissue-specific insulin resistance, plasma FFAs, plasma insulin levels, etc.). Moreover, these observational studies cannot establish causality. Even if MetS is statistically associated with NASH, it is possible that worse hepatic steatosis or increased insulin resistance are the drivers of both.[59]

Nonalcoholic fatty liver disease and dyslipidemia

We explained above how the presence of NAFLD results in elevated triglycerides, low HDL-C, and small and dense LDL particles. Available evidence suggests that these lipid changes are secondary to the degree of hepatic steatosis.[60] Specifically, Fabbrini and colleagues[61] showed that intrahepatic triglyceride content correlated well with the rate of VLDL-TG secretion. This correlation was maintained until intrahepatic triglyceride content reached approximately 10%. After this threshold, the secretion of VLDL-TG reached a plateau. In support of this finding, plasma TG and HDL-C levels were also proportionally altered with increasing intrahepatic triglyceride content until a threshold of ~8% in a different study including 352 patients.[60] Moreover, we observed that patients with NAFLD have increased levels of ApoB particles, lower ApoA1 levels, and smaller LDL particles.[62] However, these findings were associated with presence of NAFLD and/or insulin resistance, but not with worsening liver histology. As can be deduced from **Fig. 2**; **Fig. 3**, the presence of NAFLD promotes worse dyslipidemia, but there is no evidence that worse dyslipidemia has any impact on the progression of liver disease.

Nonalcoholic fatty liver disease and hypertension

Even after adjustment for other metabolic factors, NAFLD has been found to be associated with hypertension.[63,64] Whether this association is just the result of common risk factors or there is a pathophysiologic mechanism to link these conditions is unclear. Several characteristics of insulin-resistant patients can be contributing to both NAFLD and hypertension: hyperinsulinemia, subclinical inflammation, and systemic lipotoxicity. As a result of the obesity epidemic, an entity known as obesity-related glomerulopathy has been increasingly recognized.[65] It is possible that renal lipotoxicity promotes changes in kidney function that are reminiscent of hepatic lipotoxicity,

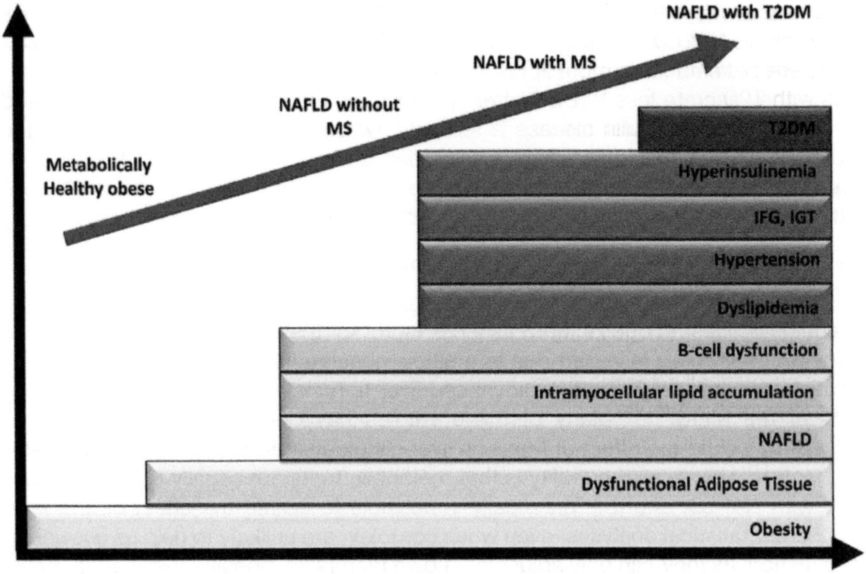

Fig. 3. Progression of metabolic abnormalities in patients with obesity.

NASH, and liver fibrosis.[66] Another potential mechanism that can explain the relation between NAFLD and hypertension is endothelial dysfunction secondary to lipotoxicity.[67] Although frequently associated, there is no strong evidence that the presence of hypertension *per se* is deleterious for the liver and contributes to the progression of NAFLD.

Nonalcoholic fatty liver disease and hyperglycemia

The relationship between NAFLD and hyperglycemia is poorly understood. There is strong evidence that the prevalence of NAFLD is increased in patients with T2D, and that patients with T2D also have a more rapid progression to severe forms of liver disease.[68] However, the mechanisms leading to worsening liver disease in these patients are unclear. Whether hyperglycemia *per se* contributes to worsening liver disease is not well-established and it is often confounded by the presence of insulin resistance. Against an important role of hyperglycemia in the development and progression of NAFLD, patients with T1D do not show a significant increase in the prevalence of NAFLD compared with BMI-matched healthy controls.[69] The authors concluded that NAFLD prevalence in patients with type 1 diabetes was at least comparable to and probably higher than in a matched general population. Heterogeneity of NAFLD prevalence in T1D was largely explained by diagnostic modality, with obesity and insulin resistance likely being the main drivers of liver disease, rather than hyperglycemia. However, this does not exclude that in T2D, obesity and insulin resistance may interact with hyperglycemia to promote the progression of NASH and liver fibrosis. However, in patients with T2D, diabetes control assessed by means of an A1c does not usually strongly correlate with the severity of the liver disease.[60] Also, treatment with medications such as insulin, sulfonylurea, metformin, and/or DPP-IV inhibitors have not been shown to improve liver disease, despite an effect on lowering hyperglycemia.[70,71] Because worse insulin resistance is associated with NAFLD and hyperglycemia, it is difficult in clinical practice to isolate the potential effect of one of these conditions from the other one. Combined they may potentiate each other to promote steatosis, and potentially steatohepatitis. For instance, elevated insulin levels drive *de novo* lipogenesis from glucose, so that hyperglycemia has a more deleterious effect to induce steatosis in the presence of hyperinsulinemia, as seen in patients with T2D.

Overall, because insulin resistance, ectopic fat deposition, and lipotoxicity often play a role in the development of NAFLD and abnormal metabolic traits, patients with worse insulin resistance typically develop NAFLD and more prominent signs of MetS. However, it currently remains difficult to establish causality and that the presence of MetS *per se* contributes to worsening liver disease.

NONALCOHOLIC FATTY LIVER DISEASE AND METABOLIC SYNDROME AS BIOMARKERS OF INSULIN RESISTANCE

MetS was originally described as a way to assist in the identification of patients at increased cardiovascular risk. However, it is important to note that many of its abnormal metabolic features develop rather late in the course of obesity, T2D or NAFLD.[59] Therefore, as a means to detect patients at risk of cardiovascular disease, MetS is a rather insensitive method. By using state-of-the-art measurements of insulin resistance (eg, hyperinsulinemic-euglycemic clamp), most patients have already significant insulin resistance in the absence (or with few or minimal) clinical metabolic abnormalities.[72] In the diagram of **Fig. 3**, we can observe that the typical clinical metabolic abnormalities of MetS only seem to develop once other metabolic abnormalities are already fully established (ie, adipose tissue dysfunction, ectopic fat deposition in organs, NAFLD, β-cell dysfunction, other). In a large study including 352 patients, intrahepatic triglyceride accumulations of ~4 to 8% were already associated with maximally impaired insulin resistance at the levels of the liver and skeletal muscle, as well as maximally impaired triglycerides and HDL-C.[60] This suggests that relatively small accumulations of intrahepatic triglyceride are already associated with metabolic abnormalities, including peripheral insulin resistance. In other words, the presence of NAFLD can be considered an early marker of metabolic disease.[73] However, no current guideline recommends screening just for hepatic steatosis as a way to identify metabolic disease. Other articles in this issue address the current strategies to screen for NAFLD and detect significant liver fibrosis in clinical practice. We refer readers to recent guidelines about the management of NAFLD in patients with or without diabetes.[43,44,56]

TARGETING INSULIN RESISTANCE IN CLINICAL PRACTICE

Lifestyle Interventions, Weight Loss Medications, and Bariatric Surgery

Strategies focused on weight loss, either through hypocaloric diets or macronutrient restriction,[74–83] intermittent calorie-restriction,[84] exercise alone or in combination with a specific diet,[85–104] bariatric surgery[105] and/or weight-loss medications including orlistat and glucagon-like peptide 1 (GLP-1) receptor agonists[106–119] have all shown to be effective for the treatment of NAFLD, and even NASH.[120,121] Whether one strategy is specifically better than others remains to be determined. In **Fig. 4**, we have plotted studies that have assessed changes in intrahepatic triglyceride content by magnetic resonance-based strategies after diverse interventions aimed at producing weight loss.[74–119] As can be observed, regardless of the strategy plotted, the relative reduction in intrahepatic triglyceride content was strongly correlated with the amount of weight loss. Moreover, by fitting the best line in the graph, it can be observed that approximately 5% of weight loss is associated with a relative reduction of ~30% of intrahepatic triglyceride content, which is considered a meaningful reduction after

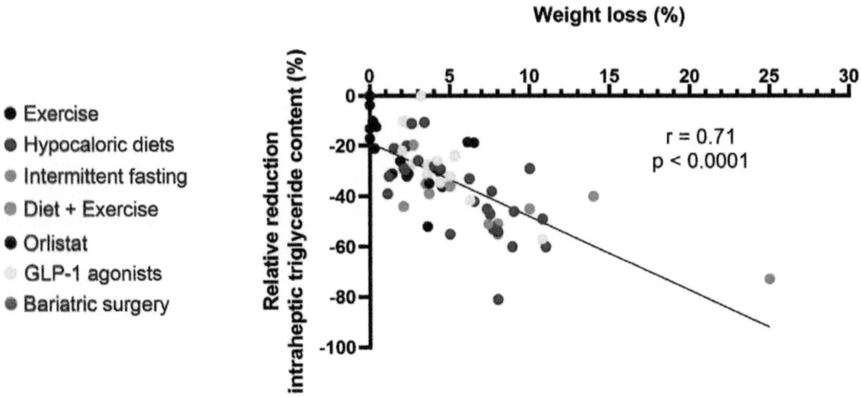

Fig. 4. Effect of weight loss on improvement of intrahepatic triglyceride accumulation based on different strategies.

an intervention. In addition, in another landmark study, Vilar-Gomez and colleagues[122] showed that the amount of weight loss was also associated with the degree of histologic improvement in patients with NASH. This study also showed that a reduction of ~5% of weight loss was needed to achieve a significant improvement in steatosis. More significant reductions in weight after follow-up were associated with improvement in lobular inflammation, ballooning, and presence of NASH (ie, ~7% weight loss) and even liver fibrosis (ie, ~10% weight loss). Studies assessing weight-loss medications, such as orlistat, suggest similar results.[123] Several guidelines have summarized current weight loss recommendations for patients with NAFLD and we refer the readership to them.[43,44,56] In summary, regardless of the strategy used to achieve weight loss, it seems that improvement of NAFLD/NASH depends directly on the amount of weight lost after the intervention.

Glucagon-Like Peptide 1 Receptor Agonists

Similarly to lifestyle interventions and other weight-loss medications, it seems that GLP-1 receptor agonists beneficial liver effects in NASH are mostly associated with the degree of weight loss (see **Fig. 4**).[107–119] Whether the incretin effect and glycemic control also play a role in NAFLD improvement with GLP-1 agonists remains unknown. Because there are no GLP-1 receptors in the liver, it is likely that improvements in NAFLD and NASH are secondary to other metabolic improvements (ie, weight loss, better glycemic control, less insulin resistance).

Although several studies have been published on the effects of exenatide and liraglutide in hepatic steatosis by MRI,[107–119] histology has only been assessed in a small study with liraglutide.[124] The larger study with GLP-1 agonists assessing histologic changes used daily injections of semaglutide.[121] In this study, the highest dose was associated with significant resolution of NASH, and although improvement in liver fibrosis did not reach statistical significance, there was a substantial slowing of fibrosis progression. Of note, the effect on liver fibrosis was confounded by the significant response observed in the placebo group (~33%). Larger and longer studies are needed to assess the effect of this class of medications in NASH. Based on the available experience from bariatric surgery studies, it is possible that long-term weight loss in the range obtained with newer GLP-1 agonists (weight loss >15%) may result in a significant improvement of liver fibrosis.

Insulin Sensitizers

Peroxisome proliferator-activated receptor agonists

Pioglitazone, a primarily peroxisome proliferator-activated receptor (PPAR)-gamma agonist with some PPAR-alpha agonism, is likely the drug with the strongest degree of evidence in patients with biopsy-proven NASH.[125,126] However, despite evidence from randomized, controlled trials showing its beneficial effects in NASH, this has not translated to global use of this drug among primary care providers or hepatologists.[127,128] Pioglitazone has been shown to significantly improve steatosis, lobular inflammation, and hepatocyte ballooning compared with placebo. This has been consistent regardless of the duration of the studies (6, 12, 18, or 24 months),[125,126,129,130] or whether patients had diabetes or not.[131] Improvement of these histologic parameters translates into a significant resolution of NASH. Moreover, when all studies were combined, pioglitazone has also shown to improve liver fibrosis stages and reverse advanced fibrosis.[132] For all of the above, current guidelines recommend the use of pioglitazone in patients with NASH and T2D.[43,44,56] It is not approved specifically for NASH, so its use in patients without diabetes would be considered off-label.

Another insulin sensitizer that has been assessed for NAFLD was saroglitazar (PPAR alpha and gamma). This drug became the first medication in the world to be specifically approved for NAFLD (ie, approved in India). In a recently published trial ($n = 106$), saroglitazar 4 mg daily (highest dose) was effective to decrease plasma aminotransferases and intrahepatic triglyceride content.[133] Ongoing studies are assessing its use to improve histology in patients with NASH. Lanifibranor, a pan-PPAR agonism (ie, alpha, delta, gamma) has also been shown to improve the resolution of NASH with no worsening of fibrosis when compared with placebo.[134] In this large, randomized, controlled trial, the higher dose of lanifibranor (1200 mg daily) also showed significant improvement in liver fibrosis without worsening of NASH compared with placebo. Ongoing phase III studies will help us see in a larger scale the effects of this new medication in patients with NASH.

These medications have been shown not only to improve liver disease, but also other metabolic parameters, such as glucose control, insulin sensitivity, and lipids. They are associated with variable degrees of weight gain, likely related to their insulin sensitizer effect.

Metformin

Despite its role in hyperglycemia management and its insulin-sensitizer effect on the liver, metformin has not shown a significant role in the treatment of NAFLD and NASH. It is safe to use in patients with T2D and NAFLD/NASH, but despite some studies showing a decrease in plasma aminotransferases, no hepatic histologic improvement has been observed with this drug.[135] In line with these results, PXL770, a novel AMPK activator, failed to improve hepatic steatosis compared with a placebo after 12 weeks of treatment.[136] However, recent observational data have suggested that compared with no medication use, metformin was associated with a lower risk of developing hepatocellular carcinoma in patients with NAFLD and T2D.[137]

Sodium-Glucose Co-Transporter 2 Inhibitors

By inhibiting sodium-glucose co-transporter 2 (SGLT-2) in the kidney, these medications induce their glucose-lowering effects independently of changes in insulin sensitivity. Studies assessing insulin sensitivity after SGLT-2 inhibitor use, have shown only minimal or no improvement in the liver and skeletal muscle insulin sensitivity.[138–141] Evidence of the role of these newer agents in NAFLD comes mainly from studies

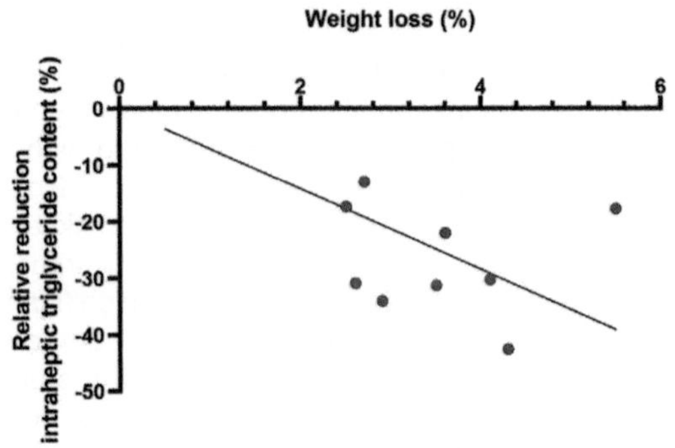

Fig. 5. Effect of weight loss on improvement of intrahepatic triglyceride accumulation in studies assessing SGLT-2 inhibitors.

that have assessed changes in hepatic steatosis compared with placebo. Although an early study with canagliflozin not targeting patients with NAFLD, but obese patients with T2D, did not observe a significant reduction in hepatic steatosis after 24 weeks of treatment,[138] other studies with empagliflozin, dapagliflozin, tofogliflozin, and ipragliflozin showed a significant reduction in hepatic steatosis by magnetic resonance techniques compared with placebo.[138,140–147] However, in relative terms, the reduction of hepatic steatosis obtained with these agents have been rather small (~20% to 30%) compared with other medications, like pioglitazone. Moreover, as can be observed in **Fig. 5**, their effect seems to be driven by weight loss. Therefore, their role in achieving histologic improvement remains to be determined. Open-label, uncontrolled studies in a small group of patients showed significant improvements in liver histology,[148,149] however randomized, controlled trials are still lacking.

SUMMARY

NAFLD has a strong correlation with steatosis and cardiometabolic risk factors, but this relationship remains incompletely understood. Insulin resistance seems to be the universal defect in people with steatosis (or steatohepatitis) and the MetS, but they may be present without features of the MetS and vice versa. Moreover, it is important to acknowledge that NASH is a complex disease with multiple molecular pathways that include insulin resistance but involve many additional defects that trigger inflammatory pathways, cell death, and fibrogenesis.[150] This review highlightedthe MetS as a cardiometabolic/insulin resistance syndrome that remains poorly understood in most aspects (from consensus about its best definition and its optimal risk factor cutoffs, to its pathways leading to cardiometabolic risk and its many phenotypes in NAFLD). That we often use the NCEP III definition for its simplicity does not mean it is the most accurate from a cardiovascular risk or biology of disease perspective. It may also not be accurate to say that NAFLD is the hepatic manifestation of MetS when it is more a reflection of insulin resistance, whether cardiometabolic features are present or not. In clinical practice, the identification of insulin resistance and its treatment should be viewed as a major target, involving lifestyle changes that promote weight loss. As discussed, when needed, the use of antiobesity medications, in particular GLP-1RAs, and some diabetes medications with cardiometabolic and liver histologic benefits should be considered key in routine clinical practice.[56] In summary, our knowledge gaps are humbling and encourage more work to deepen our understanding of the complex relationship between insulin resistance, MetS, and

NAFLD. It may also make us think twice about stating that NAFLD is the hepatic manifestation of the MetS and consider carefully the many implications to rename and/or redefine NAFLD broadly as a "metabolic dysfunction" based primarily on a diverse and poorly understood constellation of cardiometabolic features.

CLINICS CARE POINTS

- Patients with NAFLD and/or MetS almost always present some degree of insulin resistance.
- A patient can have NAFLD even in the absence of the cardiometabolic risk factors associated with the MetS.
- Targeting insulin resistance in these patients, either by weight loss or insulin sensitizers, will help NAFLD, but also all the other complications promoted by insulin resistance.

DISCLOSURES

F. Bril has nothing to disclose. A. Sanyal has stock options in Genfit, Akarna, Tiziana, Indalo, Durect Inversago, and Galmed. He has served as a consultant to Astra Zeneca, Nitto Denko, Conatus, Nimbus, Salix, Tobira, Takeda, Amgen, Genentech, Gilead, United States, Jannsen, Intercept, Regeneron, Siemens, Gilead, Terns, 89BIO, Akero, Merck, United States, Valeant, Boehringer-Ingelheim, Bristol Myers Squibb, Eli Lilly, Hemoshear, Novartis, Novo Nordisk, Pfizer, Exhalenz, and Genfit. His institution has received grant support from Gilead, Salix, Tobira, Bristol Myers, Shire, Intercept, United States, Merck, AstraZeneca, United Kingdom, Malinckrodt, Cumberland and Novartis, Switzerland. He receives royalties from Elsevier and UptoDate. He recused himself from the analysis and interpretation of NIS4. K. Cusi has received research support toward the University of Florida as principal investigator from the National Institutes of Health (NIH), United States, Echosens, Inventiva, Poxel, Labcorp, and Zydus. He is a consultant for Altimmune, Arrowhead, AstraZeneca, 89Bio, BMS, Eli Lilly, Madrigal, Merck, Myovant, Novo Nordisk, Prosciento, Quest, Sagimet, Sonic Incytes, and Terns.

REFERENCES

1. Lonardo A, Nascimbeni F, Mantovani A, et al. Hypertension, diabetes, atherosclerosis and NASH: cause or consequence? J Hepatol 2018;68:335–52.
2. Muzurovic E, Mikhailidis DP, Mantzoros C. Non-alcoholic fatty liver disease, insulin resistance, metabolic syndrome and their association with vascular risk. Metabolism 2021;119:154770.
3. Eslam M, Sanyal AJ, George J, et al. MAFLD: a consensus-driven proposed nomenclature for metabolic associated fatty liver disease. Gastroenterology 2020;158:1999–2014, e1991.
4. Eslam M, Newsome PN, Sarin SK, et al. A new definition for metabolic dysfunction-associated fatty liver disease: an international expert consensus statement. J Hepatol 2020;73:202–9.
5. Younossi ZM, Rinella ME, Sanyal AJ, et al. From NAFLD to MAFLD: implications of a premature change in terminology. Hepatology 2021;73:1194–8.
6. Samuel VT, Shulman GI. The pathogenesis of insulin resistance: integrating signaling pathways and substrate flux. J Clin Invest 2016;126:12–22.
7. Petersen MC, Shulman GI. Mechanisms of insulin action and insulin resistance. Physiol Rev 2018;98:2133–223.

8. Hudish LI, Reusch JE, Sussel L. Beta Cell dysfunction during progression of metabolic syndrome to type 2 diabetes. J Clin Invest 2019;129:4001–8.
9. Norton L, Shannon C, Gastaldelli A, et al. Insulin: the master regulator of glucose metabolism. Metabolism 2022;129:155142.
10. Caprio S, Perry R, Kursawe R. Adolescent obesity and insulin resistance: roles of ectopic fat accumulation and adipose inflammation. Gastroenterology 2017;152:1638–46.
11. Angelidi AM, Filippaios A, Mantzoros CS. Severe insulin resistance syndromes. J Clin Invest 2021;131(4):e142245.
12. Johnson AM, Olefsky JM. The origins and drivers of insulin resistance. Cell 2013;152:673–84.
13. Abbasi F, Brown BW Jr, Lamendola C, et al. Relationship between obesity, insulin resistance, and coronary heart disease risk. J Am Coll Cardiol 2002;40:937–43.
14. Gonzalez-Cantero J, Martin-Rodriguez JL, Gonzalez-Cantero A, et al. Insulin resistance in lean and overweight non-diabetic Caucasian adults: study of its relationship with liver triglyceride content, waist circumference and BMI. PLoS One 2018;13:e0192663.
15. Tay J, Goss AM, Garvey WT, et al. Race affects the association of obesity measures with insulin sensitivity. Am J Clin Nutr 2020;111:515–25.
16. Mente A, Razak F, Blankenberg S, et al. Ethnic variation in adiponectin and leptin levels and their association with adiposity and insulin resistance. Diabetes Care 2010;33:1629–34.
17. Khoo CM, Sairazi S, Taslim S, et al. Ethnicity modifies the relationships of insulin resistance, inflammation, and adiponectin with obesity in a multiethnic Asian population. Diabetes Care 2011;34:1120–6.
18. Kodama K, Tojjar D, Yamada S, et al. Ethnic differences in the relationship between insulin sensitivity and insulin response: a systematic review and meta-analysis. Diabetes Care 2013;36:1789–96.
19. Koh HE, Patterson BW, Reeds DN, et al. Insulin sensitivity and kinetics in African American and White people with obesity: insights from different study protocols. Obesity (Silver Spring) 2022;30:655–65.
20. Bril F, Portillo-Sanchez P, Liu IC, et al. Clinical and histologic characterization of nonalcoholic steatohepatitis in African American patients. Diabetes Care 2018;41:187–92.
21. Guerrero R, Vega GL, Grundy SM, et al. Ethnic differences in hepatic steatosis: an insulin resistance paradox? Hepatology 2009;49:791–801.
22. Bluher M. Metabolically healthy obesity. Endocr Rev 2020;41(3):bnaa004.
23. Unger RH. Lipotoxicity in the pathogenesis of obesity-dependent NIDDM. Genetic and clinical implications. Diabetes 1995;44:863–70.
24. Montgomery MK, De Nardo W, Watt MJ. Impact of lipotoxicity on tissue "cross talk" and metabolic regulation. Physiology (Bethesda) 2019;34:134–49.
25. Fryk E, Olausson J, Mossberg K, et al. Hyperinsulinemia and insulin resistance in the obese may develop as part of a homeostatic response to elevated free fatty acids: a mechanistic case-control and a population-based cohort study. EBioMedicine 2021;65:103264.
26. Cusi K. Role of obesity and lipotoxicity in the development of nonalcoholic steatohepatitis: pathophysiology and clinical implications. Gastroenterology 2012;142:711–725 e716.

27. Lomonaco R, Ortiz-Lopez C, Orsak B, et al. Effect of adipose tissue insulin resistance on metabolic parameters and liver histology in obese patients with nonalcoholic fatty liver disease. Hepatology 2012;55:1389–97.
28. Wu H, Ballantyne CM. Metabolic inflammation and insulin resistance in obesity. Circ Res 2020;126:1549–64.
29. Sylow L, Tokarz VL, Richter EA, et al. The many actions of insulin in skeletal muscle, the paramount tissue determining glycemia. Cell Metab 2021;33:758–80.
30. Kelley DE, Mandarino LJ. Fuel selection in human skeletal muscle in insulin resistance: a reexamination. Diabetes 2000;49:677–83.
31. Galgani JE, Moro C, Ravussin E. Metabolic flexibility and insulin resistance. Am J Physiol Endocrinol Metab 2008;295:E1009–17.
32. Fritzen AM, Lundsgaard AM, Kiens B. Tuning fatty acid oxidation in skeletal muscle with dietary fat and exercise. Nat Rev Endocrinol 2020;16:683–96.
33. Goodpaster BH. CrossTalk proposal: intramuscular lipid accumulation causes insulin resistance. J Physiol 2020;598:3803–6.
34. Kitessa SM, Abeywardena MY. Lipid-induced insulin resistance in skeletal muscle: the chase for the culprit goes from total intramuscular fat to lipid intermediates, and finally to species of lipid intermediates. Nutrients 2016;8(8):466.
35. Bril F, Lomonaco R, Cusi K. The challenge of managing dyslipidemia in patients with nonalcoholic fatty liver disease. Clin Lipidol 2012;7:471–81.
36. Bril F, Cusi K. Nonalcoholic fatty liver disease: the new complication of type 2 diabetes mellitus. Endocrinol Metab Clin North Am 2016;45:765–81.
37. Sunny NE, Bril F, Cusi K. Mitochondrial adaptation in nonalcoholic fatty liver disease: novel mechanisms and treatment strategies. Trends Endocrinol Metab 2017;28:250–60.
38. Lambert JE, Ramos-Roman MA, Browning JD, et al. Increased de novo lipogenesis is a distinct characteristic of individuals with nonalcoholic fatty liver disease. Gastroenterology 2014;146:726–35.
39. Smith GI, Shankaran M, Yoshino M, et al. Insulin resistance drives hepatic de novo lipogenesis in nonalcoholic fatty liver disease. J Clin Invest 2020;130: 1453–60.
40. Luukkonen PK, Sadevirta S, Zhou Y, et al. Saturated fat is more metabolically harmful for the human liver than unsaturated fat or simple sugars. Diabetes Care 2018;41:1732–9.
41. Ter Horst KW, Vatner DF, Zhang D, et al. Hepatic insulin resistance is not pathway selective in humans with nonalcoholic fatty liver disease. Diabetes Care 2021;44:489–98.
42. Iozzo P, Pratipanawatr T, Pijl H, et al. Physiological hyperinsulinemia impairs insulin-stimulated glycogen synthase activity and glycogen synthesis. Am J Physiol Endocrinol Metab 2001;280:E712–9.
43. European association for the study of the liver, European association for the study of diabetes, European association for the study of obesity. EASL-EASD-EASO clinical practice guidelines for the management of non-alcoholic fatty liver disease. J Hepatol 2016;64:1388–402.
44. Chalasani N, Younossi Z, Lavine JE, et al. The diagnosis and management of nonalcoholic fatty liver disease: practice guidance from the American Association for the Study of Liver Diseases. Hepatology 2018;67:328–57.
45. Sookoian S, Pirola CJ. Systematic review with meta-analysis: risk factors for nonalcoholic fatty liver disease suggest a shared altered metabolic and cardiovascular profile between lean and obese patients. Aliment Pharmacol Ther 2017;46: 85–95.

46. Ye Q, Zou B, Yeo YH, et al. Global prevalence, incidence, and outcomes of non-obese or lean non-alcoholic fatty liver disease: a systematic review and meta-analysis. Lancet Gastroenterol Hepatol 2020;5:739–52.
47. Zou B, Yeo YH, Nguyen VH, et al. Prevalence, characteristics and mortality outcomes of obese, nonobese and lean NAFLD in the United States, 1999-2016. J Intern Med 2020;288:139–51.
48. Younes R, Govaere O, Petta S, et al. Caucasian lean subjects with non-alcoholic fatty liver disease share long-term prognosis of non-lean: time for reappraisal of BMI-driven approach? Gut 2022;71:382–90.
49. Krawczyk M, Bantel H, Rau M, et al. Could inherited predisposition drive non-obese fatty liver disease? Results from German tertiary referral centers. J Hum Genet 2018;63:621–6.
50. Lin H, Wong GL, Whatling C, et al. Association of genetic variations with NAFLD in lean individuals. Liver Int 2022;42:149–60.
51. Younossi ZM, Tampi RP, Racila A, et al. Economic and clinical burden of nonalcoholic steatohepatitis in patients with type 2 diabetes in the U.S. Diabetes Care 2020;43:283–9.
52. Gancheva S, Kahl S, Pesta D, et al. Impaired hepatic mitochondrial capacity in nonalcoholic steatohepatitis associated with type 2 diabetes. Diabetes Care 2022;45:928–37.
53. Satapathy SK, Marella HK, Heda RP, et al. African Americans have a distinct clinical and histologic profile with lower prevalence of NASH and advanced fibrosis relative to Caucasians. Eur J Gastroenterol Hepatol 2021;33:388–98.
54. Hyysalo J, Gopalacharyulu P, Bian H, et al. Circulating triacylglycerol signatures in nonalcoholic fatty liver disease associated with the I148M variant in PNPLA3 and with obesity. Diabetes 2014;63:312–22.
55. Wijarnpreecha K, Scribani M, Raymond P, et al. PNPLA3 gene polymorphism and overall and cardiovascular mortality in the United States. J Gastroenterol Hepatol 2020;35:1789–94.
56. Cusi K, Isaacs S, Barb D, et al. American association of clinical endocrinology clinical practice guideline for the diagnosis and management of nonalcoholic fatty liver disease in primary care and endocrinology clinical settings: Co-sponsored by the American association for the study of liver diseases (AASLD). Endocr Pract 2022;28:528–62.
57. Kanwar P, Nelson JE, Yates K, et al. Association between metabolic syndrome and liver histology among NAFLD patients without diabetes. BMJ Open Gastroenterol 2016;3:e000114.
58. Jarvis H, Craig D, Barker R, et al. Metabolic risk factors and incident advanced liver disease in non-alcoholic fatty liver disease (NAFLD): a systematic review and meta-analysis of population-based observational studies. Plos Med 2020;17:e1003100.
59. Lonardo A, Ballestri S, Marchesini G, et al. Nonalcoholic fatty liver disease: a precursor of the metabolic syndrome. Dig Liver Dis 2015;47:181–90.
60. Bril F, Barb D, Portillo-Sanchez P, et al. Metabolic and histological implications of intrahepatic triglyceride content in nonalcoholic fatty liver disease. Hepatology 2017;65:1132–44.
61. Fabbrini E, deHaseth D, Deivanayagam S, et al. Alterations in fatty acid kinetics in obese adolescents with increased intrahepatic triglyceride content. Obesity (Silver Spring) 2009;17:25–9.

62. Bril F, Sninsky JJ, Baca AM, et al. Hepatic steatosis and insulin resistance, but not steatohepatitis, promote atherogenic dyslipidemia in NAFLD. J Clin Endocrinol Metab 2016;101:644–52.
63. Zhao YC, Zhao GJ, Chen Z, et al. Nonalcoholic fatty liver disease: an emerging driver of hypertension. Hypertension 2020;75:275–84.
64. Sung KC, Wild SH, Byrne CD. Development of new fatty liver, or resolution of existing fatty liver, over five years of follow-up, and risk of incident hypertension. J Hepatol 2014;60:1040–5.
65. de Vries AP, Ruggenenti P, Ruan XZ, et al. Fatty kidney: emerging role of ectopic lipid in obesity-related renal disease. Lancet Diabetes Endocrinol 2014;2: 417–26.
66. Musso G, Cassader M, Cohney S, et al. Fatty liver and chronic kidney disease: novel mechanistic insights and therapeutic opportunities. Diabetes Care 2016; 39:1830–45.
67. Ghosh A, Gao L, Thakur A, et al. Role of free fatty acids in endothelial dysfunction. J Biomed Sci 2017;24:50.
68. Bril F, Cusi K. Management of nonalcoholic fatty liver disease in patients with type 2 diabetes: a call to action. Diabetes Care 2017;40:419–30.
69. de Vries M, Westerink J, Kaasjager K, et al. Prevalence of nonalcoholic fatty liver disease (NAFLD) in patients with type 1 diabetes mellitus: a systematic review and meta-analysis. J Clin Endocrinol Metab 2020;105(12):3842–53.
70. Beauchamp G, Barr MM, Vergara A, et al. Treatment of hyperglycemia not associated with NAFLD improvement in children with type 2 diabetes mellitus. Int J Pediatr Adolesc Med 2022;9:83–8.
71. Godinez-Leiva E, Bril F. Nonalcoholic fatty liver disease (NAFLD) for primary care providers: beyond the liver. Curr Hypertens Rev 2021;17:94–111.
72. Sierra-Johnson J, Johnson BD, Allison TG, et al. Correspondence between the adult treatment panel III criteria for metabolic syndrome and insulin resistance. Diabetes Care 2006;29:668–72.
73. Bril F, Cusi K. Reply to: liver fat accumulation as a barometer of insulin responsiveness again points to adipose tissue as the culprit. Hepatology 2017;65(4): 1088–90.
74. Petersen KF, Dufour S, Befroy D, et al. Reversal of nonalcoholic hepatic steatosis, hepatic insulin resistance, and hyperglycemia by moderate weight reduction in patients with type 2 diabetes. Diabetes 2005;54:603–8.
75. Kirk E, Reeds DN, Finck BN, et al. Dietary fat and carbohydrates differentially alter insulin sensitivity during caloric restriction. Gastroenterology 2009;136: 1552–60.
76. Viljanen AP, Iozzo P, Borra R, et al. Effect of weight loss on liver free fatty acid uptake and hepatic insulin resistance. J Clin Endocrinol Metab 2009;94:50–5.
77. Haufe S, Engeli S, Kast P, et al. Randomized comparison of reduced fat and reduced carbohydrate hypocaloric diets on intrahepatic fat in overweight and obese human subjects. Hepatology 2011;53:1504–14.
78. Browning JD, Baker JA, Rogers T, et al. Short-term weight loss and hepatic triglyceride reduction: evidence of a metabolic advantage with dietary carbohydrate restriction. Am J Clin Nutr 2011;93:1048–52.
79. Properzi C, O'Sullivan TA, Sherriff JL, et al. Ad libitum mediterranean and low-fat diets both significantly reduce hepatic steatosis: a randomized controlled trial. Hepatology 2018;68:1741–54.

80. Ryan MC, Itsiopoulos C, Thodis T, et al. The Mediterranean diet improves hepatic steatosis and insulin sensitivity in individuals with non-alcoholic fatty liver disease. J Hepatol 2013;59:138–43.
81. Marin-Alejandre BA, Abete I, Cantero I, et al. The metabolic and hepatic impact of two personalized dietary strategies in subjects with obesity and nonalcoholic fatty liver disease: the fatty liver in obesity (FLiO) randomized controlled trial. Nutrients 2019;11(10):2543.
82. Abbate M, Mascaro CM, Montemayor S, et al. Energy expenditure improved risk factors associated with renal function loss in NAFLD and MetS patients. Nutrients 2021;13(2):629.
83. Willmann C, Heni M, Linder K, et al. Potential effects of reduced red meat compared with increased fiber intake on glucose metabolism and liver fat content: a randomized and controlled dietary intervention study. Am J Clin Nutr 2019;109:288–96.
84. Holmer M, Lindqvist C, Petersson S, et al. Treatment of NAFLD with intermittent calorie restriction or low-carb high-fat diet - a randomised controlled trial. JHEP Rep 2021;3:100256.
85. Shojaee-Moradie F, Baynes KC, Pentecost C, et al. Exercise training reduces fatty acid availability and improves the insulin sensitivity of glucose metabolism. Diabetologia 2007;50:404–13.
86. Johnson NA, Sachinwalla T, Walton DW, et al. Aerobic exercise training reduces hepatic and visceral lipids in obese individuals without weight loss. Hepatology 2009;50:1105–12.
87. Hallsworth K, Fattakhova G, Hollingsworth KG, et al. Resistance exercise reduces liver fat and its mediators in non-alcoholic fatty liver disease independent of weight loss. Gut 2011;60:1278–83.
88. Sullivan S, Kirk EP, Patterson B, et al. Effect of endurance exercise on nonalcoholic fatty liver disease. Gastroenterology 2011;140:S700.
89. Bacchi E, Negri C, Targher G, et al. Both resistance training and aerobic training reduce hepatic fat content in type 2 diabetic subjects with NAFLD (The RAED2 randomized trial). Hepatology 2013;58(4):1287–95.
90. Haus JM, Solomon TP, Kelly KR, et al. Improved hepatic lipid composition following short-term exercise in nonalcoholic fatty liver disease. J Clin Endocrinol Metab 2013;98:E1181–8.
91. Tamura Y, Tanaka Y, Sato F, et al. Effects of diet and exercise on muscle and liver intracellular lipid contents and insulin sensitivity in type 2 diabetic patients. J Clin Endocrinol Metab 2005;90:3191–6.
92. Larson-Meyer DE, Heilbronn LK, Redman LM, et al. Effect of calorie restriction with or without exercise on insulin sensitivity, beta-cell function, fat cell size, and ectopic lipid in overweight subjects. Diabetes Care 2006;29:1337–44.
93. Kantartzis K, Thamer C, Peter A, et al. High cardiorespiratory fitness is an independent predictor of the reduction in liver fat during a lifestyle intervention in non-alcoholic fatty liver disease. Gut 2009;58:1281–8.
94. Shah K, Stufflebam A, Hilton TN, et al. Diet and exercise interventions reduce intrahepatic fat content and improve insulin sensitivity in obese older adults. Obesity (Silver Spring) 2009;17:2162–8.
95. Lazo M, Solga SF, Horska A, et al. Effect of a 12-month intensive lifestyle intervention on hepatic steatosis in adults with type 2 diabetes. Diabetes Care 2010;33:2156–63.

96. Wong VW, Chan RS, Wong GL, et al. Community-based lifestyle modification programme for non-alcoholic fatty liver disease: a randomized controlled trial. J Hepatol 2013;59:536–42.
97. Cheng S, Ge J, Zhao C, et al. Effect of aerobic exercise and diet on liver fat in pre-diabetic patients with non-alcoholic-fatty-liver-disease: a randomized controlled trial. Sci Rep 2017;7:15952.
98. Keating SE, Hackett DA, Parker HM, et al. Effect of resistance training on liver fat and visceral adiposity in adults with obesity: a randomized controlled trial. Hepatol Res 2017;47:622–31.
99. Pugh CJ, Spring VS, Kemp GJ, et al. Exercise training reverses endothelial dysfunction in nonalcoholic fatty liver disease. Am J Physiol Heart Circ Physiol 2014;307:H1298–306.
100. Zhang HJ, He J, Pan LL, et al. Effects of moderate and vigorous exercise on nonalcoholic fatty liver disease: a randomized clinical trial. JAMA Intern Med 2016;176:1074–82.
101. Abdelbasset WK, Tantawy SA, Kamel DM, et al. Effects of high-intensity interval and moderate-intensity continuous aerobic exercise on diabetic obese patients with nonalcoholic fatty liver disease: a comparative randomized controlled trial. Medicine (Baltimore) 2020;99:e19471.
102. Houghton D, Thoma C, Hallsworth K, et al. Exercise reduces liver lipids and visceral adiposity in patients with nonalcoholic steatohepatitis in a randomized controlled trial. Clin Gastroenterol Hepatol 2017;15:96–102 e103.
103. Shojaee-Moradie F, Cuthbertson DJ, Barrett M, et al. Exercise training reduces liver fat and increases rates of VLDL clearance but not VLDL production in NAFLD. J Clin Endocrinol Metab 2016;101:4219–28.
104. Yaskolka Meir A, Rinott E, Tsaban G, et al. Effect of green-Mediterranean diet on intrahepatic fat: the DIRECT PLUS randomised controlled trial. Gut 2021;70: 2085–95.
105. Pooler BD, Wiens CN, McMillan A, et al. Monitoring fatty liver disease with MRI following bariatric surgery: a prospective, dual-center study. Radiology 2019; 290:682–90.
106. Ye J, Wu Y, Li F, et al. Effect of orlistat on liver fat content in patients with nonalcoholic fatty liver disease with obesity: assessment using magnetic resonance imaging-derived proton density fat fraction. Therap Adv Gastroenterol 2019; 12. 1756284819879047.
107. Smits MM, Tonneijck L, Muskiet MH, et al. Twelve week liraglutide or sitagliptin does not affect hepatic fat in type 2 diabetes: a randomised placebo-controlled trial. Diabetologia 2016;59:2588–93.
108. Petit JM, Cercueil JP, Loffroy R, et al. Effect of liraglutide therapy on liver fat content in patients with inadequately controlled type 2 diabetes: the lira-NAFLD study. J Clin Endocrinol Metab 2017;102:407–15.
109. Matikainen N, Soderlund S, Bjornson E, et al. Liraglutide treatment improves postprandial lipid metabolism and cardiometabolic risk factors in humans with adequately controlled type 2 diabetes: a single-centre randomized controlled study. Diabetes Obes Metab 2019;21:84–94.
110. Khoo J, Hsiang JC, Taneja R, et al. Randomized trial comparing effects of weight loss by liraglutide with lifestyle modification in non-alcoholic fatty liver disease. Liver Int 2019;39:941–9.
111. Frossing S, Nylander M, Chabanova E, et al. Effect of liraglutide on ectopic fat in polycystic ovary syndrome: a randomized clinical trial. Diabetes Obes Metab 2018;20:215–8.

112. Flint A, Andersen G, Hockings P, et al. Randomised clinical trial: semaglutide versus placebo reduced liver steatosis but not liver stiffness in subjects with non-alcoholic fatty liver disease assessed by magnetic resonance imaging. Aliment Pharmacol Ther 2021;54:1150–61.
113. Vanderheiden A, Harrison LB, Warshauer JT, et al. Mechanisms of action of liraglutide in patients with type 2 diabetes treated with high-dose insulin. J Clin Endocrinol Metab 2016;101:1798–806.
114. Liu L, Yan H, Xia M, et al. Efficacy of exenatide and insulin glargine on nonalcoholic fatty liver disease in patients with type 2 diabetes. Diabetes Metab Res Rev 2020;36:e3292.
115. Kuchay MS, Krishan S, Mishra SK, et al. Effect of dulaglutide on liver fat in patients with type 2 diabetes and NAFLD: randomised controlled trial (D-LIFT trial). Diabetologia 2020;63:2434–45.
116. Bizino MB, Jazet IM, de Heer P, et al. Placebo-controlled randomised trial with liraglutide on magnetic resonance endpoints in individuals with type 2 diabetes: a pre-specified secondary study on ectopic fat accumulation. Diabetologia 2020;63:65–74.
117. Dutour A, Abdesselam I, Ancel P, et al. Exenatide decreases liver fat content and epicardial adipose tissue in patients with obesity and type 2 diabetes: a prospective randomized clinical trial using magnetic resonance imaging and spectroscopy. Diabetes Obes Metab 2016;18:882–91.
118. Yan J, Yao B, Kuang H, et al. Liraglutide, sitagliptin, and insulin glargine added to metformin: the effect on body weight and intrahepatic lipid in patients with type 2 diabetes mellitus and nonalcoholic fatty liver disease. Hepatology 2019;69:2414–26.
119. Tang A, Rabasa-Lhoret R, Castel H, et al. Effects of insulin glargine and liraglutide therapy on liver fat as measured by magnetic resonance in patients with type 2 diabetes: a randomized trial. Diabetes Care 2015;38:1339–46.
120. Promrat K, Kleiner DE, Niemeier HM, et al. Randomized controlled trial testing the effects of weight loss on nonalcoholic steatohepatitis. Hepatology 2010; 51:121–9.
121. Newsome PN, Buchholtz K, Cusi K, et al. A placebo-controlled trial of subcutaneous semaglutide in nonalcoholic steatohepatitis. N Engl J Med 2021;384: 1113–24.
122. Vilar-Gomez E, Martinez-Perez Y, Calzadilla-Bertot L, et al. Weight loss through lifestyle modification significantly reduces features of nonalcoholic steatohepatitis. Gastroenterology 2015;149:367–78, e365; quiz e314-365.
123. Harrison SA, Fecht W, Brunt EM, et al. Orlistat for overweight subjects with nonalcoholic steatohepatitis: a randomized, prospective trial. Hepatology 2009;49:80–6.
124. Armstrong MJ, Gaunt P, Aithal GP, et al. Liraglutide safety and efficacy in patients with non-alcoholic steatohepatitis (LEAN): a multicentre, double-blind, randomised, placebo-controlled phase 2 study. Lancet 2016;387:679–90.
125. Sanyal AJ, Chalasani N, Kowdley KV, et al. Pioglitazone, vitamin E, or placebo for nonalcoholic steatohepatitis. N Engl J Med 2010;362:1675–85.
126. Cusi K, Orsak B, Bril F, et al. Long-term pioglitazone treatment for patients with nonalcoholic steatohepatitis and prediabetes or type 2 diabetes mellitus: a randomized trial. Ann Intern Med 2016;165:305–15.
127. Rinella ME, Lominadze Z, Loomba R, et al. Practice patterns in NAFLD and NASH: real life differs from published guidelines. Therap Adv Gastroenterol 2016;9:4–12.

128. Rinella M, Cryer DR, Articolo A, et al. Nonalcoholic steatohepatitis medical patient journey from the perspective of hepatologists, gastroenterologists and patients: a cross-sectional survey. BMC Gastroenterol 2022;22:335.
129. Belfort R, Harrison SA, Brown K, et al. A placebo-controlled trial of pioglitazone in subjects with nonalcoholic steatohepatitis. N Engl J Med 2006;355:2297–307.
130. Aithal G, Thomas J, Kaye P, et al. A randomized, double blind, placebo controlled trial of one year of pioglitazone in non-diabetic subjects with NASH. Hepatology 2007;46(suppl A#):132.
131. Bril F, Kalavalapalli S, Clark VC, et al. Response to pioglitazone in patients with nonalcoholic steatohepatitis with vs without type 2 diabetes. Clin Gastroenterol Hepatol 2018;16:558–566 e552.
132. Musso G, Cassader M, Paschetta E, et al. Thiazolidinediones and advanced liver fibrosis in nonalcoholic steatohepatitis: a meta-analysis. JAMA Intern Med 2017;177:633–40.
133. Gawrieh S, Noureddin M, Loo N, et al. Saroglitazar, a PPAR-alpha/gamma agonist, for treatment of NAFLD: a randomized controlled double-blind phase 2 trial. Hepatology 2021;74:1809–24.
134. Francque SM, Bedossa P, Ratziu V, et al. A randomized, controlled trial of the pan-PPAR agonist lanifibranor in NASH. N Engl J Med 2021;385:1547–58.
135. Lavine JE, Schwimmer JB, Van Natta ML, et al. Effect of vitamin E or metformin for treatment of nonalcoholic fatty liver disease in children and adolescents: the TONIC randomized controlled trial. JAMA 2011;305:1659–68.
136. Cusi K, Alkhouri N, Harrison SA, et al. Efficacy and safety of PXL770, a direct AMP kinase activator, for the treatment of non-alcoholic fatty liver disease (STAMP-NAFLD): a randomised, double-blind, placebo-controlled, phase 2a study. Lancet Gastroenterol Hepatol 2021;6(11):889–902.
137. Kramer JR, Natarajan Y, Dai J, et al. Effect of diabetes medications and glycemic control on risk of hepatocellular cancer in patients with nonalcoholic fatty liver disease. Hepatology 2022;75:1420–8.
138. Cusi K, Bril F, Barb D, et al. Effect of canagliflozin treatment on hepatic triglyceride content and glucose metabolism in patients with type 2 diabetes. Diabetes Obes Metab 2018;21(4):812–21.
139. Merovci A, Solis-Herrera C, Daniele G, et al. Dapagliflozin improves muscle insulin sensitivity but enhances endogenous glucose production. J Clin Invest 2014;124:509–14.
140. Kahl S, Gancheva S, Strassburger K, et al. Empagliflozin effectively lowers liver fat content in well-controlled type 2 diabetes: a randomized, double-blind, phase 4, placebo-controlled trial. Diabetes Care 2020;43:298–305.
141. Latva-Rasku A, Honka MJ, Kullberg J, et al. The SGLT2 inhibitor dapagliflozin reduces liver fat but does not affect tissue insulin sensitivity: a randomized, double-blind, placebo-controlled study with 8-week treatment in type 2 diabetes patients. Diabetes Care 2019;42:931–7.
142. Kuchay MS, Krishan S, Mishra SK, et al. Effect of empagliflozin on liver fat in patients with type 2 diabetes and nonalcoholic fatty liver disease: a randomized controlled trial (E-LIFT trial). Diabetes Care 2018;41:1801–8.
143. Eriksson JW, Lundkvist P, Jansson PA, et al. Effects of dapagliflozin and n-3 carboxylic acids on non-alcoholic fatty liver disease in people with type 2 diabetes: a double-blind randomised placebo-controlled study. Diabetologia 2018;61:1923–34.
144. Yoneda M, Honda Y, Ogawa Y, et al. Comparing the effects of tofogliflozin and pioglitazone in non-alcoholic fatty liver disease patients with type 2 diabetes

mellitus (ToPiND study): a randomized prospective open-label controlled trial. BMJ Open Diabetes Res Care 2021;9(1):e001990.
145. Inoue M, Hayashi A, Taguchi T, et al. Effects of canagliflozin on body composition and hepatic fat content in type 2 diabetes patients with non-alcoholic fatty liver disease. J Diabetes Investig 2019;10:1004–11.
146. Ohta A, Kato H, Ishii S, et al. Ipragliflozin, a sodium glucose co-transporter 2 inhibitor, reduces intrahepatic lipid content and abdominal visceral fat volume in patients with type 2 diabetes. Expert Opin Pharmacother 2017;18:1433–8.
147. Johansson L, Hockings PD, Johnsson E, et al. Dapagliflozin plus saxagliptin add-on to metformin reduces liver fat and adipose tissue volume in patients with type 2 diabetes. Diabetes Obes Metab 2020;22:1094–101.
148. Lai LL, Vethakkan SR, Nik Mustapha NR, et al. Empagliflozin for the treatment of nonalcoholic steatohepatitis in patients with type 2 diabetes mellitus. Dig Dis Sci 2020;65:623–31.
149. Akuta N, Watanabe C, Kawamura Y, et al. Effects of a sodium-glucose cotransporter 2 inhibitor in nonalcoholic fatty liver disease complicated by diabetes mellitus: preliminary prospective study based on serial liver biopsies. Hepatol Commun 2017;1:46–52.
150. Friedman SL, Neuschwander-Tetri BA, Rinella M, et al. Mechanisms of NAFLD development and therapeutic strategies. Nat Med 2018;24:908–22.

Hepatic Outcomes of Nonalcoholic Fatty Liver Disease Including Cirrhosis and Hepatocellular Carcinoma

Saleh A. Alqahtani[a,b,*], Wah-Kheong Chan[c], Ming-Lung Yu[d,e,f,g]

KEYWORDS

- Fatty liver • Hepatocellular carcinoma • Liver cancer • Liver cirrhosis
- Nonalcoholic fatty liver • Nonalcoholic steatohepatitis

KEY POINTS

- In tandem with the growing global prevalence of obesity, incidence of nonalcoholic fatty liver disease (NAFLD) is rapidly increasing.
- The progressive form of NAFLD, nonalcoholic steatohepatitis, is anticipated to overtake other liver diseases as the most common reason for liver transplantation.
- NAFLD-hepatocellular carcinoma can develop in the absence of cirrhosis or fibrosis and is typically presented at a later stage with a poor prognosis, highlighting the unmet need for the development of biomarkers for early detection.

INTRODUCTION

Nonalcoholic fatty liver disease (NAFLD) is the most common cause of chronic liver diseases in developed countries, and its prevalence and incidence are rapidly increasing worldwide.[1,2] NAFLD is a liver disease strongly associated with insulin resistance, obesity, and other metabolic risk factors, including hypertension and dyslipidemia.[1,3,4] A subgroup of patients develops NAFLD in the absence of obesity and

[a] Division of Gastroenterology and Hepatology, Johns Hopkins University, Baltimore, MD, USA; [b] Liver Transplant Center, King Faisal Specialist Hospital and Research Center, Riyadh, Saudi Arabia; [c] Gastroenterology and Hepatology Unit, Department of Medicine, Faculty of Medicine, University of Malaya, Kuala Lumpur, Malaysia; [d] School of Medicine, College of Medicine, National Sun Yat-Sen University, Kaohsiung, Taiwan; [e] Hepatitis Research Center, College of Medicine, Kaohsiung Medical University, Kaohsiung, Taiwan; [f] Hepatobiliary Section, Department of Internal Medicine, Hepatitis Center, Kaohsiung Medical University Hospital, Kaohsiung, Taiwan; [g] Division of Hepato-Gastroenterology, Department of Internal Medicine, Kaohsiung Chang Gung Memorial Hospital, Kaohsiung, Taiwan
* Corresponding author. Division of Gastroenterology and Hepatology, Johns Hopkins University, Baltimore, MD.
E-mail address: salqaht1@jhmi.edu

Clin Liver Dis 27 (2023) 211–223
https://doi.org/10.1016/j.cld.2023.01.019
liver.theclinics.com

are considered lean NAFLD, accounting for 7% in the United States and 20% in Asia.[5] Underrecognition and underdiagnosis of NAFLD is a major barrier and interferes with assessing the disease burden, its complications, as well as preventive health measures to address NAFLD/nonalcoholic steatohepatitis (NASH). Because of the asymptomatic and indolent nature of NAFLD, there is a huge gap in disease awareness from patients and health care providers[6] to society groups and policy makers.[7] This review summarizes recent key findings on the progression and regression of the various forms of the disease and highlights where we need to go to alleviate its health burden.

DISEASE SPECTRUM OF NONALCOHOLIC FATTY LIVER DISEASE

The standard definition of NAFLD is evidence of hepatic steatosis, defined by liver biopsy or imaging as the presence of greater than 5% hepatocyte triglyceride accumulation after excluding secondary causes of hepatic steatosis, such as harmful alcohol consumption, viral hepatitis, exposure to steatogenic medications, or hereditary disorders.[8] NAFLD has a broad disease spectrum, from nonalcoholic fatty liver (NAFL) or simple steatosis to NASH, which is associated with liver fibrosis and can progress to cirrhosis, hepatocellular carcinoma (HCC), and end-stage liver diseases.[9,10] **Fig. 1** describes the data on NAFLD and NASH incidence, whereas **Fig. 2** shows the fibrosis stages and progression/regression data for NASH, NASH cirrhosis, and NASH HCC.

Data from a recent phase 2 study of 1773 patients with advanced fibrosis (stage 3 or 4) from NAFLD and a median 4-year follow-up demonstrated that patients had a significantly higher risk of long-term hepatic complications, including variceal bleeding, ascites, hepatic encephalopathy, HCC, and death, when compared with patients with fibrosis stages 0 to 2.[11] Another study focused on 1135 patients with NASH having baseline histologically proven cirrhosis. Patients with baseline Ishak fibrosis stage 6 versus less than or equal to 5 had nearly a 2-fold risk of clinical events, including hepatic decompensation, the need for liver transplantation, HCC, or all-cause mortality.[12]

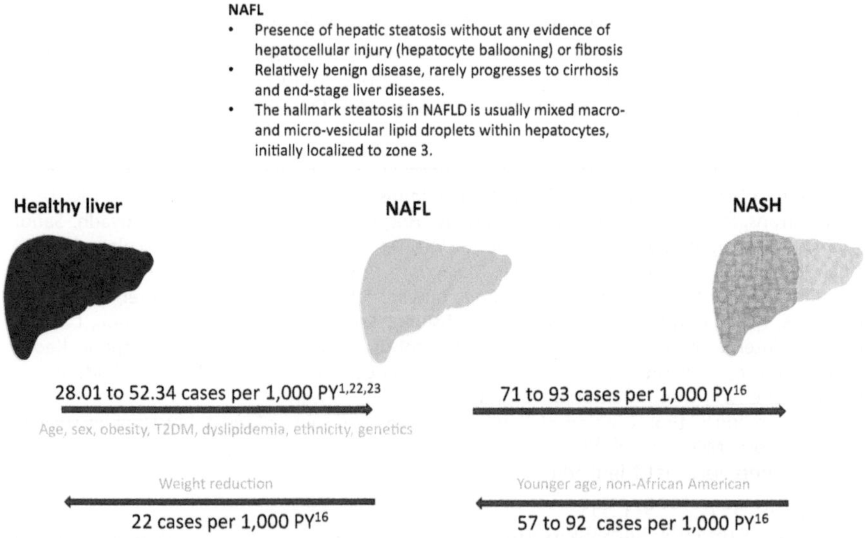
NAFL
• Presence of hepatic steatosis without any evidence of hepatocellular injury (hepatocyte ballooning) or fibrosis
• Relatively benign disease, rarely progresses to cirrhosis and end-stage liver diseases.
• The hallmark steatosis in NAFLD is usually mixed macro- and micro-vesicular lipid droplets within hepatocytes, initially localized to zone 3.
Healthy liver
NAFL
NASH
28.01 to 52.34 cases per 1,000 PY1,22,23
Age, sex, obesity, T2DM, dyslipidemia, ethnicity, genetics
71 to 93 cases per 1,000 PY16
Weight reduction
22 cases per 1,000 PY16
Younger age, non-African American
57 to 92 cases per 1,000 PY16

Fig. 1. Data on NAFLD and NASH incidence.

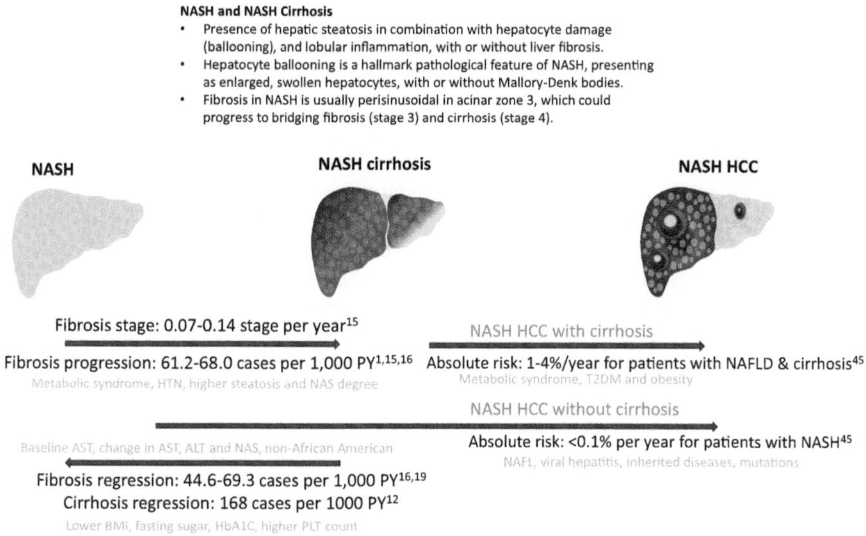

Fig. 2. Fibrosis stages and progression/regression data for NASH, NASH cirrhosis, and NASH HCC.

BIDIRECTIONAL EVOLUTION OF NONALCOHOLIC FATTY LIVER DISEASE

NAFLD is a dynamic condition that exhibits bidirectional evolution among NAFL, NASH, NASH with advanced fibrosis, and NASH cirrhosis.[13,14] Studies that evaluated the change in paired liver biopsies come from specialized centers and have observed that 30% to 40% of patients with NAFLD had fibrosis progression, whereas a substantial group of up to 25% of patients had fibrosis regression during 2 to 16 years of follow-up.[15–17] Even among the patients with NASH cirrhosis enrolled in 2 large placebo-controlled trials, regression of fibrosis could occur in 16% of patients during the follow-up (48 weeks from baseline).[12] Recent clinical trials of potential pharmacologic intervention provided better understanding of the dynamics of disease progression and regression.[18,19] It is important to keep in mind that histopathological analysis carries limitations,[20] and the availability of validated and reliable noninvasive test[21] will improve the understanding of the natural history of the disease.

BIDIRECTIONAL EVOLUTION BETWEEN NONALCOHOLIC FATTY LIVER DISEASE DEVELOPMENT AND RESOLUTION FROM NONALCOHOLIC FATTY LIVER/NONALCOHOLIC FATTY LIVER DISEASE

Nonalcoholic Fatty Liver Disease Incidence

In a meta-analysis of the global disease burden of NAFLD with a sample size of greater than 8 million from 22 countries, NAFLD incidence was only available from Japan, China, and Israel. The pooled incidence of NAFLD for Japan/China was 52.34 per 1000 (95% confidence interval [CI]: 28.31–96.77) and for Israel, 28.01 per 1000 person-years (95% CI: 19.34–40.57) (see **Fig. 1**).[1] A recent meta-analysis of 18 studies from Asia showed that the pooled incidence of NAFLD was 50.9 cases (95% CI: 44.8–57.4) per 1000 person-years in this population.[2] In a large Korean cohort of 77,425 metabolically healthy subjects without NAFLD at baseline, 10,340 subjects developed NAFLD documented by sonography during 348,193.5 person-years of follow-up, with an incidence rate of 29.7 cases per 1,000 person-years.[22] A retrospective study observed an incidence NAFLD rate of 29 cases per 100,000 person-years in a hepatology outpatient clinic in the United Kingdom.[23]

Nonalcoholic Fatty Liver Resolution

A cohort study from the NASH Clinical Research Network (NASH-CRN) explored the incidence and factors associated with progression or regression of NAFLD.[16] A total of 446 adult patients with NAFLD, including 86 (19.3%) with NAFL, were evaluated with a mean between-biopsy interval of 4.9 years. Among patients with NAFL at baseline biopsy, 12.8% (22 cases per 1000 person-year) had NAFL resolved. Factors associated with NAFLD regression included weight loss and decreasing aspartate aminotransferase (AST) levels.

BIDIRECTIONAL EVOLUTION BETWEEN NONALCOHOLIC FATTY LIVER AND NONALCOHOLIC STEATOHEPATITIS

Progression from Nonalcoholic Fatty Liver to Nonalcoholic Steatohepatitis

The estimation of NASH prevalence varies greatly depending on the population-specific reasons for obtaining a liver biopsy. For patients with NAFLD who underwent liver biopsy for a "clinical indication," 59.10% of patients had NASH; by contrast, for patients with NAFLD who underwent liver biopsy of random intent, only 6.67% to 29.85% of patients had NASH.[1] These data translated into a global NASH prevalence of 1.5% to 6.45% in the general population.[1]

In the Kleiner and colleagues' study, in patients with NAFL at baseline biopsy, 41.9% (71 cases per 1000 person-year) progressed to NASH (borderline NASH, 20.9%; definite NASH, 20.9%).[16] Among patients with borderline NASH at baseline biopsy, 46.4% (93 cases per 1000 person-year) progressed to definite NASH. Factors associated with NASH progression were higher body mass index (BMI) at baseline and higher liver enzymes.

Regression from Nonalcoholic Steatohepatitis to Nonalcoholic Fatty Liver

In the same study, in patients with borderline NASH at baseline biopsy, 28.6% (57 per 1000 person-year) had disease regression.[16] Among patients with definite NASH at baseline biopsy, 42.4% (92 per 1000 person-year) had steatohepatitis regression (20.3% to borderline NASH, 11.2% to NAFL, and 10.9% to resolved NAFLD).[16] In a recent meta-analysis including 2649 placebo-treated patients with NASH from 43 randomized controlled trials (RCTs), NASH regression was explored. Most of the study periods were between 6 and 12 months.[19] In 1066 patients assessed for NASH resolution without worsening of fibrosis, 11% achieved the endpoint of an event. In the same meta-analysis, in a set of 1287 patients with NASH treated with placebo, 21.11% even achieved a 2-point reduction in NAS without worsening fibrosis.[19] Older age and African Americans were found to be less likely to experience NASH resolution. In the same meta-analysis including 14 RCTs, disease progression defined as at least 1-point progression of fibrosis was observed in approximately 23% of 1522 placebo-treated patients with NASH.[19]

FIBROSIS PROGRESSION AND REGRESSION IN PATIENTS WITH NONALCOHOLIC STEATOHEPATITIS

Fibrosis Progression

A meta-analysis including 411 patients with NAFLD who had paired biopsies evaluated the course of fibrosis progression.[15] Overall, 33.6% of analyzed cases had fibrosis progression over 2,146 person-years follow-up, translating to an incidence of 64.4 cases per 1000 person-year. The NASH-CRN study by Kleiner and colleagues observed that of the 466 NASH patients, fibrosis progression by at least 1 stage occurred in 30% of participants with a mean between-biopsy interval of 4.9 years, translating to an incidence of 61.2 cases per 1000 person-year.[16] The annual fibrosis progression rate in patients with NAFL without baseline fibrosis was 0.07 stages but increased to 0.14 stages among those with baseline NASH, which translates to 1-stage progression of 14.3 years and 7.1 years, respectively, for patients with NAFL and those with NASH (see **Fig. 2**).[15] Another meta-analysis observed a fibrosis progression in 41% of cases with a mean annual progression rate of 0.09 among patients with histology-proven NASH at baseline. The incidence rate of progression to advanced fibrosis was 67.95 in 1000 person-years among patients with NASH.[1] Of note, of the 52 patients with NASH who had no fibrosis at baseline but had fibrosis progression at the follow-up liver biopsy with a mean interval of 5.9 years, 21.2% of patients progressed to fibrosis stage 3 or 4 and were considered rapid progressors. Contrasting this group, slow progression was considered in cases that had fibrosis stage 1 or 2 at follow-up biopsy. Patients with hypertension, a lower AST/alanine aminotransferase (ALT) ratio, higher steatosis grade, metabolic syndrome, baseline NAS, and a smaller reduction in NAS at baseline were risk factors associated with rapid fibrosis progression.[15,16] On the other hand, in the meta-analysis published by Ng CH and colleagues, no significant clinical or histologic factors were found to be associated with greater than or equal to 1-point fibrosis progression.[19]

Fibrosis Regression

In paired biopsy studies, fibrosis regression could occur in a substantial proportion of patients with NASH. Of 411 patients with NAFLD, 22.3% had fibrosis regression, defined as at least one fibrosis stage decrease as compared with baseline, during 2146 person-years follow-up, translating to an incidence of 44.6 cases per 1000 person-year.[19] Another study showed that 34% of 446 patients with NASH from NASH CRN had fibrosis regression by at least 1 stage with a mean between-biopsy interval of 4.9 years, translating to an incidence of 69.3 cases per 1000 person-year (see **Fig. 2**).[16] Baseline AST levels and changes (value at last biopsy—first biopsy) in the AST, ALT, and NAFLD activity score (NAS) were also associated with fibrosis regression.[16] Ng CH and colleagues assessed 1522 patients with NASH treated with placebo and observed that 18.82% (CI: 15.65%–22.47%) had at least a 1-point reduction of fibrosis. Patients of African American origin were less likely to have fibrosis regression.[19]

Regression of Nonalcoholic Steatohepatitis Cirrhosis

A recent large-scale study addressed if regression of documented NASH cirrhosis could occur naturally and explored its clinical relevance. Data from 2 clinical trials exploring simtuzumab and selonsertib were available to study the history in a total of 1135 patients with biopsy-proven NASH cirrhosis.[12] During a median follow-up of 16.6 months, 71 (6.3%) experienced liver-related events (decompensated cirrhosis, liver transplantation, and death). Regression of cirrhosis was observed in 176 (16%) between baseline and week 48 (estimated incidence: 168 per 1000 person-year), which was associated with a greater than 6-fold reduced risk of liver-related events (hazard ratio 0.16; 95% CI: 0.04–0.65). Patients with lower BMI, fasting glucose, hemoglobin A1c, steatosis grade, and higher platelets were more likely to have cirrhosis regression.[12]

CIRRHOSIS AND ITS COMPLICATIONS

Although cardiovascular disease is the leading cause of mortality in patients with NAFLD, patients with more advanced fibrosis are at a greater risk of liver-related mortality, with the risk increasing exponentially with increasing fibrosis stage. Patients with NAFLD and cirrhosis are more than 40 times more likely to die of liver-related causes compared with patients with NAFLD who do not have liver fibrosis.[24] The previously mentioned negative drug trials have produced the 20% rule,[25] which suggests that within the study period of 96 weeks, 20% of patients with NASH and F3 fibrosis progress to cirrhosis, and another 20% of patients with NASH and cirrhosis progress to decompensated liver disease.[26]

One of the challenges in tackling NAFLD is the high prevalence of the disease in the general population and the small yet significant proportion of patients with advanced liver fibrosis,[27] who are often asymptomatic until they start to have decompensated liver disease. For example, in a study of 81 patients with NAFLD undergoing assessment for liver transplantation, the majority (64.2%) had decompensated cirrhosis at their first diagnosis of cirrhosis.[28] Therefore, it is important that a clear assessment and referral pathway is in place to identify patients with advanced NAFLD so that they can be referred for specialist care; furthermore, this can reduce unnecessary referrals so that patients with less severe liver disease remain in primary care or endocrinology clinic, where they are best managed.[29]

The concept of compensated advanced chronic liver disease was coined to allow for noninvasive assessment of liver disease and includes the spectrum of advanced fibrosis (precirrhosis) and cirrhosis, which clinically is a continuum in asymptomatic patients. The distinction between the histologic stage F3 and compensated F4 is often not possible on clinical grounds.[30] In clinical referral pathways, simple fibrosis scores are suggested for the initial assessment, followed by liver stiffness measurement in patients with an intermediate or high risk of advanced liver fibrosis.[31]

Liver stiffness measurements are also useful to stratify patients for further management.[30] A liver stiffness measurement of less than 10 kPa had a negative predictive value of 93.8% to 96.8% for advanced liver fibrosis, whereas a liver stiffness measurement of greater than or equal to 15 kPa had a positive predictive value of 86.2% to 91.7% for cirrhosis.[32] Along with this rule of 5, screening endoscopy to identify gastroesophageal varices has been suggested in the latest Baveno VII consensus.[30] Liver stiffness measurement of less than or equal to 15 kPa plus platelet count of greater than or equal to 150 $\times$ 10^9/L is considered sufficient to exclude clinically significant portal hypertension in patients with compensated advanced chronic liver disease. In nonobese NASH-related compensated advanced chronic liver disease, liver stiffness measurement of greater than or equal to 25 kPa is considered sufficient to rule in clinically significant portal hypertension, whereas patients with liver stiffness measurement of 15 to 20 kPa and platelet count of less than 110 $\times$ 10^9/L and patients with liver stiffness measurement of 20 to 25 kPa and platelet count of less than 150 $\times$ 10^9/L have greater than or equal to 60% risk of clinically significant portal hypertension. In patients with NASH and obesity, these prediction rules may be less accurate, and the ANTICIPATE NASH model, which incorporates BMI in addition to liver stiffness measurement and platelet count, has been proposed for the prediction of clinically significant portal hypertension in these patients.[33] A meta-analysis has shown that applying these thresholds for screening endoscopy in patients with NAFLD/NASH was associated with missed varices needing treatment of 0% (0%–1.3%) and spared endoscopy rate of 38.6% (10.9%–70.8%).[34]

Sarcopenia is one of the common complications of cirrhosis and is associated with lower quality of life and a worse outcome in patients with cirrhosis.[35] The mechanism of development of sarcopenia in cirrhosis is not fully understood. Still, it is partly due to complex metabolic and hormonal changes seen in patients with cirrhosis that are not adequately addressed by nutrition and physical activity intervention alone.[36] On the other hand, lifestyle intervention, either by hypocaloric diet alone or in combination with increased physical activity, is the mainstay of treatment of NAFLD.[8]

Weight loss of greater than or equal to 10% can lead to NASH resolution in most of the patients and even fibrosis improvement, but the desired weight loss can only be achieved in a small proportion of patients.[37] Pharmacologic therapy for NASH is emerging with agents that target obesity and diabetes, such as glucagon-like peptide-1 agonist or dual and triple agonists, showing promising results. The NASH phase 2 trial showed that semaglutide at 0.1 mg, 0.2 mg, or 0.4 mg daily was associated with significantly greater NASH resolution compared with placebo; although fibrosis improvement was not significantly different between the groups, there was significantly less fibrosis progression in patients who received semaglutide.[38] In the STEP 1 study on adults with overweight or obesity, 2.4 mg of semaglutide weekly, the same dose used for the phase 3 trial for NASH, showed that 70% achieved greater than or equal to 10% weight loss, whereas 50% achieved greater than or equal to 15% weight loss.[39]

Liver transplantation in patients with NAFLD is associated with unique challenges, both pretransplantation and posttransplantation.[40] Patients with NAFLD are at a high risk of cardiovascular disease and require specific evaluation and management in the pretransplant period. Their larger body habitus may pose technical challenges during surgery. In the posttransplant period, the use of immunosuppressive therapy may worsen metabolic abnormalities and predispose a patient to early posttransplant complications. In the longer term, there may also be a higher risk of malignancy and cardiovascular events, resulting in higher mortality. Furthermore, patients may develop recurrent NAFLD posttransplant at a rate of 59% and 82% at 1- and 5-year, respectively, whereas the corresponding rates of recurrent NASH posttransplant were 53% and 38%, respectively.[41]

HEPATOCELLULAR CARCINOMA

NAFLD is becoming a common cause of HCC worldwide.[42] The prevalence of NAFLD-HCC is increasing in tandem with the increase in NAFLD. The incidence increased by 9% annually in the United States from 2004 to 2009.[43] Patients are older with more comorbidities, and NAFLD-HCC is diagnosed at more advanced stages. Together, these features adversely affect the prognosis and the likelihood of effective treatment outcome.[44] Although patients with NASH who do not have cirrhosis can still develop HCC, the absolute risk is less than 0.1% per year, whereas the risk is 1% to 4% per year for patients with NAFLD and cirrhosis.[5] Type 2 diabetes mellitus and obesity, related to NAFLD and metabolic syndrome, are implicated as independent risk factors for HCC. Both these risk factors develop hepatic steatosis and cause hepatic inflammation by steering the release of proinflammatory cytokines such as tumor necrosis factor-alpha, interleukin-6, leptin, and resistin and decreasing adiponectin. This process subsequently paves the way for HCC development.[45]

HCC surveillance is only recommended for patients with NAFLD and cirrhosis. However, liver biopsy is not routinely performed for the diagnosis of cirrhosis in clinical practice. In line with the concept of compensated advanced chronic liver disease, a liver stiffness measurement of greater than or equal to 15 kPa may be a reasonable threshold to initiate consideration for HCC surveillance.[29] Abdominal ultrasound surveillance for every 6 months has been beneficial among patients with severe fibrosis and cirrhosis but is limited by cost.[46,47] Moreover, screening for fibrosis among patients with NAFLD poses huge challenges due to a high number of at-risk populations. Therefore, efficient, cost-effective biomarkers with high predictive values are required to identify patients with advanced fibrosis and for early screening of HCC.

Noncirrhotic HCC is clinically asymptomatic at early stages, is often not subjected to surveillance, and presents at an advanced disease stage. NAFL has been shown to have a stronger association with HCC in noncirrhotic livers. The other causes of noncirrhotic HCC include viral hepatitis (hepatitis B virus and hepatitis C virus), inherited diseases (hereditary hemochromatosis, alpha-1 antitrypsin deficiency, hypercitrullinemia, Wilson disease, Alagille syndrome, Budd-Chiari syndrome, nodular regenerative hyperplasia, and glycogen storage disease), genotoxic substances (alcohol, aflatoxin B1, iron overload, chemical carcinogens, and sex hormones), and germline mutations (telomerase reverse transcriptase gene mutation).[45,48] Pathogenesis, differential diagnosis, and genomic pathways in noncirrhotic HCC vary from that of cirrhotic HCC. Differentiating hepatocellular adenoma with cytologic or architectural atypia from the noncirrhotic HCC is challenging.[49]

The GALAD score and measurements of serum inter-alpha-trypsin inhibitor heavy chain 4 (ITIH4) are among the biomarkers being developed to detect HCC more effectively. The GALAD score, a sensitive biomarker for HCC that takes into account factors such as gender, age, alpha-fetoprotein (AFP), AFP-L3, and des-gamma-carboxy-prothrombin, has shown potential in detecting HCC with an area under the receiver operating characteristic curve of 0.96.[50,51] Patients with NASH who developed HCC had higher GALAD scores than those who did not develop HCC up to 1.5 years before HCC diagnosis. Despite limited large validation studies, the US Food and Drug Administration granted breakthrough device designation to the GALAD score for the early diagnosis of HCC in March 2020, based on strong cumulative evidence.[52] Serum ITIH4 is another potential biomarker that was found to be elevated in patients with NAFLD-HCC compared with those with NASH and steatosis. More studies are required to validate its efficacy.[53]

Epigenetic markers specific to HCC have high prognostic value and can be easily isolated from peripheral blood and thus can be used as potential biomarkers for surveillance, diagnosis, and prognosis of HCC.[54–56] Further research is required to explore and validate the epigenetic markers as biomarkers of risk, diagnosis, and prognosis in HCC.

Given the growing prevalence of NAFLD worldwide, reducing the risks of HCC development needs to be prioritized. Lifestyle interventions to manage obesity and diabetes should be the primary focus of preventive strategies to reduce the risk of HCC development. Mediterranean diet can reduce the risk of HCC development among patients with NAFLD. A large European cohort study of 467,336 individuals reported an inverse association between physical activity and HCC risk, potentially driven by obesity. Multivariable-adjusted hazard ratio for developing HCC was 0.55 for active individuals compared with inactive individuals.[57] Furthermore, reports show that higher adherence to the Mediterranean diet is protective against HCC risks.[58]

SUMMARY

With the growing incidence of NAFLD on a global scale, management pathways and pharmacologic treatment options are eagerly awaited. Metabolic derangement in NAFLD associated with obesity is a key driver of disease progression and could be a useful target for pharmacologic intervention. Although NAFLD is more prevalent among individuals with obesity, an increasing prevalence among lean individuals has also been reported. The natural course of NAFLD exhibits bidirectional progression and regression between NAFL, NASH, and cirrhosis. In the future, noninvasive assessment will be the mainstay and inform referral pathways to identify patients with NAFLD and cirrhosis and adverse outcomes. Moreover, recent evidence has shown that HCC can develop in the absence of cirrhosis or severe fibrosis and is usually presented at a later stage with worse prognosis and lower response rates to curative therapies. To reduce the risk of HCC development, efficient, cost-effective biomarkers with high predictive values are required to identify patients with advanced fibrosis who can then be screened early for HCC. Currently, pharmacologic interventions for NAFLD are limited; therefore, lifestyle interventions such as diet and physical exercise remain the cornerstone of treatment and further reduce the risk of cirrhosis and HCC.

CLINICS CARE POINTS

- NAFLD is a disease spectrum ranging from NAFL or simple steatosis to NASH, which can progress to cirrhosis, HCC.
- Obesity, metabolic syndrome, age, ethnicity, and higher NAS score are associated with more rapid progression to end-stage liver disease.
- Patients with advanced liver fibrosis are at greater risk of liver-related mortality.
- Fibrosis score can be used for initial assessment, followed by liver stiffness measurement for patients with an intermediate or high risk of advanced liver fibrosis.
- Liver stiffness measurement of less than or equal to 15 kPa plus platelet count of greater than or equal to 150 $\times$ 10^9/L can reliably exclude clinically significant portal hypertension.
- HCC can develop even in the absence of cirrhosis in NAFLD.

DISCLOSURE

Dr Saleh A. Alqahtani: no competing interest to declare. Dr Wah-Kheong Chan: Advisory board member for Roche, AbbVie, Boehringer Ingelheim, and Novo Nordisk; Speaker for Hisky Medical and Viatris. Dr Ming-Lung Yu: Research support (grant) from Abbott, Abbvie, BMS, Gilead, Merck, and Roche diagnostics; Consultant of Abbvie, Abbott, BMS, Gilead, Merck, PharmaEssentia, Roche, and Roche diagnostics; Speaker of Abbvie, Abbott, BMS, Eisai, Eli Lilly, Gilead, IPSEN, Merck, Ono, Roche, and Roche diagnostics.

FUNDING

None.

REFERENCES

1. Younossi ZM, Koenig AB, Abdelatif D, et al. Global epidemiology of nonalcoholic fatty liver disease-Meta-analytic assessment of prevalence, incidence, and outcomes. Hepatology 2016;64(1):73–84.
2. Li J, Zou B, Yeo YH, et al. Prevalence, incidence, and outcome of non-alcoholic fatty liver disease in Asia, 1999-2019: a systematic review and meta-analysis. Lancet Gastroenterol Hepatol 2019;4(5):389–98.

3. Wu KT, Kuo PL, Su SB, et al. Nonalcoholic fatty liver disease severity is associated with the ratios of total cholesterol and triglycerides to high-density lipoprotein cholesterol. J Clin Lipidol 2016;10(2):420–425 e421.
4. Hsiao PJ, Kuo KK, Shin SJ, et al. Significant correlations between severe fatty liver and risk factors for metabolic syndrome. J Gastroenterol Hepatol 2007; 22(12):2118–23.
5. Fan JG, Kim SU, Wong VW. New trends on obesity and NAFLD in Asia. J Hepatol 2017;67(4):862–73.
6. Younossi ZM, Ong JP, Takahashi H, et al. A global survey of physicians knowledge about nonalcoholic fatty liver disease. Clin Gastroenterol Hepatol 2022; 20(6):e1456–68.
7. Lazarus JV, Mark HE, Anstee QM, et al. Advancing the global public health agenda for NAFLD: a consensus statement. Nat Rev Gastroenterol Hepatol 2022;19(1):60–78.
8. Chalasani N, Younossi Z, Lavine JE, et al. The diagnosis and management of nonalcoholic fatty liver disease: practice guidance from the American Association for the Study of Liver Diseases. Hepatology 2018;67(1):328–57.
9. Anstee QM, Reeves HL, Kotsiliti E, et al. From NASH to HCC: current concepts and future challenges. Nat Rev Gastroenterol Hepatol 2019;16(7):411–28.
10. Huang YH, Chan C, Lee HW, et al. Influence of nonalcoholic fatty liver disease with increased liver enzyme levels on the risk of cirrhosis and hepatocellular carcinoma. Clin Gastroenterol Hepatol 2022;S1542-3565(22):00105–7.
11. Sanyal AJ, Van Natta ML, Clark J, et al. Prospective study of outcomes in adults with nonalcoholic fatty liver disease. N Engl J Med 2021;385(17):1559–69.
12. Sanyal AJ, Anstee QM, Trauner M, et al. Cirrhosis regression is associated with improved clinical outcomes in patients with nonalcoholic steatohepatitis. Hepatology 2022;75(5):1235–46.
13. Younossi ZM. Non-alcoholic fatty liver disease - a global public health perspective. J Hepatol 2019;70(3):531–44.
14. Lin TY, Yeh ML, Huang CF, et al. Disease progression of nonalcoholic steatohepatitis in Taiwanese patients: a longitudinal study of paired liver biopsies. Eur J Gastroenterol Hepatol 2019;31(2):224–9.
15. Singh S, Allen AM, Wang Z, et al. Fibrosis progression in nonalcoholic fatty liver vs nonalcoholic steatohepatitis: a systematic review and meta-analysis of paired-biopsy studies. Clin Gastroenterol Hepatol 2015;13(4):643–54, e641-649;quiz e639-640.
16. Kleiner DE, Brunt EM, Wilson LA, et al. Association of histologic disease activity with progression of nonalcoholic fatty liver disease. JAMA Netw Open 2019;2(10): e1912565.
17. Xanthakos SA, Lavine JE, Yates KP, et al. Progression of fatty liver disease in children receiving standard of care lifestyle advice. Gastroenterology 2020;159(5): 1731–1751 e1710.
18. Huang JF, Dai CY, Huang CF, et al. First-in-Asian double-blind randomized trial to assess the efficacy and safety of insulin sensitizer in nonalcoholic steatohepatitis patients. Hepatol Int 2021;15(5):1136–47.
19. Ng CH, Xiao J, Lim WH, et al. Placebo effect on progression and regression in NASH: evidence from a meta-analysis. Hepatology 2022;75(6):1647–61.
20. Schattenberg JM, Straub BK. On the value and limitations of liver histology in assessing non-alcoholic steatohepatitis. J Hepatol 2020;73(6):1592–3.

21. Alqahtani SA, Schattenberg JM. Nonalcoholic fatty liver disease: use of diagnostic biomarkers and modalities in clinical practice. Expert Rev Mol Diagn 2021;21(10):1065–78.
22. Chang Y, Jung HS, Cho J, et al. Metabolically healthy obesity and the development of nonalcoholic fatty liver disease. Am J Gastroenterol 2016;111(8): 1133–40.
23. Whalley S, Puvanachandra P, Desai A, et al. Hepatology outpatient service provision in secondary care: a study of liver disease incidence and resource costs. Clin Med 2007;7(2):119–24.
24. Dulai PS, Singh S, Patel J, et al. Increased risk of mortality by fibrosis stage in nonalcoholic fatty liver disease: systematic review and meta-analysis. Hepatology 2017;65(5):1557–65.
25. Loomba R, Adams LA. The 20% rule of NASH progression: the natural history of advanced fibrosis and cirrhosis caused by NASH. Hepatology 2019;70(6): 1885–8.
26. Sanyal AJ, Harrison SA, Ratziu V, et al. The natural history of advanced fibrosis due to nonalcoholic steatohepatitis: data from the simtuzumab trials. Hepatology 2019;70(6):1913–27.
27. Wong VW, Chu WC, Wong GL, et al. Prevalence of non-alcoholic fatty liver disease and advanced fibrosis in Hong Kong Chinese: a population study using proton-magnetic resonance spectroscopy and transient elastography. Gut 2012;61(3):409–15.
28. Hussain A, Patel PJ, Rhodes F, et al. Decompensated cirrhosis is the commonest presentation for NAFLD patients undergoing liver transplant assessment. Clin Med 2020;20(3):313–8.
29. Chan WK, Tan SS, Chan SP, et al. Malaysian Society of Gastroenterology and Hepatology consensus statement on metabolic dysfunction-associated fatty liver disease. J Gastroenterol Hepatol 2022;37(5):795–811.
30. de Franchis R, Bosch J, Garcia-Tsao G, et al. Baveno VII - renewing consensus in portal hypertension. J Hepatol 2022;76(4):959–74.
31. Chan WK, Treeprasertsuk S, Goh GB, et al. Optimizing use of nonalcoholic fatty liver disease fibrosis score, fibrosis-4 score, and liver stiffness measurement to identify patients with advanced fibrosis. Clin Gastroenterol Hepatol 2019; 17(12):2570–80.e37.
32. Wong VW, Irles M, Wong GL, et al. Unified interpretation of liver stiffness measurement by M and XL probes in non-alcoholic fatty liver disease. Gut 2019; 68(11):2057–64.
33. Pons M, Augustin S, Scheiner B, et al. Noninvasive diagnosis of portal hypertension in patients with compensated advanced chronic liver disease. Am J Gastroenterol 2021;116(4):723–32.
34. Szakacs Z, Eross B, Soos A, et al. Baveno criteria safely identify patients with compensated advanced chronic liver disease who can avoid variceal screening endoscopy: a diagnostic test accuracy meta-analysis. Front Physiol 2019;10: 1028.
35. Tantai X, Liu Y, Yeo YH, et al. Effect of sarcopenia on survival in patients with cirrhosis: a meta-analysis. J Hepatol 2022;76(3):588–99.
36. Dasarathy S, Merli M. Sarcopenia from mechanism to diagnosis and treatment in liver disease. J Hepatol 2016;65(6):1232–44.
37. Vilar-Gomez E, Martinez-Perez Y, Calzadilla-Bertot L, et al. Weight loss through lifestyle modification significantly reduces features of nonalcoholic steatohepatitis. Gastroenterology 2015;149(2):367–78, e365; quiz e314-365.

38. Newsome PN, Buchholtz K, Cusi K, et al. A placebo-controlled trial of subcutaneous semaglutide in nonalcoholic steatohepatitis. N Engl J Med 2021;384(12): 1113–24.
39. Wilding JPH, Batterham RL, Calanna S, et al. Once-weekly semaglutide in adults with overweight or obesity. N Engl J Med 2021;384(11):989–1002.
40. Burra P, Becchetti C, Germani G. NAFLD and liver transplantation: disease burden, current management and future challenges. JHEP Rep 2020;2(6): 100192.
41. Saeed N, Glass L, Sharma P, et al. Incidence and risks for nonalcoholic fatty liver disease and steatohepatitis post-liver transplant: systematic review and meta-analysis. Transplantation 2019;103(11):e345–54.
42. Akinyemiju T, Abera S, Ahmed M, et al. The burden of primary liver cancer and underlying etiologies from 1990 to 2015 at the global, regional, and national level: results from the global burden of disease study 2015. JAMA Oncol 2017;3(12): 1683–91.
43. Younossi ZM, Otgonsuren M, Henry L, et al. Association of nonalcoholic fatty liver disease (NAFLD) with hepatocellular carcinoma (HCC) in the United States from 2004 to 2009. Hepatology 2015;62(6):1723–30.
44. Geh D, Anstee QM, Reeves HL. NAFLD-associated HCC: progress and opportunities. J Hepatocell Carcinoma 2021;8:223–39.
45. Desai A, Sandhu S, Lai JP, et al. Hepatocellular carcinoma in non-cirrhotic liver: a comprehensive review. World J Hepatol 2019;11(1):1–18.
46. Vogel A, Cervantes A, Chau I, et al. Hepatocellular carcinoma: ESMO Clinical Practice Guidelines for diagnosis, treatment and follow-up. Ann Oncol 2019; 30(5):871–3.
47. Geh D, Rana FA, Reeves HL. Weighing the benefits of hepatocellular carcinoma surveillance against potential harms. J Hepatocell Carcinoma 2019;6: 23–30.
48. Perisetti A, Goyal H, Yendala R, et al. Non-cirrhotic hepatocellular carcinoma in chronic viral hepatitis: current insights and advancements. World J Gastroenterol 2021;27(24):3466–82.
49. Rastogi A. Pathomolecular characterization of HCC in non-cirrhotic livers. Hepatoma Res 2020;6:47.
50. Yang JD, Addissie BD, Mara KC, et al. GALAD score for hepatocellular carcinoma detection in comparison with liver ultrasound and proposal of GALADUS score. Cancer Epidemiol Biomarkers Prev 2019;28(3):531–8.
51. Best J, Bechmann LP, Sowa JP, et al. GALAD score detects early hepatocellular carcinoma in an international cohort of patients with nonalcoholic steatohepatitis. Clin Gastroenterol Hepatol 2020;18(3):728–35.e724.
52. Roche - doing now what patients need next, Available at: https://www.roche.com/media/releases/med-cor-2020-03-04 Accessed January 05, 2023.
53. Nakamura N, Hatano E, Iguchi K, et al. Elevated levels of circulating ITIH4 are associated with hepatocellular carcinoma with nonalcoholic fatty liver disease: from pig model to human study. BMC Cancer 2019;19(1):621.
54. Heo MJ, Yun J, Kim SG. Role of non-coding RNAs in liver disease progression to hepatocellular carcinoma. Arch Pharm Res (Seoul) 2019;42(1):48–62.
55. Li C, Chen J, Zhang K, et al. Progress and prospects of long noncoding RNAs (lncRNAs) in hepatocellular carcinoma. Cell Physiol Biochem 2015;36(2): 423–34.

56. Xu RH, Wei W, Krawczyk M, et al. Circulating tumour DNA methylation markers for diagnosis and prognosis of hepatocellular carcinoma. Nat Mater 2017;16(11):1155–61.
57. Baumeister SE, Schlesinger S, Aleksandrova K, et al. Association between physical activity and risk of hepatobiliary cancers: a multinational cohort study. J Hepatol 2019;70(5):885–92.
58. Turati F, Trichopoulos D, Polesel J, et al. Mediterranean diet and hepatocellular carcinoma. J Hepatol 2014;60(3):606–11.

Changings and Challenges in Liver Transplantation for Nonalcoholic Fatty Liver Disease/ Steatohepatitis

Sarah Shalaby, MD, Sara Battistella, MD, Alberto Zanetto, MD, PhD, Debora Bizzaro, BS, PhD, Giacomo Germani, MD, PhD, Francesco Paolo Russo, MD, PhD, Patrizia Burra, MD, PhD*

KEYWORDS

- Liver transplant • Nonalcoholic liver disease • Nonalcoholic steatohepatitis
- Cirrhosis

KEY POINTS

- Nonalcoholic fatty liver disease/steatohepatitis (NAFLD/NASH) is increasing globally as an indication for liver transplantation (LT), in particular among patients with hepatocellular carcinoma.
- Multidisciplinary assessment and follow-up are required in candidates and transplant recipients with NAFLD/NASH.
- Model for End-Stage Liver Disease score underestimates the clinical condition of NAFLD/NASH patients and their urgency for a liver transplant.
- Recurrent NAFLD/NASH after transplant is not an infrequent event; however, its prognostic factors and treatment still need to be defined.
- Patients with NAFLD/NASH are at higher risk to develop de novo neoplasms after LT, and dedicated screening programs should be defined.

INTRODUCTION

Indications for liver transplantation (LT) are rapidly changing in the last decades,[1] facing a rapid decrease in virus-related liver disease due to the effective prevention of infection and availability of highly effective drugs. Nonetheless, the modifications in general population characteristics and lifestyle toward a higher prevalence of metabolic syndrome and obesity are happening at the same time, leading to the onset of a whole new scenario in the setting of LT.[2,3]

Gastroenterology, Multivisceral Transplant Unit, Department of Surgery, Oncology and Gastroenterology, Padua University Hospital, Via Giustiniani 2, Padua 35128, Italy
* Corresponding author.
E-mail address: burra@unipd.it

Clin Liver Dis 27 (2023) 225–237
https://doi.org/10.1016/j.cld.2023.01.003
liver.theclinics.com

This review aimed to analyze the changings and challenges in this setting, in detail the different aspects involved in the process of LT, peculiar to patients with nonalcoholic fatty liver disease/steatohepatitis (NAFLD/NASH), which are shifting the attention of transplant specialists towards different points of interest.

EPIDEMIOLOGY OF NONALCOHOLIC FATTY LIVER DISEASE/STEATOHEPATITIS IN CANDIDATES FOR LIVER TRANSPLANTATION

Although NAFLD/NASH already represents the leading indication for LT and simultaneous liver–kidney transplant in the United States,[2,4] it is still a relatively infrequent indication in Europe, possibly reflecting the lower prevalence of obesity and metabolic syndrome.[5] Nevertheless, the most recent studies display similar rates in the increase of NAFLD/NASH as an indication for LT in different countries, thus indicating that there is a common growing trend (**Table 1**).[5–17] In particular, patients affected by NAFLD/NASH-related hepatocellular carcinoma (HCC-NAFLD/NASH) seem to represent the category with the greatest growth rate in the waiting list for LT.[5–10]

Still, most of these retrospective studies either included patients with cryptogenic cirrhosis plus obesity/metabolic syndrome within the group of NAFLD/NASH patients or excluded all patients categorized as cryptogenic, introducing a significant bias in the analysis. Moreover, as we see in everyday clinical practice, there are a significant number of patients in whom NAFLD/NASH represents a co-etiological factor. In such cases, it may be difficult to assess the relative contribution of each component once cirrhosis is established, likely leading to an underestimation of NAFLD/NASH. Thus, future prospective studies are required to confirm/rescale these results.

TRANSPLANT EVALUATION

Transplant candidates with NAFLD/NASH may pose several challenges in the peritransplant setting due to their frequent multiple metabolic comorbidities, starting from the lack of suitable measuring tools to evaluate the baseline metabolic asset. The metabolic profile displayed by these patients is hardly interpretable with ranges used for the general population, and the body mass index (BMI)-based definition of obesity is not useful due to the fluid and fat redistribution status and obese sarcopenia.[18] Moreover, NAFLD/NASH can also develop in nonobese subjects (ie, "lean" NAFLD/NASH).[19] A complete pre-LT metabolic and nutritional workup should be performed by dedicated dietitians together with the multidisciplinary transplant group in all types of NAFLD/NASH, including individualized dietary supplementation and physical activity implementation.[20]

On the contrary, the management of morbid obesity in potential bariatric surgery candidates not responding to nutritional interventions is challenging. Current, low-to-moderate grade evidence suggests sleeve gastrectomy as the preferred bariatric surgical technique in LT candidates.[21] However, there is an ongoing debate on the most appropriate timing of bariatric surgery in LT candidates,[22] even when performed in centers with expertise. Future studies should investigate the comparative effectiveness of simultaneous and delayed bariatric surgery timing in the LT population.[23] In addition, if the creation of a presurgical portosystemic trans-jugular shunt in cirrhotic patients will be confirmed to be able to decrease the rate of complications of extrahepatic surgery,[24] the scenario might change in favor of the pre-LT setting.

Another challenge in patients with NAFLD/NASH is posed by the high prevalence of cardiovascular disease (CVD), which is not only secondary to the concomitant metabolic risk factors, but also to NAFLD/NASH itself.[25] Currently no gold standard exists for the pre-LT evaluation of candidates with NAFLD/NASH and the International Liver

Table 1
Changings in nonalcoholic fatty liver disease/steatohepatitis prevalence as an indication for liver transplant over the last two decades[5–17]

Study	Country	Period	Number and Type of Patients	Overall % of Patient with HCC	Trend	Note
Wong et al,[9] 2015	USA (UNOS/OPTN database)	2004 to 2013	Waitlist registrants with chronic liver Disease Number: NA	HCV: 24.6%, NAFLD/NASH: 21.0%, HCV/ALD: 13.2% ALD: 7.5%	Change in NAFLD/NASH overall: +170%	In 2013, NAFLD/NASH became the second-leading disease among liver transplant waitlist registrants, after HCV
Noureddin et al,[14] 2018	USA (UNOS/OPTN database)	2004 to 2016	127,164 waitlist registrants	NA	Change in NAFLD/NASH overall: +97% • Males: +114% • Females: +80% Change in HCC-NAFLD/NASH: +1413% • Males: +1172% • Females: +2383%	NAFLD/NASH increased as the cause in all ethnic subgroups (leading cause for liver transplant for women and the second leading cause for men, following ALD).
Goldberg et al,[7] 2017	USA (UNOS/OPTN database)	2002 to 2015	Waitlist registrants with chronic liver disease Number: NA	NA	Change in CLF- NAFLD/NASH: 12% to 23% (+92%) Change in HCC- NAFLD/NASH: 5% to 13% (+160%)	The increase in percentage was accompanied by a parallel increase in absolute number of new waitlistings
Loy et al,[11] 2018	USA (UNOS/OPTN database)	2005 to 2012	76,149 waitlist registrants with NAFLD/NASH	5.1%	Change in NAFLD/NASH overall: • Males: 3% to 8.2% (+173%) • Females: 6% to 13.3% (+121%)	NAFLD/NASH was a more frequent indication for liver transplant in women than men

(*continued on next page*)

Table 1
(continued)

Study	Country	Period	Number and Type of Patients	Overall % of Patient with HCC	Trend	Note
Holmer et al,[15] 2018	Northern Europe (Nordic Liver Transplant Registry)	1994 to 2015	4609 waitlist registrants	12.4%	Change in NAFLD/NASH overall: 2% to 6.2% (+210%)	The increase in percentage was accompanied by a parallel increase in absolute number of new waitlistings
Belli et al,[5] 2018	Europe (ELTR database)	2014 to 2017	60,527 waitlist registrants with either HCV, HBV, alcohol or NAFLD/NASH cirrhosis	28.31%	Change in CLF-NAFLD/NASH: 0.9% to 5% (+450%) Change in HCC-NAFLD/NASH: 0.2% to 1.2% (+500%)	In Northern Europe, the incidence of NAFLD/NASH as an indication for LT reached 10% in 2017
Thuluvath et al,[12] 2019	USA (UNOS/OPTN database)	2002 to 2016	33,566 waitlist registrants with wither cryptogenic, alcoholic, NAFLD/NASH or autoimmune cirrhosis	0% (exclusion criteria)	Change in NAFLD/NASH overall: 1% to 16% (+1500%)	
Younossi	USA (SRTR database)	2002 to 2016	24,431 waitlist registrants with HCC and either, HCV, HBV, alcohol and NAFLD/NASH	100%	Change in HCC-NAFLD/NASH: 2.1% to 16.2% (+670%)	The increasing trend of prevalence of HCC in liver transplant candidates with NAFLD/NASH was steeper than that for any other etiology
Haldar et al,[17] 2019	Europe (ELTR database)	2002 to 2016	68,950 waitlist registrants with end stage liver disease	Overall: 29.3% NAFLD/NASH: 39.1% Non-NAFLD/NASH: 28.9%	Change in NAFLD/NASH overall: form 1.2% to 8.4% (+600%)	A greater proportion of patients transplanted for NAFLD/NASH (39.1%) had HCC than non-NAFLD/NASH patients (28.9%, $p < 0.001$).

Cholankeril et al,[13] 2017	USA (SRTR database)	2003 to 2014	47,127 patients undergoing LT	13.74%	Change in NAFLD/NASH overall: +162%	
Young (2018)	USA (SRTR database)	2003 to 2015	47,591 waitlist registrants with either HCV, HBV, or NAFLD/NASH cirrhosis	39.2%	Change in CLF- NAFLD/NASH: +41% in PI era and +81% in DAA era, compared with IFN era Change in HCC- NAFLD/NASH: +80% in PI era and +147% in DAA era, compared with IFN era	Interferon era (IFN; 2003 to 2010), Protease inhibitor era (PI, 2011 to 2013) and direct-acting antiviral era (DAA, 2014 to 2015)
Ferrarese et al,[10] 2022	Italy (Padua University Hospital)	2006 to 2020	1491 waitlist registrants with cirrhosis		Change in NAFLD/NASH overall: 2.5% to 23% (+820%) Change in CLF- NAFLD/NASH: 1.8% to 18% (+900%) Change in HCC- NAFLD/NASH: 4% to 30% (+650%)	
Calzadilla-Bertot et al,[8] 2019	Australia and New Zealand (ANZ Liver Transplant Registry)	2003 to 2017	4666 waitlist registrants with chronic liver disease	19%	Change in NAFLD/NASH overall: 2% to 10.9% (+445%) Change in HCC- NAFLD/NASH: 4% to 9% (+115%) Change in HCC- NAFLD/NASH (2009 to 2012): 4% to 13.8% (+245%)	In 2017, NAFLD/NASH was the third leading cause of chronic liver disease among wait-list registrants and the third most frequent etiology in those with HCC

Abbreviations: ALD, alcoholic liver disease; CLF, chronic liver failure; ELTR, European Liver Transplant Registry; HBV, hepatitis B virus; HCC, hepatocellular carcinoma; HCV, hepatitis C virus; SRTR, scientific registry of transplant recipients; UNOS/OPTN, United Network for Organ Sharing/Organ Procurement and Transplantation Network; USA, United States of America.

Transplantation Society recommends a case-by-case discussion by a multidisciplinary team including a cardiologist and anesthesiologist.[20] Interestingly, Hogan and colleagues[26] suggested an algorithm for evaluation of coronary-artery disease (CAD), contemplating a coronary angiography in patients with NAFLD/NASH presenting at LT evaluation with one or more of the following risk factors: age >50 years, type 2 diabetes mellitus, hypertension, family history of CAD, smoking, or known CAD. Zorzi and colleagues[27] recently developed a non-invasive score based on standard chest computed tomography to predict severe cardiac morbidity and mortality within 1-year after LT, the coronary artery calcium score. Pending further validation, this score may be useful to identify patients at higher risk of cardiovascular mortality after LT.

In addition to CVD, patients with NAFLD/NASH are at high risk for multifactorial chronic kidney disease,[28] making the management of renal dysfunction in the peri- and post-LT settings even more challenging.[29] Moreover, even though this might favor their access to LT due to higher Model for End-Stage Liver Disease (MELD) scores compared with non-NASH patients,[30] patients needing simultaneous liver–kidney transplants have been rapidly trending up.[2] Gender disparities are also more evident in this particular population of LT candidates and need further attention.[31,32]

DROPOUT AND MORTALITY IN THE WAITING LIST

Nagai and colleagues[33] recently showed that, compared with patients with other etiologies, NAFLD/NASH patients with MELD-Na scores between 6 to 20 and 21 to 30 have a more rapid disease progression, represented by significantly higher 90-day delta MELD-Na score, a greater risk of mortality and a lower chance of recovery. Another study based on United Network for Organ Sharing (UNOS) data from 2002 to 2016 showed a higher incidence of exclusion from the waiting-list for mortality and clinical deterioration in NAFLD/NASH patients compared with patients with other indications of LT.[12] However, these results could be, at least in part, attributed to baseline demographic differences and should be confirmed.

IMMUNOSUPPRESSION

Immunosuppression should be carefully monitored in patients who undergo LT for NAFLD/NASH due to its metabolic effect. Corticosteroids promote insulin resistance, whereas calcineurin inhibitors (CNI) may favor the development of diabetes mellitus (DM), renal impairment, and hypertension.[34] Dyslipidemia is particularly affected by the mammalian target of rapamycin (mTOR) inhibitors, whereas the use of mycophenolate seems to have lesser effects on metabolic syndrome.[35] Nevertheless, the use of mTOR inhibitors with lower doses of tacrolimus has been associated with a reduction in body weight at 1 and 2 years after LT[36] and has been proposed as an alternative strategy in NAFLD/NASH recipients.[1,37] However, our study failed to show a direct association between the development of de novo metabolic syndrome and immunosuppressive therapy.[38]

OUTCOMES AFTER LIVER TRANSPLANTATION

Obese patients have a high risk of postsurgical complications, and obese NAFLD/NASH patients undergoing LT have shown a higher risk of persisting ascites, pleural effusion, dyspnea, fever, electrolyte disturbance, or wound infections compared with nonobese patients.[39] Nevertheless, in the long-term, patients and graft survival seem comparable to other indications to LT,[40] with 1- and 5-year survival rates of 85% to 90% and 70% to 80%, respectively.[41] Still, recurrence of NAFLD/NASH,[42] and cirrhosis (approximately 11% to 14% at 5 years after LT),[43] may occur. Moreover, NAFLD/NASH recipients have a significant risk of death for CVD, with rates reaching 40% at 5 years after LT in those with recurrent NAFLD/NASH,[44] and higher risk of developing posttransplant DM, which increases mortality, infections rate, and CVD.[45] Hypertriglyceridemia, high BMI, and history of alcohol abuse after LT were significantly associated with the recurrence of NAFLD/NASH.[12] Further studies are required to assess the relative contribution of these individual risk factors and propose prognostic scores for the identification of patients at higher risk for progression after transplantation.

Liver biopsy remains the gold standard for the diagnosis of recurrent NAFLD/NASH. Other potentially valuable tools such as magnetic resonance imaging, serological scores, transient elastography, and magnetic resonance elastography still require validation in the posttransplant setting.[46]

THERAPEUTICAL OPTIONS AFTER LIVER TRANSPLANTATION

The cornerstones of current treatment recommendations for obese NAFLD/NASH patients include weight loss via caloric restriction and physical activity,[47] whereas the pharmacological approach can be considered for those unable to lose weight through lifestyle modifications. In this context, Liraglutide, a glucagon-like peptide 1 (GLP-1) receptor agonist, appears to be effective, leading to histological resolution of NAFLD/NASH in 39% of patients,[48] and orlistat has shown a positive effect also on NAFLD/NASH fibrosis.[49] Nevertheless, data on LT recipients are still significantly limited and there is no current specific recommendation regarding treatment of NAFLD/NASH recurrence.[46]

For the treatment of DM and dyslipidemia in solid organ recipients, metformin, rosiglitazone, pioglitazone, sulfonylureas, GLP-1 receptor agonists, statins, and ezetimibe are considered safe,[50–53] provided that attention is paid to interactions with immunosuppressive drugs.

HEPATOCELLULAR CARCINOMA

Patients with HCC-NAFLD/NASH waitlisted for LT are less likely to undergo LT than those with non-NASH-HCC.[16,54] This might be due to the more preserved hepatic function at HCC diagnosis,[55] and the slower progression of the liver disease compared with HCV-HCC patients,[16] resulting in a lower MELD score. Furthermore, comorbidities and body habitus can delay HCC diagnosis and limit downstaging/bridge treatment options, contraindicate LT, raise chances of drop-out from the waiting list, and may affect time to HCC exception application and/or their approval of exception points.[16,54] A few clinical studies have shown that HCC-NAFLD/NASH patients might also display high-risk HCC features at diagnosis.[55,56] However, Lewin and colleagues[57] reported similar histological patterns at LT on explant pathology compared with other HCC patients.

Only a few studies describe the outcomes of LT for patients with HCC in this specific context, and in those giving data the number of recipients with HCC-NAFLD/NASH is small. The largest series comes from Sadler and colleagues[58] (929 patients transplanted for HCC, 6.5% with underlying NAFLD/NASH). The actuarial 1-, 3- and 5-year overall survival were similar, 98%, 96%, and 80% in HCC-NAFLD/NASH versus 95%, 84%, and 78% in non-NASH-HCC. Moreover, there were no significant differences in tumor recurrence rates, whereas NAFLD/NASH status appeared as a protective factor for recurrence among patients with tumors beyond Milan. Given that the pathophysiology for the development of HCC in NAFLD/NASH may be different, outcomes after LT may be different too, and these results deserve further investigation.

DE NOVO MALIGNANCIES AFTER LIVER TRANSPLANTATION

Patients with NAFLD/NASH are at high risk of cancer due to the metabolic risk factors, chronic systemic inflammation, and lifestyle habits. Indeed, malignancies are the second cause of death among non-transplanted patients with NAFLD/NASH,[59] secondary only to CVD, and the baseline high oncological risk is further raised after LT by chronic immunosuppression. An analysis of scientific registry of transplant recipients (SRTR) data of patients transplanted between 1987 and 2009 found NAFLD/NASH as one of the main etiologies associated with de novo malignancy (DNM) risk,[60] which is not surprising as obesity and diabetes are major risk factors for the development of DNM. The changings in the epidemiology of LT recipients towards a growth in the prevalence of NAFLD/NASH may therefore imply significant modifications in the epidemiology of DNM occurring in LT recipients. Therefore, it is worth considering a close monitoring of this subpopulation after LT. Recent evidences show that these patients are at higher risk to develop de novo colorectal cancer.[61] Although there is limited evidence to support strict screening guidelines, a shorter interval between post-LT colonoscopies has already been recommended.[62,63]

QUALITY OF LIFE AFTER LIVER TRANSPLANTATION

In addition to its clinical burden, NAFLD/NASH is known to have a negative impact on health-related quality of life (HRQoL), even before progression to cirrhosis has occurred. Patients with NAFLD/NASH-cirrhosis have been reported to suffer from lower HRQoL (physical health/functioning, emotional health and worry, and mental health) than patients with non-cirrhotic NAFLD/NASH and general population, with many patients reporting severe fatigue.[64,65] Currently there are no studies assessing the impact of LT on HRQoL in NAFLD/NASH patients.

PEDIATRIC POPULATION

Unlike in adults, NAFLD/NASH is a very rare indication for LT in children, and in those presenting with this diagnosis, secondary causes should be excluded, particularly inherited metabolic defects. Cananzi and colleagues[66] were not able to draw definitive recommendations on the natural history, indications, and outcome of LT for NAFLD/NASH in children due to the lack of evidence. Given the sharp increase in metabolic syndrome and associated liver disease in pediatric patients, further studies investigating the long-term effect of NAFLD/NASH and the potential need for LT in these patients are awaited. Furthermore, pediatric patients are at risk to develop metabolic syndrome with morbid obesity after LT and during the transition from pediatric to adult health care service, thus particular attention should be taken in this context and a multidisciplinary approach is recommendable.[67]

SUMMARY

LT for NAFLD/NASH is increasing rapidly worldwide; it is more frequently associated with a systemic metabolic syndrome, which significantly affects other organs, in particular cardiovascular, renal and muscular-skeletal systems. A multidisciplinary assessment and follow-up is required in candidates and transplant recipients with NAFLD/NASH. Further data to improve posttransplant protocols in these patients, particularly regarding the management of immunosuppression, treatment of recurrent NAFLD/NASH, and screening for de novo neoplasm are urgently expected.

CLINICS CARE POINTS

- Dietary and lifestyle interventions should be maintained in the pre- and post-liver transplantation (LT) settings.
- Immunosuppression should be individualized to prevent metabolic comorbidities and recurrence of nonalcoholic fatty liver disease/steatohepatitis (NAFLD/NASH).
- The safety and efficacy of pharmacological therapies for the treatment of NAFLD/NASH recurrence after LT remain to be assessed.
- A shorter interval between post-LT colonoscopies has been recommended for NAFLD/NASH patients for the high risk of de novo colorectal carcinoma.
- The impact of LT on health-related quality of life and the natural history of NAFLD/NASH in pediatric patients still needs to be assessed.

DISCLOSURE

The authors do not have any commercial or financial conflicts of interest and neither received any funding sources for this article

REFERENCES

1. Burra P, Becchetti C, Germani G. NAFLD and liver transplantation: disease burden, current management and future challenges. JHEP Rep 2020;2(6):100192.
2. Younossi Z, Anstee QM, Marietti M, et al. Global burden of NAFLD and NASH: trends, predictions, risk factors and prevention. Nat Rev Gastroenterol Hepatol 2018;15(1):11–20.
3. Singal AK, Hasanin M, Kaif M, et al. Nonalcoholic steatohepatitis is the most rapidly growing indication for simultaneous liver kidney transplantation in the United States. Transplantation 2016;100(3):607–12.
4. Younossi ZM. Nonalcoholic fatty liver disease and nonalcoholic steatohepatitis: implications for liver transplantation. Liver Transpl 2018;24(2):166–70.
5. Belli LS, Perricone G, Adam R, et al. Impact of DAAs on liver transplantation: major effects on the evolution of indications and results. An ELITA study based on the ELTR registry. J Hepatol 2018;69(4):810–7.
6. Younossi Z, Stepanova M, Ong JP, et al. Nonalcoholic steatohepatitis is the fastest growing cause of hepatocellular carcinoma in liver transplant candidates. Clin Gastroenterol Hepatol 2019;17(4):748–755 e743.
7. Goldberg D, Ditah IC, Saeian K, et al. Changes in the prevalence of hepatitis C virus infection, nonalcoholic steatohepatitis, and alcoholic liver disease among patients with cirrhosis or liver failure on the waitlist for liver transplantation. Gastroenterology 2017;152(5):1090–1099 e1091.
8. Calzadilla-Bertot L, Jeffrey GP, Jacques B, et al. Increasing incidence of nonalcoholic steatohepatitis as an indication for liver transplantation in Australia and New Zealand. Liver Transpl 2019;25(1):25–34.
9. Wong RJ, Aguilar M, Cheung R, et al. Nonalcoholic steatohepatitis is the second leading etiology of liver disease among adults awaiting liver transplantation in the United States. Gastroenterology 2015;148(3):547–55.

10. Ferrarese A, Battistella S, Germani G, et al. Nash up, virus down: how the waiting list is changing for liver transplantation: a single center experience from Italy. Medicina (Kaunas) 2022;58(2):290.
11. Loy VM, Joyce C, Bello S, et al. Gender disparities in liver transplant candidates with nonalcoholic steatohepatitis. Clin Transplant 2018;32(8):e13297.
12. Thuluvath PJ, Hanish S, Savva Y. Waiting list mortality and transplant rates for NASH cirrhosis when compared with cryptogenic, alcoholic, or AIH cirrhosis. Transplantation 2019;103(1):113–21.
13. Cholankeril G, Wong RJ, Hu M, et al. Liver transplantation for nonalcoholic steatohepatitis in the US: temporal trends and outcomes. Dig Dis Sci 2017;62(10): 2915–22.
14. Noureddin M, Vipani A, Bresee C, et al. NASH leading cause of liver transplant in women: updated analysis of indications for liver transplant and ethnic and gender variances. Am J Gastroenterol 2018;113(11):1649–59.
15. Holmer M, Melum E, Isoniemi H, et al. Nonalcoholic fatty liver disease is an increasing indication for liver transplantation in the Nordic countries. Liver Int 2018;38(11):2082–90.
16. Young K, Aguilar M, Gish R, et al. Lower rates of receiving model for end-stage liver disease exception and longer time to transplant among nonalcoholic steatohepatitis hepatocellular carcinoma. Liver Transpl 2016;22(10):1356–66.
17. Haldar D, Kern B, Hodson J, et al. Outcomes of liver transplantation for nonalcoholic steatohepatitis: a European Liver Transplant Registry study. J Hepatol 2019;71(2):313–22.
18. Kalinkovich A, Livshits G. Sarcopenic obesity or obese sarcopenia: a cross talk between age-associated adipose tissue and skeletal muscle inflammation as a main mechanism of the pathogenesis. Ageing Res Rev 2017;35:200–21.
19. Younes R, Bugianesi E. NASH in lean individuals. Semin Liver Dis 2019;39(1): 86–95.
20. Tsochatzis E, Coilly A, Nadalin S, et al. International liver transplantation consensus statement on end-stage liver disease due to nonalcoholic steatohepatitis and liver transplantation. Transplantation 2019;103(1):45–56.
21. Diwan TS, Lee TC, Nagai S, et al. Obesity, transplantation, and bariatric surgery: an evolving solution for a growing epidemic. Am J Transplant 2020;20(8): 2143–55.
22. Newsome PN, Allison ME, Andrews PA, et al. Guidelines for liver transplantation for patients with non-alcoholic steatohepatitis. Gut 2012;61(4):484–500.
23. Diwan TS, Rice TC, Heimbach JK, et al. Liver transplantation and bariatric surgery: timing and outcomes. Liver Transpl 2018;24(9):1280–7.
24. Garcia-Pagan JC, Saffo S, Mandorfer M, et al. Where does TIPS fit in the management of patients with cirrhosis? JHEP Rep 2020;2(4):100122.
25. Choudhary NS, Duseja A. Screening of cardiovascular disease in nonalcoholic fatty liver disease: whom and how? J Clin Exp Hepatol 2019;9(4):506–14.
26. Hogan BJ, Gonsalkorala E, Heneghan MA. Evaluation of coronary artery disease in potential liver transplant recipients. Liver Transpl 2017;23(3):386–95.
27. Zorzi A, Brunetti G, Cardaioli F, et al. Coronary artery calcium on standard chest computed tomography predicts cardiovascular events after liver transplantation. Int J Cardiol 2021;339:219–24.
28. Samji NS, Verma R, Keri KC, et al. Liver transplantation for nonalcoholic steatohepatitis: pathophysiology of recurrence and clinical challenges. Dig Dis Sci 2019; 64(12):3413–30.

29. Shalaby S, Burra P, Senzolo M. Renal dysfunction after liver transplantation. In: Burra P, editor. Textbook of liver transplantation: a multidisciplinary approach. Cham: Springer International Publishing; 2022. p. 373–87.
30. Park CW, Tsai NT, Wong LL. Implications of worse renal dysfunction and medical comorbidities in patients with NASH undergoing liver transplant evaluation: impact on MELD and more. Clin Transplant 2011;25(6):E606–11.
31. Burra P, Bizzaro D, Gonta A, et al. Clinical impact of sexual dimorphism in non-alcoholic fatty liver disease (NAFLD) and non-alcoholic steatohepatitis (NASH). Liver Int 2021;41(8):1713–33.
32. Burra P, Zanetto A, Germani G. Sex bias in clinical trials in gastroenterology and hepatology. Nat Rev Gastroenterol Hepatol 2022;19(7):413–4.
33. Nagai S, Safwan M, Kitajima T, et al. Disease-specific waitlist outcomes in liver transplantation - a retrospective study. Transpl Int 2021;34(3):499–513.
34. Farkas SA, Schnitzbauer AA, Kirchner G, et al. Calcineurin inhibitor minimization protocols in liver transplantation. Transpl Int 2009;22(1):49–60.
35. Watt KD. Metabolic syndrome: is immunosuppression to blame? Liver Transpl 2011;17(Suppl 3):S38–42.
36. Charlton M, Rinella M, Patel D, et al. Everolimus is associated with less weight gain than tacrolimus 2 years after liver transplantation: results of a randomized multicenter study. Transplantation 2017;101(12):2873–82.
37. De Simone P, Fagiuoli S, Cescon M, et al. Use of everolimus in liver transplantation: recommendations from a working group. Transplantation 2017;101(2):239–51.
38. Becchetti C, Ferrarese A, Zeni N, et al. A prospective longitudinal assessment of de novo metabolic syndrome after liver transplantation. Clin Transplant 2022;36(2):e14532.
39. van den Berg EH, Douwes RM, de Meijer VE, et al. Liver transplantation for NASH cirrhosis is not performed at the expense of major post-operative morbidity. Dig Liver Dis 2018;50(1):68–75.
40. Wang X, Li J, Riaz DR, et al. Outcomes of liver transplantation for nonalcoholic steatohepatitis: a systematic review and meta-analysis. Clin Gastroenterol Hepatol 2014;12(3):394–402 e391.
41. Charlton MR, Burns JM, Pedersen RA, et al. Frequency and outcomes of liver transplantation for nonalcoholic steatohepatitis in the United States. Gastroenterology 2011;141(4):1249–53.
42. Bhati C, Idowu MO, Sanyal AJ, et al. Long-term outcomes in patients undergoing liver transplantation for nonalcoholic steatohepatitis-related cirrhosis. Transplantation 2017;101(8):1867–74.
43. Saeed N, Glass L, Sharma P, et al. Incidence and risks for nonalcoholic fatty liver disease and steatohepatitis post-liver transplant: systematic review and meta-analysis. Transplantation 2019;103(11):e345–54.
44. Narayanan P, Mara K, Izzy M, et al. Recurrent or de novo allograft steatosis and long-term outcomes after liver transplantation. Transplantation 2019;103(1):e14–21.
45. Bhat V, Tazari M, Watt KD, et al. New-onset diabetes and preexisting diabetes are associated with comparable reduction in long-term survival after liver transplant: a machine learning approach. Mayo Clin Proc 2018;93(12):1794–802.
46. Germani G, Laryea M, Rubbia-Brandt L, et al. Management of recurrent and De Novo NAFLD/NASH after liver transplantation. Transplantation 2019;103(1):57–67.

47. European Association for the Study of the L, European Association for the Study of D, European Association for the Study of O. EASL-EASD-EASO Clinical Practice Guidelines for the management of non-alcoholic fatty liver disease. Diabetologia 2016;59(6):1121–40.
48. Armstrong MJ, Gaunt P, Aithal GP, et al. Liraglutide safety and efficacy in patients with non-alcoholic steatohepatitis (LEAN): a multicentre, double-blind, randomised, placebo-controlled phase 2 study. Lancet 2016;387(10019):679–90.
49. Assy N, Hussein O, Abassi Z. Weight loss induced by orlistat reverses fatty infiltration and improves hepatic fibrosis in obese patients with non-alcoholic steatohepatitis. Gut 2007;56(3):443–4.
50. Villanueva G, Baldwin D. Rosiglitazone therapy of posttransplant diabetes mellitus. Transplantation 2005;80(10):1402–5.
51. Luther P, Baldwin D Jr. Pioglitazone in the management of diabetes mellitus after transplantation. Am J Transplant 2004;4(12):2135–8.
52. Cusi K, Orsak B, Bril F, et al. Long-term pioglitazone treatment for patients with nonalcoholic steatohepatitis and prediabetes or type 2 diabetes mellitus: a randomized trial. Ann Intern Med 2016;165(5):305–15.
53. Almutairi F, Peterson TC, Molinari M, et al. Safety and effectiveness of ezetimibe in liver transplant recipients with hypercholesterolemia. Liver Transpl 2009;15(5):504–8.
54. Reddy SK, Steel JL, Chen HW, et al. Outcomes of curative treatment for hepatocellular cancer in nonalcoholic steatohepatitis versus hepatitis C and alcoholic liver disease. Hepatology 2012;55(6):1809–19.
55. Piscaglia F, Svegliati-Baroni G, Barchetti A, et al. Clinical patterns of hepatocellular carcinoma in nonalcoholic fatty liver disease: a multicenter prospective study. Hepatology 2016;63(3):827–38.
56. Ioannou GN. Epidemiology and risk-stratification of NAFLD-associated HCC. J Hepatol 2021;75(6):1476–84.
57. Lewin SM, Mehta N, Kelley RK, et al. Liver transplantation recipients with nonalcoholic steatohepatitis have lower risk hepatocellular carcinoma. Liver Transpl 2017;23(8):1015–22.
58. Sadler EM, Mehta N, Bhat M, et al. Liver transplantation for NASH-related hepatocellular carcinoma versus Non-NASH Etiologies of hepatocellular carcinoma. Transplantation 2018;102(4):640–7.
59. Sanna C, Rosso C, Marietti M, et al. Non-alcoholic fatty liver disease and extrahepatic cancers. Int J Mol Sci 2016;17(5).
60. Zhou J, Hu Z, Zhang Q, et al. Spectrum of de novo cancers and predictors in liver transplantation: analysis of the scientific registry of transplant recipients database. PLoS One 2016;11(5):e0155179.
61. Nasser-Ghodsi N, Mara K, Watt KD. De novo colorectal and pancreatic cancer in liver-transplant recipients: identifying the higher-risk populations. Hepatology 2021;74(2):1003–13.
62. Shalaby S, Burra P. De novo and recurrent malignancy. Best Pract Res Clin Gastroenterol 2020;46-47:101680.
63. Burra P, Shalaby S, Zanetto A. Long-term care of transplant recipients: de novo neoplasms after liver transplantation. Curr Opin Organ Transplant 2018;23(2):187–95.
64. McSweeney L, Breckons M, Fattakhova G, et al. Health-related quality of life and patient-reported outcome measures in NASH-related cirrhosis. JHEP Rep 2020;2(3):100099.

65. Kennedy-Martin T, Bae JP, Paczkowski R, et al. Health-related quality of life burden of nonalcoholic steatohepatitis: a robust pragmatic literature review. J Patient Rep Outcomes 2017;2:28.
66. Cananzi M, Vajro P, Rela M, et al. NAFLD and liver transplantation in children-working group report from the ILTS single topic conference on NAFLD. Transplantation 2019;103(1):68–70.
67. Ferrarese A, Germani G, Lazzaro S, et al. Short-term outcomes of paediatric liver transplant recipients after transition to Adult Healthcare Service. Liver Int 2018; 38(7):1316–21.

Extrahepatic Outcomes of Nonalcoholic Fatty Liver Disease: Cardiovascular Diseases

Angelo Armandi, MD, Elisabetta Bugianesi, MD, PhD*

KEYWORDS

• NAFLD • Cardiovascular disease • Coronary artery disease • Atherosclerosis • Cardiac remodeling • Heart failure • Gene polymorphisms • Gut dysbiosis

KEY POINTS

- Nonalcoholic fatty liver disease (NAFLD) is associated with an increased prevalence of cardiovascular disease (CVD), including hypertension, arrhythmias, atherosclerosis, coronary artery disease, ventricular remodeling with potential evolution into diastolic dysfunction, and heart failure.
- NAFLD is associated with increased incidence of fatal and nonfatal major adverse cardiovascular events and CVD represents the major cause of long-term mortality in the NAFLD population even in advanced stages of liver fibrosis.
- The deposition of ectopic fat tissue in the epicardium runs parallel to fat deposition and it is linked to myocardial insulin resistance and altered energy metabolism.
- Polymorphisms in the *TM6SF2* gene, involved in the hepatic lipid metabolism, are linked to a worse cardiovascular phenotype due to an atherogenic lipid profile.
- Gut dysbiosis promoted by the Western diet leads to alterations in the intestinal epithelial barrier and endotoxemia, favoring metabolic inflammation in both cardiac and hepatic districts.

INTRODUCTION

Nonalcoholic fatty liver disease (NAFLD) can be considered one of the protean manifestations of the metabolic syndrome (MetS). The close link and shared pathophysiology of NAFLD and visceral obesity, type 2 diabetes mellitus (T2DM), arterial hypertension, and dyslipidemia, is mirrored in the association and incidence of common adverse outcomes, with cardiovascular disease (CVD) being a major cause of morbidity and mortality in the NAFLD population. Currently, it is difficult to prove an independent role for NAFLD in the development of CVD as this liver condition is often embedded in a complex setting of insulin resistance, adipose tissue dysfunction, and gut microbiota

Department of Medical Sciences, University of Turin, Corso Dogliotti 14, Torino 10126, Italy
* Corresponding author.
E-mail address: elisabetta.bugianesi@unito.it

Clin Liver Dis 27 (2023) 239–250
https://doi.org/10.1016/j.cld.2023.01.018
1089-3261/23/

alteration. Nevertheless, some evidence suggests a reciprocal influence of MetS and NAFLD and the relative risk of CVD may vary according to the features of liver injury (steatosis, necro-inflammation, and fibrosis) and the degree of hepatic damage. Ectopic fat accumulation in the liver runs parallel to other ectopic fat depots, including the cardiac district, but a fatty liver may worsen the atherogenic profile of MetS. Local necro-inflammatory changes of nonalcoholic steatohepatitis (NASH) may significantly enhance systemic metabolic inflammation, thus increasing the risk of adverse cardiovascular outcomes. The fibrogenesis that marks the progressiveness of NAFLD can be also observed in the myocardium and precedes the development of heart failure in dysmetabolic conditions. It is crucial to investigate the effects of NAFLD on the development of cardiovascular events to organize an efficient health prevention and treatment program to identify the risk of CVD in patients with NAFLD. In this article, we summarize the association between NAFLD and CVD, highlighting the liver-centered mechanism associated with CVD and the clinical implications.

EPIDEMIOLOGY OF CARDIOVASCULAR DISEASE IN NONALCOHOLIC FATTY LIVER DISEASE INDIVIDUALS

Nonalcoholic Fatty Liver Disease, Atherosclerosis, and Ischemic Heart Disease

The increased risk of prevalent and incident cardiovascular events linked with NAFLD is well-documented across literature and mainly attributed to a reciprocal influence of NAFLD and MetS. Data extrapolated from the Framingham Heart Study showed that patients with baseline NAFLD had an increased incidence of arterial hypertension and T2DM than those without NAFLD, and that in those with metabolic comorbidities, including arterial hypertension, incident NAFLD was more prone to occur.[1] Although it is difficult to disentangle the independent contribution of each risk factor, an important clue is the increased subclinical atheromatous plaque formation in several vascular districts occurring in NAFLD subjects. A meta-analysis of 27 cross-sectional studies reported a strong association between NAFLD detected either by imaging or biopsy and markers of sub-clinical atherosclerosis (ie, impaired flow-mediated vasodilatation and increased carotid-artery intimal medial thickness) independent of classical cardiovascular risk factors and MetS features, although this finding has been not universally confirmed.[2] In a large cross-sectional study in the South Korean population, subjects with a fatty liver at ultrasound had a higher coronary calcium score (detected by coronary computed tomography angiography) than those without, and the risk for any atherosclerotic plaque was increased by 20% in NAFLD after adjustment for traditional cardiovascular risk factors (age, sex, obesity, diabetes mellitus, hypertension, hyperlipidemia, current smoking, family history of CAD, and high-sensitivity C-reactive protein).[3] The RISC (Relationship between Insulin Sensitivity and Cardiovascular disease) study showed that even healthy subjects are more prone to early carotid atherosclerosis in the presence of a fatty liver.[4] On the other hand, in high-risk groups such as diabetic subjects, the prevalence of coronary, cerebrovascular, and peripheral vascular disease is again remarkably higher in patients with NAFLD than those without, independent of traditional risk factors.[5] The impact of NAFLD in atherosclerosis is corroborated by the evidence that long-term regression of NAFLD bears a lower risk of carotid atherosclerosis development.[6]

The higher prevalence of atherosclerosis in patients with NAFLD translates into an increased risk of cardiovascular events, roughly twofold higher than in the general population. In a large prospective study of NAFLD individuals and matched population controls, CVD represented the most frequent cause of death, accounting for 36% of the total.[7] In particular, high-risk, non-calcified coronary plaques seem more frequent in NAFLD and linked to more adverse outcomes.[8] In a meta-analysis of more than 30.000 patients with a median follow-up of 7 years, the risk of incident fatal and nonfatal (myocardial infarction, stroke, angina pectoris) CVD events was increased by 64% in NAFLD compared with non-NAFLD individuals.[9] In the heterogeneous population bearing NAFLD, the presence of T2DM leads to a twofold increased risk of CVD.[10] Another meta-analysis of 34 studies found that NAFLD patients were more prone to develop coronary artery disease and hypertension (HR 2.3 and 1.16, respectively), and that the presence of NASH increased the risk of incident CVD (HR 2.97).[11] Indeed, the histological severity of NAFLD seems to have an impact on cardiovascular risk. Although cirrhosis is the strongest determinant for liver-related death, advanced fibrosis is associated with the strongest hazards for CVD.[12] NAFLD is significantly associated with increased CVD incidence more than 14 years of follow-up, but only NAFLD with advanced hepatic fibrosis (assessed by noninvasive scores) has a 70% increased risk of mortality due to CVD.[13] The aforementioned meta-analysis[9] reported a higher incidence of cardiovascular events as well as higher mortality due to CVD (odds ratio [OR] 3.28) in a subgroup of patients with severe NAFLD (defined as altered liver biochemistry, increased noninvasive scores of fibrosis or advanced fibrosis at histology). A large Swedish population-based cohort study assessed the risk for incident major adverse cardiovascular events (MACE) (including ischemic heart disease, stroke, congestive heart failure, or cardiovascular mortality) in about 10.000 patients with histologically confirmed NAFLD compared with matched population controls without NAFLD by age, sex, calendar year and country (n = 46.517).[14] Over a median of 13.6 years, patients with NAFLD had a higher incidence of MACE than controls (aHR 1.63), including higher rates of ischemic heart disease (aHR 1.64), congestive heart failure (aHR 1.75), stroke (aHR 1.58) and cardiovascular mortality (aHR 1.37). Rates of incident MACE increased progressively with worsening NAFLD severity, with the highest incidence observed in cirrhosis. Although the parallel increase of CV risk and liver fibrosis has been confirmed in other studies, the association with cirrhosis has not been universally confirmed and might be biased by International Classification of Disease (ICD) codes. In a multi-center prospective study of biopsied patients, the incidence of CVD was more pronounced in pre-cirrhosis (fibrosis stage F3), whereas in cirrhosis a major incidence of liver-related events was observed.[15]

Overall, the main message delivered by the above data is that, whatever the reason might be, a subject with NAFLD has an increased risk of CV events and should be managed accordingly.

Nonalcoholic Fatty Liver Disease, Cardiac Dysfunction, and Arrhythmias

NAFLD is associated with abnormalities in cardiac function, both in diabetic and nondiabetic populations. In a community-based cohort of 1.886 Korean adults, ultrasound-diagnosed NAFLD was associated with left ventricular diastolic dysfunction, independently of established cardiovascular risk factors.[16] In diabetic patients with known coronary artery disease, the presence of ultrasound-proven NAFLD was associated with reduced coronary functional capacity.[17] Diastolic dysfunction, an early predictive sign of heart failure with preserved ejection fraction, has been linked to impaired myocardial energy metabolism. Perseghin and colleagues[18] showed that otherwise healthy individuals with fatty liver have an increased amount of fat in the epicardial area and display an abnormal cardiac energy metabolism despite normal left ventricle morphological features and systolic/diastolic functions. Similar findings have been confirmed also in pediatric NAFLD, where overweight or obese children with NAFLD had echocardiographic features of early left ventricular dysfunction independent of multiple CVD risk factors; some functional cardiac alterations were more pronounced in subjects with NASH.[19] Moreover, recent evidence links NAFLD to cardiac valve disease, including aortic valve sclerosis and mitral annulus calcifications, which contribute to left ventricular hypertrophy and the development of heart failure.[20]

Finally, an increased prevalence of arrhythmias, such as atrial fibrillation and atrioventricular blocks, further links NAFLD to cardiac complications. A meta-analysis of 9 cross-sectional studies found an association between NAFLD and persistent atrial fibrillation in middle-aged and elderly individuals with T2DM.[21] In a prospective study of 400 diabetic patients with a 10-year follow-up, atrial fibrillation occurred more frequently in patients with concomitant NAFLD.[22] In a retrospective study based on 24-h Holter monitoring, NAFLD resulted also significantly associated with ventricular arrhythmias (nonsustained ventricular tachycardia and premature ventricular complexes), independent of multiple risk factors and comorbidities.[23] These additional CV complications of NAFLD are less documented and certainly require additional evidence.

Nonalcoholic Fatty Liver Disease and Cerebrovascular Disease

The pathophysiological link between atherosclerosis and NAFLD can also translate into an increased risk of stroke, but the evidence is controversial so far. A recent meta-analysis estimated a 5.04% prevalence of stroke in individuals with NAFLD, significantly higher when compared with non-NAFLD individuals (OR 1.88), with a stepwise increase following the severity of liver steatosis.[24] The incidence of ischemic stroke linked to the presence of NAFLD has also been found to increase in a longitudinal study (HR 1.21 over 10 years)[25] and NAFLD has been potentially identified as an independent risk factor for the severity and progression of brain infarctions.[26] However, another meta-analysis of 20 observational studies involving more than 17 million individuals found only a mild susceptibility to stroke (OR 1.18), without a strong association with liver fibrosis.[27] In the noninvasive assessment of liver fibrosis, the variables included in simple scores may change the association with stroke; for instance, in one study brain infarction was associated with liver fibrosis assessed by Fibrosis-4 (FIB-4) score, but not by NAFLD Fibrosis Score (NFS).[28] A large European population-based study involving 18 million individuals confirmed the lack of association between NAFLD and incident ischemic or unspecified stroke after adjusting for metabolic cofactors (including T2DM, hypertension, and dyslipidemia), with HR ranging from 0.99 to 1.09.[29] These conflicting results may partially be explained by the complex and heterogeneous etiology of cerebrovascular disease. In one study evaluating the stroke subtypes, only large artery atherosclerosis and small vessel occlusion were causally linked to NAFLD.[30]

Overall, the association between NAFLD and stroke appears largely driven by the presence of other metabolic comorbidities, although NAFLD may be an additional risk factor for large vessel atherosclerotic disease, ultimately leading to a major susceptibility to cerebrovascular disease.

PATHOPHYSIOLOGY

The Deposition of Ectopic Fat Tissue as Key Driver of Metabolic Dysfunctions

The accumulation of adipose tissue in ectopic sites is linked to the most adverse cardiometabolic outcomes of MetS (**Fig. 1**). The accumulation of ectopic fat in the epicardium shapes the epicardial adipocytes into a pro-inflammatory, pro-thrombotic phenotype and modulates the heart function through its anatomical proximity and shared microcirculation with the myocardium.[31,32] The reduction in the adiponectin

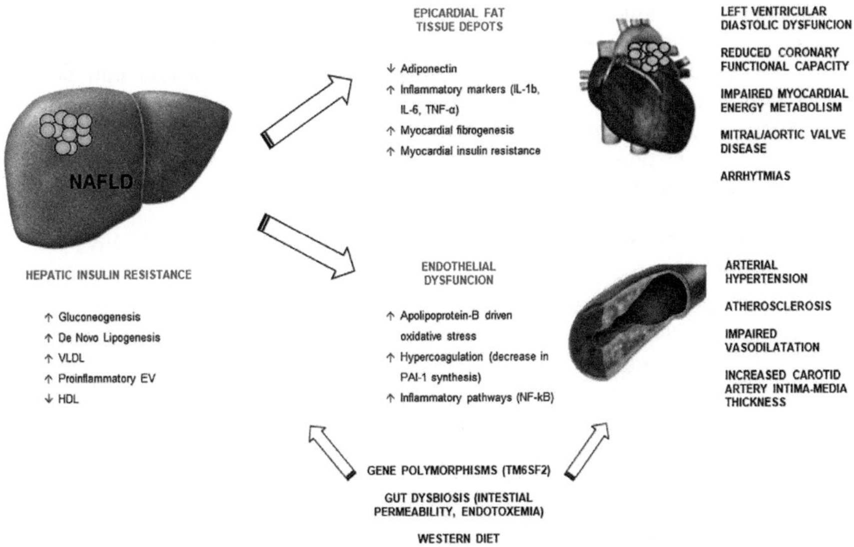

Fig. 1. Pathophysiology pathways and clinical manifestations of cardiovascular dysfunctions in NAFLD. EV, extracellular vesicles; HDL, high-density lipoproteins; IL, interleukin; NF-kB, nuclear factor-kB; PAI-1, plasminogen activator inhibitor-1; TNF, tumor necrosis factor; VLDL, very-low-density lipoproteins.

synthesis, the infiltration of pro-inflammatory macrophages, and the increased synthesis of tumor necrosis-alpha, interleukin-1b, and interleukin-6 promote a chronic, low-grade inflammation that alter the microvascular system and activate fibrogenesis processes. The effect of this metabolically altered microenvironment upon the myocardium translates into coronary artery disease, chronic ischemic heart disease, and cardiac dysfunction due to ventricular fibrosis, which ultimately leads to heart failure.[33] Insulin resistance in the cardiac muscle largely contributes to deranged myocardial energy metabolism and perfusion. In uncomplicated T2DM, Rijzewijk and colleagues[34] showed a positive association between intramyocardial and intrahepatic fat contents detected by proton magnetic resonance spectroscopy, but liver steatosis was the strongest predictor of myocardial insulin sensitivity and perfusion. In this complex picture of "metabolic" inflammation, the interconnection between different affected tissues exerts pleiotropic effects and may lead to synergic effects than deserve to be better investigated.

Hepatic Insulin Resistance and Altered Metabolism

The hepatic insulin resistance arising in a fatty liver can affect heart function through impaired lipid and glucose metabolism. The excessive fat accumulation in the liver enhances the synthesis of very low-density lipoproteins (VLDL) through activation of lipogenic transcription factors (including the sterol regulatory element-binding protein 1c), inducing a systemic condition of atherogenic dyslipidemia, characterized by high triglycerides and low high-density lipoprotein (HDL) cholesterol. The apolipoprotein-B in these particles undergoes oxidative processes and acts as damage-associated molecular patterns (DAMPs) in the subendothelial vascular space. In parallel, both increased intake of sugars, particularly fructose, and increased gluconeogenesis foster *de novo* lipogenesis. The activation of the innate immune system promotes intravascular inflammation via toll-like receptors.[35–37] The increased synthesis of plasminogen activator inhibitor-1 by the liver affects fibrinolysis and increases susceptibility to microvascular thrombosis.[38] Moreover, steatotic hepatocytes can secrete extracellular vesicles containing specific miRNA (including miR-1) which promotes a pro-inflammatory phenotype of the endothelium via activation of Nuclear Factor kappa-B.[39] All these processes induce the formation of vulnerable atherosclerotic plaques, which are key drivers of cardiovascular outcomes.

Genetic Determinants of Cardiovascular Disease Susceptibility in Nonalcoholic Fatty Liver Disease

Mutations of targeted genes associated with a more aggressive course of liver disease, including PNPLA3 (Patatin-like phospholipase domain-containing protein 3) or *TM6SF2* (Transmembrane 6 Superfamily Member 2), are mainly involved in the regulation of lipid metabolism. Carriage of single nucleotide polymorphisms in these genes causes impaired lipid export and lipid-derived oxidative stress in the liver. In contrast, this might translate into a lower circulating lipid burden that reduces the risk factors of CVD. However, PNPLA3 polymorphisms have no proven effect on CVD,[40,41] whereas *TM6SF2* polymorphisms have a differential impact on liver disease and CVD. Carriage of the *TM6SF2* T allele is linked to more severe hepatic inflammation and fibrosis, whereas carriage of the more common C allele leads to enhanced VLDL excretion, dyslipidemia, and a higher risk for CVD.[42,43] Finally, variants in the glucokinase regulatory protein (GCKR) may predispose to CVD risk through a more atherogenic lipid profile.[44]

Role of Nutrition and Gut Microbiota

The Western diet is the most relevant environmental factor for the development of NAFLD and metabolic comorbidities.[45] High consumption of saturated fats, sucrose-sweetened beverages, high glycemic index nutrients, and processed meats, shape the gut microbiota into a less favorable profile (including reduced diversity and rise in Gram-negative strains) and affect the integrity of the epithelial intestinal barrier. The rise in Gram-negative strains induced by a high-fat diet is linked to enhanced synthesis of lipopolysaccharide (LPS), which is responsible for the endotoxemia that contributes to the systemic inflammation observed in NAFLD patients.[46] A specific gut microbiome signature has been suggested for NAFLD.[47] For instance, individuals with coronary artery disease and additional NAFLD showed a significant increase in the abundance of *Coprococcus* and *Veillonella*, and reduction in the abundance of *Parabacteroides*, *Bacteroides*, and *Ruminococcus*, which was well-distinguished from individuals without NAFLD.[48] A diet rich in red meats and dairy products has a more pronounced impact on CVD outcomes via the gut microbiota. This type of diet is particularly rich in L-carnitine, which is converted by gut commensals into trimethylamine (TMA) and then metabolized in the liver to TMA N-oxide (TMAO).[49] Circulating levels of TMAO have been associated with incident fatal and nonfatal CVD events, with markedly increased levels in patients with ischemic stroke.[50] In particular, TMAO seems to upregulate Nuclear Factor kappa-B, inducing endothelial dysfunction and vascular calcifications.[51] In addition, preclinical models have shown a prothrombotic effect of TMAO through the modulation of calcium signaling pathways in platelets.[52] However, the association between NAFLD and TMAO is less clear, as only one study conducted on 61 biopsy-based NAFLD reported higher levels of TMAO in individuals with severe liver injury.[53] This complex crosstalk between diet, microbiome shaping, and inflammatory pathways may contribute to the interconnection between liver and cardiac affections.

CLINICAL IMPLICATIONS AND MANAGEMENT

The current evidence supports a strong relationship between NAFLD and both prevalent and incident CVD through shared pathophysiology and risk factors and suggests an independent role of NAFLD on the risk of multiple cardiac complications. It is still unclear whether the inclusion of NAFLD-based parameters would help improve the prediction ability for future CVD events. The Framingham risk equation has been validated for patients with NAFLD, but it includes only the traditional risk factors for CVD.[54] Current guidelines for NAFLD management remark on the importance of treating the underlying metabolic co-factors (including T2DM, arterial hypertension, and dyslipidemia), which help improve both liver and cardiovascular health.[55] No clear referral pathways or strong diagnostic pathways have been developed to help clinicians in a comprehensive metabolic evaluation of patients with NAFLD. The same dialogue that currently exists between diabetologists and cardiologists is not established yet for the hepatology setting.

Whatever the reason might be the strong association between NAFLD and CVD poses attention to careful screening for early, preclinical signs of cardiovascular involvement in NAFLD patients, followed by management according to current CVD guidelines (**Fig. 2**). NAFL (nonalcoholic fatty liver) does not seem to affect significantly the cardiovascular compartment, but the presence of NASH and fibrosis are clearly linked to adverse cardiovascular outcomes. In this perspective, the identification of liver fibrosis through invasive or noninvasive modalities could improve the screening for subclinical cardiac and vascular dysfunction.

In the follow-up of patients with NAFLD, a comprehensive assessment of the glucose and lipid profile is warranted, to detect early signs of insulin resistance and atherogenic dyslipidemia. Regular domiciliary monitoring of arterial blood pressure, followed by management according to current CV guidelines, would prevent systemic and organ complications of arterial hypertension. Carotid artery ultrasound is a useful tool to detect early carotid plaques and their calcification rate. Echocardiography is a strong tool to detect early signs of diastolic dysfunctions, which predispose to heart failure with preserved ejection fraction.

The advice for a healthy lifestyle including dietary changes and physical exercise represents the cornerstone of NAFLD management, aiming at weight loss and improvement of metabolic dysregulations. The American Heart Association stated that replacing saturated fat with polyunsaturated vegetable oil reduces the incidence of CVD by 30%.[56] Importantly, this shift toward more unsaturated fats occurs when a Westernized diet containing processed foods is replaced by the Mediterranean diet. It is beyond the scope of this article to discuss the many potential mechanisms of benefit by which a Mediterranean Diet may benefit NAFLD and CVD, but a reduction in saturated fats and red meat consumption may also help prevent the intestinal dysbiosis and improve an altered liver–gut axis with important cardiovascular implications.

Finally, as NAFLD is associated with extra-hepatic complications such as T2DM and chronic kidney disease that also increase the risk of CVD, effective treatment strategies are urgently required. Crucially, similar proportions of people with NAFLD die from CVD as from liver disease and when patients with NAFLD develop T2DM, the presence of diabetes further increases the risk of CVD, creating a vicious spiral of ill health. Consequently, an ideal treatment of NAFLD might be expected not only to reduce the risk of chronic liver disease-related complications but also to decrease the risk of T2DM and CVD. Statins are known to be safe in patients with NAFLD and should be prescribed for increased cardiovascular risk. Further, statin use is probably associated with a lower risk of hepatic decompensation and

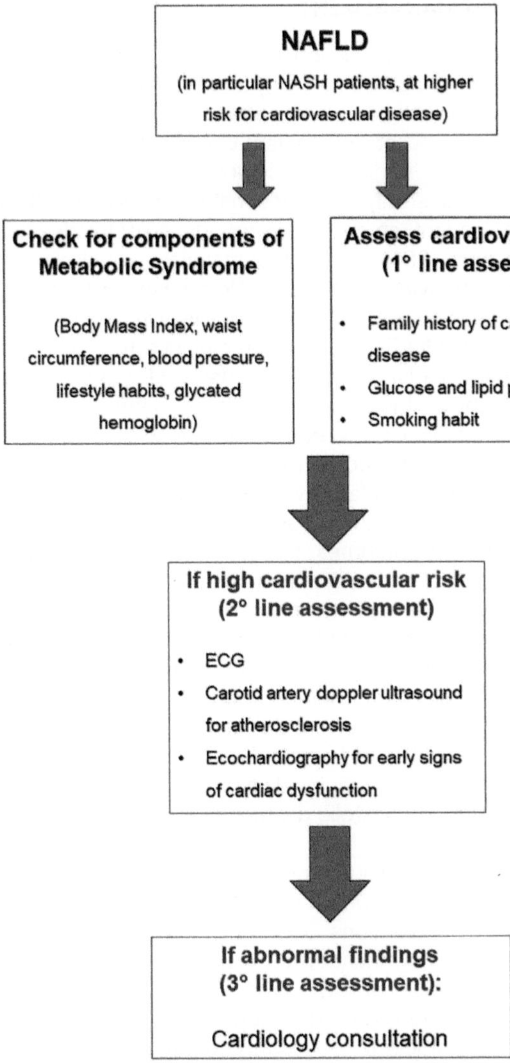

Fig. 2. Suggested clinical management for cardiovascular risk in NAFLD. ECG, electrocardiogram; NASH, nonalcoholic steatohepatitis.

mortality and might reduce portal hypertension, in patients with advanced chronic liver disease.[57]

SUMMARY

In conclusion, the strong association between NAFLD and CVD demands a comprehensive evaluation of metabolic dysfunctions in multiple districts. Cardiovascular health represents the main target of screening strategies to prevent adverse outcomes in the NAFLD population. Improved referral policies and the development of shared pathways of management will help reduce the burden of cardiovascular mortality in this population.

CLINICS CARE POINTS

- A comprehensive clinical evaluation is advisable in the NAFLD setting, due to the multidimensional impact of the liver disease.
- A combined evaluation of metabolic risk factors and cardiovascular risk is useful for a better risk strafication of patients with NAFLD.
- In the presence of high cardiovascular risk factors, second-line examination would be required (including ECG, carotid artery doppler ultrasound, ecocardiography).
- Although patients with chronic liver disease and liver transplant recipients may have an impaired response to COVID-19 vaccination, vaccination in these patients has still been proven to be safe and effective at preventing morbidity and mortality due to COVID-19.
- Patients with NAFLD may have ultrasound-based signs of pre-clinical cardiac dysfuncion; a cardiology referral would help for screening strategies/early treatment options.

REFERENCES

1. Ma J, Hwang SJ, Pedley A, et al. Bi-directional analysis between fatty liver and cardiovascular disease risk factors. J Hepatol 2017;66(2):390–7.
2. Oni ET, Agatston AS, Blaha MJ, et al. A systematic review: burden and severity of subclinical cardiovascular disease among those with nonalcoholic fatty liver; should we care? Atherosclerosis 2013;230(2):258–67.
3. Lee SB, Park GM, Lee JY, et al. Association between non-alcoholic fatty liver disease and subclinical coronary atherosclerosis: an observational cohort study. J Hepatol 2018;68(5):1018–24.
4. Gastaldelli A, Kozakova M, Højlund K, et al. Fatty liver is associated with insulin resistance, risk of coronary heart disease, and early atherosclerosis in a large European population. Hepatology 2009;49(5):1537–44.
5. Targher G, Bertolini L, Padovani R, et al. Prevalence of nonalcoholic fatty liver disease and its association with cardiovascular disease among type 2 diabetic patients. Diabetes Care 2007;30(5):1212–8.
6. Sinn DH, Cho SJ, Gu S, et al. Persistent nonalcoholic fatty liver disease increases risk for carotid atherosclerosis. Gastroenterology 2016;151(3):481–8.e1.
7. Hagström H, Nasr P, Ekstedt M, et al. Fibrosis stage but not NASH predicts mortality and time to development of severe liver disease in biopsy-proven NAFLD. J Hepatol 2017;67(6):1265–73.
8. Osawa K, Miyoshi T, Yamauchi K, et al. Nonalcoholic hepatic steatosis is a strong predictor of high-risk coronary-artery plaques as determined by multidetector CT. PLoS One 2015;10(6):e0131138.
9. Targher G, Byrne CD, Lonardo A, et al. Non-alcoholic fatty liver disease and risk of incident cardiovascular disease: a meta-analysis. J Hepatol 2016;65(3):589–600.
10. Zhou YY, Zhou XD, Wu SJ, et al. Synergistic increase in cardiovascular risk in diabetes mellitus with nonalcoholic fatty liver disease: a meta-analysis. Eur J Gastroenterol Hepatol 2018;30(6):631–6.
11. Wu S, Wu F, Ding Y, et al. Association of non-alcoholic fatty liver disease with major adverse cardiovascular events: a systematic review and meta-analysis. Sci Rep 2016;6:33386.
12. Ekstedt M, Hagström H, Nasr P, et al. Fibrosis stage is the strongest predictor for disease-specific mortality in NAFLD after up to 33 years of follow-up. Hepatology 2015;61(5):1547–54.

13. Kim D, Kim WR, Kim HJ, et al. Association between noninvasive fibrosis markers and mortality among adults with nonalcoholic fatty liver disease in the United States. Hepatology 2013;57(4):1357–65.
14. Simon TG, Roelstraete B, Hagström H, et al. Non-alcoholic fatty liver disease and incident major adverse cardiovascular events: results from a nationwide histology cohort. Gut 2022;71(9):1867–75.
15. Vilar-Gomez E, Calzadilla-Bertot L, Wai-Sun Wong V, et al. Fibrosis severity as a determinant of cause-specific mortality in patients with advanced nonalcoholic fatty liver disease: a multi-national cohort study. Gastroenterology 2018;155(2):443–57.e17.
16. Kim NH, Park J, Kim SH, et al. Non-alcoholic fatty liver disease, metabolic syndrome and subclinical cardiovascular changes in the general population. Heart 2014;100(12):938–43.
17. Lautamäki R, Borra R, Iozzo P, et al. Liver steatosis coexists with myocardial insulin resistance and coronary dysfunction in patients with type 2 diabetes. Am J Physiol Endocrinol Metab 2006;291(2):E282–90.
18. Perseghin G, Lattuada G, De Cobelli F, et al. Increased mediastinal fat and impaired left ventricular energy metabolism in young men with newly found fatty liver. Hepatology 2008;47(1):51–8.
19. Pacifico L, Di Martino M, De Merulis A, et al. Left ventricular dysfunction in obese children and adolescents with nonalcoholic fatty liver disease. Hepatology 2014;59(2):461–70.
20. Anstee QM, Mantovani A, Tilg H, et al. Risk of cardiomyopathy and cardiac arrhythmias in patients with nonalcoholic fatty liver disease. Nat Rev Gastroenterol Hepatol 2018;15(7):425–39.
21. Mantovani A, Dauriz M, Sandri D, et al. Association between non-alcoholic fatty liver disease and risk of atrial fibrillation in adult individuals: an updated meta-analysis. Liver Int 2019;39(4):758–69.
22. Targher G, Valbusa F, Bonapace S, et al. Non-alcoholic fatty liver disease is associated with an increased incidence of atrial fibrillation in patients with type 2 diabetes. PLoS One 2013;8(2):e57183.
23. Mantovani A, Rigamonti A, Bonapace S, et al. Nonalcoholic fatty liver disease is associated with ventricular arrhythmias in patients with type 2 diabetes referred for clinically indicated 24-hour holter monitoring. Diabetes Care 2016;39(8):1416–23.
24. Tang ASP, Chan KE, Quek J, et al. Non-alcoholic fatty liver disease increases risk of carotid atherosclerosis and ischemic stroke: an updated meta-analysis with 135,602 individuals. Clin Mol Hepatol 2022;28(3):483–96.
25. Xu J, Dai L, Zhang Y, et al. Severity of nonalcoholic fatty liver disease and risk of future ischemic stroke events. Stroke 2021;52(1):103–10.
26. Li H, Hu B, Wei L, et al. Non-alcoholic fatty liver disease is associated with stroke severity and progression of brainstem infarctions. Eur J Neurol 2018;25(3):577-e34.
27. Wang M, Zhou BG, Zhang Y, et al. Association between non-alcoholic fatty liver disease and risk of stroke: a systematic review and meta-analysis. Front Cardiovasc Med 2022;9:812030.
28. Parikh NS, VanWagner LB, Elkind MSV, et al. Association between nonalcoholic fatty liver disease with advanced fibrosis and stroke. J Neurol Sci 2019;407:116524.

29. Alexander M, Loomis AK, van der Lei J, et al. Non-alcoholic fatty liver disease and risk of incident acute myocardial infarction and stroke: findings from matched cohort study of 18 million European adults. BMJ 2019;367:l5367.
30. Wu M, Zha M, Lv Q, et al. Non-alcoholic fatty liver disease and stroke: a Mendelian randomization study. Eur J Neurol 2022;29(5):1534–7.
31. Packer M. Epicardial adipose tissue may mediate deleterious effects of obesity and inflammation on the myocardium. J Am Coll Cardiol 2018;71(20):2360–72.
32. Tsaban G, Wolak A, Avni-Hassid H, et al. Dynamics of intrapericardial and extrapericardial fat tissues during long-term, dietary-induced, moderate weight loss. Am J Clin Nutr 2017;106(4):984–95.
33. Gruzdeva O, Uchasova E, Dyleva Y, et al. Adipocytes directly affect coronary artery disease pathogenesis via induction of adipokine and cytokine imbalances. Front Immunol 2019;10:2163.
34. Rijzewijk LJ, Jonker JT, van der Meer RW, et al. Effects of hepatic triglyceride content on myocardial metabolism in type 2 diabetes. J Am Coll Cardiol 2010;56(3): 225–33.
35. Lechner K, McKenzie AL, Kränkel N, et al. High-risk atherosclerosis and metabolic phenotype: the roles of ectopic adiposity, atherogenic dyslipidemia, and inflammation. Metab Syndr Relat Disord 2020;18(4):176–85.
36. Goulopoulou S, McCarthy CG, Webb RC. Toll-like receptors in the vascular system: sensing the dangers within. Pharmacol Rev 2016;68(1):142–67.
37. Armandi A, Rosso C, Caviglia GP, et al. Insulin resistance across the spectrum of nonalcoholic fatty liver disease. Metabolites 2021;11(3):155.
38. Anand SS, Yi Q, Gerstein H, et al. Relationship of metabolic syndrome and fibrinolytic dysfunction to cardiovascular disease. Circulation 2003;108(4):420–5.
39. Jiang F, Chen Q, Wang W, et al. Hepatocyte-derived extracellular vesicles promote endothelial inflammation and atherogenesis via microRNA-1. J Hepatol 2020;72(1):156–66.
40. Romeo S, Kozlitina J, Xing C, et al. Genetic variation in PNPLA3 confers susceptibility to nonalcoholic fatty liver disease. Nat Genet 2008;40(12):1461–5.
41. Valenti L, Al-Serri A, Daly AK, et al. Homozygosity for the patatin-like phospholipase-3/adiponutrin I148M polymorphism influences liver fibrosis in patients with nonalcoholic fatty liver disease. Hepatology 2010;51(4):1209–17.
42. Holmen OL, Zhang H, Fan Y, et al. Systematic evaluation of coding variation identifies a candidate causal variant in TM6SF2 influencing total cholesterol and myocardial infarction risk. Nat Genet 2014;46(4):345–51.
43. Kahali B, Liu YL, Daly AK, et al. TM6SF2: catch-22 in the fight against nonalcoholic fatty liver disease and cardiovascular disease? Gastroenterology 2015; 148(4):679–84.
44. Brouwers MCGJ, Simons N, Stehouwer CDA, et al. Non-alcoholic fatty liver disease and cardiovascular disease: assessing the evidence for causality. Diabetologia 2020;63(2):253–60.
45. Armandi A, Schattenberg JM. Beyond the paradigm of weight loss in nonalcoholic fatty liver disease: from pathophysiology to novel dietary approaches. Nutrients 2021;13(6):1977.
46. Pendyala S, Walker JM, Holt PR. A high-fat diet is associated with endotoxemia that originates from the gut. Gastroenterology 2012;142(5):1100–1.e2.
47. Caussy C, Tripathi A, Humphrey G, et al. A gut microbiome signature for cirrhosis due to nonalcoholic fatty liver disease. Nat Commun 2019;10(1):1406.

48. Zhang Y, Xu J, Wang X, et al. Changes of intestinal bacterial microbiota in coronary heart disease complicated with nonalcoholic fatty liver disease. BMC Genomics 2019;20(1):862.
49. Koeth RA, Lam-Galvez BR, Kirsop J, et al. l-Carnitine in omnivorous diets induces an atherogenic gut microbial pathway in humans. J Clin Invest 2019;129(1):373–87.
50. Schiattarella GG, Sannino A, Toscano E, et al. Gut microbe-generated metabolite trimethylamine-N-oxide as cardiovascular risk biomarker: a systematic review and dose-response meta-analysis. Eur Heart J 2017;38(39):2948–56.
51. Zhang X, Li Y, Yang P, et al. Trimethylamine-N-Oxide promotes vascular calcification through activation of NLRP3 (Nucleotide-Binding domain, leucine-rich-containing family, pyrin domain-containing-3) inflammasome and NF-κB (nuclear factor κB) signals. Arterioscler Thromb Vasc Biol 2020;40(3):751–65.
52. Zhu W, Gregory JC, Org E, et al. Gut microbial metabolite TMAO enhances platelet hyperreactivity and thrombosis risk. Cell 2016;165(1):111–24.
53. Chen YM, Liu Y, Zhou RF, et al. Associations of gut-flora-dependent metabolite trimethylamine-N-oxide, betaine and choline with non-alcoholic fatty liver disease in adults. Sci Rep 2016;6:19076.
54. Treeprasertsuk S, Leverage S, Adams LA, et al. The Framingham risk score and heart disease in nonalcoholic fatty liver disease. Liver Int 2012;32(6):945–50.
55. European Association for the Study of the Liver (EASL), European Association for the Study of Diabetes (EASD), European Association for the Study of Obesity (EASO). EASL-EASD-EASO clinical practice guidelines for the management of non-alcoholic fatty liver disease. J Hepatol 2016;64(6):1388–402.
56. Sacks FM, Lichtenstein AH, Wu JHY, et al. Dietary fats and cardiovascular disease: a presidential advisory from the American heart association. Circulation 2017;136(3):e1–23.
57. Kim RG, Loomba R, Prokop LJ, et al. Statin use and risk of cirrhosis and related complications in patients with chronic liver diseases: a systematic review and meta-analysis. Clin Gastroenterol Hepatol 2017;15(10):1521–30.e8.

Extrahepatic Outcomes of Nonalcoholic Fatty Liver Disease: Nonhepatocellular Cancers

Maryam K. Ibrahim, MD[a,b], Tracey G. Simon, MD[b,c,d], Mary E. Rinella, MD[e,f,*]

KEYWORDS

- Cancer • Carcinogenesis • Cancer outcomes • Cancer therapy • Diabetes
- Insulin resistance • inflammation • Nonalcoholic fatty liver

INTRODUCTION

Nonalcoholic fatty liver disease (NAFLD) encompasses the entire spectrum of fatty liver disease in individuals without significant alcohol consumption, including isolated steatosis, steatohepatitis, and cirrhosis. The overall global prevalence of NAFLD is estimated to be 30%,[1] and the associated clinical and economic burden will continue to increase.[2] NAFLD is a multisystemic disease with established links to cardiovascular disease, type 2 diabetes (T2DM), metabolic syndrome, chronic kidney disease, polycystic ovarian syndrome, and intra- and extrahepatic malignancies.[3] Increased mortality in patients with NAFLD, compared with the general population, is often attributable to extrahepatic cancer,[4] suggesting that adequate disease treatment or attenuation of progression could positively affect outcomes. NAFLD may also increase the risk of cancer-specific and all-cause mortality among cancer survivors.[5] The mechanisms underpinning this link are diverse and incompletely understood. Obesity and diabetes, both tightly linked with NAFLD, are important risk factors for malignancy, especially gastrointestinal and hormone-related malignancies.[6–8] Therefore, whether NAFLD is an independent predictor or a mediator of extrahepatic cancer development is still unclear.[9] Here the authors review the potential mechanisms and current evidence for the association between NAFLD and extrahepatic cancers and the resultant impact on clinical outcomes.

[a] Department of Medicine, Massachusetts General Hospital, Boston, MA, USA; [b] Harvard Medical School, Boston, MA, USA; [c] Division of Gastroenterology and Hepatology, Massachusetts General Hospital, Boston, MA, USA; [d] Clinical and Translational Epidemiology Unit (CTEU), Massachusetts General Hospital, Boston, MA, USA; [e] University of Chicago Pritzker School of Medicine; [f] University of Chicago Hospitals
* Corresponding author. The University of Chicago Medicine, 5841 South Maryland Avenue, Chicago, IL 60637.
E-mail address: mrinella@bsd.uchicago.edu

Clin Liver Dis 27 (2023) 251–273
https://doi.org/10.1016/j.cld.2023.01.004 liver.theclinics.com

Potential Mechanisms for Extrahepatic Carcinogenesis in Nonalcoholic Fatty Liver Disease

Adipose tissue expansion and dysfunction

Increased adiposity and associated chronic inflammation results in increased secretion of tumor necrosis factor alpha (TNF-α) and leptin and decreased secretion of adiponectin[10] (**Fig. 1**). Chronic inflammation and altered adipocytokine signaling exacerbates insulin resistance.[11] Inflammatory cytokines can stimulate cell proliferation, tumor progression, cancer angiogenesis, and metastasis.[12–14] The relationship between colorectal cancer and TNF-α has been demonstrated in animal models, whereas IL-6 has been linked to renal cell carcinoma, gastric, and colorectal cancer.[15] Adiponectin has anticarcinogenic effects and can inhibit TNF-α; thus reduced levels in the context of NAFLD may contribute to an increased risk of malignancy. Leptin, especially in the presence of low adiponectin levels, has procarcinogenic effects.[15] For example, high plasma leptin concentrations are associated with increased risk of colorectal cancer,[16] in part by increasing motility and invasiveness of colon cancer cells.[17] Elevated leptin and low adiponectin have also been linked to an increased risk of Barrett esophagus and esophageal adenocarcinoma[18,19] as well as more aggressive breast cancer with the propensity to metastasize.[15,20]

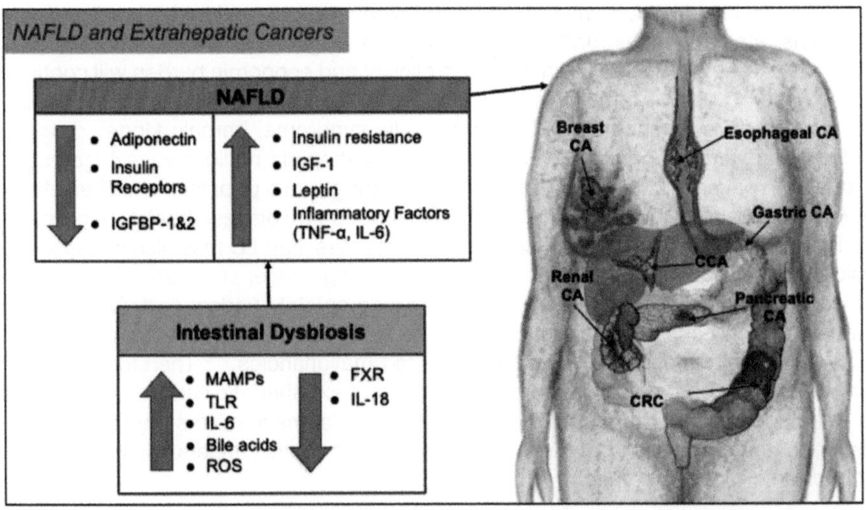

Fig. 1. Potential mechanisms for extrahepatic carcinogenesis in nonalcoholic fatty liver disease (NAFLD). Adipose tissue dysfunction results in increased secretion of inflammatory factors (TNF-α, IL-6) and leptin, and decreased secretion of adiponectin, which can potentially drive carcinogenesis in NAFLD. Insulin resistance in NAFLD leads to hyperinsulinemia, which reduces liver synthesis of IGFBP-1 and -2, and resultant increased levels of IGF-1, which drives carcinogenesis. Dysbiosis leads to increased intestinal permeability and activation of TLRs via MAMPs, which can promote carcinogenesis. Dysbiosis is also associated with reduced IL-18, increased IL-6, and ROS, which promotes carcinogenesis. Secondary bile acids and decreased FXR is another potential driver of carcinogenesis in NAFLD. CA, cancer; CCA, cholangiocarcinoma; CRC, colorectal cancer; FXR, farnesoid X receptor; IGF-1, insulin-like growth factor 1; IGFBP, insulin-like growth factor-binding protein; IL-18, interleukin-18; IL-6, interleukin-6; MAMPs, microorganism-associated molecular patterns; ROS, reactive oxygen species; TLR, Toll-like receptors; TNF-α, tumor necrosis factor alpha.

Insulin resistance

Insulin resistance–induced chronic inflammation leads to stimulation of the insulin-like growth factor 1 (IGF-1) axis, fostering a suitable microenvironment for cancer development.[15] Insulin resistance leads to compensatory chronic hyperinsulinemia, which leads to reduced liver synthesis and secretion of IGF-binding protein 1 and 2 (IGFBP-1 and -2); this results in increased levels of bioavailable IGF-1, which along with insulin accelerate the accumulation of mutations, promote cellular proliferation, and inhibit apoptosis in many tissue types, fostering carcinogenesis.[21] In fact, elevated levels of IGF-1 have been associated with prostate, colorectal, lung, breast, and potentially esophageal cancer.[15]

Intestinal dysbiosis

Intestinal dysbiosis may play an important role in the pathogenesis of NAFLD and disease progression[22] and may also foster the development of extrahepatic malignancy.[15,23] Dysbiosis can also lead to increased intestinal permeability, resulting in increased levels of bacterial products in the systemic circulation and activation of Toll-like receptors (TLRs) via the recognition of microorganism-associated molecular patterns, which can drive carcinogenesis.[15] Quantitative or qualitative changes in the gut microbiome can promote carcinogenesis through chronic inflammation, reduced inflammasome-derived IL-18, and increased IL-6 signaling, which protects premalignant cells from apoptosis.[15,24] Changes in gut metabolism provide another potential link between NAFLD and malignancy.[25] Several bacterial metabolites such as hydrogen sulfide, secondary bile acids, polyamines, and reactive oxygen species can cause DNA damage or inflammation through TNF-α and IL-6 production, which promotes carcinogenesis.[24] Dysbiosis-associated changes in bile acids and decreased farnesoid X receptor expression could potentially facilitate carcinogenesis in NAFLD. Changes in microbiota profiles and the associated systemic inflammation could also contribute to a carcinogenic milieu in the setting of NAFLD.[26] Dysbiosis has also been described in colon cancer.[27,28] Further research is still needed to better define the mechanisms linking NAFLD to extrahepatic cancers.

Gastrointestinal Malignancies

Cholangiocarcinoma

Available data suggest that NAFLD is associated with an increased risk of cholangiocarcinoma (CCA). The ongoing inflammatory milieu in NAFLD, particularly in the context of cirrhosis, alters the microenvironment, which can promote the development of CCA.[29,30] Specifically, the aberrant expression of proinflammatory cytokines such as IL-6 and TNF-α[31] induce cholangiocyte proliferation.[32] TNF-α activates inducible nitric oxide synthase (iNOS), leading to nitric oxide production, which consequently inhibits DNA repair mechanisms and promotes DNA damage.[29,33] iNOS activation also upregulates COX2 expression, promoting the growth of cholangiocytes.[29,34] Another potential mechanism is through insulin resistance and the resulting increase in IGF-1,[35] which is also highly expressed in CCA.[36]

Data from case-control studies and metanalyses suggest that NAFLD (with and without cirrhosis) is associated with an increased risk of intra- and extrahepatic CCA.[29,35,37,38] However, the associated risk of extrahepatic CCA has been called into question by subsequent metanalysis and trial sequential analyses[35] (**Table 1**). Further data from longitudinal prospective studies are needed to better understand the potential risk of CCA in patients with NAFLD.

Table 1
Studies evaluating the association between nonalcoholic fatty liver disease and cholangiocarcinoma

Study	Country	Study Design	Study Population	Diagnosis of NAFLD	Main Findings
Petrick et al,[37] 2017	United States	Case control	2092 iCCA and 2981 eCCA cases and 323,615 controls identified using the SEER-Medicare database	ICD-9 codes	• NAFLD associated with ~ 3-fold increased risks of iCCA (OR = 3.52, 95% CI: 2.87–4.32) and eCCA (OR = 2.93, 95% CI: 2.42–3.55) • Similar to risk in other forms of liver disease (viral hepatitis, alcohol related, and nonspecific cirrhosis)
Wongjarupong et al,[29] 2017	United States China Taiwan South Korea Japan 10 European countries	Metanalysis of case-control studies	7 case-control studies included 9102 CCA patients (5067 iCCA and 4035 eCCA) and 129,111 controls	ICD9, imaging, histology, or hepatic steatosis index	• NAFLD associated with increased risk for all CCAs, iCCA, and eCCA, with overall pooled adjusted ORs 1.97 (95% CI: 1.41–2.75, I^2 = 71%), 2.09 (95% CI, 1.49–2.91, I^2 = 42%) and 2.05 (95% CI, 1.59–2.64, I^2 = 0%), respectively
Liu et al,[38] 2020	US Japan Europe South Korea China	Metanalysis of case-control studies	7 case-control studies	ICD-9, histology, imaging, hepatic steatosis index	• Pooled OR of risk of iCCA and eCCA in NAFLD were 2.46 (95% CI: 1.77–3.44) and 2.24 (95% CI: 1.58–3.17), respectively
Corrao et al,[35] 2021	South Korea China US Japan Europe	Cumulative meta-analyses with trial sequential analyses	7 case-control studies	Imaging, ICD-9, histology, hepatic steatosis index	• NAFLD associated with increased risk of total CCA and iCCA, OR 1.88 (95% CI: 1.25–2.83), OR 2.19 (95% CI:1.48–3.25)

Abbreviations: CI, confidence interval; eCCA, extrahepatic cholangiocarcinoma; iCCA, intrahepatic cholangiocarcinoma; OR, odds ratio.

Colorectal cancer and adenomas

The association between NAFLD and colorectal cancer (CRC) has been well studied. Several cross-sectional studies as well as meta-analyses showed an increased risk of colorectal lesions (adenomas and CRC) among patients with NAFLD[15,38–44] (**Table 2**). Longitudinal studies have similarly shown an increased risk of adenomatous polyps or CRC in patients with NAFLD,[45,46] with a higher risk of adenoma formation when NAFLD co-existed with other risk factors such as metabolic syndrome, smoking, or hypertension (compared with patients without NAFLD and these comorbidities).[46] However, having NAFLD did not influence CRC prognosis or disease recurrence during follow-up.[45]

Another longitudinal cohort study identified 2224 incident cancers after NAFLD diagnosis during a median follow-up of 8 years. Colon CA was among the top 3 most common types of cancer in NAFLD. Interestingly, the effect of NAFLD on cancer risk varied by sex, whereby men with NAFLD were 90% more likely to develop colon cancer as compared with women[9]; this was higher than the estimated increased incidence of CRC in men as compared with women (incidence rate of CRC in men is 45% higher compared with women worldwide).[47] Also, colon CA occurred more commonly in NAFLD at a young age.[9] Some data suggest that the risk of CRC increases in the setting of advanced fibrosis.[40,44] Severe NAFLD (defined either by the presence of steatosis on imaging studies plus a high Fibrosis-4 score or by NASH on liver histology) was associated with an increased risk of incident adenomas/CRC as compared with mild/moderate NAFLD.[41] However, several of these studies were limited by the sample size of each cancer endpoint or being mostly from Asian countries where body fat distribution and other risk factors are different from the US/European populations. The poor sensitivity of ultrasound in detecting mild hepatic steatosis or underreporting of NAFLD in clinical records may also bias the effect estimates. Most recently, in a study from the UK Biobank, with a total of 2869 incident CRC, patients with high NAFLD risk (defined by the Dallas Steatosis Index DSI) had an increased risk of CRC. Interestingly, stronger associations were observed for cancers of earlier onset (defined as <60 years old).[48] Although many studies have shown an association with NAFLD and CRC, others have not,[15] including a recent population-based cohort study of 8892 Swedish adults with histologically defined NAFLD after adjusting for several factors including age, sex, cardiovascular disease, diabetes, hypertension, dyslipidemia, obesity, end-stage renal disease, family history of cancer at age of less than 50 years, and alcohol misuse.[49] However, this study was limited by lack of laboratory values or data regarding smoking, alcohol consumption, body mass index, or absence of viral hepatitis. Moreover, NAFLD was defined histologically, as these findings may not extend to patients with NAFLD who do not undergo biopsy.[49]

Colorectal cancer outcomes

Prior studies have looked at the outcomes of CRC in patients with chronic liver disease (CLD). In a Danish population–based cohort study of patients undergoing CRC surgery, the 30-day mortality after CRC surgery was significantly higher in patients with CRC with any preexisting liver disease (including NAFLD) compared with patients who had CRC without liver disease. Among patients with cirrhosis, mortality was 24.1%.[50] Other data showed that patients with cirrhosis had a significant risk of postoperative morbidity and mortality after colectomy,[51–54] possibly due to increased bleeding or hepatic decompensation.[55]

Lee and colleagues found that in patients with CRC who underwent colorectal surgery, those with coexisting CLD (excluding cirrhosis) had a significantly longer duration of hospital stay compared with patients without CLD. The presence of CLD was

Table 2
Studies evaluating the association between nonalcoholic fatty liver disease and colorectal lesions

	Country	Study Design	Study Population	Diagnosis of NAFLD and Colorectal Lesions	Factors Adjusted For	Main Findings
Hwang et al,[42] 2010	South Korea	Cross-sectional study	2917 participants undergoing routine colonoscopy (556 subjects with adenomatous polyps and 2361 without)	Ultrasound; colonoscopy	Age, sex, smoking, hypertension, diabetes, and metabolic syndrome	• Higher prevalence of NAFLD in adenomatous polyp group vs control group: 41.5% vs 30.2% ($p < 0.001$). • NAFLD associated with increased risk of developing colorectal adenomatous polyps (OR 1.28; 95% CI 1.03–1.60; $p = 0.029$)
Wong et al,[44] 2011	China	Cross-sectional study	380 community patients undergoing screening colonoscopy (199 patients with NAFLD and 181 patients without NAFLD)	Liver biopsy or proton magnetic resonance spectroscopy; colonoscopy	Age, gender, smoking, BMI, diabetes, hypertension, CRC in first-degree relatives	• Higher prevalence of colorectal adenomas in NAFLD vs control group: 34.7% vs 21.5% ($p = 0.043$). • Higher Prevalence of advanced colorectal neoplasms in NAFLD vs control group: 18.6% vs 5.5% ($p = 0.002$). • In biopsy-proven NAFLD, patients with NASH had higher prevalence of adenomas (51.0% vs 25.6%) and advanced neoplasms (34.7% vs 14.0%) as compared with simple steatosis.

						• NASH associated with colorectal adenomas (adjusted OR 4.89; 95% CI 2.04–11.70; $p < 0.001$) and advanced colorectal neoplasms. (adjusted OR 5.34; 95% CI 1.92–14.84; $p = 0.001$)
Stadlmayr et al,[43] 2011	Austria	Cross-sectional study	1211 patients undergoing colonoscopy (632 patients with NAFLD and 579 without NAFLD)	Ultrasound; colonoscopy	Age, sex, BMI, and glucose intolerance	• Higher prevalence of colorectal lesions in NAFLD vs control group: 34% vs 21.7%; $p < 0.001$. • Among men, prevalence of rectal adenomas (NAFLD vs control group: 11 vs 3.4%, $p = 0.004$) and CRC prevalence (NAFLD vs control group: 1.6% vs 0.4%; $p < 0.001$). • Hepatic steatosis independently associated with increased risk of developing colorectal adenomas (adjusted OR 1.47; 95% CI 1.079–2.003, $p = 0.015$).

(*continued on next page*)

Table 2
(*continued*)

	Country	Study Design	Study Population	Diagnosis of NAFLD and Colorectal Lesions	Factors Adjusted For	Main Findings
Lee et al,[45] 2012	South Korea	Retrospective cohort study	5517 women undergoing life insurance health examinations (831 participants with NAFLD and 4686 without)	Ultrasound; colonoscopy	Age, smoking, BMI, hypertension, high fasting plasma glucose, high total cholesterol, high triglyceride, and low HDL	• NAFLD independently associated with increased risk of developing colorectal adenomatous polyps (aRR 1.94; 95% CI 1.11–3.40) and CRC (aRR 3.08; 95% CI 1.02–9.34)
Huang et al,[46] 2013	Taiwan	Retrospective cohort study	1522 participants undergoing 2 consecutive colonoscopies (216 individuals with colorectal adenomas and 1306 without colorectal adenomas after a negative baseline colonoscopy	Ultrasound; colonoscopy	Age, BMI, gender, smoking, hypertension, diabetes, and metabolic syndrome	• Higher NAFLD prevalence in adenoma vs nonadenoma group (55.6 vs 38.8%; $p < 0.05$). • NAFLD was an independent risk factor for developing colorectal adenomas after a negative baseline colonoscopy (aOR 1.45; 95% CI 1.07–1.98; $p = 0.016$)

Ahn et al,[40] 2017	South Korea	Cross-sectional study	26,540 participants undergoing colonoscopy and abdominal US as part of health check-up program (9501 with NAFLD and 17,039 without NAFLD)	Ultrasound; colonoscopy	Age, sex, BMI, smoking, alcohol intake, first-degree family history of colorectal cancer, aspirin use, fasting plasma glucose, total cholesterol, triglycerides, systolic blood pressure, use of any hypoglycemic, antihypertensive drugs or use of statins	• Higher prevalence of colorectal tumors in NAFLD vs non-NAFLD group (38% vs 28.9%; $p < 0.001$). • Higher prevalence of advanced colorectal neoplasia in NAFLD vs non-NAFLD group (2.8% vs 1.9%; $p < 0.001$). • NAFLD independently associated with increased risk of developing any colorectal neoplasia (adjusted OR, 1.10; 95% CI, 1.03–1.17; $p = 0.002$), but not advanced colorectal neoplasia (adjusted OR, 1.21; 95% CI, 0.99–1.47; $p = 0.053$)
Mantovani et al,[39] 2018	Asia	Metanalysis	11 observational studies (8 cross-sectional and 3 longitudinal) with aggregate data on 91,124 asymptomatic adults (32.1% with NAFLD) of predominantly Asian descent accounting for a total of 14,911 colorectal adenomas and 1684 cancers	Imaging or biopsy	Age, sex, and metabolic factors	• NAFLD associated with increased risk of prevalent colorectal adenomas and cancer. • NAFLD associated with increased risk of incident colorectal adenomas and cancer. • Risks independent of age, sex, smoking, BMI, and diabetes (or metabolic syndrome)

(continued on next page)

Table 2
(continued)

	Country	Study Design	Study Population	Diagnosis of NAFLD and Colorectal Lesions	Factors Adjusted For	Main Findings
Chen et al,[41] 2019	US Korea Austria China Korea Turkey Taiwan	Metanalysis	21 eligible studies including 124,206 participants	Liver biopsy or MRI or ultrasound; colonoscopy	Age, sex, and metabolic factors	• NAFLD associated with increased risk of any incident CRA (aOR: 1.30, 95% CI: 1.19–1.43) and advanced incident CRA/CRC (aOR: 1.57, 95% CI: 1.21–2.04). • Compared with mild and/or moderate NAFLD, severe NAFLD associated with increased risk of incident CRA/CRC (aOR: 2.19, 95% CI: 1.33–3.60). • Although pooled cOR revealed that NAFLD was associated with an increased risk of recurrent CRA/CRC (cOR = 1.73; 95% CI: 1.12–2.68), after adjustment for confounding factors, NAFLD had less correlation with the risk of recurrent CRA/CRC (aOR: 1.81, 95% CI: 0.70–4.65).

Allen et al,[9] 2019	US	Retrospective cohort study	19,163 subjects (4722 subjects with NAFLD and 14,441 age- and sex-matched referent individuals)	HCIDA/ICD-codes; ICD-9	N/A	• NAFLD associated with increased colon cancer risk (IRR, 1.8; 95% CI, 1.1–2.8)
Liu et al,[38] 2020	China, South Korea, US, Austria, Japan	Systematic review and metanalysis	10 studies for CRC and 9 studies for colorectal adenoma	Ultrasound, liver biopsy, magnetic resonance spectroscopy, HCIDA/ ICD-9 codes, computed tomography; colonoscopy, ICD-9, pathology	Age, sex, metabolic factors	• Pooled OR values of risk of colorectal cancer and adenomas in patients with NAFLD were 1.72 (95% CI: 1.40–2.11) and 1.37 (95% CI: 1.29–1.46), respectively
Simon et al,[49] 2021	Sweden	Prospective cohort	All adults with histologically defined NAFLD in Sweden from 1966 to 2016 (N = 8,892)	Histopathology	Age, sex, cardiovascular disease, diabetes, hypertension, dyslipidemia, obesity, end-stage renal disease, family history of cancer at age <50 y, and alcohol misuse	• No significant associations between NAFLD and colon cancer (aHR 1.05, 95% CI [0.85–1.28])
McHenry et al,[48] 2022	US	Prospective cohort	319,290 participants in the UK Biobank (2006–2019)	NAFLD risk estimated by the Dallas Steatosis Index; ICD-10 Code	Age, sex, education, the Townsend Deprivation index, physical activity, smoking status and intensity, family history of CRC, and alcohol frequency	• Compared with participants at low risk of NAFLD, individuals at high NAFLD risk had 13% increased risk of colorectal cancer (RR 1.13; 95% CI 1.03–1.24) (P-trend <0.001)

Abbreviations: aHR, adjusted hazard ratio; BMI, body mass index; CI, confidence interval; CRA, colorectal adenoma; CRC, colorectal carcinoma; IRR, incidence rate ratio; OR, odds ratio; RR, relative risk.

associated with a higher risk of postoperative bleeding and higher risk of in-hospital mortality. In the CLD group, 28.36% had NAFLD; this could be due to impairment of hepatic functions such as drug metabolism, detoxification, and production of plasma proteins.[55] As such, in patients with liver disease, careful preoperative and postoperative monitoring, as well as assessment of Child-Pugh classification and Model for End-Stage Liver Disease score are essential to improve outcomes.[56,57]

Few studies have specifically evaluated the association between NAFLD and outcomes in CRC, with mixed results (**Table 3**).[58–61] The differences in the definition of NAFLD, study population, and sample size might account for the inconsistent conclusions between these studies. Further large-scale, prospective cohort studies with well-defined NAFLD are needed to elucidate the association between NAFLD and outcomes in CRC.

Liver metastasis

The impact of NAFLD on CRC metastasis remains controversial. Although some studies suggested that CRC liver metastasis was less frequent in the setting of NAFLD, other studies suggest that patients with NAFLD have a higher risk of liver metastasis and postoperative recurrence.[62–67] A study by Yan and colleagues found that NAFLD was associated with an increased incidence of synchronous liver metastasis, detected concurrently on or before the primary CRC; this could be explained through the "seed-soil" hypothesis, which suggests that metastatic cancer cells will migrate to an area where the local microenvironment is favorable. The "soil" has unique biological characteristics and microenvironment with molecular components and cell populations that promote metastasis.[68] Earlier studies suggested that cirrhosis is associated with a lower risk of liver metastasis.[54,69] This concept was supported by a study demonstrating that as NAFLD progressed to advanced fibrosis or cirrhosis, fewer synchronous CRC liver metastasis were noted. Compression and distortion of intrahepatic blood vessels and parenchyma in the context of advanced fibrosis or cirrhosis could impede the entry of tumor cells into the liver.[68] More research is still needed to better understand this association in populations with well-phenotyped NAFLD and accounting for different fibrosis stages.

Esophageal and gastric cancer

This association between NAFLD and gastrointestinal malignancies may be mediated by several mechanisms. For instance, insulin resistance and the upregulation of the IGF axis as well as the altered hormonal action of adipocytes in patients with NAFLD could stimulate the formation of gastric cancer.[15,70,71] The steatotic and inflamed liver may secrete growth-promoting factors into the systemic circulation, which could contribute to metastasis and cancer progression.[72]

Several studies have shown an association between NAFLD and the risk of esophageal or gastric cancer; however, the extent to which this is primarily mediated by obesity remains unclear.[9,70] A metanalysis by Liu and colleagues[38] of 3 high-quality studies (assessed according to the Newcastle-Ottawa Scale [NOS]) showed that patients with NAFLD had a higher risk of developing gastric cancer, with a pooled odds ratio (OR) of 1.74. Similarly, an association between NAFLD and the risk of developing esophageal cancer has been suggested, with an OR of 1.77 in the same metanalysis.[38]

Lee and colleagues[72] found that NAFLD (defining NAFLD as fatty liver index [FLI] $\geq$60) was significantly associated with the development of esophageal and gastric cancer as well as all-cause mortality. However, most studies have been limited by few cancer outcomes, the ability to accurately phenotype NAFLD, and its severity.[73] In addition, generalizability of existing data may be limited, as it has largely been

Table 3
Studies evaluating the association between nonalcoholic fatty liver disease and colorectal cancer outcomes

Study	Study Design	Study Population	NAFLD Definition	Main Findings	Additional Comments
Wu et al,[58] 2019	Retrospective cohort study	Caucasians	ICD codes from EMRs	• Patients with CRC and preexisting NAFLD had a worse prognosis (overall and CRC-specific mortality) than those without NAFLD before CRC diagnosis	• Finding independent of BMI • Limitation is identification of NAFLD using ICD codes, which underestimates prevalence
Chen et al,[59] 2018	Retrospective cohort study	Chinese women	Significant NAFLD defined as moderate and severe NAFLD as determined by hepatic ultrasound scan	• Significant NAFLD was an independent risk factor for CRC-specific mortality • Significant NAFLD and metabolic syndrome had synergistic effect on promoting CRC-specific mortality	Limitation is short follow-up period and data collection from only one center
You et al,[60] 2015	Retrospective cohort Study	Chinese patients with CRC	Abdominal ultrasonography	• Cumulative 1-, 3-, and 5-year OS rates were significantly higher in the NAFLD group • No difference in the DFS rates between CRC patients with and without NAFLD	Study limited by the small number of patients with NAFLD
Min et al,[61] 2012	Retrospective cohort study	South Korea	Patients diagnosed with CRC underwent abdominal ultrasonography within 6 months before diagnosis	• No statistically significant difference in the cumulative 1-,3-, and 5-year survival rates in CRC patients with NAFLD as compared with CRC patients without NAFLD • No difference in freedom from recurrence between CRC patients with and without NAFLD	Study limited by small sample size

Abbreviations: BMI, body mass index; CRC, colorectal carcinoma; DFS, disease-free survival; OS, overall survival.

derived from Asian populations. In their study from the UK Biobank (a predominantly White population), McHenry and colleagues showed that individuals at intermediate or high NAFLD risk (defined by DSI) had a 21% and 51% increased risk of esophageal cancer, respectively. Similarly, those with high-risk NAFLD had a 21% increased risk of gastric cancer. Stronger associations were observed for cancers of earlier onset.[48] Although the study by Simon and colleagues[49] of biopsy-confirmed NAFLD found no association between NAFLD and incident gastric or esophageal cancer, it was limited by few esophageal or gastric cancer events.

Pancreatic cancer

Emerging epidemiologic and translational data support the role of local ectopic fat as a paracrine mechanism for the development of pancreatic cancer, where the local adipose tissue microenvironment affects tumor progression.[9,74] Release of proinflammatory cytokines, systemic inflammation,[75–77] as well as the altered microbiome in patients with hepatic steatosis can potentially increase the risk of pancreatic cancer.[22,75,78]

Allen and colleagues[9] found a 2-fold increase in the risk of pancreatic cancer in patients with NAFLD, which occurred more commonly in NAFLD at a young age. Another observational study found that NAFLD was an independent risk factor for pancreatic cancer (after controlling for diabetes, smoking, aspirin and statin use) and that patients with pancreatic cancer and NAFLD had poorer overall survival than patients without NAFLD.[79] Although Kim and colleagues[80] did not find a significant increase in the incidence rate of pancreatic cancer in patients with NAFLD, a recent metanalysis of 3 high-quality cohort studies (according to their NOS scores) found that patients with NAFLD had an elevated risk of pancreatic cancer, with a pooled OR of 2.12.[38] Similarly, Simon and colleagues[49] showed a significantly higher rate of pancreatic cancer with an adjusted HR (aHR) of 2.15. These previous studies were performed in hospitals, thus not accounting for the asymptomatic NAFLD, and had a limited number of pancreatic cancer cases. A recent cohort study of the Korean general population with 8 million adults whereby 10,470 participants were newly diagnosed with pancreatic cancer found that NAFLD (assessed using the fatty liver index) was independently associated with an increased risk of pancreatic cancer regardless of obesity. The risk of pancreatic cancer increased with increasing fatty liver index scores. The combination of NAFLD and smoking further increased the risk of pancreatic cancer. These findings could suggest that NAFLD may be a modifiable risk factor for pancreatic cancer.[75] Finally, McHenry and colleagues recently showed that individuals at intermediate or high NAFLD risk (defined by DSI) had a 30% and 51% increased risk of pancreatic cancer, respectively[48]

Nongastrointestinal Malignancies

Renal cell carcinoma

TNF-α can promote the progression of renal cell carcinoma (RCC) by enhancing tumor invasion and epithelial-mesenchymal transition.[81] Moreover, lower serum adiponectin and higher serum leptin are associated with higher aggressiveness of RCC.[82,83] Insulin resistance and the associated increase in IGF and insulin levels are also associated with tumor development and progression of RCC.[84] Clinical data support this potential association with an increased incidence of RCC in large retrospective cohort studies, with only 2 studies showing a statistically significant risk.[49,80,85,86] Simon and colleagues[49] found that patients with NAFLD had significantly higher risk of developing kidney/bladder cancer (aHR 1.41, 95% confidence interval [CI] 1.07–1.86). One Japanese study found hepatic steatosis was associated with more aggressive forms of RCC and shorter overall survival.[10]

Prostate cancer

Large studies have evaluated the association between NAFLD and the risk of prostate cancer, with inconsistent results. In a large cohort study from Korea of more than 10 million men, NAFLD (defined by a FLI $\geq$60 or hepatic steatosis index $\geq$ 36) was associated with the development of prostate cancer even in the absence of obesity.[87] In a metanalysis by Liu and colleagues of 3 large cohort studies, patients with NAFLD had a high risk of developing prostate cancer (OR = 1.36, 95% CI: 1.03–1.79),[9,80,87] whereas other studies failed to show such an association.[49] One study showed that the presence of NAFLD was an independent negative predictor for biochemical recurrence (BCR) after radical prostatectomy, and NAFLD fibrosis score was a single independent negative predictor for BCR, with higher BCR-free survival rate at 5 years in the higher NAFLD fibrosis score group. However, this study was limited by the small number of patients with NAFLD; this could be explained in part by the association between low serum testosterone levels in men with NAFLD as well as insulin resistance, which limits the growth effects of insulin on the prostate.[88] As such, the existence and direction of an association between NAFLD and prostate cancer needs further evaluation.

Breast cancer

Several studies have evaluated the association between NAFLD and breast cancer with some mixed results. A large retrospective study showed an almost 70% increase in the incidence of breast cancer among patients with NAFLD after adjusting for age and sex.[9] A subsequent metanalysis of 4 high-quality studies showed that patients with NAFLD are more susceptible to breast cancer (pooled OR of breast cancer in NAFLD was 1.69).[38] However, most of these studies did not control for traditional (including menopausal and reproductive) risk factors for breast cancer. On the other hand, other studies found no significant association between NAFLD and breast cancer.[49]

Kim and colleagues found an almost 90% increase in the incidence of breast cancer among patients with NAFLD after adjusting for demographic and metabolic factors (age, gender, smoking status, diabetes, hypertension, γ-glutamyl transpeptidase, high-density lipoprotein cholesterol, low-density lipoprotein cholesterol, and triglycerides). They found an association between NAFLD and the development of breast cancer in nonobese female subjects, whereas no association between them was found in obese female subjects with NAFLD (defined as BMI $\geq$25 kg/m^2). One potential explanation is that the increased incidence rate of breast cancer is driven by obesity-related metabolic or hormonal derangements such as disruption in insulin metabolism, adipokines, and inflammation. The presence of NAFLD per se did not increase the incidence rate of breast cancer in obese subjects. However, the increased breast cancer incidence in nonobese patients with NAFLD could be due to similar hormonal or metabolic derangements caused by NAFLD instead of obesity.[80] Another case control study also found that NAFLD was significantly associated with breast cancer independent of traditional risk factors, and this association existed in the nonobese subgroup but not in the obese subgroup in a subgroup analysis.[89] On the other hand, although other studies showed that NAFLD was significantly higher in patients with breast cancer, a significant proportion of patients with breast cancer were obese and fatty liver in patients with breast cancer was associated with being overweight.[90] The preponderance of current data shows that obesity is an important driver of this association, and the increased risk in nonobese women may be driven by other risk factors that were not well controlled for.

Outcomes in breast cancer

Limited data exist on breast cancer outcomes related to prognosis, cancer progression, or response to endocrine therapy in the context of NAFLD, and the results are mixed.[91–94]

A case control study showed that NAFLD was more prevalent in women with breast cancer compared with healthy controls and that the overall survival did not differ significantly between the groups with and without NAFLD. However, patients without NAFLD had a significantly higher recurrence-free survival as compared with those with NAFLD, although obesity was not controlled for. Among patients receiving endocrine treatment (ET), a higher cumulative incidence of significant liver injury was found in the NAFLD group. Compared with other endocrine drugs, tamoxifen significantly increased the risk of aminotransferase elevation.[95] Therefore, careful attention to liver tests is needed in patients with NAFLD receiving ET, especially tamoxifen. A metanalysis of 6 studies found that NAFLD was significantly associated with lymph node metastases and hormone receptor positivity in patients with breast cancer. NAFLD had no significant impact on disease-free survival (DFS) and overall survival (OS). Interestingly, ET-associated NAFLD had no significant impact on DFS and OS, whereas preexisting NAFLD before ET was significantly correlated with poor overall survival.[96] Recently, a study evaluating HR+/HER2– patients with nonmetastatic breast cancer found that those who developed NAFLD during treatment had longer DFS.[97] It is unclear if this is related to tamoxifen use. Based on available data, the impact of NAFLD on breast cancer outcomes remains unclear.

Other malignancies

Some evidence suggests an association between other extrahepatic cancers and NAFLD; however, this association is not clear, as studies are contradictory (gynecologic cancers such as uterine, ovarian, cervical,[9,39,49,80] lung cancer,[39,49] hematologic malignancies,[49,80,86] head and neck cancers[85,86]). No significant difference was found in the incidence rate of thyroid cancer in patients with NAFLD.[80,86] Further research is needed to better evaluate these relationships and determine the extent of causality.

Nonalcoholic fatty liver disease and cancer therapy

CLD and cirrhosis can affect the management and prognosis of patients with cancer. It can limit treatment options, influence the pharmacokinetics, increase the side effects of anticancer drugs, and increase the risk of hepatotoxicity as well as morbidity and mortality.[98] A significant number of patients receiving chemotherapy develop hepatic steatosis, indicating altered lipid metabolism and lipoprotein synthesis in hepatocytes. Patients with a higher hepatocellular lipid content are more vulnerable to severe hepatocellular injury with repeated cycles of chemotherapy through recruitment of inflammatory cells.[99] Certain chemotherapies have been associated with "chemotherapy-induced acute steatohepatitis" known as "CASH"[100–103] (**Box 1**). As such, physicians need to pay careful attention and monitor liver tests during cancer treatment in patients with CLD, including patients with NAFLD.

Emerging evidence suggests difference in clinical outcomes of patients with NAFLD receiving cancer therapy. A recent retrospective study compared the clinical outcomes of patients with non–small cell lung cancer who underwent immune checkpoint inhibitor–based treatment. They found no significant difference in response, disease control rate, or progression-free survival between patients with and without NAFLD. Interestingly, in patients with liver metastasis, there was a significant difference in response, disease control rate, and median progression-free survival between patients with and without NAFLD. The disease control rate of liver metastasis was

Box 1
Chemotherapy drugs associated with steatosis and steatohepatitis

Chemotherapy Drugs
- Fluorouracil (5-FU)
- Irinotecan L-asparaginase
- Methotrexate
- Tamoxifen
- Oxaliplatin
- Capecitabine
- Gemcitabine
- Cisplatin (rare)

significantly higher in patients with NAFLD.[104] More studies are still needed to better evaluate this potential difference in clinical outcomes and its implications on treatment options.

Cancer screening in patients with nonalcoholic fatty liver disease

More data are needed to confirm and quantify the risk of extrahepatocellular cancers among patients with NAFLD. Although plausible mechanistic links support an independent association between NAFLD and several malignancies, there is insufficient evidence to alter general screening recommendations. Clinicians must assure that patients with NAFLD adhere to age-appropriate cancer screening and limit modifiable risk factors for cancer such as smoking and alcohol.[3]

Managing cancer risk in nonalcoholic fatty liver disease

The cornerstone of management in patients with NAFLD remains weight loss, modification of diet, and physical activity.[3] In a recent retrospective cohort study of patients with severe obesity and NAFLD, bariatric surgery reduced the overall risk of any cancer and mostly obesity-related cancer. This effect was higher in patients with cirrhosis, and bariatric surgery was associated with a significantly lower risk of cancers of the colon, hepatocellular, pancreatic, endometrial, thyroid, and multiple myeloma.[105] It would be interesting to evaluate the effect of pharmacologic interventions on the risk of extrahepatic cancer in patients with NAFLD.

SUMMARY

NAFLD is inextricably linked to many metabolic comorbidities, including obesity and T2DM, which are clearly associated with an increased incidence of many malignancies. Increasing evidence suggests that NAFLD may contribute independently to an increased risk of some nonhepatocellular cancers. Prospective data from large cohorts with well-phenotyped NAFLD and long-term follow-up are needed to better define and quantify the risk at the population level. A clearer understanding of the risk of malignancies attributable to NAFLD would affect counseling, screening, and surveillance strategies.

DISCLOSURE

M.K. Ibrahim, M.E. Rinella, and T.G. Simon have no commercial or financial conflicts of interest or funding sources to disclose.

CLINICS CARE POINTS

- There is an association between NAFLD and extrahepatocellular cancers, especially intrahepatic CCA, colorectal, and pancreatic cancer.

- In patients with cirrhosis including NASH cirrhosis, treatment approaches that include surgery, careful patient selection, and monitoring are essential to reduce the risk of hepatic decompensation.
- Careful attention and monitoring of liver chemistries during cancer treatment is needed in patients with CLD, including NAFLD.
- Although there is insufficient evidence to warrant targeted cancer screening, patients with NAFLD should undergo age-appropriate cancer screening.

ACKNOWLEDGMENT

We would like to acknowledge Dana Coons for her outstanding work on the medical illustrations in the manuscript.

REFERENCES

1. Younossi ZM, Golabi P, Paik JM, et al. The global epidemiology of nonalcoholic fatty liver disease (NAFLD) and nonalcoholic steatohepatitis (NASH): a systematic review [published online ahead of print, 2023 Jan 3], Hepatology, 2023, https://doi.org/10.1097/HEP.0000000000000004.
2. Younossi ZM, Blissett D, Blissett R, et al. The economic and clinical burden of nonalcoholic fatty liver disease in the United States and Europe. Hepatology 2016;64(5):1577–86.
3. Wijarnpreecha K, Aby ES, Ahmed A, et al. Evaluation and management of extrahepatic manifestations of nonalcoholic fatty liver disease. Clin Mol Hepatol 2021;27(2):221–35.
4. Simon TG, Roelstraete B, Khalili H, et al. Mortality in biopsy-confirmed nonalcoholic fatty liver disease. Gut 2021;70(7):1375–82.
5. Brown JC, Harhay MO, Harhay MN. Nonalcoholic fatty liver disease and mortality among cancer survivors. Cancer Epidemiol 2017;48:104–9.
6. Kyrgiou M, Kalliala I, Markozannes G, et al. Adiposity and cancer at major anatomical sites: umbrella review of the literature. BMJ 2017;356:j477.
7. Ling S, Brown K, Miksza JK, et al. Association of type 2 diabetes with cancer: a meta-analysis with bias analysis for unmeasured confounding in 151 cohorts comprising 32 million people. Diabetes Care 2020;43(9):2313–22.
8. Bjornsdottir HH, Rawshani A, Rawshani A, et al. A national observation study of cancer incidence and mortality risks in type 2 diabetes compared to the background population over time. Sci Rep 2020;10(1):17376.
9. Allen AM, Hicks SB, Mara KC, et al. The risk of incident extrahepatic cancers is higher in non-alcoholic fatty liver disease than obesity - a longitudinal cohort study. J Hepatol 2019;71(6):1229–36.
10. Watanabe D, Horiguchi A, Tasaki S, et al. Clinical implication of ectopic liver lipid accumulation in renal cell carcinoma patients without visceral obesity. Sci Rep 2017;7(1):12795.
11. Kwon H, Pessin JE. Adipokines mediate inflammation and insulin resistance. Front Endocrinol 2013;4:71.
12. Codoñer-Franch P, Resistin AIE. Insulin resistance to malignancy. Clin Chim Acta Int J Clin Chem 2015;438:46–54.
13. Hursting SD, Dunlap SM. Obesity, metabolic dysregulation, and cancer: a growing concern and an inflammatory (and microenvironmental) issue. Ann N Y Acad Sci 2012;1271:82–7.

14. Yadav A, Kumar B, Datta J, et al. IL-6 promotes head and neck tumor metastasis by inducing epithelial-mesenchymal transition via the JAK-STAT3-SNAIL signaling pathway. Mol Cancer Res MCR 2011;9(12):1658–67.
15. Sanna C, Rosso C, Marietti M, et al. Non-alcoholic fatty liver disease and extra-hepatic cancers. Int J Mol Sci 2016;17(5):E717.
16. Ho GYF, Wang T, Gunter MJ, et al. Adipokines linking obesity with colorectal cancer risk in postmenopausal women. Cancer Res 2012;72(12):3029–37.
17. Jaffe T, Schwartz B. Leptin promotes motility and invasiveness in human colon cancer cells by activating multiple signal-transduction pathways. Int J Cancer 2008;123(11):2543–56.
18. Chandar AK, Devanna S, Lu C, et al. Association of serum levels of adipokines and insulin with risk of Barrett's esophagus: a systematic review and meta-analysis. Clin Gastroenterol Hepatol Off Clin Pract J Am Gastroenterol Assoc 2015; 13(13):2241–55, e1-4;[quiz e179].
19. Francois F, Roper J, Goodman AJ, et al. The association of gastric leptin with oesophageal inflammation and metaplasia. Gut 2008;57(1):16–24.
20. Delort L, Rossary A, Farges MC, et al. Leptin, adipocytes and breast cancer: focus on inflammation and anti-tumor immunity. Life Sci 2015;140:37–48.
21. Pérez-Hernández AI, Catalán V, Gómez-Ambrosi J, et al. Mechanisms linking excess adiposity and carcinogenesis promotion. Front Endocrinol 2014;5:65.
22. Lang S, Schnabl B. Microbiota and fatty liver disease—the known, the unknown, and the future. Cell Host Microbe 2020;28(2):233–44.
23. Wegermann K, Hyun J, Diehl AM. Molecular mechanisms linking nonalcoholic steatohepatitis to cancer. Clin Liver Dis 2021;17(1):6–10.
24. Vanni E, Marengo A, Mezzabotta L, et al. Systemic complications of nonalcoholic fatty liver disease: when the liver is not an innocent bystander. Semin Liver Dis 2015;35(3):236–49.
25. Song Q, Zhang X. The role of gut–liver axis in gut microbiome dysbiosis associated NAFLD and NAFLD-HCC. Biomedicines 2022;10(3):524.
26. Said I, Ahad H, Said A. Gut microbiome in non-alcoholic fatty liver disease associated hepatocellular carcinoma: current knowledge and potential for therapeutics. World J Gastrointest Oncol 2022;14(5):947–58.
27. Cheng Y, Ling Z, Li L. The intestinal microbiota and colorectal cancer. Front Immunol 2020;11:615056.
28. Wong SH, Yu J. Gut microbiota in colorectal cancer: mechanisms of action and clinical applications. Nat Rev Gastroenterol Hepatol 2019;16(11):690–704.
29. Wongjarupong N, Assavapongpaiboon B, Susantitaphong P, et al. Non-alcoholic fatty liver disease as a risk factor for cholangiocarcinoma: a systematic review and meta-analysis. BMC Gastroenterol 2017;17(1):149.
30. Welzel TM, Graubard BI, El-Serag HB, et al. Risk factors for intrahepatic and extrahepatic cholangiocarcinoma in the United States: a population-based case-control study. Clin Gastroenterol Hepatol 2007;5(10):1221–8.
31. Duan Y, Pan X, Luo J, et al. Association of inflammatory cytokines with non-alcoholic fatty liver disease. Front Immunol 2022;13:880298.
32. Wehbe H, Henson R, Meng F, et al. Interleukin-6 contributes to growth in cholangiocarcinoma cells by aberrant promoter methylation and gene expression. Cancer Res 2006;66(21):10517–24.
33. Jaiswal M, LaRusso NF, Shapiro RA, et al. Nitric oxide-mediated inhibition of DNA repair potentiates oxidative DNA damage in cholangiocytes. Gastroenterology 2001;120(1):190–9.

34. Ishimura N, Bronk SF, Gores GJ. Inducible nitric oxide synthase upregulates cyclooxygenase-2 in mouse cholangiocytes promoting cell growth. Am J Physiol Gastrointest Liver Physiol 2004;287(1):G88–95.
35. Corrao S, Natoli G, Argano C. Nonalcoholic fatty liver disease is associated with intrahepatic cholangiocarcinoma and not with extrahepatic form: definitive evidence from meta-analysis and trial sequential analysis. Eur J Gastroenterol Hepatol 2021;33(1):62–8.
36. Alvaro D, Barbaro B, Franchitto A, et al. Estrogens and insulin-like growth factor 1 modulate neoplastic cell growth in human cholangiocarcinoma. Am J Pathol 2006;169(3):877–88.
37. Petrick JL, Yang B, Altekruse SF, et al. Risk factors for intrahepatic and extrahepatic cholangiocarcinoma in the United States: a population-based study in SEER-Medicare. PLoS One 2017;12(10):e0186643.
38. Liu SS, Ma XF, Zhao J, et al. Association between nonalcoholic fatty liver disease and extrahepatic cancers: a systematic review and meta-analysis. Lipids Health Dis 2020;19(1):118.
39. Mantovani A, Dauriz M, Byrne CD, et al. Association between nonalcoholic fatty liver disease and colorectal tumours in asymptomatic adults undergoing screening colonoscopy: a systematic review and meta-analysis. Metabolism 2018;87:1–12.
40. Ahn JS, Sinn DH, Min YW, et al. Non-alcoholic fatty liver diseases and risk of colorectal neoplasia. Aliment Pharmacol Ther 2017;45(2):345–53.
41. Chen J, Bian D, Zang S, et al. The association between nonalcoholic fatty liver disease and risk of colorectal adenoma and cancer incident and recurrence: a meta-analysis of observational studies. Expert Rev Gastroenterol Hepatol 2019; 13(4):385–95.
42. Hwang ST, Cho YK, Park JH, et al. Relationship of non-alcoholic fatty liver disease to colorectal adenomatous polyps. J Gastroenterol Hepatol 2010;25(3): 562–7.
43. Stadlmayr A, Aigner E, Steger B, et al. Nonalcoholic fatty liver disease: an independent risk factor for colorectal neoplasia. J Intern Med 2011;270(1):41–9.
44. Wong VWS, Wong GLH, Tsang SWC, et al. High prevalence of colorectal neoplasm in patients with non-alcoholic steatohepatitis. Gut 2011;60(6):829–36.
45. Lee YI, Lim YS, Park HS. Colorectal neoplasms in relation to non-alcoholic fatty liver disease in Korean women: a retrospective cohort study. J Gastroenterol Hepatol 2012;27(1):91–5.
46. Huang KW, Leu HB, Wang YJ, et al. Patients with nonalcoholic fatty liver disease have higher risk of colorectal adenoma after negative baseline colonoscopy. Colorectal Dis 2013;15(7):830–5.
47. Abancens M, Bustos V, Harvey H, et al. Sexual dimorphism in colon cancer. Front Oncol 2020;10:607909.
48. McHenry S, Zong X, Shi M, et al. Risk of nonalcoholic fatty liver disease and associations with gastrointestinal cancers. Hepatol Commun 2022. https://doi.org/10.1002/hep4.2073.
49. Simon TG, Roelstraete B, Sharma R, et al. Cancer risk in patients with biopsy-confirmed nonalcoholic fatty liver disease: a population-based cohort study. Hepatol Baltim Md 2021;74(5):2410–23.
50. Montomoli J, Erichsen R, Christiansen CF, et al. Liver disease and 30-day mortality after colorectal cancer surgery: a Danish population-based cohort study. BMC Gastroenterol 2013;13:66.

51. Nguyen GC, Correia AJ, Thuluvath PJ. The impact of cirrhosis and portal hypertension on mortality following colorectal surgery: a nationwide, population-based study. Dis Colon Rectum 2009;52(8):1367–74.
52. Meunier K, Mucci S, Quentin V, et al. Colorectal surgery in cirrhotic patients: assessment of operative morbidity and mortality. Dis Colon Rectum 2008; 51(8):1225–31.
53. Metcalf AM, Dozois RR, Wolff BG, et al. The surgical risk of colectomy in patients with cirrhosis. Dis Colon Rectum 1987;30(7):529–31.
54. Gervaz P, Pak-art R, Nivatvongs S, et al. Colorectal adenocarcinoma in cirrhotic patients. J Am Coll Surg 2003;196(6):874–9.
55. Lee KC, Chung KC, Chen HH, et al. Short-term postoperative outcomes of colorectal cancer among patients with chronic liver disease: a national population-based study. BMJ Open 2018;8(7):e020511.
56. Hanje AJ, Patel T. Preoperative evaluation of patients with liver disease. Nat Clin Pract Gastroenterol Hepatol 2007;4(5):266–76.
57. Friedman LS. Surgery in the patient with liver disease. Trans Am Clin Climatol Assoc 2010;121:192–204 [discussion: 205].
58. Wu K, Zhai MZ, Weltzien EK, et al. Non-alcoholic fatty liver disease and colorectal cancer survival. Cancer Causes Control CCC 2019;30(2):165–8.
59. Chen ZF, Dong XL, Huang QK, et al. The combined effect of non-alcoholic fatty liver disease and metabolic syndrome on colorectal carcinoma mortality: a retrospective in Chinese females. World J Surg Oncol 2018;16:163.
60. You J, Huang S, Huang GQ, et al. Nonalcoholic fatty liver disease: a negative risk factor for colorectal cancer prognosis. Medicine (Baltim) 2015;94(5):e479.
61. Min YW, Yun HS, Chang WI, et al. Influence of non-alcoholic fatty liver disease on the prognosis in patients with colorectal cancer. Clin Res Hepatol Gastroenterol 2012;36(1):78–83.
62. Murono K, Kitayama J, Tsuno NH, et al. Hepatic steatosis is associated with lower incidence of liver metastasis from colorectal cancer. Int J Colorectal Dis 2013;28(8):1065–72.
63. Hayashi S, Masuda H, Shigematsu M. Liver metastasis rare in colorectal cancer patients with fatty liver. Hepato-Gastroenterology 1997;44(16):1069–75.
64. Cai B, Liao K, Song XQ, et al. Patients with chronically diseased livers have lower incidence of colorectal liver metastases: a meta-analysis. PLoS One 2014;9(9):e108618.
65. Kondo T, Okabayashi K, Hasegawa H, et al. The impact of hepatic fibrosis on the incidence of liver metastasis from colorectal cancer. Br J Cancer 2016; 115(1):34–9.
66. Hamady ZZR, Rees M, Welsh FK, et al. Fatty liver disease as a predictor of local recurrence following resection of colorectal liver metastases. Br J Surg 2013; 100(6):820–6.
67. Brouquet A, Nordlinger B. Metastatic colorectal cancer outcome and fatty liver disease. Nat Rev Gastroenterol Hepatol 2013;10(5):266–7.
68. Lv Y, Zhang HJ. Effect of non-alcoholic fatty liver disease on the risk of synchronous liver metastasis: analysis of 451 consecutive patients of newly diagnosed colorectal cancer. Front Oncol 2020;10:251.
69. Dahl E, Rumessen J, Gluud LL. Systematic review with meta-analyses of studies on the association between cirrhosis and liver metastases. Hepatol Res Off J Jpn Soc Hepatol 2011;41(7):618–25.
70. Hamaguchi M, Hashimoto Y, Obora A, et al. Non-alcoholic fatty liver disease with obesity as an independent predictor for incident gastric and colorectal

cancer: a population-based longitudinal study. BMJ Open Gastroenterol 2019;6(1):e000295.
71. Fan JH, Wang JB, Wang SM, et al. Body mass index and risk of gastric cancer: a 30-year follow-up study in the Linxian general population trial cohort. Cancer Sci 2017;108(8):1667–72.
72. Lee JM, Park YM, Yun JS, et al. The association between nonalcoholic fatty liver disease and esophageal, stomach, or colorectal cancer: national population-based cohort study. PLoS One 2020;15(1):e0226351.
73. Ahmed OT, Allen AM. Extrahepatic malignancies in nonalcoholic fatty liver disease. Curr Hepatol Rep 2019;18(4):455–72.
74. Hori M, Takahashi M, Hiraoka N, et al. Association of pancreatic fatty infiltration with pancreatic ductal adenocarcinoma. Clin Transl Gastroenterol 2014;5(3):e53.
75. Park JH, Hong JY, Han K, et al. Increased risk of pancreatic cancer in individuals with non-alcoholic fatty liver disease. Sci Rep 2022;12(1):10681.
76. Hausmann S, Kong B, Michalski C, et al. The role of inflammation in pancreatic cancer. Adv Exp Med Biol 2014;816:129–51.
77. Ren R, Yu J, Zhang Y, et al. Inflammation promotes progression of pancreatic cancer through WNT/β-catenin pathway-dependent manner. Pancreas 2019;48(8):1003–14.
78. Wei MY, Shi S, Liang C, et al. The microbiota and microbiome in pancreatic cancer: more influential than expected. Mol Cancer 2019;18(1):97.
79. Chang CF, Tseng YC, Huang HH, et al. Exploring the relationship between nonalcoholic fatty liver disease and pancreatic cancer by computed tomographic survey. Intern Emerg Med 2018;13(2):191–7.
80. Kim GA, Lee HC, Choe J, et al. Association between non-alcoholic fatty liver disease and cancer incidence rate. J Hepatol. Published online November 2017;2. S0168-8278(17)32294-8.
81. Al-Lamki RS, Mayadas TN. TNF receptors: signaling pathways and contribution to renal dysfunction. Kidney Int 2015;87(2):281–96.
82. Pinthus JH, Kleinmann N, Tisdale B, et al. Lower plasma adiponectin levels are associated with larger tumor size and metastasis in clear-cell carcinoma of the kidney. Eur Urol 2008;54(4):866–73.
83. Horiguchi A, Sumitomo M, Asakuma J, et al. Increased serum leptin levels and over expression of leptin receptors are associated with the invasion and progression of renal cell carcinoma. J Urol 2006;176(4 Pt 1):1631–5.
84. Solarek W, Czarnecka AM, Escudier B, et al. Insulin and IGFs in renal cancer risk and progression. Endocr Relat Cancer 2015;22(5):R253–64.
85. Sørensen HT, Mellemkjaer L, Jepsen P, et al. Risk of cancer in patients hospitalized with fatty liver: a Danish cohort study. J Clin Gastroenterol 2003;36(4):356–9.
86. Sun LM, Lin MC, Lin CL, et al. Nonalcoholic cirrhosis increased risk of digestive tract malignancies: a population-based cohort study. Medicine (Baltim) 2015;94(49):e2080.
87. Choi YJ, Lee DH, Han KD, et al. Is nonalcoholic fatty liver disease associated with the development of prostate cancer? A nationwide study with 10,516,985 Korean men. PLoS One 2018;13(9):e0201308.
88. Choi WM, Lee JH, Yoon JH, et al. Nonalcoholic fatty liver disease is a negative risk factor for prostate cancer recurrence. Endocr Relat Cancer 2014;21(2):343–53.

89. Kwak MS, Yim JY, Yi A, et al. Nonalcoholic fatty liver disease is associated with breast cancer in nonobese women. Dig Liver Dis 2019;51(7):1030–5.
90. Chu CH, Lin SC, Shih SC, et al. Fatty metamorphosis of the liver in patients with breast cancer: possible associated factors. World J Gastroenterol WJG 2003; 9(7):1618–20.
91. Zheng Q, Xu F, Nie M, et al. Selective estrogen receptor modulator-associated nonalcoholic fatty liver disease improved survival in patients with breast cancer: a retrospective cohort analysis. Medicine (Baltim) 2015;94(40):e1718.
92. Wu W, Chen J, Ye W, et al. Fatty liver decreases the risk of liver metastasis in patients with breast cancer: a two-center cohort study. Breast Cancer Res Treat 2017;166(1):289–97.
93. Lee JI, Yu JH, Anh SG, et al. Aromatase inhibitors and newly developed nonalcoholic fatty liver disease in postmenopausal patients with early breast cancer: a propensity score-matched cohort study. Oncol 2019;24(8):e653–61.
94. Yan M, Wang J, Xuan Q, et al. The relationship between tamoxifen-associated nonalcoholic fatty liver disease and the prognosis of patients with early-stage breast cancer. Clin Breast Cancer 2017;17(3):195–203.
95. Lee YS, Lee HS, Chang SW, et al. Underlying nonalcoholic fatty liver disease is a significant factor for breast cancer recurrence after curative surgery. Medicine (Baltim) 2019;98(39):e17277.
96. Wang C, Zhou Y, Huang W, et al. The impact of pre-existed and SERM-induced non-alcoholic fatty liver disease on breast cancer survival: a meta-analysis. J Cancer 2020;11(15):4597–604.
97. Taroeno-Hariadi KW, Putra YR, Choridah L, et al. Fatty liver in hormone receptor-positive breast cancer and its impact on patient's survival. J Breast Cancer 2021;24(5):417–27.
98. Pinter M, Trauner M, Peck-Radosavljevic M, et al. Cancer and liver cirrhosis: implications on prognosis and management. ESMO Open 2016;1(2):e000042.
99. Ramadori G, Cameron S. Effects of systemic chemotherapy on the liver. Ann Hepatol 2010;9(2):133–43.
100. Lee MCM, Kachura JJ, Vlachou PA, et al. Evaluation of adjuvant chemotherapy-associated steatosis (CAS) in colorectal cancer. Curr Oncol Tor Ont 2021;28(4): 3030–40.
101. White MA, Fong Y, Singh G. Chemotherapy-associated hepatotoxicities. Surg Clin North Am 2016;96(2):207–17.
102. West S, Gunnerson C, Komar M, et al. An unintended consequence: chemotherapy associated steatohepatitis: 844. J Am Coll Gastroenterol ACG 2015; 110:S366. Available at: https://journals.lww.com/ajg/Fulltext/2015/10001/An_Unintended_Consequence__Chemotherapy_Associated.844.aspx. Accessed October 17, 2022.
103. Meunier L, Larrey D. Chemotherapy-associated steatohepatitis. Ann Hepatol 2020;19(6):597–601.
104. Zhou J, Zhou F, Chu X, et al. Non-alcoholic fatty liver disease is associated with immune checkpoint inhibitor-based treatment response in patients with non-small cell lung cancer with liver metastases. Transl Lung Cancer Res 2020;9(2).
105. Rustgi VK, Li Y, Gupta K, et al. Bariatric surgery reduces cancer risk in adults with nonalcoholic fatty liver disease and severe obesity. Gastroenterology 2021;161(1):171–84.e10.

Clinics in Liver Disease: Update on Nonalcoholic Steatohepatitis

Sarcopenia and Nonalcoholic Fatty Liver Disease

Takumi Kawaguchi, MD, PhD[a], Hirokazu Takahashi, MD, PhD[b], Lynn H. Gerber, MD[c,*]

KEYWORDS

- Steatosis • Sarcopenia • Loss of muscle strength • Non–liver-related mortality
- Myokines • Myosteatosis • Lifestyle modification • Exercise

KEY POINTS

Definition for sarcopenia varies among the studies depending on the following criteria and data availability:

- Sarcopenia has a significant negative impact on survival through an increase in both liver-related and non–liver-related mortality in patients with nonalcoholic fatty liver disease (NAFLD).
- Sarcopenia is associated with loss of type 2 muscle fibers and infiltration of fat, myosteatosis, thought to be a significant risk factor for severe liver disease.
- Muscle is critical for metabolic homeostasis and reduction of chronic inflammation associated with the dual diagnoses of sarcopenia and NAFLD, through insulin resistance, lipolysis, reduction in vitamin D, testosterone, and growth hormone.
- Treatment of the condition includes weight loss, increased activity/exercise, and dietary modification to increase protein intake while reducing energy consumption.
- Efforts to educate patients and health care providers about the importance of sarcopenia in the NAFLD setting is needed for good health outcomes.

T. Kawaguchi received honoraria (lecture fees) from Janssen Pharmaceutical K.K., Taisho Pharmaceutical Co., Ltd., Otsuka Pharmaceutical Co., Ltd., and EA Pharma Co., Ltd.

[a] Department of Medicine, Division of Gastroenterology, Kurume University, School of Medicine, 67 Asahi-machi, Kurume 830-0011, Japan; [b] Department of Laboratory Medicine, Liver Center, Saga University Hospital, 5-1-1 Nabeshima, Saga 849-8501, Japan; [c] Department of Medicine, Betty and Guy Beatty Center for Integrated Research, Inova Health System, Center for Liver Disease, Inova Fairfax Hospital, Claude Moore Health Education and Research Building, 3rd Floor, 3300 Gallows Road, Falls Church, VA 22042, USA

* Corresponding author. Claude Moore Health Education and Research Building, 3rd Floor, 3300 Gallows Road, Falls Church, VA 22042, USA

E-mail address: lynn.gerber@inova.org

Clin Liver Dis 27 (2023) 275–286
https://doi.org/10.1016/j.cld.2023.01.005

DEFINITION OF SARCOPENIA

Irwin Rosenberg first described the term sarcopenia, which had been derived from the Greek words "sarx" meaning muscle/flesh, and "penia" meaning loss/poverty.[1] Sarcopenia originally was the term designated for age-related skeletal muscle loss. Recently, evidence has accumulated that supports an association between sarcopenia and several chronic conditions including obesity and nonalcoholic fatty liver disease (NAFLD), independent of age. In fact, the term "sarcopenic obesity" has been accepted to reflect this association. Impaired muscle strength and a standardized measure of physical performance, such as ambulation or chair stand test, are also required for the diagnosis of sarcopenia. Although the diagnostic criteria for sarcopenia have varied, a consensus has emerged: loss of skeletal muscle mass is the essential qualification and either muscle strength or physical performance should be evaluated for the diagnosis of sarcopenia (**Table 1**).

On the other hand, methodology and cut-off points vary among the individual criteria. European Working Group on Sarcopenia in Older People (EWGSOP2) recommends measuring appendicular skeletal muscle mass (ASM) using dual-energy X-ray absorptiometry (DEXA), and the cut-off of ASM for sarcopenia is 20 kg for men and 15 kg for women, or ASM divided by height squared (m^2) is 7.0 kg/m^2 for men and 5.5 kg/m^2 for women.[2] Asian Working Group for Sarcopenia (AWGS2019) recommends using DEXA and defines the cut-off of ASM divided by height squared (m^2) as 7.0 kg/m^2 for men and 5.4 kg/m^2 for women. Skeletal muscle index (SMI), which is defined as ASM/body mass index (BMI), is also described in AWGS2019, and the cut-off is 0.789 kg/BMI for men and 0.512 kg/BMI for women.[3] SMI was originally provided in Foundation of Nutritional Institutes of Health (FNIH)[4] to normalize the effect of obesity, and the cut-off for sarcopenia is the same as AWGS2019. Sarcopenia defined by SMI was more closely related to insulin resistance than ASM/height squared in the Korean population.[5] AWGS2019 defined the cut-off for ASM/height $(m)^2$ obtained by bioelectrical impedance analysis as 7.0 kg/m^2 for men and 5.7 kg/m^2 for women.[3] Imaging modalities including abdominal computed tomography (CT) scan and MRI are used to measure muscle mass. The Japan Society of Hepatology guideline, which was generated to define sarcopenia in chronic liver disease, includes the cut-off of the iliopsoas muscle area at the level of the third lumbar vertebra (measured by CT with the manual trace method) divided by height squared (m^2) as 42 cm^2/m^2 for men and 38 cm^2/m^2 for women.[6] This CT imaging–based procedure is strongly correlated to SMI.[7] For the evaluation of muscle strength, hand dynamometry or grip

Table 1
Recent diagnostic criteria for sarcopenia

	Skeletal Muscle	Strength	Physical Performance
EWGSOP2[2]	✓	✓	+
AWGS2019[3]	✓	✓ (either)	
FNIH[4]	✓	✓	+
JSH[6]	✓	✓	×

Note. Check mark, plus mark, and cross mark individually indicates essential qualification, additional requirement, and not necessary condition.

Abbreviations: AWGS2019, Asian Working Group for Sarcopenia; EWGSOP2, European Working Group on Sarcopenia in Older People; FNIH, Foundation for Nutritional Institutes of Health; JSH, the Japan society of Hepatology.

strength is generally measured. The cut-off for sarcopenia of EWGSOP2 is 27 kg for men and 16 kg for women.[2] In EWGSOP2, the chair stand test (5 times sit-to-stand) can be also used for evaluation of skeletal muscle strength, and the cut-off is 15 seconds. The cut-off of the grip test of AWGS2019 is 28 kg for men and 18 kg for women.[3] For the evaluation of physical performance, gate speed is mostly measured and the cut-off is 0.8 m/s, 1.0 m/s, and 0.8 m/s for EWGSOP2,[2] AWGS2019,[3] and FNIH.[4] EWGSOP2[2] and AWGS2019[3] use the short physical performance battery test, which consists of balance, gait speed, muscle strength, and endurance tests.[8] To date, there is no unified definition for sarcopenia.

The definition of sarcopenia in the studies for NAFLD is inconsistent or incomplete. In the epidemiological studies that retrospectively investigated relatively large cohorts, data availability is limited and either skeletal muscle mass[9] or strength[10] or physical performance[11] is evaluated. At times, skeletal mass was determined using different assessments (eg, DEXA, CT, MRI, or bioimpedance). Therefore, subjects included in these studies never met the full criteria for the diagnosis of sarcopenia. Methodology and the cut-off point for the evaluation of individual qualifications vary among the studies. Moreover, demographics including age, gender, and race are different among the studies. In order to test the pathological association between “conventional sarcopenia” and NAFLD in the research field, a study including the subjects who met the full criteria is probably required. On the other hand, recent studies indicate that hepatic outcome and mortality of NAFLD could be predicted by a single qualification such as skeletal muscle mass or muscle strength.[9,10] Moreover, a recent study identified that not sarcopenia but myosteatosis evaluated by CT imaging and considered to be fat infiltration in the skeletal muscle is highly correlated with liver fibrosis in NAFLD.[12] Efforts to generate sensitive and specific measures for sarcopenia in people with NAFLD that have prognostic value, are feasible, and can be easily used in the clinical setting are needed.

AN ASSOCIATION BETWEEN SARCOPENIA AND MORTALITY

Skeletal muscle plays a crucial role in energy metabolism, and sarcopenia is known as a risk factor for NAFLD. Moreover, several studies including a meta-analysis demonstrated that sarcopenia is associated with significant fibrosis independently of hepatic and metabolic risk factors in patients with NAFLD.[13–16] In addition, Petermann-Rocha and colleagues performed a prospective study of UK Biobank participants and demonstrated that sarcopenia was associated with a higher risk of developing severe NAFLD.[10] These studies suggest that sarcopenia is associated with a poor prognosis in patients with NAFLD.

Recently, several studies have examined the impact of sarcopenia on mortality in patients with NAFLD. By using public data files of the National Health and Nutrition Examination Survey (NHANES), Golabi and colleagues examined the impact of sarcopenia on mortality in patients with NAFLD.[17] Of 4611 participants, a total of 586 subjects died, of whom 251 had NAFLD during a median follow-up of 13.5 years. Among those who died with NAFLD, 33.0% had sarcopenia. Compared with nonsarcopenic NAFLD, sarcopenic NAFLD was significantly associated with a higher risk of all-cause (hazard ratio [HR] 1.78 [1.16–2.73]), cardiac-specific (HR 3.19 [1.17–8.74]), and cancer-specific mortality (HR 2.12 [1.08–4.15]). Sun and colleagues[18] also used the NHANES database. They performed a multivariate model analysis using participants with no NAFLD and no sarcopenia as the reference group. In subjects with both NAFLD and sarcopenia, risks of all-cause and cardiovascular mortality were 1.69 times (95% confidence interval [CI] 1.23–2.31) and 2.17 times (95% CI 1.33–3.54) higher than the reference group, respectively. However, subjects with nonsarcopenic NAFLD had HRs for all-cause and cardiovascular mortality similar to those of the reference group (no NAFLD and no sarcopenia).[18] Furthermore, Kim and colleagues[19] examined all-cause and cause-specific mortality from sarcopenia using the NHANES database. They found that only in subjects with NAFLD sarcopenia was associated with a higher risk for all-cause mortality, whereas this association was absent in subjects with no NAFLD. Furthermore, sarcopenia was associated with a higher risk for cancer- and diabetes-related mortality among subjects with NAFLD. This association was not noted in subjects with no NAFLD.

In the Asian population, Moon and colleagues[9] investigated the association of sarcopenia and/or NAFLD with mortality using the database of Korean National Health and Nutrition Examination Surveys. They found that NAFLD and sarcopenia additively increased the risk of mortality on an ordinal scale (HR 1.46, 95% CI 1.18–1.81, P for trend = 0.001). The coexistence of NAFLD and sarcopenia increased mortality risk by almost twice as much, even after adjustment for advanced fibrosis (HR 2.18, 95% CI 1.38–3.44). Thus, the results of recent studies indicate that sarcopenia has a significant negative impact on survival through an increase in both liver-related and non–liver-related mortality (**Fig. 1**).

Histopathology of Sarcopenic Muscle

Studies of tissue pathology in patients with sarcopenia have shown a significant loss of type 2 muscle fibers, more than type 1 fibers. Type 2, or fast-twitch fibers, are associated with muscles that generate bursts of power and fatigue faster than type 1. Data comparing the morphometry of fiber loss in people with osteoporosis (OP), who are likely to have drop out of type 2 muscle fibers and likely to have sarcopenia, as compared with people with osteoarthritis (OA), show significant differences between the 2 groups. Patients with OA showed about 30.00% atrophic fibers with a diameter of less than 30 μm (16.81 ± 1.21% type I and 18.90 ± 1.24% type II), whereas, people with OP had 50.00% atrophic fibers with prevalence of type II fibers affected (19.13 ± 2.07% type I and 29.41 ± 2.56% type II). Controls (CTRL) showed less than 15% atrophic fibers. Similar differences among the 3 groups were found when

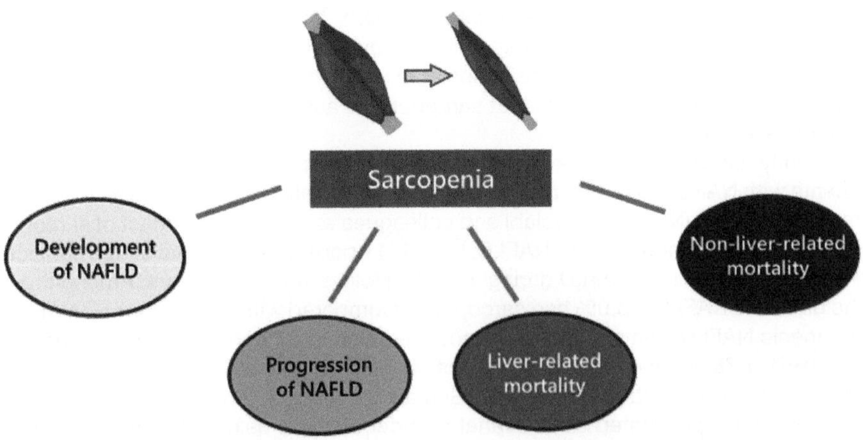

Fig. 1. An association between sarcopenia and NAFLD. Sarcopenia is associated with the development of and progression of NAFLD. Sarcopenia is also associated with both liver-related and non–liver-related mortalities in patients with NAFLD.

immunostaining and other histopathological techniques were used.[20] There was a decrease of BMP2, 4, and 7 expression in patients with OP compared with both OA group and CTRL, suggesting metabolic changes in affected muscle. Others have also found a strong association between sarcopenia and metabolic abnormalities of muscle.[21]

Biochemical and Metabolic Markers Associated with Sarcopenic Nonalcoholic Fatty Liver Disease

Linkages between sarcopenia and NAFLD, NASH, and cirrhosis and other liver diseases are many and complex. Some of this complexity is due to different definitions of sarcopenia and criteria for diagnosis. The earlier discussion in this article has identified a variety of definitions for sarcopenia and the various diagnostic criteria used throughout the world. The field has not yet designated a single set of criteria for diagnosis but there is agreement that a necessary condition for diagnosis of sarcopenia includes loss of skeletal mass. Reports of several investigators suggest there is an inverse correlation between skeletal mass and NAFLD[14] and that this is true even when controlling for obesity (odds ratios [ORs] = 1.55–3.02) or metabolic syndrome (ORs = 1.63–4.00) with p values less than 0.001.[22] Although some report that this relationship holds independent of insulin resistance, many have shown that the loss of skeletal mass is associated with decreased insulin signaling and decreased insulin response (insulin resistance), which has been discussed in recent reviews.[23,24]

There is evidence that people with sarcopenic NAFLD more frequently demonstrate significant liver fibrosis (F2, 46.0 vs 25.0%, $p < 0.001$).[25] Those with sarcopenia have a 2-fold increase in risk for NASH (OR 2.46; 95% CI, 1.35–4.48) and significant fibrosis (OR 2.01; 95% CI, 1.12–3.61).[14] The risk of fibrosis was slightly reduced when adjusted for HOMA-IR and high-sensitivity C-reactive protein but remain significant and supports the view that IR and chronic inflammation are contributors to the severity of liver disease.

Muscle has been shown to be a paracrine, autocrine, and endocrine organ. In its endocrine capacity, it secretes hormone-like products that influence the behavior of several organs. These hormonelike substances are called myokines and have been shown to exert substantial effect on metabolism in the brain, adipose tissue, bone, liver, gut, pancreas, and the vascular bed, among others. They do not always act as proinflammatory cytokines.[26] In its paracrine capacity, these molecules have direct impact on all components of muscle and mitochondria. Investigators recently identified that muscles release cytokines, challenging the belief that adipose tissue is the main source of cytokines, and further, that myokines act directly on organs such as liver and adipose, without having to invoke the central nervous system as the sole source and regulator of hormonal release. The identification of interleukin-6 (IL-6) in plasma during exercise, followed by the presence of IL-1 receptor antagonist and the antiinflammatory cytokine IL-10 supported the hypothesis, which has been confirmed, that humoral factors are released during exercise and are not inflammatory cytokines.[26] In fact, IL-6 may function as an energy sensor during exercise because plasma levels of IL-6 drop if one consumes glucose during exercise.

IL-6 has a significant impact on glucose metabolism.[27,28] IL-6 increased basal glucose uptake and increased insulin-stimulated glucose uptake in vitro. In fact, IL-6 knockout mice have been shown to develop maturity onset diabetes, glucose intolerance, and obesity.[29] The role of IL-6 is still being studied because chronic persistent elevation of IL-6 is associated with inflammation and has been associated with hyperinsulinemia, impaired glucose uptake by skeletal muscle.[30] Explanations for the various roles of IL-6 include the fact that in exercise-induced IL-6 release, levels of

IL-6 increase acutely to up to 100-fold and return to baseline, whereas in chronic conditions, the levels do not increase as steeply or as high and often do not return to baseline. This latter condition is thought to originate from the release of IL-6 from macrophages. In skeletal muscle, however, during exercise IL-6 acts intramuscularly to increase skeletal muscle glucose uptake and fat oxidation and to increase hepatic glucose production and lipolysis in adipose, hence IL-6 does not act as inflammatory myokine, as it is when released from macrophages.[31]

If the data presented earlier are valid, and exercising muscle does release high levels of IL-6, which in its capacity as a hormone facilitates skeletal muscle glucose uptake and promotes insulin sensitivity and fat oxidation, it is plausible that conditions that favor inactivity, sedentary behavior, lack of muscle contraction, and nonexercising muscle promote the opposite. Namely, a low skeletal mass status likely is associated with inefficient glucose uptake by skeletal muscle, insulin resistance, and decreased fatty acid oxidation. This hypothesis may be the link between activity (or lack thereof) and metabolic and inflammatory regulation. Data suggest that sedentary behaviors are also associated with the development of visceral adiposity, myo- and hepatic steatosis.[32]

Myosteatosis, the analogue to fatty liver in muscle, has been identified as a risk factor for more severe liver disease.[33] Muscle composition and specifically muscle fat infiltrate are associated with all-cause mortality in people with NAFLD.[34] Perimuscular fat also affects muscle atrophy. In vitro studies also support an association between inflammation and lipid metabolism as a likely pathogenesis of insulin resistance in skeletal muscle.[35] The perilipin family of proteins is embedded in lipid droplets and functions as a regulator of skeletal muscle lipid metabolism and mitochondrial oxidation. In cultured myocytes, a lipid droplet–associated protein perilipin 2 increases expression of NLRP3 inflammasome, resulting in impaired insulin-stimulated glucose uptake. These results suggest that increased fat accumulation in muscle impairs energy metabolism as well as glucose homeostasis, leading to catabolic status and atrophy of the skeletal muscle. Muscle composition, in particular muscle fat infiltration, also called myosteatosis, is a major determinant not only for muscle strength and function but also for metabolic and liver-related clinical outcomes.[24]

Inflow of fat into muscle may accumulate and thereby exceed oxidative capacity, hence fat accumulates, which blocks GLUT4. GLUT4 is critical for the entry of glucose into cells. When glucose entry is blocked, and fat accumulates in mitochondria, it inhibits mitochondrial respiration, increases reactive oxygen species formation and myocyte toxicity, and may lead to the development of sarcopenia. Intermyocellular adipose tissue (IMAT) and IMCL secrete myostatin, CCL2, TNF-α, IL-1β, and IL-6, thus inducing IR and lipotoxicity, all of which affects liver function.[36]

Fig. 2 displays contributing interactions among visceral fat, hepatic, and muscle factors relevant to the development of the inflammatory and metabolic imbalances seen in sarcopenic NAFLD. The relevant changes in liver physiology are associated with its evolution from normal, healthy tissue to steatosis and steatohepatitis, fibrosis, and cirrhosis; the role of adipose tissues, especially visceral adipose, in promoting sarcopenia and NAFLD, both metabolic and inflammatory; and the profound changes in muscles associated with the development of sarcopenia.

Functional Measures Used in Assessing Sarcopenic Nonalcoholic Fatty Liver Disease

The definition of sarcopenia includes measures of function as well as skeletal mass, and NAFLD is frequently associated with fatigue and low levels of activity.[2] Although

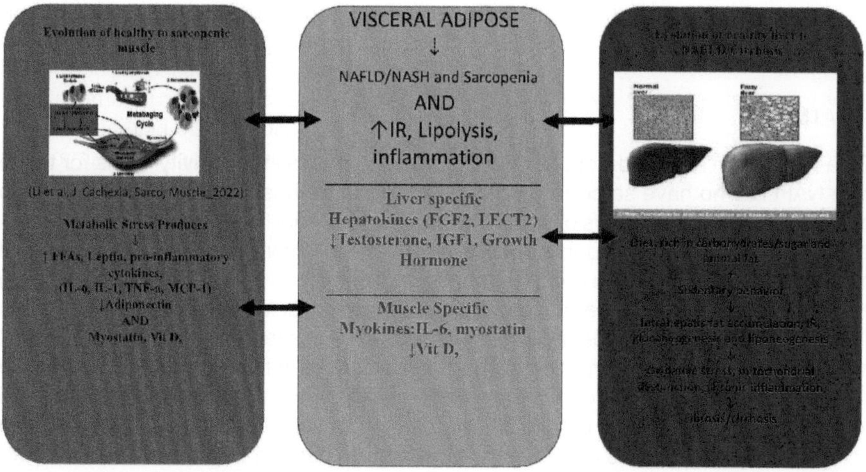

Fig. 2. Contributing interactions among visceral fat, hepatic, and muscle factors relevant to the development of the inflammatory and metabolic imbalances seen in sarcopenic NAFLD.

there is not universal agreement on which functional measures are best used to assess function, many studies include measures of strength and physical performance. Strength measures usually rely on hand dynamometry, used in assessing grip strength and overall physical performance of batteries, such as the Short Form Physical Performance Battery, gait speed, timed up-and-go, and the stair climb power test, among others.[2] These instruments are frequently used both as diagnostic criteria for sarcopenia and also to provide important information about fall risks, which is an important clinical consideration for all with sarcopenia, not only the frail elderly.

The combination of NAFLD and sarcopenia pose substantial risks. Among patients with NAFLD, the presence of sarcopenia was associated with a 78% increase in all-cause mortality. More strikingly, in the NAFLD population, sarcopenia was associated with a 320% increase in cardiac-specific deaths.[17] Furthermore, sarcopenia was associated with a higher risk for cancer- and diabetes-related mortality among those with NAFLD.[19]

It is accepted that dual diagnoses of sarcopenia and NAFLD have impact on mortality. Equally important is that it has significant impact on function and life activity. The relative risk for incident disability in sarcopenic obese subjects was 2.63 (95% confidence interval, 1.19 to 5.85), adjusting for age, sex, physical activity level, length of follow-up, and prevalent morbidity.[37] Compared with women with a healthy body composition and after adjustment for confounders, purely sarcopenic women had no increased odds of having difficulties for all of the physical functions assessed, purely obese women had a 44% to 79% higher odds of having difficulties with most of the physical functions assessed ($P < 0.05$), and sarcopenic-obese women had a 2.60 higher odds of having difficulty climbing stairs and a 2.35 higher odds of having difficulty going down stairs (all $P < 0.05$). These deficits may pose a safety risk to people with sarcopenic obesity.[38]

Additional data have been reported that suggest there is a link among insulin resistance, dementia, sarcopenia, and visceral adiposity.[39] Data have been gathered using a variety of cognitive batteries including the Mini-Mental Status Examination. The hypothetical mechanism for this is that insulin modulates glucose use in the central nervous system through receptors located in the hippocampus and frontal cortex, which has been shown to be proposed to be associated with executive functioning and poor visual scanning (TMT-A) ($\beta = 11.005$; $P = .02$), poor visual scanning with added cognitive flexibility (TMT-B) ($\beta = 28.379$; $P < .001$), and poor cognitive efficiency.[40,41]

TREATMENT

Data have been reported from NHANES studies that show the activity levels for those with NAFLD who have sarcopenia, as contrasted with those who do not. Among the participants with a diagnosis of NAFLD without sarcopenia, 42% reported being physically inactive and 43% reported practicing the recommended level of activity for a healthy lifestyle. Among the group that had sarcopenia and NAFLD 64% were inactive and only 24% practiced the recommended level of physical activity.[17]

Both NAFLD and sarcopenia are conditions likely to respond to interventions that target weight loss and increased activity. Interventions for treating sarcopenia have been tested mainly in those with age-related sarcopenia; these include aerobic and resistance exercise and nutritional supplements, which has been shown and confirmed over the past 3 decades.[42] Many reports confirm the value of diet and exercise in the treatment of NAFLD. A recent publication of clinical practice guidelines for treatment of NAFLD summarizes the current evidence-based interventions for lifestyle modification in the treatment of NAFLD and provides best practice advice statements to address key issues in clinical management.[43] Recommendations include weight loss and reduction of total carbohydrate, fat, and sugar consumption, coupled with an increase in physical activity.

Although exercise is not an effective strategy for weight loss, it has been shown to help maintain weight loss. It is thought that exercise contributes to improvements in NAFLD and sarcopenia outcomes via a variety of different pathways. It is likely that exercise reduces visceral fat. In a 12-week controlled trial comparing an aerobic exercise intervention with no exercise, as expected, exercise training led to a reduction in visceral adipose tissue mass (probably through lipolysis) and is mediated by the myokine IL-6, which is secreted directly by muscle as a result of exercise. In this setting, IL-6 functions as a hormone, does not function as an inflammatory cytokine, but stimulates glucose uptake and lipolysis. It may also facilitate mobilization of myosteatosis.[44] The outcome of the study was a reduction in NAFLD and improvement in sarcopenia. The combination of progressive resistance training and aerobic exercise results in maximum benefits to weight loss, increase in skeletal muscle mass and strength gain, and improvements in insulin resistance in trials of older individuals aged 60 to –80 years with obesity. The highest muscle gains of up to about 1 kg after 6 months were observed in the resistance exercise group.

Resistance exercise is effective and safe to prevent muscle loss even in old (mean age 87 years) and frail individuals, potentially by also decreasing skeletal muscle apoptosis and improving mitochondrial function and diminishing muscle apoptosis.[45] Treatments for sarcopenia have been shown to be useful, but many investigators indicate that prevention of sarcopenia is more effective. Critical to both treatment and prevention is assessment of what is referred to as "good" protein intake. The issue of what is "good" (or best) source of protein is as yet unresolved. Many believe animal protein is optimal because it is easily digested and absorbed. Many studies have supplemented diet with animal protein (whey) but others believe plant-sourced protein is best. Nonetheless, optimal dietary protein intake, daily 1.0 to 1.2 g/kg with 25 to 30 g of high-quality protein per meal, is what is recommended to prevent sarcopenia. All studies indicate the importance of complete amino acids, branch chain amino acids, and in particular, leucine and cheese and milk protein (whey).[46] Recent studies have demonstrated the value of adding vitamin D to this regimen. A review of several controlled trials for dietary interventions effective for treating sarcopenia has recently been published.[47]

As of this writing, specific trials to evaluate the best regiment for diet, exercise, and functional outcomes have not yet been reported, but it is very likely that interventions targeting treatment of NAFLD focus on weight loss and increased activity, and efforts to increase muscle mass using resistance and aerobic exercise are likely to have good outcomes in people with sarcopenic obesity.

The substantial challenges to improved health and functional outcomes that face the health care community and patients with this disorder are the following: (1) educating stakeholders about the health risks of sarcopenic NAFLD; (2) establishing generally acceptable diagnostic criteria and readily available tools with which to determine these; and (3) making a commitment to instituting the demonstrated effective lifestyle changes.

CLINICS CARE POINTS

- Definition of sarcopenia: focuses on low muscle strength as a key characteristic of sarcopenia, uses detection of low muscle quantity and quality to confirm the sarcopenia diagnosis, and identifies poor physical performance as indicative of severe sarcopenia.
- Evaluation of sarcopenia should consist of measures of muscle strength, physical function, such as ambulation or sit-to-stand, and appendicular muscle mass.
- The combination of NAFLD and sarcopenia is a risk for all cause mortality and associated with high risk for cancer and diabetes-related mortality. This combination should be screened for.
- Treatment for sarcopenic obesity includes aerobic and resistance exercise, 25-30 g high quality protein per meal and control(if present) of pre-diabetes/diabetes.

REFERENCES

1. Rosenberg IH. Summary comments. Am J Clin Nutr 1989;50(5):1231–3.
2. Cruz-Jentoft AJ, Bahat G, Bauer J, et al. Sarcopenia: revised European consensus on definition and diagnosis. Age Ageing 2019;48(1):16–31.
3. Chen LK, Woo J, Assantachai P, et al. Asian working group for sarcopenia: 2019 consensus update on sarcopenia diagnosis and treatment. J Am Med Dir Assoc 2020;21(3):300–307 e302.
4. McLean RR, Shardell MD, Alley DE, et al. Criteria for clinically relevant weakness and low lean mass and their longitudinal association with incident mobility impairment and mortality: the foundation for the National Institutes of Health (FNIH) sarcopenia project. J Gerontol A Biol Sci Med Sci 2014;69(5):576–83.
5. Kim TN, Park MS, Lee EJ, et al. Comparisons of three different methods for defining sarcopenia: an aspect of cardiometabolic risk. Sci Rep 2017;7(1):6491.
6. Nishikawa H, Shiraki M, Hiramatsu A, et al. Japan Society of Hepatology guidelines for sarcopenia in liver disease (1st edition): recommendation from the working group for creation of sarcopenia assessment criteria. Hepatol Res 2016; 46(10):951–63.
7. Hamaguchi Y, Kaido T, Okumura S, et al. Proposal for new diagnostic criteria for low skeletal muscle mass based on computed tomography imaging in Asian adults. Nutrition 2016;32(11–12):1200–5.
8. Guralnik JM, Simonsick EM, Ferrucci L, et al. A short physical performance battery assessing lower extremity function: association with self-reported disability

and prediction of mortality and nursing home admission. J Gerontol 1994;49(2): M85–94.
9. Moon JH, Koo BK, Kim W. Non-alcoholic fatty liver disease and sarcopenia additively increase mortality: a Korean nationwide survey. J Cachexia Sarcopenia Muscle 2021;12(4):964–72.
10. Petermann-Rocha F, Gray SR, Forrest E, et al. Associations of muscle mass and grip strength with severe NAFLD: a prospective study of 333,295 UK Biobank participants. J Hepatol 2022;76(5):1021–9.
11. Chun HS, Lee M, Lee HA, et al. Association of Physical Activity With Risk of Liver Fibrosis, Sarcopenia, and Cardiovascular Disease in Nonalcoholic Fatty Liver Disease. Clin Gastroenterol Hepatol 2023;21(2):358–69.e12.
12. Hsieh YC, Joo SK, Koo BK, et al. Innovative Target Exploration of NAFLD (ITEN) Consortium. Myosteatosis, but not Sarcopenia, Predisposes NAFLD Subjects to Early Steatohepatitis and Fibrosis Progression. Clin Gastroenterol Hepatol 2023;21(2):388–97.e10.
13. Lee YH, Kim SU, Song K, et al. Sarcopenia is associated with significant liver fibrosis independently of obesity and insulin resistance in nonalcoholic fatty liver disease: nationwide surveys (KNHANES 2008-2011). Hepatology 2016;63(3): 776–86.
14. Koo BK, Kim D, Joo SK, et al. Sarcopenia is an independent risk factor for nonalcoholic steatohepatitis and significant fibrosis. J Hepatol 2017;66(1):123–31.
15. Petta S, Ciminnisi S, Di Marco V, et al. Sarcopenia is associated with severe liver fibrosis in patients with non-alcoholic fatty liver disease. Aliment Pharmacol Ther 2017;45(4):510–8.
16. Pan X, Han Y, Zou T, et al. Sarcopenia contributes to the progression of nonalcoholic fatty liver disease- related fibrosis: a meta-analysis. Dig Dis 2018;36(6): 427–36.
17. Golabi P, Gerber L, Paik JM, et al. Contribution of sarcopenia and physical inactivity to mortality in people with non-alcoholic fatty liver disease. JHEP Rep 2020; 2(6):100171.
18. Sun X, Liu Z, Chen F, et al. Sarcopenia modifies the associations of nonalcoholic fatty liver disease with all-cause and cardiovascular mortality among older adults. Sci Rep 2021;11(1):15647.
19. Kim D, Wijarnpreecha K, Sandhu KK, et al. Sarcopenia in nonalcoholic fatty liver disease and all-cause and cause-specific mortality in the United States. Liver Int 2021;41(8):1832–40.
20. Scimeca M, Piccirilli E, Mastrangeli F, et al. Bone Morphogenetic Proteins and myostatin pathways: key mediator of human sarcopenia. J Transl Med 2017; 15(1):34.
21. Tarantino U, Scimeca M, Piccirilli E, et al. Sarcopenia: a histological and immunohistochemical study on age-related muscle impairment. Aging Clin Exp Res 2015;27(Suppl 1):S51–60.
22. Lee YH, Jung KS, Kim SU, et al. Sarcopaenia is associated with NAFLD independently of obesity and insulin resistance: nationwide surveys (KNHANES 2008-2011). J Hepatol 2015;63(2):486–93.
23. Batsis JA, Villareal DT. Sarcopenic obesity in older adults: aetiology, epidemiology and treatment strategies. Nat Rev Endocrinol 2018;14(9):513–37.
24. Zambon Azevedo V, Silaghi CA, Maurel T, et al. Impact of sarcopenia on the severity of the liver damage in patients with non-alcoholic fatty liver disease. Front Nutr 2021;8:774030.

25. Guo W, Zhao X, Miao M, et al. Association between skeletal muscle mass and severity of steatosis and fibrosis in non-alcoholic fatty liver disease. Front Nutr 2022;9:883015.
26. van Hall G, Steensberg A, Sacchetti M, et al. Interleukin-6 stimulates lipolysis and fat oxidation in humans. J Clin Endocrinol Metab 2003;88(7):3005–10.
27. Pedersen BK, Febbraio MA. Muscle as an endocrine organ: focus on muscle-derived interleukin-6. Physiol Rev 2008;88(4):1379–406.
28. Febbraio MA, Steensberg A, Keller C, et al. Glucose ingestion attenuates interleukin-6 release from contracting skeletal muscle in humans. J Physiol 2003;549(Pt 2):607–12.
29. Wallenius V, Wallenius K, Ahren B, et al. Interleukin-6-deficient mice develop mature-onset obesity. Nat Med 2002;8(1):75–9.
30. Krook A, Wallberg-Henriksson H, Zierath JR. Sending the signal: molecular mechanisms regulating glucose uptake. Med Sci Sports Exerc 2004;36(7):1212–7.
31. Pedersen BK, Fischer CP. Beneficial health effects of exercise–the role of IL-6 as a myokine. Trends Pharmacol Sci 2007;28(4):152–6.
32. Olsen RH, Krogh-Madsen R, Thomsen C, et al. Metabolic responses to reduced daily steps in healthy nonexercising men. JAMA 2008;299(11):1261–3.
33. Nachit M, Lanthier N, Rodriguez J, et al. A dynamic association between myosteatosis and liver stiffness: results from a prospective interventional study in obese patients. JHEP Rep 2021;3(4):100323.
34. Linge J, Petersson M, Forsgren MF, et al. Adverse muscle composition predicts all-cause mortality in the UK Biobank imaging study. J Cachexia Sarcopenia Muscle 2021;12(6):1513–26.
35. Cho KA, Kang PB. PLIN2 inhibits insulin-induced glucose uptake in myoblasts through the activation of the NLRP3 inflammasome. Int J Mol Med 2015;36(3):839–44.
36. Kwon Y, Jeong SJ. Relative skeletal muscle mass is an important factor in non-alcoholic fatty liver disease in non-obese children and adolescents. J Clin Med 2020;9(10):3355–64.
37. Baumgartner RN, Wayne SJ, Waters DL, et al. Sarcopenic obesity predicts instrumental activities of daily living disability in the elderly. Obes Res 2004;12(12):1995–2004.
38. Rolland Y, Lauwers-Cances V, Cristini C, et al. Difficulties with physical function associated with obesity, sarcopenia, and sarcopenic-obesity in community-dwelling elderly women: the EPIDOS (EPIDemiologie de l'OSteoporose) Study. Am J Clin Nutr 2009;89(6):1895–900.
39. Whitmer RA, Gustafson DR, Barrett-Connor E, et al. Central obesity and increased risk of dementia more than three decades later. Neurology 2008;71(14):1057–64.
40. Karakousis ND, Chrysavgis L, Chatzigeorgiou A, et al. Frailty in metabolic syndrome, focusing on nonalcoholic fatty liver disease. Ann Gastroenterol 2022;35(3):234–42.
41. Scarpecci F, Cannas A, Sanniti B, et al. [Operation "Provide Comfort": use of techniques of locoregional anesthesia]. Minerva Anestesiol 1991;57(12):1684.
42. Fiatarone MA, O'Neill EF, Ryan ND, et al. Exercise training and nutritional supplementation for physical frailty in very elderly people. N Engl J Med 1994;330(25):1769–75.
43. Younossi ZM, Corey KE, Lim JK. AGA clinical practice update on lifestyle modification using diet and exercise to achieve weight loss in the management of nonalcoholic fatty liver disease: expert review. Gastroenterology 2021;160(3):912–8.

44. Severinsen MCK, Pedersen BK. Muscle-organ crosstalk: the emerging roles of myokines. Endocr Rev 2020;41(4):594–609.
45. Davidson LE, Hudson R, Kilpatrick K, et al. Effects of exercise modality on insulin resistance and functional limitation in older adults: a randomized controlled trial. Arch Intern Med 2009;169(2):122–31.
46. Yanai H. Nutrition for sarcopenia. J Clin Med Res 2015;7(12):926–31.
47. Cereda E, Pisati R, Rondanelli M, et al. Whey protein, leucine- and vitamin-D-enriched oral nutritional supplementation for the treatment of sarcopenia. Nutrients 2022;14(7):1524–44.

Nonalcoholic Fatty Liver Disease in Asia, Africa, and Middle East Region

Janus Ong, MD[a], Khalid Alswat, MD[b], Saeed Hamid, MD[c], Mohamed El-Kassas, MD[d,*]

KEYWORDS

- Nonalcoholic steatohepatitis (NASH) • Nonalcoholic fatty liver disease (NAFLD)
- Africa • MENA • Asia • Epidemiology • Prevalence

KEY POINTS

- Nonalcoholic fatty liver disease (NAFLD) is one of the leading causes of chronic hepatic disease worldwide.
- Southeast Asia had the highest prevalence of NAFLD by subregion in Asia (42.04%).
- NAFLD is highly prevalent in South Asia reaching 32.74% in India, 33.86% in Bangladesh, and 24.74% in Sri Lanka.
- There is scant evidence and conflicting data on the prevalence of NAFLD in the Middle East and North Africa ranging from 3 to 44 %.
- There are little data on the incidence and prevalence of NAFLD in sub-Saharan Africa ranging from 9.0% in Nigeria to 20.0% in Sudan.

INTRODUCTION

Nonalcoholic fatty liver disease (NAFLD) is one of the leading causes of chronic hepatic disease worldwide.[1] It consists of a histopathological spectrum that encompasses nonalcoholic fatty liver (NAFL), nonalcoholic steatohepatitis (NASH), fibrosis, cirrhosis, and hepatocellular carcinoma (HCC).[2] The global prevalence of the disease differs, ranging from 6% to 35%.[3] In a meta-analysis of the worldwide epidemiological data of NAFLD, the African, Asian, and Middle Eastern countries had variable prevalence rates of the said disorder despite being distinct models from the western patterns of NAFLD (**Fig. 1**).[4] Furthermore, with an upsurge in NAFLD and NASH predisposing factors such as obesity, metabolic syndrome (MetS), and type 2 diabetes mellitus (T2DM), the prevalence is expected to rise even more.

[a] College of Medicine, University of the Philippines, Manila, Philippines; [b] Department of Medicine, Liver Disease Research Centre, College of Medicine, King Saud University, Riyadh, Saudi Arabia; [c] Department of Medicine, Aga Khan University, Karachi, Pakistan; [d] Endemic Medicine Department, Faculty of Medicine, Helwan University, Ain Helwan, Cairo 11795, Egypt
* Corresponding author.
E-mail address: m_elkassas@hq.helwan.edu.eg

Clin Liver Dis 27 (2023) 287–299
https://doi.org/10.1016/j.cld.2023.01.014
liver.theclinics.com

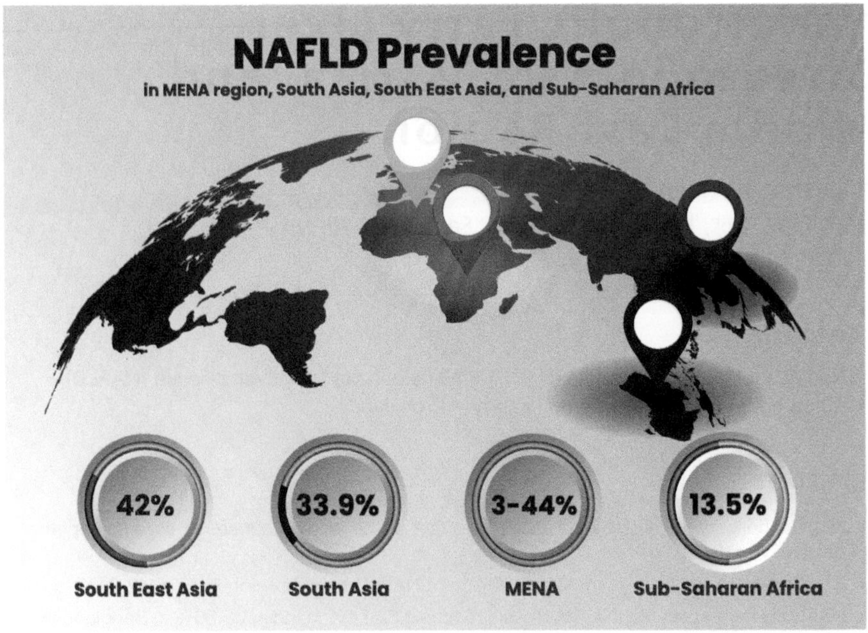

Fig. 1. NAFLD prevalence in MENA region, South Asia, South East Asia, and Sub-Saharan Africa.

Owing to the apparent rising prevalence of NAFLD, its management has become one of the world's most pressing concerns. Because the pathophysiology of NAFLD is uncertain, NAFLD preventative approaches are confined to reducing associated risk factors. As a result, preventing NAFLD risk factors such as obesity, insulin resistance, T2DM, and MetS is the most effective strategy for lowering the global prevalence of NAFLD.[5]

The widely known chronic liver disease in the Western world is NAFLD, which is yet to be researched in most Asian, African, and Middle Eastern regions. As a result, an effort has been made to depict the epidemiology, associated predictors and risk factors, management, and challenges connected with preventing the stated disease in these regions.

NONALCOHOLIC FATTY LIVER DISEASE AND NONALCOHOLIC STEATOHEPATITIS IN SOUTHEAST ASIA

Southeast Asia (SEA) is situated south of China, east of the Indian subcontinent, and northwest of Australia. It comprises 11 countries distributed into continental (Cambodia, Laos, Myanmar, Malaysia, Thailand, and Vietnam) and maritime SEA (Brunei, East Timor, Indonesia, Philippines, and Singapore). The region has significant diversity in religion, culture, history, and economy, which impacts the presentation and management of NAFLD.

Epidemiology of Nonalcoholic Fatty Liver Disease in Southeast Asia

The prevalence of NAFLD in SEA is less studied than in other countries in the Asia-Pacific region. In a large meta-analysis that evaluated the epidemiology of NAFLD in Asia, only seven studies from four Southeast Asian countries were included.[6]

Nevertheless, in this meta-analysis, SEA had the highest prevalence of NAFLD by subregion in Asia (42.04% vs 29.62% overall NAFLD prevalence in Asia), and Indonesia had the highest prevalence (51%) among all countries. Other Southeast Asian countries also had NAFLD prevalence higher than the overall prevalence in Asia (Malaysia 38% and Singapore 40%). The prevalence was higher in patients with risk factors for NAFLD, including T2DM, overweight and obesity, and MetS. However, NAFLD and NASH can be observed in lean or nonobese patients and accounts for 22% of all NAFLD patients.[7] This was observed in an extensive international NAFLD registry in Asian countries wherein 34% of the patients were from SEA.[2] The variation in the prevalence of NAFLD among Southeast Asian countries and even within Southeast Asian countries can be attributed to differences in ethnicity, socioeconomic status, lifestyle, and diet.[8,9] Of concern is the finding that the prevalence of NAFLD in Asia and SEA has increased and is expected to increase in the coming years.[10] The increase in the prevalence of NAFLD and NASH was shown to be highest in Singapore in a modeling study that included four countries in Asia.[11] This increase has been attributed to the ongoing epidemic of obesity and T2DM in the region.[10,12]

Clinical Presentation of Nonalcoholic Fatty Liver Disease in Southeast Asia

Patients with NAFLD in SEA were younger (43 years vs 53 years for Western Pacific and 48 years for Eastern Mediterranean) compared with other subregions in Asia.[13] There were, however, no differences in the mean body mass index (BMI), and alanine transaminase (ALT) and aspartate transaminase (AST) levels among the subregions in Asia. The mean ALT and AST levels were only slightly higher than normal.[13] These characteristics highlight the lack of utility of age or abnormal serum transaminases as criteria to screen for NAFLD. In a registry of biopsy-proven NAFLD patients, of which 44% were from SEA, 63% had NASH, and 17% had advanced fibrosis.[14] Predictors of NASH were body mass index $\geq$30 kg/m^2, T2DM, dyslipidemia, and elevated ALT and AST. Age $\geq$55 years, T2DM, and platelet count <150 $\times$ 10^9/L were predictors of advanced fibrosis. An Asia-Pacific NAFLD advanced fibrosis risk score was developed, and a low score had a negative predictive value of 96% for advanced fibrosis.[14] Among non-obese NAFLD patients in SEA, a substantial number had NASH (50%) and significant fibrosis (14%); however, these proportions were lower compared with obese NAFLD patients suggesting that nonobese NAFLD patients belong to the less severe spectrum of NAFLD.[7]

One unique aspect of the presentation of NAFLD in SEA is the presence of concurrent chronic hepatitis B (CHB). SEA has one of the highest Hepatitis B prevalence rates at 6.2%,[15]; therefore, concurrent NAFLD and CHB are not uncommon.[9] NAFLD is observed in 30% to 34% of patients with CHB.[9] The increase in the prevalence of NAFLD among CHB is paralleled by the rise in the prevalence of metabolic comorbidities among NAFLD patients.[16] Metabolic comorbidities and NAFLD in patients with CHB are associated with a higher likelihood of advanced fibrosis, cirrhosis, HCC, and liver-related mortality, which is more pronounced in patients with low viral load.[17,18] Patients with NAFLD and CHB should have aggressive management of their metabolic comorbidities.

NAFLD is the fastest growing cause of HCC in the West.[19] In Asia, NAFLD is also becoming a significant risk factor for HCC as the risk for HBV- and HCV-related HCC has decreased.[20] Screening for HCC is recommended in NAFLD patients with cirrhosis. For those who do not have apparent signs of cirrhosis, the use of noninvasive tests of fibrosis such as AST to Platelet Ratio Index (APRI) and liver stiffness measurement by elastography can identify patients with cirrhosis who should undergo screening and surveillance.[21]

Awareness

There is limited awareness about NAFLD in SEA. A survey conducted in Singapore showed that awareness about NAFLD and its risk factors and complications is suboptimal in the general population.[22] The same findings were observed in other countries in SEA in a more extensive study that looked at an overall liver index.[23] Even among physicians, a significant knowledge gap has been observed in identifying, diagnosing, and managing NAFLD. This was shown in a global survey that included specialists (gastroenterologists, hepatologists, and endocrinologists) and primary care physicians. Specialists had greater knowledge about NAFLD than primary care physicians.[24] In a global survey of 102 countries on NAFLD preparedness, no country had a national strategy for NAFLD, and only 32 had a national guideline on NAFLD.[25] None of the Southeast Asian countries surveyed had a national strategy or guidelines. However, most of the countries in SEA had an overall NAFLD policy score better than half of the countries in the survey. Only Thailand in SEA had a government-funded campaign on liver health, and only Malaysia had a civil society group focused on NAFLD. There is a pressing need to develop education programs to raise awareness among the general public and health care providers and to develop a comprehensive public health response to NAFLD.[26]

Management of Nonalcoholic Fatty Liver Disease in Southeast Asia

Lifestyle modification that includes dietary adjustments and structured exercise to achieve weight loss is recommended and is considered the cornerstone of the treatment of NAFLD by the APASL Guidelines on NAFLD.[27] For pharmacologic therapy, The Asian Pacific Association for the Study of the Liver (APASL) guidelines state that pioglitazone can be considered in prediabetic and diabetic patients with steatohepatitis for short-term use with careful consideration of other comorbid conditions such as osteoporosis and heart disease.[23] For Vitamin E and the other antidiabetic medications, such as the glucagon-like peptide 1 agonist (GLP-1a) and sodium-glucose cotransporter 2 inhibitors (SGLT2i), whereas there are promising studies of their benefit, no firm recommendations have been given pending further studies.[27,28] There are limited studies on pharmacologic treatment of NAFLD in SEA, and Asian patients, in general, are underrepresented in clinical trials.[29] Silymarin, which has antioxidant, anti-inflammatory, antifibrotic, as well as metabolic effects, was shown in one study to improve fibrosis in Malaysian patients with NASH.[30] The results will need confirmation in a larger trial. Dapagliflozin, a highly selective SGLT2i, was shown in a Thai study to lead to hepatic and visceral fat reduction and improved liver enzymes in diabetic patients with NAFLD.[31] The GLP-1a, liraglutide, was found to be as effective as an intensive combined diet and exercise regimen in decreasing weight as well as improving serum aminotransferases, liver fat, and liver stiffness among patients with NAFLD in Singapore.[32] In a modeling study done for Thai patients, weight reduction was the preferred treatment over Pioglitazone and Vitamin E and was shown to be cost-saving.[33] It is concerning that in a study of Asian patients with biopsy-proven NAFLD, of which more than half had NASH and close to one-fifth of the patients had advanced fibrosis; only 1.7% were referred for a structured lifestyle program.[14] This is especially important since, in a sizeable multicenter study of NAFLD patients, the majority had an unhealthy lifestyle and physical inactivity.[34]

NONALCOHOLIC FATTY LIVER DISEASE IN SOUTH ASIA

According to the South Asian Association for Regional Cooperation (SAARC) membership, South Asia comprises the following countries: Afghanistan, Bangladesh, Bhutan,

India, Maldives, Nepal, Pakistan, and Sri Lanka. The population of the region stood at 1.94 billion in 2020, nearly a quarter of the world's population, with a gross domestic product per capita of $2,260 (nominal) in 2022 and purchasing power parity of $8,000.[35]

Epidemiology and Risk Factors for Nonalcoholic Fatty Liver Disease in South Asia

A systematic review of NAFLD prevalence, incidence, and outcome between 1999 and 2019 shows that the overall prevalence of NAFLD increased from 25.28% to 33.90% between 1999 and 2017 (2). In South Asia currently, NAFLD prevalence is 32.74% in India, 33.86% in Bangladesh, and 24.74% in Sri Lanka, based on an ultrasound diagnosis.[36]

The significant risk factors attributed to the development of NAFLD are prevalent in the South Asian populations. However, there are essential differences in the prevalence and manifestations of these patient-related factors. For example, the prevalence of T2DM and prediabetes is approximately 25% in South Asians, which is one of the highest prevalences globally. For Pakistan, the comparative T2DM prevalence (prevalence standardized to the world population (aged 20 to 79) for the respective year) is suggested to be 30.8% in 2021.[37] T2DM, in particular, is on the rise in South Asians. In comparison, people from South Asian communities living in the western world are six times more likely to have T2DM than the general population, coupled with poorer diabetes management.

Obesity is also rising in South Asia, both among young children and adults, due mainly to changing lifestyles and eating patterns. South Asians are more likely to have central obesity, which is strongly associated with T2DM and NAFLD. According to the Indian Council of Medical Research (ICMR)-India Diabetes (INDIAB) study 2015, obesity and central obesity prevalence rates vary from 11.8% to 31.3% and 16.9% to 36.3%, respectively.[38] Lower BMI values are suggested as ideal for South Asians, as complications of obesity, particularly cardiovascular disease, occur much more frequently at a lower BMI level compared with western white populations, for example,

Obesity in the South Asian context has several important differences contributing to the pathophysiology of body fat. For example, for an equivalent BMI, body fat level is higher, particularly in South Asians, compared with white Caucasians.[39] This leads to a high prevalence of abdominal obesity, with more intra-abdominal and truncal subcutaneous adiposity and a more significant accumulation of fat in the liver.[40] These changes can cause a higher level of insulin resistance, with its accompanying features of the MetS, including dyslipidemia.

Clinical Features of Nonalcoholic Fatty Liver Disease in South Asia

A longitudinal study from India of 4313 followed at 23 centers shows that 10.6% of the patients were lean, 16.2% overweight, and 72.7% obese. MetS in 42.7%, and at least one metabolic risk factor was present in 92.6% of patients. Of the various components of MetS, central obesity (83.9%) was the most common. Fibrosis measurement using multiple modalities showed that 20% of patients have evidence of significant fibrosis, and 10% had evidence of cirrhosis with a Fibroscan value of > 13 kPa.[41] Both hepatic and extrahepatic outcomes were worse in patients with compensated NASH cirrhosis than those with and without significant fibrosis. Patients with compensated cirrhosis (Liver Stiffness Measurement [LSM] ‡ 13 kPa, $n = 71$ [5.2%]), 26 (36.7%) had hepatic events (jaundice 3, upper Gastrointestinal [UGI] bleed 3, HCC 2, hepatic encephalopathy [HE] 8, and ascites 10), and 8 (11.3%) had extrahepatic events (chronic kidney disease [CKD] 5, myocardial infarction 2, and bone fracture). South Asian patients have higher cardiac events, CKD, and bone fractures, compared with reports from the west.

Lean/Nonobese Nonalcoholic Fatty Liver Disease in South Asia

Lean and nonobese NAFLD was considered more prevalent, particularly in South Asian populations, but recent meta-analyses suggest it is a global phenomenon. Still, the prevalence of lean NAFLD was higher at 12% in Asians compared with other regions. Asians are, however, considered to be lean at lower BMIs (<23 kg/m^2) and overweight if they have a BMI of 23.0 to 27.5 kg/m^2, compared with non-Asian populations. On the basis of these parameters, the prevalence of nonobese NAFLD was estimated at 40.9% in South Asia, with 47.7% on average in India, 31.3% in Sri Lanka, 25.6% in Bangladesh, and 22.5% in Pakistan.[36]

Lean/nonobese NAFLD is closely associated with MetS. Patients with lean NAFLD have a higher mean systolic and diastolic blood pressure, hemoglobin A1C, and HOMA-IR when compared with obese NAFLD patients. Insulin resistance may be similar in lean versus obese NAFLD. However, compared with healthy subjects who were lean without NAFLD, subjects with lean NAFLD had higher mean BMI, diastolic blood pressure, hemoglobin A1C, and insulin resistance. Some association is suggested with the presence of a PNPLA3 variant in lean NAFLD patients from a Sri Lankan study.[42] Overall, Lean NAFLD is associated with better outcomes when compared with obese NAFLD patients.[43]

NONALCOHOLIC FATTY LIVER DISEASE IN THE MIDDLE EAST AND NORTH AFRICA REGION

Epidemiology of Nonalcoholic Fatty Liver Disease in the Middle East and North Africa Region

There is scant evidence from limited investigations with various classifications and significant design flaws on the prevalence of NAFLD in the Middle East and North Africa (MENA). The prevalence ranges from 3% to 44%.[44,45] According to estimates, the prevalence of this disease in Saudi Arabia will rise to 31.7% by 2030, whereas in the United Arab Emirates, it is estimated to expand to 30.2% by 2030.[46] Because of multiple major drivers such as obesity and T2DM, the incidence of the disease in the territory is significant and expected to rise by more than 30% within the next years.[4] According to Sohrabpour and colleagues,[47] the prevalence rate was 33.3%, 21.5%, and 43.8% in Kuwait, South Iran, and northern Iran, respectively, but research was undertaken in 2018 assessed the prevalence to be 25% in both KSA and UAE.[46] Between 2009 and 2019, death rates owing to NAFLD increased significantly in the United Arab Emirates and Syria, which were the dominating nations in this category; whereas, countries like Oman, Kuwait, and Afghanistan showed better mortality patterns.[48]

Disease Burden

Until 2030, the occurrence of NAFLD is expected to rise in tandem with the incidence of obesity and diabetes. According to Alswat and colleagues,[46] there will be approximately 12,534,000 NAFLD occurrences in Saudi Arabia by 2030 and 372,000 cases in the UAE.

It is well known that the rise of NASH coincides with rising obesity and T2DM preponderance, and Middle Eastern countries have some of the highest percentages of adult obesity and T2DM in the world. According to one estimate, each Middle Eastern country will need to spend more than 5% of its yearly health budget to tackle the NASH epidemic and its consequences. Most of the expenditures associated with NASH maintenance are associated with the disease's latter stages. The need for quick attention and action is clear, with the proportion of early fibrosis episodes and HCC cases expected to rise considerably across three Middle Eastern countries (Saudi

Arabia, United Arab Emirates, and Kuwait) by the year 2030 if patient management remains unchanged.[49]

Risk factors of nonalcoholic fatty liver disease in the Middle East and North Africa region

Although obesity and T2DM are reported to be the root drivers of NAFLD, the vast plurality of nations in the MENA area experienced a >25% spike in the prevalence of NAFLD in a decade, notably between the years 2009 and 2019, with the United Arab Emirates, Syria, and Sudan at the forefront.[46,50] Numerous factors, including excessive fast food and carbohydrate intake, high-calorie energy intake, a decline in the consumption of fresh fruits and vegetables, a decline in physical activity, a tendency toward sedentary behavior, and others, may be to blame for the high prevalence of fatty liver disease in Middle East countries.[51,52]

Challenges to the disease in the Middle East and North Africa region

Despite the significant prevalence of NAFLD in these nations, no appropriate observational studies or localized clinical practice guidelines exist. MENA region countries will be unable to cope with the dearth of inexpensive, precise, reliable, and sensitive biochemical indicators, as well as the enormous financial expenses involved with the burden of NAFLD. The inability to conduct mass population monitoring, rising rates of obesity and diabetes in the community, insufficient health education in the population, and a shortage of health practitioners all contribute to the disease's incidence.[53]

NONALCOHOLIC FATTY LIVER DISEASE IN SUB-SAHARAN AFRICA

There are little data on the incidence and prevalence of NAFLD in Africa. According to a published meta-analysis, the prevalence of NAFLD was 13.5%, ranging from 9.0% in Nigeria to 20.0% in Sudan.[3,4,54] Sub-Saharan Africa is seeing a shift from the infectious illnesses of tuberculosis, malaria, and human immunodeficiency virus (HIV) to a rising burden of noncommunicable diseases (NCDs).[55] Therefore, it is expected that the highest worldwide rise in NCD-related mortality will occur in sub-Saharan Africa.[56] In sub-Saharan Africa, women were more likely than males to have MetS, whereas semi-urban and urban regions tended to have higher rates than rural ones. Southern Africa had the most significant prevalence of MetS, which is consistent with the region's higher rates of obesity. Eastern, western, and central Africa were next in line.[57,58]

Risk factors and prognostic indicators for nonalcoholic fatty liver disease in Sub-Saharan Africa

A high estimated pooled prevalence of significant metabolic risk factors among individuals with food insecurity (41.8%) is supported by a meta-analysis focused on the association between food insecurity and metabolic risk factors in sub-Saharan Africa.[59] The most common risk factors were overweight (15.8%), dyslipidemia (27.6%), and hypertension (24.7%). According to estimates based on GBD data (1990 to 2017), the age-standardized prevalence of NAFLD varied from 5.0 to 7.5% to 10.1% to 12.5% in sub-Saharan Africa, with 20.0% to 25.0% in Mauritius. The most significant estimated yearly percentage change of 1.26 to 1.5 was seen in Ghana and Benin.[60]

Obesity and T2DM are two risk factors for NAFLD that are rising in the region.[61,62] In Nigeria, the prevalence of NAFLD has been estimated to be between 1.2% and 4.5% in those who do not have T2DM and between 9.5% and 16.7% in those who have.[63,64] Central obesity (waist circumference >88 cm in women and >102 cm in men) and dyslipidemia was linked to NAFLD.[63] Over the last 10 years, the prevalence of obesity in

Ghana—as an example—has risen from 5% to 25%, with an associated probable increase in the incidence of NAFLD.[65,66]

High NAFLD prevalence has also been seen in central parts of sub-Saharan Africa. In urban-dwelling persons with MetS, the prevalence of NAFLD was 37.2% in Burundi and 38.7% in Congo Brazzaville.[67,68] Over the last 20 years, obesity has gradually grown in central Africa. For instance, it rose from 26% to 54% in Burundi and from 44% to 67% in the Democratic Republic of the Congo.[69]

The most significant rates of obesity may be seen in southern sub-Saharan Africa. Estimates of obesity based on age range from 11.7% in males to 37% in females.[70] The most afflicted countries in 2016 were Botswana and South Africa, where 26.5% to 38.6% of men and 50.7% to 64% of women were overweight, whereas 7% to 14.5% of men and 25.5% to 38.5% of women were obese.[71] Notably, NAFLD prevalence may be influenced by other variables that may impact HIV prevalence in southern sub-Saharan Africa, the area with the highest HIV prevalence worldwide, including HIV infection, its treatments, and its metabolic effects.[72]

A similar situation is present in the Eastern parts of the continent. In 2020, in a comprehensive review and meta-analysis of 16 studies including 19 527 individuals, adult Ethiopians were found to have a pooled prevalence of overweight and obesity of 19% and 5.4%, respectively.[73] A population-based NAFLD study from 2014 estimated a prevalence of 20% among Sudanese.[74]

Management of Nonalcoholic Fatty Liver Disease in Africa

Prevention must be the main focus of NAFLD care in sub-Saharan Africa. Despite the little information on NASH in sub-Saharan Africa currently available, metabolic conditions associated with NAFLD are widely distributed and becoming more common there. Through actively pursuing primary care and preventative efforts, sub-Saharan Africa is in a unique location to possibly balance the burden of NAFLD, which is now on the rise. A diagnosis must be made initially, and NAFLD screening is necessary. Targeted groups, such as those with obesity or T2DM, might benefit from using a straightforward, noninvasive, and affordable test like the Fibrosis-4 (FIB-4) index in nations with limited resources.[61]

CLINICS CARE POINTS

- Prevention must be the main focus of NAFLD care in Asia and Africa.
- A diagnosis of NAFLD must be made initially, and NAFLD screening is necessary.
- Targeted groups for screening , such as those with T2DM, might benefit from using a non-invasive, and affordable tests in limited resource countries.

DISCLOSURE

None related to this work.

REFERENCES

1. Musso G, Gambino R, Cassader M, et al. A meta-analysis of randomized trials for the treatment of nonalcoholic fatty liver disease. Hepatology 2010;52:79–104.
2. Perumpail BJ, Khan MA, Yoo ER, et al. Clinical epidemiology and disease burden of nonalcoholic fatty liver disease. World J Gastroenterol 2017;23:8263–76.

3. Sayiner M, Koenig A, Henry L, et al. Epidemiology of nonalcoholic fatty liver disease and nonalcoholic steatohepatitis in the United States and the rest of the world. Clin Liver Dis 2016;20:205–14.
4. Younossi ZM, Koenig AB, Abdelatif D, et al. Global epidemiology of nonalcoholic fatty liver disease—meta-analytic assessment of prevalence, incidence and outcomes. Hepatology 2016;64:73–84.
5. Zelber-Sagi S, Lotan R, Shlomai A, et al. Predictors for incidence and remission of NAFLD in the general populationpopulation during a seven-year prospective follow-up. J Hepatol 2012;56:1145–51.
6. Li J, Zou B, Yeo YH, et al. prevalence, incidence, and outcome of nonalcoholic fatty liver disease in Asia, 1999–2019: a systematic review and meta-analysis. Lancet Gastroenterology Hepatology 2019;4(5):389–98.
7. Tan EXX, Lee JWJ, Jumat NH, et al. Non-obese nonalcoholic fatty liver disease (NAFLD) in Asia: an international registry study. Metabolis 2022;126:154911.
8. Roza MAD, Goh GBB. The increasing clinical burden of NAFLD in Asia. Lancet Gastroenterology Hepatology 2019;4(5):333–4.
9. Wong SW, Chan WK. Epidemiology of nonalcoholic fatty liver disease in Asia. Indian J Gastroenterology 2020;39(1):1–8.
10. Koh JC, Loo WM, Goh KL, et al. Asian consensus on the relationship between obesity and gastrointestinal and liver diseases. J Gastroenterol Hepatol 2016; 31(8):1405–13.
11. Estes C, Razavi H, Loomba R, et al. Modeling the epidemic of nonalcoholic fatty liver disease demonstrates an exponential increase in burden of disease. Hepatology Baltim Md 2018;67(1):123–33.
12. Teufel F, Seiglie JA, Geldsetzer P, et al. Body-mass index and diabetes risk in 57 low-income and middle-income countries: a cross-sectional study of nationally representative, individual-level data in 685 616 adults. Lancet 2021; 398(10296):238–48.
13. Kam LY, Huang DQ, Teng MLP, et al. Clinical profiles of asians with NAFLD: a systematic review and meta-analysis. Digest Dis 2021;1–11. https://doi.org/10.1159/000521662.
14. Chan WK, Treeprasertsuk S, Imajo K, et al. Clinical features and treatment of nonalcoholic fatty liver disease across the Asia Pacific region-the GO ASIA initiative. Aliment Pharmacol Ther 2018;47(6):816–25.
15. Collaborators PO. Global prevalence, treatment, and prevention of hepatitis B virus infection in 2016: a modelling study. The lancet Gastroenterology & Hepatology 2018;3(6):383–403.
16. Wong GL, Wong VW, Yuen BW, et al. An Aging Population of Chronic Hepatitis B With Increasing Comorbidities: A Territory-Wide Study From 2000 to 2017. J Hepatol 2020;71(2):444–55.
17. Choi HSJ, Brouwer WP, Zanjir WMR, et al. Nonalcoholic steatohepatitis is associated with liver-related outcomes and all-cause mortality in chronic hepatitis B. Hepatology 2020;71(2):539–48.
18. Yu MW, Lin CL, Liu CJ, et al. Influence of metabolic risk factors on risk of hepatocellular carcinoma and liver-related death in men with chronic hepatitis B: a large cohort study. Gastroenterology 2017;153(4):1006–17.e5.
19. Younossi Z, Stepanova M, Ong JP, et al. Nonalcoholic steatohepatitis is the fastest growing cause of hepatocellular carcinoma in liver transplant candidates. Clinical gastroenterology and hepatology : the official clinical practice. Journal of the American Gastroenterological Association 2019;17(4):748–55.e3.

20. Zhang C, Cheng Y, Zhang S, et al. Changing epidemiology of hepatocellular carcinoma in Asia. Liver Int 2022. https://doi.org/10.1111/liv.15251.
21. Cheuk-Fung YT, Won LH, Kheong CW, et al. Asian perspective on NAFLD-associated HCC. J Hepatol 2021;76(3):726–34.
22. Tan C, Goh GB, Youn J, et al. Public awareness and knowledge of liver health and diseases in Singapore. J Gastroenterol Hepatol 2021;36(8):2292–302.
23. Lee MH, Ahn SH, Chan HLY, et al. Contextual and individual factors associated with knowledge, awareness and attitude on liver diseases: a large-scale Asian study. J Viral Hepatitis 2021. https://doi.org/10.1111/jvh.13636.
24. Younossi ZM, Ong JP, Takahashi H, et al. A global survey of physicians knowledge about nonalcoholic fatty liver disease. Clin Gastroenterol H 2022;20(6): e1456–68.
25. Lazarus JV, Mark HE, Villota-Rivas M, et al. The global NAFLD policy review and preparedness index: are countries ready to address this silent public health challenge? J Hepatol 2022;76(4):771–80.
26. Lazarus JV, Mark HE, Anstee QM, et al. Advancing the global public health agenda for NAFLD: a consensus statement. Nat Rev Gastroentero 2021;1–19. https://doi.org/10.1038/s41575-021-00523-4.
27. Eslam M, Sarin SK, Wong VWS, et al. The Asian Pacific Association for the study of the Liver clinical practice guidelines for the diagnosis and management of metabolic associated fatty liver disease. Hepatology International 2020; 5(1511–1520):1–31.
28. Chitturi S, Wong VWS, Chan WK, et al. The asia-pacific working party on nonalcoholic fatty liver disease guidelines 2017-part 2: management and special groups. J Gastroenterol Hepatol 2018;33(1):86–98.
29. Nakatsuka T, Tateishi R, Koike K. Changing clinical management of NAFLD in Asia. Liver Int 2021. https://doi.org/10.1111/liv.15046.
30. Kheong CW, Mustapha NRN, Mahadeva S. A randomized trial of silymarin for the treatment of nonalcoholic steatohepatitis. Clin Gastroenterol H 2017;15(12): 1940–9.e8.
31. Phrueksotsai S, Pinyopornpanish K, Euathrongchit J, et al. The effects of dapagliflozin on hepatic and visceral fat in type 2 diabetes patients with nonalcoholic fatty liver disease. J Gastroenterol Hepatol 2021;36(10):2952–9.
32. Khoo J, Hsiang J, Taneja R, et al. Comparative effects of liraglutide 3 mg vs structured lifestyle modification on body weight, liver fat and liver function in obese patients with nonalcoholic fatty liver disease: a pilot randomized trial. Diabetes Obes Metab 2017;19(12):1814–7.
33. Chongmelaxme B, Phisalprapa P, Sawangjit R, et al. Weight reduction and pioglitazone are cost-effective for the treatment of nonalcoholic fatty liver disease in Thailand. Pharmacoeconomics 2019;37(2):267–78.
34. Zhang X, Goh GB-B, Chan W, et al. Unhealthy lifestyle habits and physical inactivity among Asian patients with nonalcoholic fatty liver disease. Liver Int 2020; 40(11):2719–31.
35. Available at: https://mfasia.org/mfa_programs/advocacy/south-asian-association-for-regional-cooperation/. Accessed August 8, 2022.
36. Ye Q, Zou B, Yeo YH, et al. Global prevalence, incidence, and outcomes of non-obese or lean nonalcoholic fatty liver disease: a systematic review and meta-analysis. Lancet Gastroenterol Hepatol 2020. https://doi.org/10.1016/S2468-1253(19)30039-1.

37. Sun H, Saeedi P, Karuranga S, et al. IDF Diabetes Atlas: global, regional and country-level diabetes prevalence estimates for 2021 and projections for 2045. Diabetes Res Clin Pract 2022;183:109119.
38. Pradeepa R, Mohan Anjana R, Joshi SR, et al. Prevalence of generalized & abdominal obesity in urban & rural India- the ICMR - INDIAB Study. Indian J Med Res 2015;142(2):139–50.
39. Misra A, Khurana L. Obesity related non-communicable diseases: south Asians vs white Caucasians. Int J Obes 2011;35:167–87.
40. Misra A, Shrivastava U. Obesity and dyslipidemia in South Asians. Nutrients 2013;5:2708–33.
41. Duseja A, Singh SP, Mehta M, et al. Clinicopathological profile and outcome of a large cohort of patients with nonalcoholic fatty liver disease from south asia: interim results of the indian consortium on nonalcoholic fatty liver disease. Metab Syndr Relat Disord 2022;20(3):166–73.
42. Niriella MA, Kasturiratne A, Pathmeswaran A, et al. Lean nonalcoholic fatty liver disease (lean NAFLD): characteristics, metabolic outcomes and risk factors from a 7-year prospective, community cohort study from Sri Lanka. Hepatology International 2019;13:314–22.
43. Young S, Tariq R, Provenza J, et al. Prevalence and profile of nonalcoholic fatty liver disease in lean adults: systematic review and meta-analysis. Hepatology Communications 2020;4(7).
44. Al-Quorain A, Satti M, al-Hamdan AR, et al. Pattern of chronic liver disease in the eastern province of Saudi Arabia. A hospital-based clinicopathological study. Trop Geogr Med 1994;46:358–60, 79.
45. Ostovaneh MR, Zamani F, Ansari-Moghaddam A, et al. Nonalcoholic fatty liver: the association with metabolic abnormalities, body mass index and central obesity—a population-based study. Metab Syndr Relat Disord 2015;13:304–11.
46. Alswat K, Aljumah AA, Sanai FM, et al. Nonalcoholic fatty liver disease burden–Saudi Arabia and United Arab Emirates, 2017–2030. Saudi J Gastroenterol 2018;24:211–9 [Erratum appears in Saudi J Gastroenterol 2018;24(4):255].
47. Sohrabpour A, Rezvan H, Amini-Kafiabad S, et al. Prevalence of nonalcoholic steatohepatitis in Iran: a populationpopulation based study. Middle East J. Dig. Dis. 2010;2:14–9.
48. Golabi P, Paik JM, AlQahtani S, et al. Burden of nonalcoholic fatty liver disease in asia, the Middle East and North Africa: data from global burden of disease 2009-2019. J Hepatol 2021 Oct;75(4):795–809.
49. Sanai FM, Abaalkhail F, Hasan F, et al. Management of nonalcoholic fatty liver disease in the Middle East. World J Gastroenterol 2020;26(25):3528–41.
50. Anushiravani A, Ghajarieh Sepanlou S. Burden of liver diseases: a review from Iran. Middle East J Dig Dis 2019;11:189–91.
51. Inoue Y, Qin B, Poti J, et al. Epidemiology of obesity in adults: latest trends. Curr Obes Rep 2018 Dec;7(4):276–88.
52. Guthold R, Stevens GA, Riley LM, et al. Worldwide trends in insufficient physical activity from 2001 to 2016: a pooled analysis of 358 population-based surveys with 1.9 million participants. Lancet Glob Health 2018;6:1077–86.
53. Ahmed MH, Woodward C, Mital D. Metabolic clinic for individuals with HIV/AIDS: a commitment and vision to the future of HIV services. Cardiovascular Endocrinology 2017;6:109–12.
54. Younossi Z, Anstee QM, Marietti M, et al. Global burden of NAFLD and NASH: trends, predictions, risk factors and prevention. Nat Rev Gastroenterol Hepatol 2018;15:11–20.

55. Gouda HN, Charlson F, Sorsdahl K, et al. Burden of non-communicable diseases in sub-Saharan Africa, 1990–2017: results from the Global Burden of Disease Study 2017. Lancet Glob Health 2019;7:e1375–87.
56. Ezzati M, Pearson-Stuttard J, Bennett JE, et al. Acting on non-communicable diseases in low- and middle-income tropical countries. Nature 2018;559:507–16.
57. Jaspers Faijer-Westerink H, Kengne AP, Meeks KAC, et al. Prevalence of metabolic syndrome in sub-Saharan Africa: a systematic review and meta-analysis. Nutr Metab Cardiovasc Dis 2020;30:547–65.
58. NCD Risk Factor Collaboration (NCD-RisC)—Africa Working Group. Trends in obesity and diabetes across Africa from 1980 to 2014: an analysis of pooled population-based studies. Int J Epidemiol 2017;46:1421–32.
59. Nkambule SJ, Moodley I, Kuupiel D, et al. Association between food insecurity and key metabolic risk factors for diet-sensitive non-communicable diseases in sub-Saharan Africa: a systematic review and meta-analysis. Sci Rep 2021;11:5178.
60. Ge X, Zheng L, Wang M, et al. Prevalence trends in nonalcoholic fatty liver disease at the global, regional and national levels, 1990–2017: a population-based observational study. BMJ Open 2020;10:e036663.
61. Paruk IM, Pirie FJ, Motala AA. Nonalcoholic fatty liver disease in Africa: a hidden danger. Glob Health Epidemiol Genom 2019;4:e3.
62. Afolabi BI, Ibitoye BO, Ikem RT, et al. The relationship between glycaemic control and nonalcoholic fatty liver disease in Nigerian type 2 diabetic patients. J Natl Med Assoc 2018;110:256–64.
63. Olusanya TO, Lesi OA, Adeyomoye AA, et al. Non alcoholic fatty liver disease in a Nigerian population with type II diabetes mellitus. Pan Afr Med J 2016;24:20.
64. Onyekwere CA, Ogbera AO, Balogun BO. Nonalcoholic fatty liver disease and the metabolic syndrome in an urban hospital servingan African community. Ann Hepatol 2011;10:119–24.
65. Ofori-Asenso R, Agyeman AA, Laar A, et al. Overweight and obesity epidemic in Ghana-a systematic review and meta-analysis. BMC Public Health 2016;16:1239.
66. Biritwum R, Gyapong J, Mensah G. The epidemiology of obesity in Ghana. Ghana Med J 2005;39:82–5.
67. Ntagirabiri R, Cikomola J, Baransaka E, et al. Hepatic steatosis and metabolic syndrome in black African adult: Burundi case. J Afr Hepato Gastroenterol 2014;8:195–9.
68. Ahoui-Apendi C, Itoua-Ngaporo NA, Mongo-Onkouo A, et al. Hepatic steatosis in patients with metabolic syndrome at the Brazzaville university hospital center. Open J Gastroenterol 2020;10:119–27.
69. Agyemang C, Boatemaa S, Frempong GA, et al. Obesity in sub-Saharan Africa. In: Ahima R, editor. Metabolic syndrome. Cham: Springer; 2015. p. 1–33.
70. Ng M, Fleming T, Robinson M, et al. Global, regional, and national prevalence of overweight and obesity in children and adults during 1980–2013: a systematic analysis for the Global Burden of Disease Study 2013. Lancet 2014;384:766–81.
71. Global Health Data Exchange, Global burden of disease study 2019 (GBD 2019) socio-demographic index (SDI) 1950–2019, Available at: http://ghdx.healthdata.org/record/ihme-data/gbd-2019-sociodemographic-index-sdi-1950-2019. Accessed August 8, 2022.
72. Mac as J, Pineda JA, Real LM. Nonalcoholic fatty liver disease in HIV infection. AIDS Rev 2017;19:35–46.

73. Kassie AM, Abate BB, Kassaw MW. Prevalence of overweight/obesity among the adult population in Ethiopia: a systematic review and meta-analysis. BMJ Open 2020;10:e039200.
74. Almobarak AO, Barakat S, Khalifa MH, et al. Non alcoholic fatty liver disease (NAFLD) in a Sudanese population: what is the prevalence and risk factors? Arab J Gastroenterol 2014;15:12–5.

Nonalcoholic Fatty Liver Disease in Latin America and Australia

Marlen Ivon Castellanos-Fernandez, MD[a], Shreya C. Pal, MD[b,c], Marco Arrese, MD[d,e], Juan Pablo Arab, MD[d,f,g], Jacob George, MD[h], Nahum Méndez-Sánchez, MD, MSc, PhD[b,c,*]

KEYWORDS

• Fatty liver • Steatosis • Liver diseases • Cirrhosis • Mortality

KEY POINTS

- Prevalence of nonalcoholic fatty liver disease (NAFLD) in Latin America and Caribbean (LAC) varies subregionally, whereas in Australia, it is much homogenous.
- South America exhibiting the most rapid increase in the prevalence of NAFLD in recent years.
- Risk factors for NAFLD are continuously increasing in the LAC, Australia, and New Zealand.
- Differences in socioeconomic conditions, lifestyles, diets, and cultural traditions influence on the increasing incidence of NAFLD.
- Disparity in availability and accessibility to health care affects the outcomes.

INTRODUCTION

Lifestyle transformation during the past decades has had a large impact in the increasing incidence of noncommunicable disease. Since 1990, there has been a marked shift toward a greater proportion of disease burden from such diseases and injuries. Ischemic heart disease, diabetes, stroke, and chronic kidney disease have

[a] Institute of Gastroenterology, University of Medical Sciences of Havana, Cuba; [b] Faculty of Medicine, National Autonomous University of Mexico, Av. Universidad 3000, Coyoacán, Mexico City, Mexico; [c] Liver Research Unit, Medica Sur Clinic & Foundation, Mexico City, Mexico; [d] Departamento de Gastroenterologia, Escuela de Medicina, Pontificia Universidad Catolica de Chile, Santiago, Chile; [e] Centro de Envejecimiento y Regeneración (CARE), Facultad de Ciencias Biológicas, Pontificia Universidad Católica de Chile, Santiago, Chile; [f] Division of Gastroenterology, Department of Medicine, Schulich School of Medicine, Western University & London Health Sciences Centre, London, Ontario, Canada; [g] Alimentiv, London, Ontario, Canada; [h] Storr Liver Centre, The Westmead Institute for Medical Research, Westmead Hospital and University of Sydney, New South Wales, Australia
* Corresponding author. Liver Research Unit, Medica Sur Clinic & Foundation and Faculty of Medicine, National Autonomous University of Mexico, Mexico City, Mexico.
E-mail address: nmendez@medicasur.org.mx

Clin Liver Dis 27 (2023) 301–315
https://doi.org/10.1016/j.cld.2023.01.015
liver.theclinics.com

seen the largest absolute increases in number of disability-adjusted life-years lost between 1990 and 2019 and have been the major contributors to this disease shift.[1] In this context, due to parallel increases in the rates of obesity and type 2 diabetes (T2D) mellitus, chronic liver disease (CLD) related to nonalcoholic fatty liver disease (NAFLD) is also increasing globally with NAFLD now being the most prevalent liver disease worldwide.[2–4]

NAFLD comprises a spectrum of liver lesions spanning from isolated steatosis to nonalcoholic steatohepatitis (NASH).[5] This entity can lead to serious liver disease, including cirrhosis, cancer, and death. NAFLD and is considered a "silent" epidemic because most people with NAFLD are asymptomatic for many years until they develop advanced disease.[6] Of note, NAFLD is associated with substantial morbidity and mortality resulting in substantial health-care costs and economic losses[7,8]

Recently, an international expert panel recommended renaming NAFLD to metabolic-dysfunction-associated fatty liver disease[9,10] and suggested adopting a set of positive criteria to diagnose the disease that includes metabolic abnormalities and do not consider a limit for alcohol intake or the exclusion of other liver diseases.[9] To address the appropriate terminology for fatty liver disease, a global multisociety consensus group was recently created (recognized as NAFLD Nomenclature Consensus Task Force). Since a consensus about the new name has not been finalized, we will keep the acronym NAFLD throughout this article.

The global incidence of liver cirrhosis caused by NASH, the more progressive from of NAFLD, increased 106.12% from 1990 to 2017.[11] The highest age-standardized incidence rate was noted in Central Latin America where the maximum rate was in Mexico (19.67 per 1,000,000), followed by El Salvador (16.07 per 1,000,000) and Guatemala (15.97 per 1,000,000).[11]

The vast geographic spread of the Latin America and Caribbean (LAC) area, the regional diversity in terms of ethnics, social inequalities and fragmented health-care systems, disparities on diet and lifestyle among different countries and within countries along with possible genetic influences are factors that account for the wide variation of NAFLD prevalence among different countries.[6,12] However, there is not strong data regarding the natural history of NAFLD patients currently living in LAC.[13] In fact, most studies investigating the impact of Latino ethnicity on NAFLD were conducted on persons living in the United States where there are very different environmental and socioeconomic conditions that can affect the course of this liver disease.[14–16] Therefore, our current knowledge of NAFLD, by ethnicity from persons living in their respective LAC countries, is important for further understanding of the interplay between environment and genetic makeup in the development of this metabolically related liver disease. In the present review, we will review available data on epidemiology of fatty liver disease in LAC examining the current evidence regarding potential regional and/or racial peculiarities in Latin America. At the other end, we will examine data for fatty liver disease related to metabolic risk factors from Australia.

BACKGROUND CONCEPTS ON LATIN AMERICA AND CARIBBEAN AND AUSTRALIA

Latin America comprises the entire continent of South America in addition to Mexico, Central America, and the islands of the Caribbean whose inhabitants speak a Romance language. The people of this area were conquered and colonized by the Spaniards, Portuguese, and French during a period ranging from the late fifteenth century through the eighteenth century. Although many of the nations have experienced similar trends and have a common heritage, there are also enormous social and cultural differences among them. In addition to the ethnic admixture from Europe and the native indigenous population during the colonization period, LAC has also experienced a very large import from slave trading from Africa.[17] The slave trade between Africa and the Caribbean (Cuba and Dominican), Brazil, and other countries began soon after the conquest and grew in scale during the seventeenth century with the development of crop plantations most notably sugar cane.[18] Together these factors have created a very diverse ethnic makeup of the LAC region.

Lifestyle in LAC also historically differs among regions and is based on the living conditions in the regions. Related to sedentarism, one large section of the indigenous American population, the most numerous, based in Mesoamerica (central and southern Mexico and Guatemala) and the central Andes, were sedentary due to living in nations and districts with distinct borders and permanent intensive agriculture. This sustained people whether they lived in either an urban or rural community. These people and the Europeans tend to have more in common with each other than with other indigenous peoples of the LAC. Semisedentary is a descriptor used to define the group of indigenous peoples who are frequently moving to obtain their sources of food. This group is usually found in relatively temperate forested areas. The third category of indigenous people are defined as nonsedentary peoples because they have little or no stable food source and so move annually in small bands over large territories while hunting and gathering. This group is located in the plains and dense tropical forests.[17]

Despite these patterns of obtaining food, there has been a nutrition transition in LAC with easier access to less healthy food sources, which had led to the increase in obesity and other diet-related health problems. This transition began slowly in the late nineteenth century but rapidly increased in the 1960s. This shifting is particularly recognizable in the Caribbean region, which became dependent on food imports to provide food to its enslaved labor force, which seems to have started as early as the seventeenth century. Areas with extractive industries and export agriculture have also been major drivers of the nutritional transformation.[19]

The population composition legacy for NAFLD in Australia and New Zealand has many parallels to that in LAC. Australia is home to the world's oldest living continuous civilization in the Australian Indigenous peoples, while New Zealand is home to the Māori population. Since the arrival of Captain Cook and European settlement, traditional nomadic lifestyles among the indigenous people have been supplanted by urbanized populations reliant on food sources from both domestic and imported sources. During the past decades, Australia and New Zealand have also witnessed successive waves of immigration, not only from Asia, particular from Southeast Asia, but also from the Pacific Islands, the Middle East, South Asia, and more generally from across the globe. Thus, both nations today are truly multicultural and multiethnic, with distinct differences in food patterns and social behaviors. This has resulted in differences in the natural history and outcomes of fatty liver diseases ascribed to metabolic risks.

The current population of Latin America and the Caribbean is 664,658,655 as of Wednesday, May 4, 2022, based on the latest United Nations estimates. Thus, LAC represents 8.42% of the world population, ranking fourth among the regions of the world. The population density is 32/km^2, 82.5% of the population is urban, and the median age is 31 years.[20]

The populations of the countries in the region are of very unequal size. Almost 80% of the population lives in just 5 countries: Brazil, Mexico, Colombia, Argentina, and Peru. According to July 2015 estimates, Brazil and Mexico alone account for more than half of the region's population, with 204 and 121 million inhabitants, respectively. At the other extreme, the 20 or so Caribbean countries represent hardly ~ 7% of the total (https://population.un.org/wpp/).

LAC is the region of the world with the largest income disparities with no signs of expected substantial change in the short term or medium term. Poverty levels are highest among rural communities, among the indigenous populations and those of African origin (https://www.cepal.org/en/work-areas/population-and-development). Aging patterns vary substantially across the region but, regardless, the aged populations are projected to increase. Specifically, the aged populations of Bolivia, Guatemala, Haiti, Honduras, Nicaragua, and Paraguay are expected to reach 15% to 18% by 2050 while Belize, Colombia, Costa Rica, Ecuador, El Salvador, Guyana, Mexico, Peru, the Dominican Republic, and Venezuela will exceed 20%. Others such as the Bahamas, Brazil, Chile, Jamaica, Suriname, and Trinidad and Tobago sited the "advanced aging" countries were expected to grow rapidly, reaching 25% to 30% of their population by 2050. Argentina, Uruguay, Cuba, and several Caribbean islands (Netherlands Antilles, Barbados, Guadeloupe, Martinique, and Puerto Rico) are also experiencing a growth in the "very advanced aged" reaching more than 30% of the population by 2050[21] (CELADE: Latin-American and Caribbean Demographic Center [Centro Latinoamericano y caribeño de Demografia] – Population Division of ECLAC: http://www.eclac.cl/celade/default.asp)

LAC, as the result of its' complex history, political, and economics on country and subregion levels has resulted in high levels of violence, growing political instability, and great inequality. The region's health systems are deeply fragmented and segmented, which limits the region's capacity to provide equitable access to quality health-care and public health services.[22] In addition, income disparities, lack of clinically oriented medical training, and insufficient availability of research funding among others has also hindered medical research in the region.[23] This is especially true for study on NAFLD although some steps have been taken toward addressing these barriers, more coordinated efforts are needed to address the peculiarities of the NAFLD disease burden in the region.[23]

The political and social landscape for Australia and New Zealand is different to that of the LAC countries, with both having liberal democracies, stable political systems, and nationalized equitable health care. According to the United Nations, Australia had a population of 26,107, 467 as of July 24, 2022, whereas that of New Zealand was smaller at 4,822,233. Both nations have a high standard of living. According to the Human Development index, Australia's HDI value for 2019 was 0.944, in the very high human development category, positioning it at 8 out of 189 countries and territories. For New Zealand, this was 0.931, positioning it at number 15.[24] As expected, life expectancy is long, more than 82 years for both Australia and New Zealand.

EPIDEMIOLOGY OF NONALCOHOLIC FATTY LIVER DISEASE IN LATIN AMERICA AND CARIBBEAN

Prevalence

The global prevalence of NAFLD in LAC was first estimated in as reaching 25.24% using a meta-analytic assessment.[13] In this highly cited report, NAFLD exhibited a high prevalence in all continents, with the highest reported in the Middle East (31.78%) and South America (30.45%), whereas the lowest is in Africa (13.48%).[13] Data suggested that severity of NAFLD also may be greater in people from Latin American origin although no primary data regarding this is available. A more recent report suggests that current prevalence may reach up to 34.5% with South America showing the most rapid increase in prevalence in recent years (2.7% per year).[4,25] The estimated prevalence of NAFLD in LAC is likely inaccurate as primary data from most countries are lacking.[7,12,26] However, among Hispanics residing in the United States, it has been documented that the prevalence of NAFLD varies by Hispanic/Latino background, with a higher prevalence among those of Mexican and Central American background compared with the other groups.[14,15] In the multiethnic study of atherosclerosis cohort including 788 Hispanic participants, Fleischman and colleagues[14] found 29% of NAFLD prevalence, those of Mexican descent had a significantly higher prevalence of NAFLD (33%), compared with Dominican descent (16%), and Puerto Rican descent (18%). After controlling for age, sex, body mass index, waist circumference, hypertension, serum HDL cholesterol, triglyceride, high-sensitivity C-reactive protein level and insulin resistance, Mexican descent remained significantly more likely to have NAFLD than those of Dominican and Puerto Rican origin.[14]

Similarly, Kallwitz and colleagues[15] showed that NAFLD is not equally present in Hispanic/Latino subgroups, with individuals from Central American, South American, or Mexican heritage being more affected than subjects with Cuban, Puerto Rican, and Dominican backgrounds. In multivariate analysis compared with persons of Mexican heritage, persons of Cuban (odds ratio [OR], 0.69; 95% confidence interval [CI], 0.57 to 0.85), Puerto Rican (OR, 0.67; 95% CI, 0.52–0.87), and Dominican backgrounds (OR, 0.71; 95% CI, 0.54–0.93) had lower rates of suspected NAFLD. Persons of Central American and South American heritage had a similar prevalence of suspected NAFLD compared with persons of Mexican heritage.

During the past 15 years, the prevalence of NAFLD in Latin American population-based studies ranged from 14.3% to 35.2%.[6] Studies from Mexico and Brazil reported a wide variation in prevalence, ranging from 14.3%[27] to 34.6%[28] and 18.0% to 35.2%,[29] respectively, with higher prevalence in risk populations (see also López-Velázquez et al.[30] and references therein), whereas Chile reported 23%,[31] Colombia 26.6%,[32] and more recently Cuba 16.3%.[33]

Some epidemiologic studies demonstrated higher rates of NAFLD prevalence in South America.[25] According to one study, out of 5743 healthy Brazilian subjects (43 ± 10 years, 79% men) without clinical coronary heart, 36% were diagnosed with NAFLD using ultrasound.[34] When other comorbidities were included such as MetS and Obesity, NAFLD prevalence increased to 74% and 73%, respectively. In other study, among 60 obese Brazilians individuals undergoing bariatric surgery, the histologic evaluation detected NAFLD in 95% and NASH prevalence of 66.7%.[35]

A recent meta-analysis in Latin America found the prevalence of NAFLD to be 24%.[36] This figure is similar to the global prevalence of NAFLD reported by Younossi and colleagues.[13] Among high-risk groups (T2D mellitus or obesity), the prevalence increases up to 68%.[13,36] Although there is a lack of primary data, using the information available it seems that the prevalence of NAFLD is lower in the Caribbean compared with Central and South American countries. However, more studies need to be done to validate these data.

For Australia, a commissioned report by the Gastroenterological Society in 2013 noted that NAFLD is the most common liver disease, affecting about a third of the population (5.5 million people, including 15% of schoolchildren), and 13% of the population of New Zealand.[37] This is not surprising because Australia and New Zealand have one of the highest burdens of overweight and obesity. Temporal changes in adult obesity data can be gleaned from the Australian National Health Survey[38] and the Non-Communicable Risk Factor Collaboration meta-analysis for Australia.[39] The former reported obesity prevalence at 21.6% in 1995, increasing to 31.8% in 2015. The Risk Factor Collaboration adjusted obesity was 11.4% in 1975, increasing to 32.0% in 2014. A more recent Australian population-based survey of 9447 individuals reported that NAFLD is the most common cause of abnormal liver tests with nearly half the population having an elevated alanine aminotransferase attributable to truncal obesity.[40] According to the Australian Bureau of Statistics (ABS), as of July 2021,[41] 27.6% of the Australian population was born overseas; 81% were of European ancestry and 5.5% of Chinese ancestry. Of these, according to the ABS, 67% of adults were overweight or obese, an increase from 63% in 2014 to 2015. A greater proportion of men were overweight or obese than women (75% compared with 60%) while 25% of children were overweight or obese. More concerning, 1 in 20 Australians had diabetes (5.3% or 1.3 million people) with men and women having similar rates (5.7% and 4.9%, respectively).

Recently, there have been modeled projections of NAFLD burden across Australia from 2019 to 2030 by the Center for Disease analysis, United States.[42] In that study, prevalent cases were projected to increase 25% from 5.5 million in 2019 to 7 million by 2030. The expected increase in the number of cases of steatohepatitis was 40%. Consequently, incident cases of advanced liver disease were projected to increase 85% by 2030, and incident NAFLD-related liver deaths were estimated to increase 85% from 1900 deaths in 2019 to 3500 deaths by 2030. Similarly, cases of incident liver cancer were forecast to increase 75% from 420 in 2019 to 730 by 2030. As expected, cumulative incident cases of primary liver cancer between 2019 and 2030 were estimated to be 6800.

Racial differences in prevalence of NAFLD have been most marked in multiethnic studies population from United States. In general, Hispanic Americans have the highest prevalence of NAFLD followed by Americans of European descent and African Americans having the lowest prevalence.[43–46] More recent meta-analysis in population-based cohorts showed that 23% of Hispanics have NAFLD versus 14% of Caucasians and 13% of African Americans.[46]

There is a heterogeneous genetic among different LAC countries, with a greater contribution of African genetic ancestry in the Caribbean and Tropical America population and of native American ancestry in Central, Andean, and Southern America (Bolivia, Peru, Mexico, Ecuador, Chile, and Colombia). The higher Hispanic ancestralism in Latin American population would which causes more risk to NAFLD development and progression.[47]

Although ethnicity is an important aspect in NAFLD heterogeneity, there is presently insufficient evidence to confidently conclude that race, per se, plays a role in the progression of NAFLD and its associations.[48,49] The cause for these ethnicity differences is probably multifactorial, explained by genetic and sociocultural factors including diet, exercise, alcohol consumption, education, family income, and quality of life. More research is needed to understand why NAFLD progresses in some groups while not others.

The admixture of Native Americans, Europeans, and Africans varies throughout Latin America. African genetic ancestry contribution has been found more frequently in the Caribbean and Brazilian population, whereas the contribution of Native American ancestry is higher in Bolivia, Peru, Mexico, Ecuador, Chile, and Colombia. The lower prevalence of NAFLD among African Americans than Hispanics despite higher prevalence of obesity among non-Hispanics brings into focus the complexities on the pathogenesis of NAFLD. The role of genetics as well as epigenetic influences operating through diet, lifestyle, and other environmental factors are key to understanding this development. It is also important to recognize that intraethnic differences exist particularly among Hispanics according to their country of origin.

NAFLD is known to occur between the fourth and sixth decades of life, although older age is related to higher rates of developing the disease.[13] Traditionally, it was thought that NAFLD occurred more in men, although some studies dispute this sex bias.[6] The median age of women who develop NAFLD is also higher than that of men. Our understanding of sex differences in NAFLD is expanding. In a recent review summarizing the current knowledge of sex differences in NAFLD, NAFLD prevalence and incidence were reported higher in men than in premenopausal women (or age $\leq$ 50–60 years) but was found to be more common in women after menopause (or age $\geq$ 50–60 years) probably due to the result of the loss of the protective estrogen effect, which then caused body fat redistribution to the abdomen.[50] Sex differences do exist in the prevalence, risk factors, fibrosis, and clinical outcomes of NAFLD.[51]

Many factors, including diagnostic modalities used and intercountry variation in obesity prevalence by sex, could contribute to the sex discrepancies found among studies. Studies from LAC have no uniform data regarding sex prevalence but NAFLD seems to be higher among women.[36]

Risk Factors of Nonalcoholic Fatty Liver Disease

The LAC region shows the worst indices of all risk factors related to NAFLD, particularly obesity and its consequences, sedentary lifestyle, and unhealthy diets.

There is a great variability in the age-standardized obesity prevalence by wealth and education socioeconomic measures in LAC. The prevalence of obesity has been increasing not only among the poor, least educated, rural populations but also among the rich, highly educated, and urban populations.[52] According to Federación Latinoamericana de Sociedades de Obesidad consensus statement in 2016, 3 countries of the region (Bolivia, Mexico, and Guatemala) were at the higher prevalence of obesity above 30%, whereas Ecuador had the lowest prevalence of 14.2%.[53] Central Latin America has one of the highest rates of obesity with an increase of 0·95 kg/m^2 per decade (0·64-1·25).[2] In the region, there is more variation in the rate of BMI increase in children and adolescents than in adults, girls gained more weight than boys, and the age-standardized mean BMI is more than 20 kg/m^2.[2]

The LAC region faces a major diet-related health problem accompanied by enormous economic and social costs. The rapid increasing overweight and obese in LAC is probably associated with changes in food systems and living environments characterized by increased availability, accessibility, and affordability of ultraprocessed foods, which deteriorates overall nutritional dietary quality and promotes excessive energy intake.[54] There are major shifts in intake of less-healthful low-nutrient-density foods, sugary beverages, and more eating and snacking away from home. Sugar is a major element in all Latin American foods and beverages, particularly coffee, pastries, packaged foods, and sugar-sweetened beverages.[37]

How the variations and similarities in the standard diet within a geographic region or among individuals of a particular ethnic background promote hepatic steatosis and the progression of NAFLD are still unclear. As well as whether a specific diet affects disease progression differently in patients of various backgrounds.[55,56]

Parallel to obesity, T2D is one of the most critical public health problems in LAC. The region has one of the highest prevalence rates of T2D. The prevalence of T2D in the region in 2017 ranges 1.2% to 8% in the Caribbean, Puerto Rico reported 15.4% and Cuba's prevalence is 10.6%, whereas the highest in Central America was found in Mexico (13.6%) and Nicaragua (10%).[57,58]

Regarding to sedentarism, a pooled analysis of 358 surveys across 168 countries, including 1.9 million participants found a global age-standardized prevalence of insufficient physical activity of 27.5% (95% uncertainty interval 25.0–32.2) in 2016 but in LAC was 39.1% (37.8–40.6), highest levels were in women (43.7%, 42.9–46.5).[59]

For Australia, metabolic risk factors for fatty liver disease remain much the same across the community except among Indigenous Australians. According to the Australian Institute of Health and Welfare[60] about 1 million adults (5.3% of those aged 18 years and older) had T2D in 2017 to 2018 with age-specific rates for men higher than for women from age 45 years. Relatively similar rates were reported across major cities (4.8%), inner regional (4.2%), and outer regional and remote areas (6.0%). As would be expected, diabetes risk was twice as high among those living in the lowest socioeconomic areas (7.0%) compared with the highest socioeconomic areas (3.3%). Around 7.9% of Indigenous Australians (64,100 people) had diabetes according to the ABS 2018 to 2019 National Aboriginal and Torres Strait Islander Health Survey.[61] This is similar to the 7.7% reported in the 2012 to 2013. After controlling for differences in the age structures, Indigenous Australians were almost 3 times as likely to have diabetes as their non-Indigenous counterparts (12.6% compared with 4.3%).

For overweight and obesity, in 2017 to 2018, 2 in 3 (67%) Australian adults were overweight or obese (36% were overweight but not obese, and 31% were obese) affecting 12.5 million adults. Men had higher rates of overweight and obesity than women (75% of men and 60% of women), and higher rates of obesity (33% of men and 30% of women). Obesity was more common in older age groups comprising 41% of adults aged 65 to 74 years. A quarter of children and adolescents aged 2 to 17 years was overweight or obese. This amounted to 17% being overweight but not obese, and 8.2% being obese. Rates varied across age groups but were similar for men and women.[38] In 2018 to 2019, 71% (381,800) of Indigenous Australians aged 15 years and older were overweight or obese, higher than in 2012 to 2013 (66%). The increase was driven by an increase in nonremote areas.[62]

Regarding genetic factors, common polymorphisms associated to NAFLD[63] have not been studied at population level neither in LAC nor Australia regions. Patatin-like phospholipase domain-containing protein (PNPLA3) nonsynonymous gene variant (rs738409 c.444 C > G p.I148 M) is the most notable genetic polymorphism shown to be robustly associated with steatosis, steatohepatitis, and fibrosis in patients with NAFLD.[64] The rs738409 variant, which resulted of substitution of methionine for isoleucine, causing a loss of function in the PNPLA3 protein, contributes to increased accumulation of triglycerides in lipid droplets within hepatocytes as compared with cells with functional PNPLA3.[64,65] This variant has been associated with increased susceptibility to NAFLD in a variety of different ethnicities. The frequency of the (G) risk allele is 23.1% in the general population but the frequency of PNPLA3-G is higher in Hispanics with American ancestry (Mexican American, Central American, and South American) may reach up to 60%.[66–69] More studies analyzing the prevalence of NAFLD genes in different populations in both LAC and Australia are needed.

Clinical Outcomes

Liver fibrosis is associated with the risk of mortality and liver-related morbidity in patients with NAFLD, and the evidence suggest that Hispanics have higher rates of disease progression and fibrosis.[43,70]

In a multinational cohort study with 458 patients with biopsy confirmed that patients with NAFLD of Spain, Australia, Hong Kong, and Cuba demonstrated during a mean follow-up time of 5.5 years (range, 2.7–8.2 years) that annual incidence of vascular events and nonhepatic cancer were 0.9% and 1.2%, respectively in patients with bridging fibrosis (F3).[71] However, patients with cirrhosis were more likely than patients with F3 fibrosis to have hepatic decompensation (44%; 95% CI, 32%–60% vs 6%, 95% CI, 2%–13%) or hepatocellular carcinoma (HCC) (17%; 95% CI, 8%–31% vs 2.3%, 95% CI, 1%–12%).[71]

Hispanic individuals have a greater risk of HCC mortality, and this may be attributed to increased exposures to well-known risk factors, such as excessive alcohol consumption, obesity, hyperlipidemia, and diabetes mellitus, in turn resulting in the development of NAFLD/NASH.[72,73] In a retrospective study with 296,707 patients with NAFLD, Hispanics were found to have an annual incidence rate of 23.76 per 1000 person-years compared with those of white and African Americans, where both races were found to have an annual incidence rate of 11.94 per 1000 person years.[74] Cohorts of HCC studies from South America found up to 5% to 9% of HCC was attributable to NAFLD.[75,76]

Despite the higher propensity of metabolic risk factors among Hispanic recent studies found lower overall risk of mortality among Hispanic than non-Hispanic whites in the United States, it is called as "the Hispanic mortality paradox."[77,78] Regarding NAFLD, the analysis of Kim and colleagues[79] found on the total US mortality captured in the latest National Vital Statistics database, that Hispanics with a diagnosis of NAFLD have lower mortality than Caucasians. Notwithstanding critics about the limitations of the Kim study, the reasons for these results are not completely understood, further investigations are needed to elucidate these disparities.[80]

Studies including Australian populations have highlighted the role of diabetes as a risk factor for clinical outcomes in people with steatohepatitis. For example, a study including patients from Spain, Australia, and Hong Kong examined outcomes among biopsy-proven Child-Pugh A steatohepatitis cirrhosis cases from April 1995 to December 2016.[81] Of these, 212 had T2D at baseline and 8 of 87 patients developed diabetes during a median follow-up time of 5.1 years. As expected, higher proportions with diabetes had hepatic decompensation (51% vs 26% of patients with no diabetes) and HCC (25% vs 7% of patients with no diabetes). Consistent with several other reports, metformin use was associated with a significant reduction in risk of death or liver transplantation, hepatic decompensation, and HCC. Interestingly, metformin reduced the risk of decompensation and HCC only in subjects with HbA1c levels greater than 7.0%, whereas T2D increased the risk of death and liver-related outcomes, including HCC. In another study comprising patients from Spain, Australia, Hong Kong, Cuba and the United States, the ABIDE model comprising routine clinical parameters (Aspartate aminotransferase/alanine aminotransferase ratio, Bilirubin, International normalized ratio T2D, and Esophageal varices) was a good predictor of risk of decompensation, 5-year cumulative incidence of decompensation and shorter mean duration to decompensation. This model was more accurate than the NAFLD fibrosis score, fibrosis-4 (FIB-4), Model for End-Stage Liver Disease (MELD), Child-Turcotte-Pugh (CTP), and albumin-bilirubin (ALBI)-FIB-4 (all $P < .001$).[82]

SUMMARY AND OUTLOOK

As in other regions of the world, NAFLD had become the most prevalent CLD in LAC and Australia. Current epidemiologic data is imperfect and need to be refined but the projected health burden is significant and urgent measures are needed. Major challenges to tackle NAFLD in these regions are the following: lack of disease awareness, health system fragmentation, limited educational opportunities for health-care personnel and public, and lack of effective strategies for the prevention and effective treatment of NAFLD and common comorbidities, namely obesity and T2DM.[23] Public health approaches to address NAFLD are limited and require extensive collaboration between scientific societies, governments, nongovernmental organizations, pharmaceutical industry, and other stakeholders.[23,83] Development of an effective public health policies agenda that allows us to address this disease through a societal approach is indeed urgently needed.[84,85]

CLINICS CARE POINTS

- Non-alcoholic fatty liver disease (NAFLD) is the most common cause of chronic liver disease in Western countries as well as in Latin American countries and Australia
- There are few studies epidemiological studies in the general population in Latin America
- Environment and genetics play an important role in the prevalence of NAFLD in Latin America and Australia
- The prevalence of obesity and T2D are very high in Latin American countries and those account for the high prevalence of NAFLD
- Latin American people are very susceptible for the fibrosis progression due to metabolic risk and high prevalence of the PNPLA3

DISCLOSURE

M.I. Castellanos Fernandez: Nothing to declare. J. George: He is supported by the Robert W. Storr Bequest to the Sydney Medical Foundation, University of Sydney; a National Health and Medical Research Council of Australia (NHMRC) Program Grant (APP1053206), Project, Ideas, and Investigator grants (APP2001692, APP1107178, APP1108422, APP1196492) and a Cancer Institute NSW grant (2021/ATRG2028). M. Arrese: He received support of Chilean government through the Fondo Nacional de Desarrollo Científico y Tecnológico (FONDECYT 1200227 to J.P. Arab and 1191145 to M. Arrese) and the Agencia Nacional de Investigación y desarrollo (ANID) through ANID ACE 210009 grant.

REFERENCES

1. Diseases GBD, Injuries C. Global burden of 369 diseases and injuries in 204 countries and territories, 1990-2019: a systematic analysis for the Global Burden of Disease Study 2019. Lancet 2020;396(10258):1204–22.
2. Collaboration NCDRF. Worldwide trends in body-mass index, underweight, overweight, and obesity from 1975 to 2016: a pooled analysis of 2416 population-based measurement studies in 128.9 million children, adolescents, and adults. Lancet 2017;390(10113):2627–42.
3. Collaborators GBDO, Afshin A, Forouzanfar MH, et al. Health effects of overweight and obesity in 195 countries over 25 years. N Engl J Med 2017;377(1):13–27.
4. Henry L, Paik J, Younossi ZM. Review article: the epidemiologic burden of non-alcoholic fatty liver disease across the world. Aliment Pharmacol Ther 2022;56(6):942–56.
5. Powell EE, Wong VW, Rinella M. Non-alcoholic fatty liver disease. Lancet 2021;397(10290):2212–24.
6. Arab JP, Dirchwolf M, Alvares-da-Silva MR, et al. Latin American Association for the study of the liver (ALEH) practice guidance for the diagnosis and treatment of non-alcoholic fatty liver disease. Ann Hepatol 2020;19(6):674–90.
7. Younossi Z, Tacke F, Arrese M, et al. Global perspectives on nonalcoholic fatty liver disease and nonalcoholic steatohepatitis. Hepatology 2019;69(6):2672–82.

8. O'Hara J, Finnegan A, Dhillon H, et al. Cost of non-alcoholic steatohepatitis in Europe and the USA: the GAIN study. JHEP Rep 2020;2(5):100142.
9. Eslam M, Newsome PN, Sarin SK, et al. A new definition for metabolic dysfunction-associated fatty liver disease: an international expert consensus statement. J Hepatol 2020;73(1):202–9.
10. Eslam M, Sanyal AJ, George J, et al. MAFLD: a consensus-driven proposed nomenclature for metabolic associated fatty liver disease. Gastroenterology 2020;158(7):1999–2014 e1.
11. Zhai M, Liu Z, Long J, et al. The incidence trends of liver cirrhosis caused by nonalcoholic steatohepatitis via the GBD study 2017. Sci Rep 2021;11(1):5195.
12. Diaz LA, Ayares G, Arnold J, et al. Liver diseases in Latin America: current status, unmet needs, and opportunities for improvement. Curr Treat Options Gastroenterol 2022;20(3):261–78.
13. Younossi ZM, Koenig AB, Abdelatif D, et al. Global epidemiology of nonalcoholic fatty liver disease-Meta-analytic assessment of prevalence, incidence, and outcomes. Hepatology 2016;64(1):73–84.
14. Fleischman MW, Budoff M, Zeb I, et al. NAFLD prevalence differs among hispanic subgroups: the Multi-Ethnic Study of Atherosclerosis. World J Gastroenterol 2014;20(17):4987–93.
15. Kallwitz ER, Daviglus ML, Allison MA, et al. Prevalence of suspected nonalcoholic fatty liver disease in Hispanic/Latino individuals differs by heritage. Clin Gastroenterol Hepatol 2015;13(3):569–76.
16. Velasco-Mondragon E, Jimenez A, Palladino-Davis AG, et al. Hispanic health in the USA: a scoping review of the literature. Public Health Rev 2016;37:31.
17. Kittleson RA, Lockhart J, Bushnell D. History of Latin America. 2021 [Encyclopedia Britannica]. Available at: https://www.britannica.com/place/Latin-America.
18. Fernandez Prieto L. Islands of knowledge: science and agriculture in the history of Latin America and the Caribbean. Isis 2013;104(4):788–97.
19. Ablard JD. Framing the Latin American nutrition transition in a historical perspective, 1850 to the present. Hist Cienc Saude Manguinhos 2021;28(1):233–53.
20. Latin Worldometer. America and the caribbean population 2022. Available at: https://www.worldometers.info/world-population/latin-america-and-the-caribbean-population/.
21. Guzmán JM, Rodríguez J, Martínez J, et al. La démographie de l'Amérique latine et de la Caraïbe depuis 1950. Population 2006;61(5):623–734.
22. Ruano AL, Rodriguez D, Rossi PG, et al. Understanding inequities in health and health systems in Latin America and the Caribbean: a thematic series. Int J Equity Health 2021;20(1):94.
23. Arab JP, Diaz LA, Dirchwolf M, et al. NAFLD: challenges and opportunities to address the public health problem in Latin America. Ann Hepatol 2021;24:100359.
24. Center UNHDD. Developed countries list 2022. 2022. Available at: https://worldpopulationreview.com/country-rankings/developed-countries.
25. Le MH, Yeo YH, Li X, et al. 2019 global NAFLD prevalence: a systematic review and meta-analysis. Clin Gastroenterol Hepatol 2021;20(12):2809–17.e28.
26. Pinto Marques Souza de Oliveira C, Pinchemel Cotrim H, Arrese M. Nonalcoholic fatty liver disease risk factors in Latin American populations: current scenario and perspectives. Clin Liver Dis 2019;13(2):39–42.
27. Lizardi-Cervera J, Becerra-Laparra I, Chavez-Tapia NC, et al. Prevalence of nonalcoholic fatty liver and metabolic syndrome in asymptomatic population. Rev Gastroenterol México 2006;71(4):453–9.

28. Sepulveda-Villegas M, Roman S, Rivera-Iniguez I, et al. High prevalence of nonalcoholic steatohepatitis and abnormal liver stiffness in a young and obese Mexican population. PLoS One 2019;14(1):e0208926.
29. Karnikowski M, Cordova C, Oliveira RJ, et al. Non-alcoholic fatty liver disease and metabolic syndrome in Brazilian middle-aged and older adults. Sao Paulo Med J 2007;125(6):333–7.
30. Lopez-Velazquez JA, Silva-Vidal KV, Ponciano-Rodriguez G, et al. The prevalence of nonalcoholic fatty liver disease in the Americas. Ann Hepatol 2014; 13(2):166–78.
31. Riquelme A, Arrese M, Soza A, et al. Non-alcoholic fatty liver disease and its association with obesity, insulin resistance and increased serum levels of C-reactive protein in Hispanics. Liver Int 2009;29(1):82–8.
32. Perez M, Gonzales L, Olarte R, et al. Nonalcoholic fatty liver disease is associated with insulin resistance in a young Hispanic population. Prev Med 2011;52(2): 174–7.
33. Castellanos-Fernandez MI, Crespo-Ramirez E, Del Valle-Diaz S, et al. Non-alcoholic fatty liver disease in Cuba. MEDICC Rev 2021;23(1):64–71.
34. Oni ET, Kalathiya R, Aneni EC, et al. Relation of physical activity to prevalence of nonalcoholic Fatty liver disease independent of cardiometabolic risk. Am J Cardiol 2015;115(1):34–9.
35. Feijo SG, Lima JM, Oliveira MA, et al. The spectrum of non alcoholic fatty liver disease in morbidly obese patients: prevalence and associate risk factors. Acta Cir Bras 2013;28(11):788–93.
36. Rojas YAO, Cuellar CLV, Barron KMA, et al. Non-alcoholic fatty liver disease prevalence in Latin America: a systematic review and meta-analysis. Ann Hepatol 2022;27(6):100706.
37. Popkin BM, Reardon T. Obesity and the food system transformation in Latin America. Obes Rev 2018;19(8):1028–64.
38. Australian Government AIoHaWA. Overweight and obesity. 2022. Available at: https://www.aihw.gov.au/reports/australias-health/overweight-and-obesity.
39. Collaboration NCDRF. Trends in adult body-mass index in 200 countries from 1975 to 2014: a pooled analysis of 1698 population-based measurement studies with 19.2 million participants. Lancet 2016;387(10026):1377–96.
40. Mahady SE, Wong G, Turner RM, et al. Elevated liver enzymes and mortality in older individuals: a prospective cohort study. J Clin Gastroenterol 2017;51(5): 439–45.
41. Statistics ABo. People and communities 2022 [ABS Website]. Available at: https://www.abs.gov.au/statistics/people/people-and-communities.
42. Adams LA, Roberts SK, Strasser SI, et al. Nonalcoholic fatty liver disease burden: Australia, 2019-2030. J Gastroenterol Hepatol 2020;35(9):1628–35.
43. Browning JD, Szczepaniak LS, Dobbins R, et al. Prevalence of hepatic steatosis in an urban population in the United States: impact of ethnicity. Hepatology 2004; 40(6):1387–95.
44. Balakrishnan M, Kanwal F, El-Serag HB, et al. Acculturation and nonalcoholic fatty liver disease risk among hispanics of Mexican origin: findings from the national health and nutrition examination survey. Clin Gastroenterol Hepatol 2017;15(2): 310–2.
45. Saab S, Manne V, Nieto J, et al. Nonalcoholic fatty liver disease in latinos. Clin Gastroenterol Hepatol 2016;14(1):5–12, quiz e9-0.
46. Rich NE, Oji S, Mufti AR, et al. Racial and ethnic disparities in nonalcoholic fatty liver disease prevalence, severity, and outcomes in the United States: a

systematic review and meta-analysis. Clin Gastroenterol Hepatol 2018;16(2): 198–210 e2.
47. Yang C, Hallmark B, Chai JC, et al. Impact of Amerind ancestry and FADS genetic variation on omega-3 deficiency and cardiometabolic traits in Hispanic populations. Commun Biol 2021;4(1):918.
48. Szanto KB, Li J, Cordero P, et al. Ethnic differences and heterogeneity in genetic and metabolic makeup contributing to nonalcoholic fatty liver disease. Diabetes Metab Syndr Obes 2019;12:357–67.
49. Bonacini M, Kassamali F, Kari S, et al. Racial differences in prevalence and severity of non-alcoholic fatty liver disease. World J Hepatol 2021;13(7):763–73.
50. Ye ZL, Guo WQ, Li L. Sex-based differences in the association between nonalcoholic fatty liver disease and mortality. Clin Gastroenterol Hepatol 2019;17(1): 211–2.
51. Lonardo A, Nascimbeni F, Ballestri S, et al. Sex differences in nonalcoholic fatty liver disease: state of the art and identification of research gaps. Hepatology 2019;70(4):1457–69.
52. Jiwani SS, Carrillo-Larco RM, Hernandez-Vasquez A, et al. The shift of obesity burden by socioeconomic status between 1998 and 2017 in Latin America and the Caribbean: a cross-sectional series study. Lancet Glob Health 2019;7(12): e1644–54.
53. (FLASO) LAFoOS. II Consenso Latino-Americano de Obesidad. 2017. In: (FLASO) LAFoOS, editor. 2017.
54. Aviles-Santa ML, Hsu L, Lam TK, et al. Funding of hispanic/latino health-related research by the national institutes of health: an analysis of the portfolio of research Program grants on six health topic areas. Front Public Health 2020; 8:330.
55. Rodriguez LA, Kanaya AM, Shiboski SC, et al. Does NAFLD mediate the relationship between obesity and type 2 diabetes risk? evidence from the multi-ethnic study of atherosclerosis (MESA). Ann Epidemiol 2021;63:15–21.
56. Yoshida H, Maddock JE. Relationship between health behaviors and obesity in a sample of hawai'i's 4 most populous ethnicities. Hawaii J Health Soc Welf 2020; 79(4):104–11.
57. Gallardo-Rincon H, Cantoral A, Arrieta A, et al. Review: type 2 diabetes in Latin America and the Caribbean: regional and country comparison on prevalence, trends, costs and expanded prevention. Prim Care Diabetes 2021;15(2):352–9.
58. Sinisterra-Loaiza L, Cardelle-Cobas A, Abraham AG, et al. Diabetes in Latin America: prevalence, complications, and socio-economic impact. International Journal of Diabetes and Clinical Research 2019;6:112.
59. Guthold R, Stevens GA, Riley LM, et al. Worldwide trends in insufficient physical activity from 2001 to 2016: a pooled analysis of 358 population-based surveys with 1.9 million participants. Lancet Glob Health 2018;6(10):e1077–86.
60. Statistics ABo. Diabetes 2022 [ABS website]. Available at: https://www.aihw.gov.au/reports/diabetes/diabetes/contents/how-many-australians-have-diabetes/type-2-diabetes.
61. Statistics ABo. National aboriginal and Torres Strait Islander health survey (2018-2019). 2022 [ABS Website]. Available at: https://www.aihw.gov.au/reports/diabetes/diabetes/contents/how-many-australians-have-diabetes/type-2-diabetes.
62. Australian Government AIoHaWA. Determinants of health for indigenous Australians 2022. Available at: https://www.aihw.gov.au/reports/australias-health/social-determinants-and-indigenous-health.

63. Trepo E, Valenti L. Update on NAFLD genetics: from new variants to the clinic. J Hepatol 2020;72(6):1196–209.
64. Sookoian S, Pirola CJ. Meta-analysis of the influence of I148M variant of patatin-like phospholipase domain containing 3 gene (PNPLA3) on the susceptibility and histological severity of nonalcoholic fatty liver disease. Hepatology 2011;53(6): 1883–94.
65. Tepper CG, Dang JHT, Stewart SL, et al. High frequency of the PNPLA3 rs738409 [G] single-nucleotide polymorphism in Hmong individuals as a potential basis for a predisposition to chronic liver disease. Cancer 2018;124(Suppl 7):1583–9.
66. Kallwitz ER, Tayo BO, Kuniholm MH, et al. American ancestry is a risk factor for suspected nonalcoholic fatty liver disease in hispanic/latino adults. Clin Gastroenterol Hepatol 2019;17(11):2301–9.
67. Walker RW, Belbin GM, Sorokin EP, et al. A common variant in PNPLA3 is associated with age at diagnosis of NAFLD in patients from a multi-ethnic biobank. J Hepatol 2020;72(6):1070–81.
68. Arrese M, Arab JP, Riquelme A, et al. High prevalence of PNPLA3 rs738409 (I148M) polymorphism in Chilean latino population and its association to non-alcoholic fatty liver disease risk and histological disease severity. Hepatology 2015;62:1285A.
69. Pontoriero AC, Trinks J, Hulaniuk ML, et al. Influence of ethnicity on the distribution of genetic polymorphisms associated with risk of chronic liver disease in South American populations. BMC Genet 2015;16:93.
70. Taylor RS, Taylor RJ, Bayliss S, et al. Association between fibrosis stage and outcomes of patients with nonalcoholic fatty liver disease: a systematic review and meta-analysis. Gastroenterology 2020;158(6):1611–1625 e12.
71. Vilar-Gomez E, Calzadilla-Bertot L, Wai-Sun Wong V, et al. Fibrosis severity as a determinant of cause-specific mortality in patients with advanced nonalcoholic fatty liver disease: a multi-national cohort study. Gastroenterology 2018;155(2): 443–457 e17.
72. Venepalli NK, Modayil MV, Berg SA, et al. Features of hepatocellular carcinoma in Hispanics differ from African Americans and non-Hispanic Whites. World J Hepatol 2017;9(7):391–400.
73. Ha J, Chaudhri A, Avirineni A, et al. Burden of hepatocellular carcinoma among hispanics in South Texas: a systematic review. Biomark Res 2017;5:15.
74. Kanwal F, Kramer JR, Mapakshi S, et al. Risk of hepatocellular cancer in patients with non-alcoholic fatty liver disease. Gastroenterology 2018;155(6): 1828–18237 e2.
75. Debes JD, Chan AJ, Balderramo D, et al. Hepatocellular carcinoma in South America: evaluation of risk factors, demographics and therapy. Liver Int 2018; 38(1):136–43.
76. Fassio E, Diaz S, Santa C, et al. Etiology of hepatocellular carcinoma in Latin America: a prospective, multicenter, international study. Ann Hepatol 2010; 9(1):63–9.
77. Cortes-Bergoderi M, Goel K, Murad MH, et al. Cardiovascular mortality in Hispanics compared to non-Hispanic whites: a systematic review and meta-analysis of the Hispanic paradox. Eur J Intern Med 2013;24(8):791–9.
78. Ruiz JM, Steffen P, Smith TB. Hispanic mortality paradox: a systematic review and meta-analysis of the longitudinal literature. Am J Public Health 2013;103(3): e52–60.

79. Kim D, Li AA, Perumpail RB, et al. Disparate trends in mortality of etiology-specific chronic liver diseases among hispanic subpopulations. Clin Gastroenterol Hepatol 2019;17(8):1607–16015 e2.
80. Callahan KE, Pinheiro PS. Hepatocellular carcinoma among hispanics: an understudied public health priority. Clin Gastroenterol Hepatol 2019;17(8):1649–50.
81. Vilar-Gomez E, Calzadilla-Bertot L, Wong VW, et al. Type 2 diabetes and metformin use associate with outcomes of patients with nonalcoholic steatohepatitis-related, child-pugh A cirrhosis. Clin Gastroenterol Hepatol 2021;19(1):136–145 e6.
82. Calzadilla-Bertot L, Vilar-Gomez E, Wong VW, et al. ABIDE: an accurate predictive model of liver decompensation in patients with nonalcoholic fatty liver-related cirrhosis. Hepatology 2021;73(6):2238–50.
83. Lazarus JV, Mark HE, Anstee QM, et al. Advancing the global public health agenda for NAFLD: a consensus statement. Nat Rev Gastroenterol Hepatol 2022;19(1):60–78.
84. Diaz LA, Fuentes-Lopez E, Ayares G, et al. The establishment of public health policies and the burden of non-alcoholic fatty liver disease in the Americas. Lancet Gastroenterol Hepatol 2022;7(6):552–9.
85. Lazarus JV, Mark HE, Colombo M, et al. A sustainable development goal framework to guide multisectoral action on NAFLD through a societal approach. Aliment Pharmacol Ther 2022;55(2):234–43.

Pathogenetic Pathways in Nonalcoholic Fatty Liver Disease: An Incomplete Jigsaw Puzzle

Qin Pan, MD[a,b], Jian-Gao Fan, MD, PhD[b,c,*], Yusuf Yilmaz, MD[d,e,*]

KEYWORDS

• Nonalcoholic fatty liver disease • Nonalcoholic steatohepatitis • Liver fibrosis
• Signaling pathways • Pathophysiology

KEY POINTS

- Non-alcoholic fatty liver disease (NAFLD) has become the most prevalent chronic liver disease worldwide.
- Multiple pathways regulate hepatic steatosis, including Insulin signaling pathway, MAPK signaling pathway, GLP-1R signaling, nuclear receptors, and non-coding RNAs.
- Oxidative stress, endoplasmic reticulum stress, cytokines, gut microbiota contribute to lobular inflammation.
- TGF-beta signaling pathway, nuclear receptors, autophagy, and apoptosis of HSCs involve in the pathogenesis of liver fibrosis.

INTRODUCTION

Nonalcoholic fatty liver disease (NAFLD) is characterized by excess liver fat infiltration (steatosis in $\geq$ 5% of hepatocytes) in the absence of significant alcohol consumption or other causes of hepatic steatosis.[1] This condition is regarded as a disease spectrum encompassing different stages, from nonalcoholic fatty liver (NAFL), through nonalcoholic steatohepatitis (NASH), to liver fibrosis, cirrhosis, and even hepatocellular carcinoma.[1] NAFL is the initial stage of NAFLD, which is generally considered benign due to its limited or subclinical impact on hepatic function. According to currently accepted models of disease pathophysiology, NAFL represents the first of the "two-hit system" used to describe the natural history of NAFLD over time. Although

[a] Research Center, Zhoupu Hospital Affiliated to the Shanghai University of Medicine & Health Sciences, Shanghai 201318, China; [b] Department of Gastroenterology, Xinhua Hospital Affiliated to the Shanghai Jiao Tong University School of Medicine, Shanghai 200092, China; [c] Shanghai Key Lab of Pediatric Gastroenterology and Nutrition, Shanghai 200092, China; [d] Department of Gastroenterology, School of Medicine, Recep Tayyip Erdoğan University, Rize 53200, Turkey; [e] Liver Research Unit, Institute of Gastroenterology, Marmara University, İstanbul 34840, Turkey
* Corresponding authors.
E-mail addresses: fanjiangao@xinhuamed.com.cn (J.-G.F.); dryusufyilmaz@gmail.com (Y.Y.)

Clin Liver Dis 27 (2023) 317–332
https://doi.org/10.1016/j.cld.2023.01.013
liver.theclinics.com

accumulation of lipids in the liver is considered benign, it can increase the production of reactive oxygen species (ROS), which in turn elicits an inflammatory response. This second hit can potentially result in the development of lobular inflammation and hepatocellular ballooning (NASH).[1] Thereafter, if the pathogenetic damage continues to persist and/or accumulate, the disease may progress into more advanced stages, namely liver fibrosis and cirrhosis, with the possible concomitant risk of hepatic carcinogenesis.

From an epidemiological standpoint, the burden associated with NAFLD is currently recognized as one of the most pressing issues in public health, with around 32.4% of the global population having this condition.[2] Currently, NAFLD represents the most prevalent cause of chronic liver diseases worldwide and, with the increasing prevalence of unhealthy lifestyles, an epidemic of this condition is anticipated.[1,2] Remarkably, the adverse impact of NAFLD is not limited to liver-related morbidity and mortality but extends over a wide spectrum of extrahepatic manifestations—including cardiometabolic complications and chronic and extrahepatic tumour.[1] Although an international consensus panel has recently recommended metabolic-associated fatty liver disease as a more appropriate term to describe fatty liver disease associated with metabolic dysfunction, a multisociety consensus process concerning disease naming is currently underway.[3] Until the process is completed, the term NAFLD is still being used. Unfortunately, as of now, only modestly effective pharmacological therapies exist for this condition. The uncomplete understanding of the pathophysiology underlying the heterogeneous disease spectrum known as NAFLD remains one of the major obstacles to the development of novel therapeutic approaches. However, growing evidence indicates that NAFLD advances through the interaction between different liver cell types and pathogenic cell-to-cell communication through a host of signaling pathways. The present review compiles current knowledge on the principal pathogenic mechanisms of NAFLD, which are analyzed in relation to the main pathological hallmarks of the spectrum (ie, steatosis, steatohepatitis, and fibrosis). The following sections are not intended to be exhaustive but are aimed to highlight those aspects most relevant to developing effective methods of treatment. It is hoped that these data may inform the identification of novel therapeutic targets and can pave the way for breakthrough treatments of NAFLD.

SIGNALING PATHWAYS INVOLVED IN THE PATHOGENESIS OF HEPATOCYTE STEATOSIS

The liver is a central hub for lipid metabolism, and hepatic steatosis may emerge as an expected consequence whenever this delicate equilibrium is disrupted. Under physiologic conditions, the hepatic fatty acid pool is the result of a balance between fatty acid influx from the diet and adipose tissue lipolysis, *de novo* lipogenesis, and disposal of fatty acid through very-low-density lipoprotein (VLDL) secretion or β-oxidation. Disturbances in these processes can precipitate intracellular lipid accumulation as a result of excess fatty acid content with respect to the oxidative needs of the hepatocytes. Although several different pathways have been involved in hepatic fat deposition and lipid toxicity, the most extensively investigated include insulin signaling, mitogen-activated protein kinase (MAPK) signaling, glucagon-like peptide-1 (GLP-1) signaling, nuclear receptors (NRs) signaling, and noncoding RNA (ncRNA) (**Fig. 1**).

Insulin Signaling Pathway

Hepatic insulin resistance is a key mechanism in the pathogenesis of NAFLD and closely connected to excess lipid accumulation in hepatocytes. Under physiologic

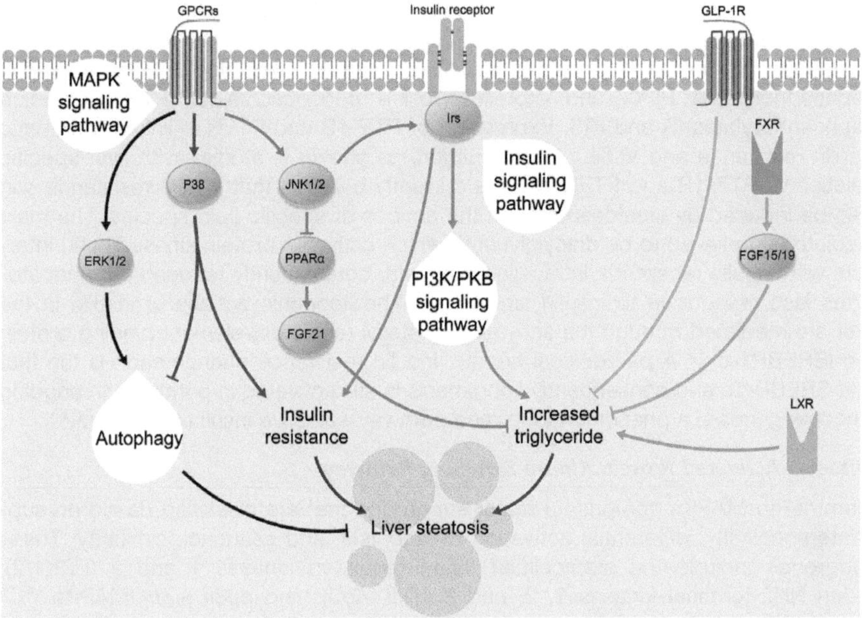

Fig. 1. Pathways associate with hepatocyte steatosis in nonalcoholic fatty liver disease (NAFLD). ERK1/2 of MAPK signaling pathway promotes autophagy of hepatocytes to attenuate liver steatosis. P38 of MAPK signaling pathway simultaneously inhibit autophagy and induce insulin resistance. JNK1/2, another subgroup of MAPKs, increases triglyceride concentration by the downregulation of PPARα-induced FGF21 expression. JNK1 also mediates inhibitory phosphorylation of Irs, leading to the insulin resistance. Insulin signaling pathway cooperates with PI3K/PKB signaling pathway to upregulate TG level, whereas hepatic insulin resistance is thought to involve serine phosphorylation of Irs. In addition, nuclear receptors of LXR and FXR regulate the hepatic triglyceride content in positive and negative manner, respectively. Ligand-activated GLP-1R functions to prevent the triglyceride accumulation in liver. Integration of these pathways finally results in liver steatosis by insulin resistance, autophagy inhibition, and increased triglyceride level. ERK, extracellular signal-regulated kinase; FGF21, fibroblast growth factor 21; FXR, farnesoid X receptor; GLP-1R, glucagon-like peptide-1 receptor; GPCR, G protein–coupled receptor; Irs, insulin receptor substrate; JNK, c-Jun N-terminal kinase; LXR, liver X receptor; PI3K, phosphatidylinositol 3-kinase; PKB, PI3K/protein kinase B; PPARα, peroxisome proliferator–activated receptor α.

conditions, insulin signaling starts with insulin binding to the insulin receptor on the cell surface. On binding, receptor autophosphorylation leads to activation of tyrosine kinase activity—resulting in tyrosine phosphorylation of intracellular insulin receptor substrates (IRS).[4] These effectors bind to a signaling protein complex to activate the MAPK pathway that mediates the mitogenic effects of insulin.[5] IRS is also capable of binding to the regulatory subunit of phosphatidylinositol 3-kinase (PI-3K), which activates the PI-3K/protein kinase B pathway to mediate the metabolic responses to insulin. This signaling arm results in the production of phosphatidylinositol-3,4,5-trisphosphate (PIP3), which recruits both phosphoinositide-dependent kinase (PDK)1/2 and Akt to the plasma membrane, where PDK1/2 phosphorylates and activates Akt.[6] Induction of hepatic insulin resistance is thought to involve serine phosphorylation of IRS proteins[7]; this is deemed to play a role in insulin resistance by decreasing PI-3K interaction with IRS proteins and can also result in IRS1 degradation.[8] In addition to inactivation by serine phosphorylation, the metabolic arm of insulin signaling is also reversibly modulated by dephosphorylation of the signal mediators by downstream regulatory phosphatases, particularly phosphatase and tensin homolog (PTEN), which dephosphorylates PIP3, and protein tyrosine phosphatase-1B (PTP-1B), which dephosphorylates IR and IRS. Expression of PTP-1B and PTEN is linked to hepatic insulin resistance and VLDL overproduction, as shown in studies with liver-specific deletion of PTP-1B and PTEN.[9,10] It is currently believed that insulin resistance can also be induced by steatosis through the actions of specific lipid species. The main mediator is believed to be diacylglycerol, which activates protein kinase C and interacts with insulin receptor's intracellular domain, consequently rendering the hepatocytes less responsive to insulin signaling.[11] The lipogenic actions of insulin in the liver are mediated through the activation of sterol regulatory element binding protein 1-c (SREBP1-c).[12] A paradoxical hepatic insulin resistance phenomenon is the fact that SREBP-1c and consequently lipogenesis is still activated in parallel with ongoing gluconeogenesis, a phenomenon termed pathway-selective insulin resistance.[13]

Mitogen-Activated Protein Kinase Signaling Pathway

Mammalian MAPKs comprise 3 major subgroups that are classified based on substrate specificity, differential activation by agonists, and sequence similarity. These subgroups include the extracellular signal-regulated kinases 1 and 2 (ERK1/2); c-Jun NH2-terminal kinases 1, 2, and 3 (JNK1/2/3); and p38α/β/δ/γ MAPKs.[14–16] The MAPK signaling pathway is a cascade of protein kinases that play a key role in the regulation of hepatic metabolism. ERK1/2 activity has been shown to be compromised in livers of leptin receptor–deficient (db/db) mice, and it may protect against steatosis by promoting autophagy. Activated autophagy could attenuate liver steatosis by sequestering lipid droplets, which are eventually eliminated.[14] MAPK phosphatase-1 is overexpressed in mice with hepatic steatosis fed a high-fat diet (HFD), suggesting that hepatic p38α/β MAPK declines in states of obesity.[17] Similar findings have been reported for JNK. The first evidence implicating JNK signaling in steatosis was JNK1-mediated inhibitory phosphorylation of IRS-1 on the serine-307, which results in insulin resistance.[15] JNK1-null mice have significantly lower degree of steatosis and liver injury than wild-type counterpart.[18] JNK1/2 activation was also observed in liver biopsies from obese patients with hepatic steatosis.[19] Mechanistically, JNK1/2 represses the nuclear hormone receptor peroxisome proliferator–activated receptor α (PPARα) and fibroblast growth factor 21 (FGF21) signaling, in part through regulating nuclear receptor corepressor 1.[20] Hepatic p38α/β expression decreases in livers of HFD-fed mice, leading to increased transcription of lipogenic genes, which is a driver of increased triglyceride levels.[16] Notably, p38γ promotes the phosphorylation of AKT, which in turn phosphorylates AMPK on the inhibitory residues S485 and S491, driving insulin resistance. Insulin resistance is also induced by p38γ/δ activation of p62-mTORC1-S6K1-IRS signaling, which inhibits autophagy.[21] Insulin resistance, autophagy inhibition, and increased triglyceride levels converge to induce hepatic steatosis.

Glucagon-Like Peptide-1 Receptor Signaling

The GLP-1 receptor (GLP-1R) is a G protein–coupled receptor expressed on the surface of many cell types. Its cognate ligand is a 30-residue peptide hormone, GLP-1, which stimulates glucose-mediated insulin production by pancreatic beta cells.[22] Studies have shown a decrease in endogenous GLP-1 secretion in patients with NAFLD.[23] GLP-1R agonists are analogues of GLP-1 and fall under the class of incretin mimetics. In obese mice and in humans, administration of GLP-1R agonists reduces hepatic steatosis.[24] Apart from its effects on weight loss, GLP-1R agonists might play a direct role in improving hepatic steatosis through upregulation of insulin signaling pathways, fatty acid metabolism, and autophagy-dependent lipid degradation.[25] For example, liraglutide, as an agonist of GLP-1R, has been shown to restore autophagic flux, specifically the transcription factor EB–mediated autophagy-lysosomal pathway.[26] Liu and colleagues[27] have also shown a critical role of liver-derived FGF 21 in mediating the effects of GLP-1, and Farnesoid-X-receptor (FXR) is a multipurpose NR that plays an important role in regulating bile acid homeostasis, glucose and lipid metabolism, and hepatic regeneration.[28]

Nuclear Receptors

NRs comprise a superfamily of ligand-activated transcription factors that act as important cellular sensors. They primarily function through DNA binding and can be activated by several lipid soluble signals. Farnesoid X receptor (FXR) is a multipurpose NR that plays an important role in regulating bile acid homeostasis, glucose and lipid metabolism, and hepatic regeneration. FXR activation represses hepatic lipogenesis via the FXR-SHP-SREBP-1c pathway.[29] In addition, it reduces hepatic fatty acid uptake and promotes lipid oxidation.[30] Obeticholic acid, an agonist of FXR, has been shown to improve histological hepatic steatosis, suggesting a key role of FXR in the pathogenesis of NAFLD.[31] Interestingly, the therapeutic actions of FXR agonism may involve FGF15 and FGF19 as downstream effectors.[32] Other NRs, including liver X receptors (LXRs), are important regulators of intracellular cholesterol and lipids homeostasis. Differently from FXR agonists, LXR agonists can cause hepatic steatosis and dysfunction in part by increasing expression of SREBP1-c, a transcription factor that upregulates fatty acid synthesis.[33] Therefore, FXR- and LXR-related pathways are involved in the pathogenesis of hepatic steatosis in an opposite fashion.

Noncoding Ribonucleic Acid (RNAs)

ncRNAs constitute a vast and diverse family of non–protein-coding transcripts. Through their interaction with DNA, RNA, and proteins, ncRNAs may regulate various biological processes, such as gene transcription, RNA turnover, and mRNA translation that can affect intrahepatic fat accumulation. An increase of the adipocyte-secreted microRNA-34a (miR-34a) is responsible for the decrease of PPAR-α expression and consequent steatosis development.[34] In addition, inhibition of hepatic miR-24 leads to an increase in the Insig1 target, a lipogenesis inhibitor, preventing hepatic lipid accumulation.[35] Another study showed that miR-141/200c deficiency in mice reduced triglyceride accumulation via AMPK activation to promote PPARα-mediated fatty acid β-oxidation.[36] Circular RNA Circ_0057558,[37] LncRNA Blnc1,[38] lncRNA H19,[39] miR-137-3p,[40] circRNA_0046366,[41] and NEAT1/miR-140[42] have all been identified in the literature as potential mediators of hepatic lipogenesis. In general, miRNA expression patterns are complex and dynamic. Emerging data encourage further analysis and characterization of specific miRNAs that may be either downregulated or upregulated aberrantly in hepatic steatosis.

SIGNALING PATHWAYS INVOLVED IN THE PATHOGENESIS OF NONALCOHOLIC STEATOHEPATITIS

In general, accumulation of fat in the liver is not *per se* sufficient to cause parenchymal inflammation, and a "second-hit" is required to trigger liver injury. When different triggers are present concomitantly, the risk of NASH development increases markedly. Currently, the most common triggers of inflammatory changes include oxidative

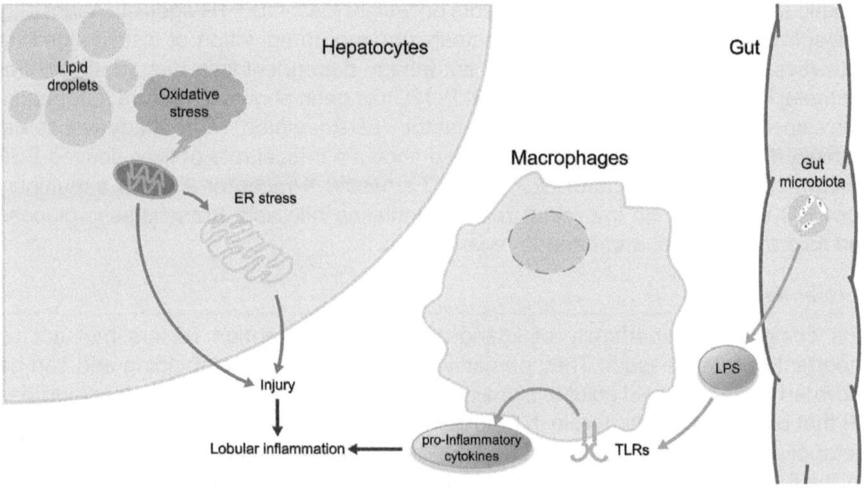

Fig. 2. Pathways regulate lobular inflammation in NAFLD. Liver steatosis provokes lipid peroxidation and successively ER stress, both of which lead to hepatocyte injury. Injured hepatocytes initiate the lobular inflammation in NAFLD. On dysbiosis, endotoxin (eg, LPS) derived from gram-negative gut bacteria activates resident and recruited macrophages via pattern recognition receptors (eg, TLRs). Activated macrophages release proinflammatory cytokines, which disrupt the balance between pro- and antiinflammatory factors, to promote inflammatory response in hepatic lobule. ER, endoplasmic reticulum; LPS, lipopolysaccharide; TLR, Toll-like receptor.

stress, endoplasmic reticulum stress, cytokines, and/or bacterial endotoxin. It has been estimated that 15% to 25% of cases of NAFL will ultimately progress to NASH. The development of NASH is thus a complex phenomenon in which Kupffer cells seem to play a major role.

Oxidative Stress

Oxidative stress occurs when ROS are produced in excess of antioxidant defenses. In the liver, oxidative stress can be generated through mechanisms involving mitochondrial dysfunction (leading to progressive impairment of β-oxidation, respiratory chain, and Adenosine Triphosphate synthesis) and increased fatty acid oxidation in either peroxisomes by acyl-CoA oxidase[43] or the endoplasmic reticulum by cytochrome P450 (CYP) enzymes 2E1 and CYP4A isoforms (**Fig. 2**).[44] Mitochondrial structure can also play a role in its dysfunction; in patients with NASH, at least 40% of mitochondria are structurally abnormal. These abnormalities (enlarged mitochondria, loss of mitochondrial cristae, and paracrystalline inclusions) impair the electron transport chain enzyme activity and lead to uncoupling of oxidation from phosphorylation and production of ROS.[45]

Endoplasmic Reticulum Stress

Endoplasmic reticulum (ER) stress (ie, disruption of ER function leading to complex signaling cascades that attempt to ameliorate the stress) can lead to generation of ROS. Two CYP enzymes, CYP2E1 and CYP4A, are found in the ER and are responsible for a variety of detoxification reactions.[46] CYP2E1 catalyzes the ω-1 hydroxylation of long-chain fatty acids, whereas CYP4A catalyzes the ω and ω-1 hydroxylation of medium chain fatty acids (C6-C12). Moreover, CYP2E1 catalyzes the NADH-dependent reduction of oxygen, leading to lipid peroxidation. Hepatic CYP2E1 expression has been shown to be increased in both rat dietary models of steatohepatitis as well as in patients with NASH.[47] In mice fed a methionine choline–deficient (MCD) diet, steatohepatitis was induced as well as CYP2E1 expression and catalysis of lipid peroxides by hepatic microsomes.[48] This study showed that CYP2E1 can act as an initiator of oxidative stress in steatotic livers; however, when CYP2E1 knockout mice were fed a MCD diet, steatohepatitis and lipid peroxidation were still induced,[48] suggesting there are other catalysts to lipid peroxidation involved in the progression of steatohepatitis. One such alternative catalyst is CYP4A, which was discovered in vitro to play a role in lipid peroxidation in the absence of CYP2E1. In this scenario, targeting a specific enzyme involved in lipid peroxidation may be futile due to the redundant nature of microsomal enzyme expression in lipid store management under conditions of NAFLD. Hanada and colleagues[49] used human hepatoma cells and hepatocytes to show that oxidative stress coupled with limited proteosome inhibition induced ER dysfunction and inclusion formation. Inclusion formations (or Mallory bodies) in hepatocytes are significant markers of many liver diseases, including NASH. Prevention or alleviation of oxidative stress may prevent or reduce Mallory body formation and ER dysfunction in NAFLD.

Cytokines

Cytokines are pleiotropic molecules responsible for the propagation of immune response signal. The liver plays a secretory role in the development of NASH in the context of cytokine release from Kupffer cells.[50] For example, tumor necrosis factor alpha (TNF-α) production occurs early and triggers production of other cytokines that recruit inflammatory cells, kill hepatocytes, and initiate fibrogenesis. Proinflammatory cytokines can upregulate the synthesis of secondary mediators and proinflammatory cytokines by macrophages and mesenchymal cells, stimulate production of acute phase proteins, and attract inflammatory cells.[51] In the context of liver injury, TNF-α production occurs early and triggers production of other cytokines that recruit inflammatory cells, kill hepatocytes, and initiate fibrogenesis.[52] Antiinflammatory cytokines counteract inflammation through direct inhibition of proinflammatory cytokines or through other means. From an anatomical standpoint, both the liver and visceral adipose tissue share proximal associations between metabolic cells (hepatocytes and adipocytes, respectively), immune cells, Kupffer cells, hepatic stellate cells, endothelial cells, or macrophages, with each tissue having immediate access to an extensive network of blood vessels for continuous or dynamic immune and metabolic responses.[53] Data in the fatty livers of Zucker diabetic (fa/fa) rats and leptin-deficient ob/ob mice showed abnormal basal cytokine production after a Kupffer cell–activating endotoxin challenge, which resulted in the development of severe NASH.[54] TNF-α has consistently shown to be increased in patients with NASH and correlates with NASH severity.[55]

Gut Microbiota

Bacterial endotoxin, such as lipopolysaccharides (LPS) derived from gram-negative bacteria, are glycolipids that have the ability to induce an inflammatory response in infected organisms. The liver functions to restrict the entry of LPS from the gut into the systemic circulation. The activation of Kupffer cells in the liver plays a critical role in the hepatic clearance of LPS. Specifically, this activation is mediated through LPS binding protein (LBP), CD14, and Toll-like receptor 4 (TLR-4). LPS binds to LBP in the serum, which transfers LPS to the peripheral monocyte membrane-bound

CD14.[56,57] In Kupffer cells, CD14 expression is relatively low normally but is rapidly upregulated on exposure to agents such as LPS. TLR-4 is a downstream component of CD14 and required for Kupffer cell activation. On activation, Kupffer cells release proinflammatory cytokines.[51] This inflammatory response can induce liver injury, perhaps not via a single cytokine alone but rather through disruption of the balance between pro- and antiinflammatory factors. The composition of gut microflora can have a profound impact on caloric intake in both mice and humans. There are 2 predominant populations of microbiota in both the mouse and human, *Firmicutes* and *Bacteroidetes*. In obese individuals, the proportion of *Firmicutes* is higher than that of lean individuals.[58] The significance of this observation lies in the ability of Firmicutes to encode enzymes that can break down otherwise indigestible dietary polysaccharides, thus increasing caloric absorption. When chronic, this enhanced caloric absorption may lead to increased body weight. Alterations in the composition of gut microflora can influence the integrity of the liver. In one study, Sprague-Dawley rats received either saline, probiotics, *Escherichia coli*, *Salmonella enteritidis*, or gentamicin orally for 7 days. On the eighth day, acute liver damage was induced by intraperitoneal injection of D-galactosamine in all but the control saline group. The probiotic, *Escherichia coli* and gentamicin groups had attenuated liver damage, decreased bacterial translocation, and decreased circulating levels of TNF-α, interleukin-6 (IL-6), IL-10, and IL-12.[59] Overall, the study showed that alterations in gut microflora acted through modifications of bacterial translocation, local gut cytokine expression, and endotoxin to prevent (eg, probiotic, , and gentamicin) or exacerbate (eg, *Salmonella enteritidis*) acute liver injury. The composition of gut microbiota can also influence gut permeability. In a study done by Cani and colleagues, ob/ob mice were treated with a control diet or a control diet fortified with either prebiotic or nonprebiotic carbohydrates. Prebiotic treatment involved incorporation of fermentable dietary fiber (oligofructose), whereas nonprebiotic treatment involved incorporation of nonfermentable dietary fiber (cellulose). Prebiotic treated mice exhibited lower circulating LPS, cytokines, and decreased hepatic expression of inflammatory and oxidative stress biomarkers when compared with nonprebiotic controls.[60]

SIGNALING PATHWAYS INVOLVED IN THE PATHOGENESIS OF LIVER FIBROSIS

The onset and severity of liver fibrosis is the most important predictor of hepatic and extrahepatic outcomes in patients with NAFLD. The main acknowledged cell mediators of profibrotic mechanisms in NAFLD are hepatic stellate cells (HSCs). Activation and transdifferentiation of HSCs toward myofibroblasts and, to a lesser extent, other mesenchymal cells (eg, portal fibroblasts, mesothelia fibroblasts, vascular smooth muscle cells, and scar-associated mesenchymal cells) plays a key role in the deposition of extracellular matrix (ECM) of the liver.

Transforming Growth Factor Beta Signaling Pathway of Hepatic Stellate Cells

The exposure of HSCs to profibrotic mediators, such as Hh, OPN, DAMP, transforming growth factor beta (TGF-β), platelet-derived growth factor, TNFSF12, and IL-1β locating in the sinusoidal space adjacent to Kupffer cells, pit cells, and endothelial cells, function to deposit vitamin A in cytoplasmic lipid droplets.[61] They experience the quiescent-to-activated transition of phenotype after exposing to several fibrogenic agents derived from injured or dead hepatocytes and immune cells. Although lots of pathways exhibit implication in the activation of HSCs, TGF-β signaling pathway has widely been accepted to play a central role. TGF-β_1, one of the key drivers of liver fibrogenesis, released initially in the latent form undergoes activation by local integrin

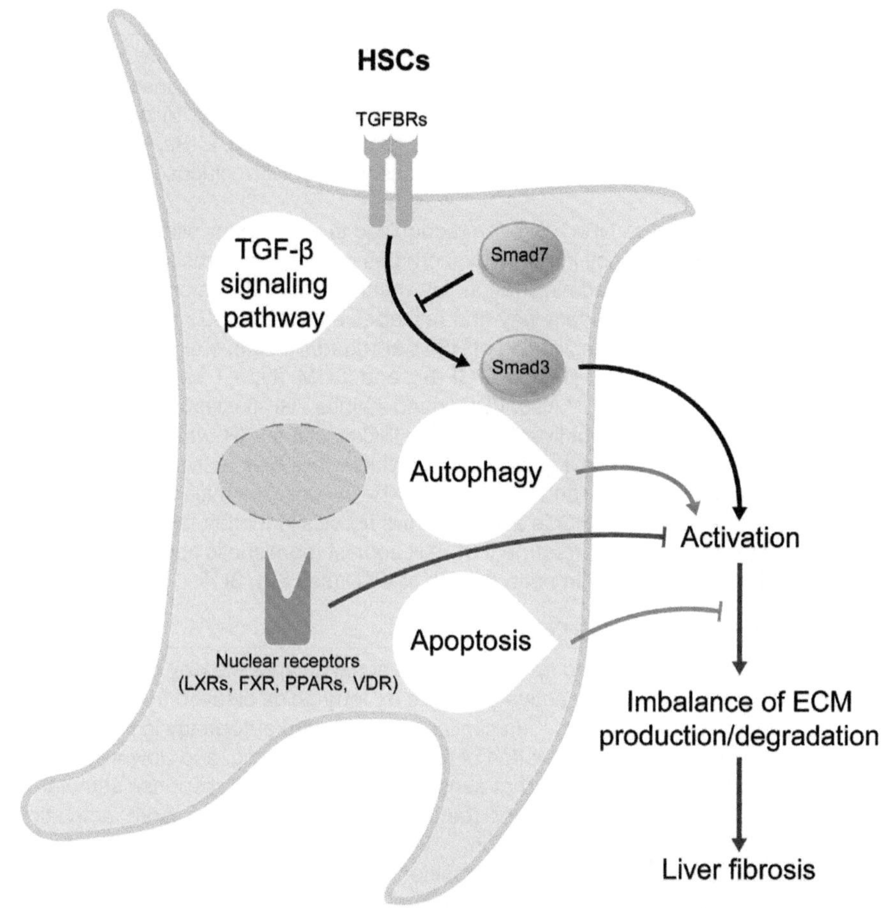

Fig. 3. Pathogenetic pathways underlying hepatic stellate cell (HSC)-induced liver fibrosis in NAFLD. Ligands of TGFBRs activate HSCs through TGF-beta signaling pathway in Smad3-dependent manner, whereas Smad7 antagonizes the process. In similar, autophagy of HSCs promotes their activation. However, nuclear receptors (eg, LXRs, FXR, PPARs, VDR) exert inhibitory role in HSC activation. HSCs apoptosis decreases the population of activated HSCs. Activation of HSCs disrupts the balance of ECM production/degradation and resultantly induces liver fibrosis. ECM, extracellular matrix; ER, endoplasmic reticulum; FXR, farnesoid X receptor; LXR, liver X receptor; PPAR, peroxisome proliferator–activated receptor; TGFBR, transforming growth factor beta receptor.

aV. Then it phosphorylates type I TGF-β receptor to activate the TGF-β signaling pathway in a Smad-dependent way. Phosphorylation of SMAD family member 3 (Smad3) further promotes the transcription of ECM comprising 20 types of fibrillary and nonfibrillar collagen, especially type I and type III collagen. ECM overproduction, together with inhibited degradation, by activated HSCs disrupts the dynamic balance in ECM metabolism and leads to liver fibrosis. Conversely, Smad7 acts as negative regulator to block the fibrogenic response induced by TGF-β signaling pathway (**Fig. 3**).[62] miR-29b, which shows expressive deficiency in activated murine HSCs, exerts inhibitory effect on collagen expression.[63]

Nuclear Receptors of Hepatic Stellate Cells

Except for the imbalanced ECM metabolism, activated HSCs demonstrate phenotypic changes in proliferation, apoptosis, epithelial-to-mesenchymal transition (EMT), chemotaxis, contractility, and so forth. Most of them are revealed to be under the modulation, mainly in the negative pattern, of a group of NRs (eg, LXRs, FXR, PPARs, vitamin D receptor, retinoid X receptor α) associated with glucose and/or lipid metabolism.

Downregulation of these NRs has been recognized in accompany with the activation of HSCs.[64] PPAR-γ deficiency in HSCs exacerbates rodent liver fibrosis in response to carbon tetrachloride (CCl_4) administration. By contrast, miR-16 restores the PPAR-γ expression in a Wnt3a-dependent way and reshapes activated HSCs to the quiescent phenotype.[64] Phenotypic normalization of HSCs abrogates their overexpression of EMT marker (α-SMA), fibrogenic cytokine (TGF-β), and ECM (type I collagen), with an outcome of fibrosis alleviation.[64] Also, VDR ligand inhibits TGF-β–stimulated HSCs activation and subsequently rodent liver fibrosis.[65] HSCs lacking LXR-α/LXR-β suffer from increased cholesterol and retinyl esters, both of which drive their activation through the retinoic acid receptor signaling and predispose LXR-α/β-deficient mice to liver fibrogenesis.[66] Similar phenomena of HSCs activation and fibrosis induction take place in condition of FXR loss.[67] However, treatment of FXR agonist (obeticholic acid) confers clear improvement of fibrosis stage in patients with NAFLD (see **Fig. 3**).[68]

Autophagy of Hepatic Stellate Cells

The pathways of autophagy and apoptosis often act in an antergic way to regulate the activation of HSCs. Autophagy activates HSCs by fatty acids cleaved from retinyl esters of cytoplasmic lipid droplets.[69] In similar, LPS-induced autophagy in HSCs leads to the loss of lipid droplets, dysfunction of retinoic acid signaling, and downregulation of TGF-β pseudoreceptor (Bambi) that sensitize them to fibrotic response stimulated by TGF-β.[70] But autophagy inhibitor (bafilomycin A1) decreases both activation marker of HSCs and their proliferation.[71] HSC-specific deficiency of autophagy-related protein 7 reduces the ECM deposition and fibrogenesis in mice with CCl_4 exposure.[72] Consistently, autophagic inhibition in HSCs and mice attenuates matrix accumulation and live fibrosis (see **Fig. 3**).[73] CircRNA608-miR-222-PINK1 axis has been verified an epigenetic regulation underlying the mitophagy of HSCs in NASH-related liver fibrosis.[74]

Apoptosis of Hepatic Stellate Cells

Compared with their quiescent phenotype, activated HSCs are featured by the resistance to apoptosis.[75] The enhanced proliferation and suppressed apoptosis integrate to expand the population of activated HSCs, which takes essential part in the progression of liver fibrosis (see **Fig. 3**). The activation-related apoptotic insensitivity of HSCs is partly attributed to the significant reduction of miR-130a-3p and resultantly the reactivation of TGF-β signaling pathway by TGFBR1 and TGFBR2 rescue.[76] Expressive loss of miR-16 and miR-15b represents another important mechanism of apoptotic resistance *via* the upregulated level of B-cell lymphoma-2 that prevents mitochondrial apoptosis.[77] Nevertheless, low-level expression of signal transducer and activator of transcription 1 may contribute to this phenotypic characteristics.[78]

SUMMARY

Multiple pathways including insulin signaling, JNK1/2 of MAPK signaling, GLP-1R signaling, and NRs affect to maintain the homeostasis of lipid metabolism in normal liver. ERK1/2 and P38 of MAPK signaling pathway antagonistically regulate the autophagy of hepatocytes. Functional imbalance of these pathways leads to hepatic steatosis by triglyceride increase and autophagy inhibition, together with insulin resistance based on inhibitory phosphorylation of Irs. Liver steatosis provokes lipid peroxidation and ER stress, which result in hepatocyte injury and lobular inflammation. Besides, gut-derived microbial metabolite (eg, LPS) stimulates the TLR-dependent production of proinflammatory cytokines by macrophages. Both hepatic injury and cytokine-induced inflammatory response initiate the occurrence and development of NASH and related fibrosis. On ligand-based TGFBRs activation, HSCs obtain activated phenotype through the TGF-β signaling pathway. But the activation and population of HSCs can be inhibited by NRs and apoptosis, respectively. Abnormalities in these pathways disrupt the balance of ECM production and degradation of the liver, with an outcome of advanced fibrosis and cirrhosis. Despite the present knowledge of pathogenic pathways, further researches are needed to highlight other ones underlying NAFLD effector cells and related pathological characteristics. Finishing this jigsaw puzzle could make access to the effective prevention and treatment of NAFLD, and keep patients free for NASH and related cirrhosis, and hepatocellular carcinoma.

CLINICS CARE POINTS

- Dysregulation and functional imbalance of pathways (e.g., JNK, ERK, P38, GLP-1R, and insulin signaling) lead to hepatic steatosis.
- Liver steatosis, dysbiosis, and microbial metabolite provokes hepatocyte injury and lobular inflammation.
- Both hepatic injury and inflammatory response induce NASH.
- Quiescent-to-activation transition of hepatic stellate cells results in liver fibrosis and cirrhosis.

FINANCIAL SUPPORT

This work was supported by the National Natural Science Foundation of China (grants 82170588 and 81470859 to Q. Pan; grants 81873565 and 82170593 to J-G. Fan) and the National Key Research and Development Program of China (grant 2021YFC2700802 to J-G. Fan). People's Livelihood Project of PuDong Committee on Science and Technology (PKJ2022-Y44) to Q. Pan.

CONFLICTS OF INTEREST

The authors have no conflicts of interest to declare.

REFERENCES

1. Fan JG, Wei L, Zhuang H. National workshop on fatty liver and alcoholic liver disease, Chinese society of hepatology, Chinese medical association; fatty liver disease expert committee, Chinese medical doctor association. Guidelines of prevention and treatment of nonalcoholic fatty liver disease (2018, China). J Dig Dis 2019;20(4):163–73.
2. Riazi K, Azhari H, Charette JH, et al. The prevalence and incidence of NAFLD worldwide: a systematic review and meta-analysis. Lancet Gastroenterol Hepatol 2022. https://doi.org/10.1016/S2468-1253(22)00165-0. S2468-1253(22)00165-0.

3. Kaya E, Yilmaz Y. Epidemiology, natural history, and diagnosis of metabolic dysfunction-associated fatty liver disease: a comparative review with nonalcoholic fatty liver disease. Ther Adv Endocrinol Metab 2022;13. https://doi.org/10.1177/20420188221139650. 20420188221139650.
4. Matsuzaka T, Kuba M, Koyasu S, et al. Hepatocyte ELOVL fatty acid elongase 6 determines ceramide Acyl-Chain length and hepatic insulin sensitivity in mice. Hepatology 2020;71(5):1609–25.
5. Cordero-Herrera I, Martín MA, Goya L, et al. Cocoa flavonoids protect hepatic cells against high-glucose-induced oxidative stress: relevance of MAPKs. Mol Nutr Food Res 2015;59(4):597–609.
6. Jeong S-H, Kim H-B, Kim M-C, et al. Hippo-mediated suppression of IRS2/AKT signaling prevents hepatic steatosis and liver cancer. J Clin Investig 2018;128(3):1010–25.
7. Yue X, Han T, Hao W, et al. SHP2 knockdown ameliorates liver insulin resistance by activating IRS-2 phosphorylation through the AKT and ERK1/2 signaling pathways. FEBS Open Bio 2020;10(12):2578–87.
8. Jeong O, Kim H-S. Dietary chokeberry and dried jujube fruit attenuates high-fat and high-fructose diet-induced dyslipidemia and insulin resistance via activation of the IRS-1/PI3K/Akt pathway in C57BL/6 J mice. Nutr Metab 2019;16:38.
9. Elchebly M, Payette P, Michaliszyn E, et al. Increased insulin sensitivity and obesity resistance in mice lacking the protein tyrosine phosphatase-1B gene. Science (New York, NY) 1999;283(5407):1544–8.
10. Yamamoto-Kataoka S, Ebihara K, Aizawa-Abe M, et al. Leptin improves fatty liver independently of insulin sensitization and appetite suppression in hepatocyte-specific Pten-deficient mice with insulin hypersensitivity. Horm Metab Res 2015;47(3):168–75.
11. Lyu K, Zhang Y, Zhang D, et al. A membrane-bound diacylglycerol species induces PKCε-mediated hepatic insulin resistance. Cell Metab 2020;32(4):654–64.e5.
12. Linden AG, Li S, Choi HY, et al. Interplay between ChREBP and SREBP-1c coordinates postprandial glycolysis and lipogenesis in livers of mice. J Lipid Res 2018;59(3):475–87.
13. Laplante M, Sabatini DM. mTORC1 activates SREBP-1c and uncouples lipogenesis from gluconeogenesis. Proceedings of the National Academy of Sciences of the United States of America 2010;107(8):3281–2.
14. Xiao Y, Liu H, Yu J, et al. Activation of ERK1/2 ameliorates liver steatosis in leptin receptor-deficient (db/db) mice via stimulating ATG7-dependent autophagy. Diabetes 2016;65(2):393–405.
15. Kim T, Wayne Leitner J, Adochio R, et al. Knockdown of JNK rescues 3T3-L1 adipocytes from insulin resistance induced by mitochondrial dysfunction. Biochem Biophys Res Commun 2009;378(4):772–6.
16. Tang P, Low HB, Png CW, et al. Protective function of mitogen-activated protein kinase phosphatase 5 in aging- and diet-induced hepatic steatosis and steatohepatitis. Hepatol Commun 2019;3(6):748–62.
17. Lawan A, Zhang L, Gatzke F, et al. Hepatic mitogen-activated protein kinase phosphatase 1 selectively regulates glucose metabolism and energy homeostasis. Mol Cell Biol 2015;35(1):26–40.
18. Schattenberg JM, Singh R, Wang Y, et al. JNK1 but not JNK2 promotes the development of steatohepatitis in mice. Hepatology 2006;43(1):163–72.

19. Bertran L, Portillo-Carrasquer M, Aguilar C, et al. Deregulation of secreted Frizzled-related protein 5 in nonalcoholic fatty liver disease associated with obesity. Int J Mol Sci 2021;22(13):6895.
20. Vernia S, Cavanagh-Kyros J, Garcia-Haro L, et al. The PPARα-FGF21 hormone axis contributes to metabolic regulation by the hepatic JNK signaling pathway. Cell Metab 2014;20(3):512–25.
21. Duran A, Amanchy R, Linares JF, et al. p62 is a key regulator of nutrient sensing in the mTORC1 pathway. Mol Cell 2011;44(1):134–46.
22. Yang H, Wang S, Ye Y, et al. GLP-1 preserves β cell function via improvement on islet insulin signaling in high fat diet feeding mice. Neuropeptides 2021;85: 102110.
23. Liu Y, Wei R, Hong T-P. Potential roles of glucagon-like peptide-1-based therapies in treating non-alcoholic fatty liver disease. World J Gastroenterol 2014;20(27): 9090–7.
24. Dong Y, Lv Q, Li S, et al. Efficacy and safety of glucagon-like peptide-1 receptor agonists in non-alcoholic fatty liver disease: a systematic review and meta-analysis. Clinics and Research In Hepatology and Gastroenterology 2017;41(3): 284–95.
25. Gupta NA, Mells J, Dunham RM, et al. Glucagon-like peptide-1 receptor is present on human hepatocytes and has a direct role in decreasing hepatic steatosis in vitro by modulating elements of the insulin signaling pathway. Hepatology 2010;51(5):1584–92.
26. Fang Y, Ji L, Zhu C, et al. Liraglutide alleviates hepatic steatosis by activating the TFEB-regulated autophagy-lysosomal pathway. Front Cell Dev Biol 2020;8: 602574.
27. Liu D, Pang J, Shao W, et al. Hepatic Fibroblast Growth Factor 21 Is Involved in mediating functions of liraglutide in mice with dietary challenge. Hepatology 2021;74(4):2154–69.
28. Xi Y, Li H. Role of farnesoid X receptor in hepatic steatosis in nonalcoholic fatty liver disease. Biomedicine & Pharmacotherapy = Biomedecine & Pharmacotherapie 2020;121:109609.
29. Carino A, Cipriani S, Marchianò S, et al. BAR502, a dual FXR and GPBAR1 agonist, promotes browning of white adipose tissue and reverses liver steatosis and fibrosis. Sci Rep 2017;7:42801.
30. Gai Z, Krajnc E, Samodelov SL, et al. Obeticholic acid ameliorates valproic acid-induced hepatic steatosis and oxidative stress. Mol Pharmacol 2020;97(5): 314–23.
31. Gai Z, Visentin M, Gui T, et al. Effects of farnesoid X receptor activation on arachidonic acid metabolism, NF-kB signaling, and hepatic inflammation. Mol Pharmacol 2018;94(2):802–11.
32. Han X, Cui Z-Y, Song J, et al. Acanthoic acid modulates lipogenesis in nonalcoholic fatty liver disease via FXR/LXRs-dependent manner. Chem Biol Interact 2019;311:108794.
33. Wen F, An C, Wu X, et al. MiR-34a regulates mitochondrial content and fat ectopic deposition induced by resistin through the AMPK/PPARα pathway in HepG2 cells. Int J Biochem Cell Biol 2018;94:133–45.
34. Ng R, Wu H, Xiao H, et al. Inhibition of microRNA-24 expression in liver prevents hepatic lipid accumulation and hyperlipidemia. Hepatology 2014;60(2):554–64.
35. Tran M, Lee S-M, Shin D-J, et al. Loss of miR-141/200c ameliorates hepatic steatosis and inflammation by reprogramming multiple signaling pathways in NASH. JCI Insight 2017;2(21):e96094.

36. Chen X, Tan Q-Q, Tan X-R, et al. Circ_0057558 promotes nonalcoholic fatty liver disease by regulating ROCK1/AMPK signaling through targeting miR-206. Cell Death Dis 2021;12(9):809.
37. Zhao X-Y, Xiong X, Liu T, et al. Long noncoding RNA licensing of obesity-linked hepatic lipogenesis and NAFLD pathogenesis. Nat Commun 2018;9(1):2986.
38. Liu C, Yang Z, Wu J, et al. Long noncoding RNA H19 interacts with polypyrimidine tract-binding protein 1 to reprogram hepatic lipid homeostasis. Hepatology 2018; 67(5):1768–83.
39. Yu Y, He C, Tan S, et al. MicroRNA-137-3p improves nonalcoholic fatty liver disease through activating AMPK. Analytical Cellular Pathology (Amsterdam) 2021; 2021:4853355.
40. Guo X-Y, Sun F, Chen J-N, et al. circRNA_0046366 inhibits hepatocellular steatosis by normalization of PPAR signaling. World J Gastroenterol 2018;24(3):323–37.
41. Sun Y, Song Y, Liu C, et al. LncRNA NEAT1-MicroRNA-140 axis exacerbates nonalcoholic fatty liver through interrupting AMPK/SREBP-1 signaling. Biochem Biophys Res Commun 2019;516(2):584–90.
42. Moreto F, Ferron AJT, Francisqueti-Ferron FV, et al. Differentially expressed proteins obtained by label-free quantitative proteomic analysis reveal affected biological processes and functions in Western diet-induced steatohepatitis. J Biochem Mol Toxicol 2021;35(6):1–11.
43. Liu Y, Liao L, Chen Y, et al. Effects of daphnetin on lipid metabolism, insulin resistance and oxidative stress in OA-treated HepG2 cells. Mol Med Rep 2019;19(6): 4673–84.
44. Vecchione G, Grasselli E, Cioffi F, et al. The nutraceutic silybin counteracts excess lipid accumulation and ongoing oxidative stress in an model of nonalcoholic fatty liver disease progression. Front Nutr 2017;4:42.
45. Song B-J, Akbar M, Jo I, et al. Translational implications of the alcohol-metabolizing enzymes, including cytochrome P450-2E1, in alcoholic and nonalcoholic liver disease. Adv Pharmacol 2015;74:303–72.
46. Ma H-L, Chen S-D, Zheng KI, et al. TA allele of rs2070673 in the CYP2E1 gene is associated with lobular inflammation and nonalcoholic steatohepatitis in patients with biopsy-proven nonalcoholic fatty liver disease. J Gastroenterol Hepatol 2021;36(10):2925–34.
47. Gopal T, Kumar N, Perriotte-Olson C, et al. Nanoformulated SOD1 ameliorates the combined NASH and alcohol-associated liver disease partly via regulating CYP2E1 expression in adipose tissue and liver. Am J Physiol Gastrointest Liver Physiol 2020;318(3):G428–38.
48. Leclercq IA, Farrell GC, Field J, et al. CYP2E1 and CYP4A as microsomal catalysts of lipid peroxides in murine nonalcoholic steatohepatitis. J Clin Investig 2000;105(8):1067–75.
49. Hanada S, Harada M, Kumemura H, et al. Oxidative stress induces the endoplasmic reticulum stress and facilitates inclusion formation in cultured cells. J Hepatol 2007;47(1):93–102.
50. Song K, Kwon H, Han C, et al. Yes-associated protein in kupffer cells enhances the production of proinflammatory cytokines and promotes the development of nonalcoholic steatohepatitis. Hepatology 2020;72(1):72–87.
51. Wree A, McGeough MD, Inzaugarat ME, et al. NLRP3 inflammasome driven liver injury and fibrosis: roles of IL-17 and TNF in mice. Hepatology 2018;67(2): 736–49.

52. Carranza-Trejo AM, Vetvicka V, Vistejnova L, et al. Hepatocyte and immune cell crosstalk in non-alcoholic fatty liver disease. Expet Rev Gastroenterol Hepatol 2021;15(7):783–96.
53. Li H, Zhou Y, Wang H, et al. Crosstalk between liver macrophages and surrounding cells in nonalcoholic steatohepatitis. Front Immunol 2020;11:1169.
54. Diehl AM. Nonalcoholic steatosis and steatohepatitis IV. Nonalcoholic fatty liver disease abnormalities in macrophage function and cytokines. Am J Physiol Gastrointest Liver Physiol 2002;282(1):G1–5.
55. Kugelmas M, Hill DB, Vivian B, et al. Cytokines and NASH: a pilot study of the effects of lifestyle modification and vitamin E. Hepatology 2003;38(2):413–9.
56. Ciesielska A, Matyjek M, Kwiatkowska K. TLR4 and CD14 trafficking and its influence on LPS-induced pro-inflammatory signaling. Cell Mol Life Sci 2021;78(4): 1233–61.
57. Tsukamoto H, Takeuchi S, Kubota K, et al. Lipopolysaccharide (LPS)-binding protein stimulates CD14-dependent Toll-like receptor 4 internalization and LPS-induced TBK1-IKKε-IRF3 axis activation. J Biol Chem 2018;293(26):10186–201.
58. Magne F, Gotteland M, Gauthier L, et al. The firmicutes/bacteroidetes ratio: a relevant marker of gut dysbiosis in obese patients? Nutrients 2020;12(5):1474.
59. Li Y-T, Wang L, Chen Y, et al. Effects of gut microflora on hepatic damage after acute liver injury in rats. J Trauma 2010;68(1):76–83.
60. Cani PD, Possemiers S, Van de Wiele T, et al. Changes in gut microbiota control inflammation in obese mice through a mechanism involving GLP-2-driven improvement of gut permeability. Gut 2009;58(8):1091–103.
61. Zhang J, Li Y, Liu Q, et al. Sirt6 alleviated liver fibrosis by deacetylating conserved lysine 54 on Smad2 in hepatic stellate cells. Hepatology 2021;73(3): 1140–57.
62. Mu M, Zuo S, Wu R-M, et al. Ferulic acid attenuates liver fibrosis and hepatic stellate cell activation via inhibition of TGF-β/Smad signaling pathway. Drug Des Dev Ther 2018;12:4107–15.
63. Gong X, Wang X, Zhou F. Liver microRNA-29b-3p positively correlates with relative enhancement values of magnetic resonance imaging and represses liver fibrosis. J Biochem 2020;168(6):603–9.
64. Pan Q, Guo C-J, Xu Q-Y, et al. miR-16 integrates signal pathways in myofibroblasts: determinant of cell fate necessary for fibrosis resolution. Cell Death Dis 2020;11(8):639.
65. Wan L-Y, Zhang Y-Q, Li J-M, et al. Liganded Vitamin D receptor through its interacting repressor inhibits the expression of type I collagen α1. DNA Cell Biol 2016; 35(9):498–505.
66. Endo-Umeda K, Makishima M. Liver X receptors regulate cholesterol metabolism and immunity in hepatic nonparenchymal cells. Int J Mol Sci 2019;20(20):5045.
67. Yang R, Hu Z, Zhang P, et al. Probucol ameliorates hepatic stellate cell activation and autophagy is associated with farnesoid X receptor. J Pharmacol Sci 2019; 139(2):120–8.
68. Younossi ZM, Ratziu V, Loomba R, et al. Obeticholic acid for the treatment of non-alcoholic steatohepatitis: interim analysis from a multicentre, randomised, placebo-controlled phase 3 trial. Lancet 2019;394(10215):2184–96.
69. Trivedi P, Wang S, Friedman SL. The power of plasticity-metabolic regulation of hepatic stellate cells. Cell Metab 2021;33(2):242–57.
70. Chen M, Liu J, Yang W, et al. Lipopolysaccharide mediates hepatic stellate cell activation by regulating autophagy and retinoic acid signaling. Autophagy 2017;13(11):1813–27.

71. Wu L, Zhang Q, Mo W, et al. Quercetin prevents hepatic fibrosis by inhibiting hepatic stellate cell activation and reducing autophagy via the TGF-β1/Smads and PI3K/Akt pathways. Sci Rep 2017;7(1):9289.
72. Chen W, Zhang Z, Yao Z, et al. Activation of autophagy is required for Oroxylin A to alleviate carbon tetrachloride-induced liver fibrosis and hepatic stellate cell activation. Int Immunopharm 2018;56:148–55.
73. Meng D, Li Z, Wang G, et al. Carvedilol attenuates liver fibrosis by suppressing autophagy and promoting apoptosis in hepatic stellate cells. Biomedicine & Pharmacotherapy = Biomedecine & Pharmacotherapie 2018;108:1617–27.
74. Xu Z-X, Li J-Z, Li Q, et al. CircRNA608-microRNA222-PINK1 axis regulates the mitophagy of hepatic stellate cells in NASH related fibrosis. Biochem Biophys Res Commun 2022;610:35–42.
75. Bian M, Chen X, Zhang C, et al. Magnesium isoglycyrrhizinate promotes the activated hepatic stellate cells apoptosis via endoplasmic reticulum stress and ameliorates fibrogenesis in vitro and in vivo. Biofactors 2017;43(6):836–46.
76. Wang Y, Du J, Niu X, et al. MiR-130a-3p attenuates activation and induces apoptosis of hepatic stellate cells in nonalcoholic fibrosing steatohepatitis by directly targeting TGFBR1 and TGFBR2. Cell Death Dis 2017;8(5):e2792.
77. Guo C-J, Pan Q, Xiong H, et al. Therapeutic potential of microRNA: a new target to treat intrahepatic portal hypertension? BioMed Res Int 2014;2014:797898.
78. Martí-Rodrigo A, Alegre F, Moragrega ÁB, et al. Rilpivirine attenuates liver fibrosis through selective STAT1-mediated apoptosis in hepatic stellate cells. Gut 2020;69(5):920–32.

Genetic Markers Predisposing to Nonalcoholic Steatohepatitis

Aalam Sohal, MD[a], Hunza Chaudhry, MD[b],
Kris V. Kowdley, MD[a,c,*]

KEYWORDS

• NASH • Progression • Genetic markers • *PNPLA3* • *TM6SF2* • *GCKR* • *MARC1*
• *HSD17B13*

KEY POINTS

- A better understanding of the genetic markers playing a role in the progression of nonalcoholic fatty liver disease (NAFLD) is needed.
- *PNPLA3* gene was the first gene identified to be associated with NAFLD via genome-wide association studies.
- Other genes that have been studied in association with NAFLD include *TM6SF2*, *MBOAT7*, *HSD17B13*, *GCKR*, and *HFE*.
- Assessment of polygenic scores can be beneficial in identifying patients at risk of NAFLD and increased risk of severe liver injury.

INTRODUCTION

Nonalcoholic fatty liver disease (NAFLD) has emerged as one of the most common causes of liver disease worldwide. The pooled prevalence of NAFLD worldwide has been estimated to be approximately 25%, with wide geographical variability.[1] Studies have projected that cases of NAFLD and nonalcoholic steatohepatitis (NASH) will continue to increase in the coming years. Based on current estimates, the prevalence of NAFLD will increase to 100 million cases, and NASH will increase to 27 million cases in the United States by 2030.[2] Given the estimated prevalence, there has been a growing interest in understanding the pathophysiology and natural history of this disease.

[a] Liver Institute Northwest, 3216 Northeast 45th Place Suite 212, Seattle, WA 98105, USA; [b] Department of Internal Medicine, UCSF Fresno, 155 North Fresno Street, Fresno, CA 93722, USA; [c] Elson S. Floyd College of Medicine, Washington State University, WA, USA
* Corresponding author. Liver Institute Northwest, 3216 Northeast 45th Place Suite 212, Seattle, WA 98105.
E-mail address: kkowdley@liverinstitutenw.org

Clin Liver Dis 27 (2023) 333–352
https://doi.org/10.1016/j.cld.2023.01.006 liver.theclinics.com

NAFLD can range from simple steatosis to NASH. NAFLD alone has not been associated with progression to more advanced stages of liver disease; however, the small proportion of patients with NAFLD who develop NASH[1] may be at increased risk of fibrosis, cirrhosis, and hepatocellular carcinoma (HCC).[3–5] The reasons for the differences in disease progression between individuals are largely unknown. In recent years, genetic differences have been considered to play a role in influencing the progression of the disease.

Previous epidemiological, familial, and twin studies have found that NAFLD is an inheritable disease.[6,7] Initial studies focused on select candidate genes, but the landscape has changed as genome-wide association studies (GWAS) have become more prevalent. GWAS has reduced limitations previously encountered, such as small size, false-positive associations due to cryptic population stratification, and reliance on prior knowledge for gene selection.[8–10] GWAS has led to the identification of genetic markers associated with NAFLD, with *PNPLA3* being the first identified genetic marker.[11] Since then, multiple other genetic markers have been identified.

Identifying these genetic markers can be an essential tool for the clinical management of patients with NAFLD. It could aid in risk stratification and identify potential therapeutic targets for NAFLD. In this review, we discuss the genetic markers that contribute to disease progression and the therapeutic targets currently being studied.

Genetic Markers Associated with the Progression of Steatosis to Nonalcoholic Steatohepatitis

PNPLA3 gene

PNPLA3 gene encodes the enzyme adiponutrin and is highly expressed in hepatocytes, stellate cells, and sinusoidal cells. *PNPLA3* protein has been shown to possess triacylglycerol lipase and acylglycerol transacylase activity (**Fig. 1**).[12] A single nucleotide mutation from isoleucine to methionine at position 148 (I148 M) is associated with loss of function of lipid remodeling in lipid droplets. This genetic variant was the first to be identified and associated with NAFLD.[11]

The prevalence of this genetic variant in the general population was 23% in the Dallas Heart Study; however, significant interethnic variations were reported. Hispanics had the highest prevalence of the I148 M allele (49%), whereas European Americans had a 23% prevalence. The lowest prevalence was noted in African Americans (17%).[11] These findings revealed that genetic makeup might explain the interethnic differences in the prevalence of NAFLD. In this study of 2111 individual patients from different ethnic backgrounds, the I148 M variant was associated with increased steatosis on GWAS, determined by magnetic resonance spectroscopy irrespective of alcohol or metabolic factors.[11] A subgroup analysis in the African American population identified a genetic variant rs6006460, associated with a lower hepatic fat in this ethnic group.[11] I148 M has also been associated with higher hepatic lipid content in the Finnish population.[13] This genetic variant has been associated with a higher risk of fatty liver and histological severity of NASH.

A study of 103 patients in Argentina identified an association between I148 M and NAFLD severity, determined by liver biopsy.[14] Dai and colleagues[15] reported that rs738409 polymorphism is associated with increased susceptibility to NAFLD and aggressive disease. Histological studies have shown that the I148 M is associated with higher odds of the portal and lobular inflammation and fibrosis.[16] The results of these studies were also confirmed in a meta-analysis performed by Sookian and Pirola.[17] It was found that I148 M is associated with an increased risk of steatosis, NASH, and fibrosis.

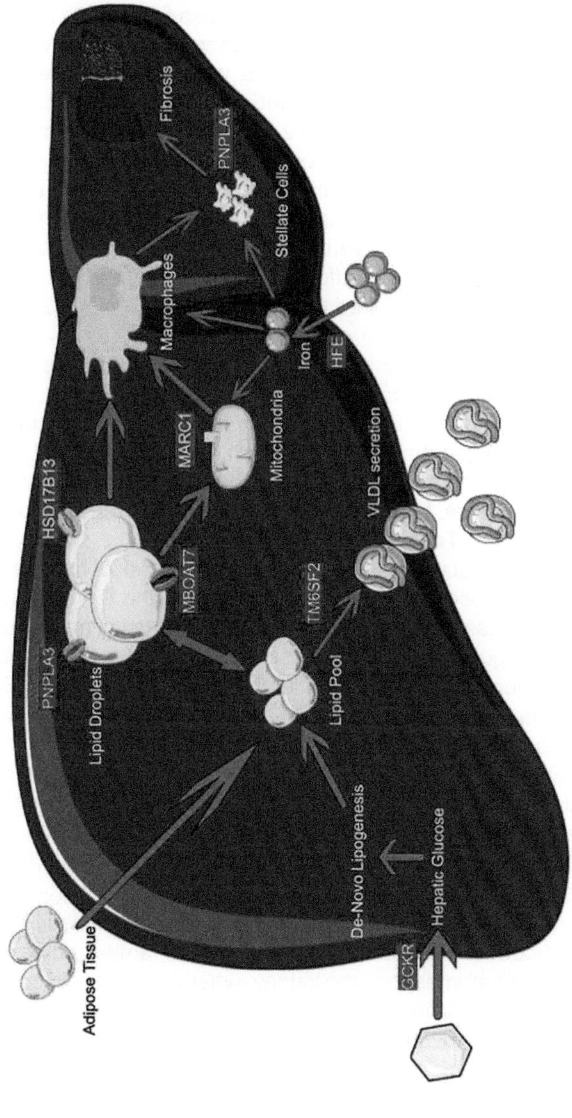

Fig. 1. Genetic markers associated with the progression of steatosis to NASH.

The I148 M variant has also been studied in the pediatric population. A study by Valenti and colleagues[18] on 149 pediatric patients with NAFLD pointed out that the I148 M determines the degree of hepatic steatosis. Interestingly, all patients in the study who were homozygous for this variant were diagnosed with NASH. A study on Mexican children aged 6 to 12 reported that the I148 M is associated with increased serum alanine transaminase (ALT) levels.[19] Similar results were reported in German children aged 5 to 9 years.[20] These findings are of clinical importance as identifying these patients early and tailoring weight-loss treatments may be beneficial in delaying disease progression. As an association was noted between I148 M and steatosis, inflammation, and fibrosis in patients with NAFLD, researchers studied the association of I148 M with HCC. Valenti and colleagues[21] reported that homozygosity for the I148 M was associated with a 2.2 higher risk of developing HCC in patients with chronic hepatitis C. This association was also noted in patients with alcoholic liver disease.[22] In a prospective study by Burza and colleagues[23] on 4000+ obese patients, an association was found between HCC and I148 M. However, it is currently unclear if the genetic variant confers a higher risk of HCC or if the increased risk of HCC is due to the effect of this genetic variant on inflammation and fibrosis. Further research is required to study the role of *PNPLA3* as a carcinogen in patients with NAFLD.

Weight loss has been shown to improve the outcomes in patients with the I148 M variant. A study by Marzuillo and colleagues[24] revealed that weight loss can improve steatosis in patients carrying the I148 M allele. In their study of 129 patients, weight loss was associated with a greater degree of serum ALT reduction and steatosis in patients homozygous for I148 M as compared with those who were heterozygous or homozygous for the major allele. Information on the effect and function of PNPLA3 and other genes is presented in **Tables 1** and **2**.

Owing to the known association between genes and the risk of NAFLD in the general population, studies have been conducted to investigate the therapeutic potential of *PNPLA3*. *PNPLA3* gene has been targeted in mice studies using antisense oligonucleotide. Linden and colleagues[25] reported that silencing this gene using antisense oligonucleotide reduces hepatic steatosis, inflammation, and fibrosis. BasuRay and colleagues[26] used small hairpin RNA (shRNA) against *PNPLA3* knock-in mice and reported a reduction in the hepatic triglyceride content. They also found that increasing proteolysis of the *PNPLA3* I148 M variant reduced the hepatic triglyceride content.[26] Clinical trials in humans have not yet targeted this variant. Prospective studies targeting I148 M may be beneficial in developing strategies against NAFLD.

Transmembrane 6 superfamily member 2 genes

The transmembrane 6 superfamily member 2 (*TM6SF2*) gene is located on chromosome 19, and it encodes a protein that contains 351 amino acids and is highly expressed in the liver, small intestine, and kidney, whereas a lower expression is noted in other organs.[27,28] Mahdessian and colleagues[28] observed that *TM6SF2* is primarily located in the endoplasmic reticulum (ER) and ER-Golgi intermediate compartment in hepatoma cells. A single nucleotide point mutation leads to the substitution of lysine instead of glutamate at codon 167. This genetic variant is referred to as the E167 K variant.[29] The mutation results in protein misfolding, further leading to increased protein degradation and reduced protein levels in the body.

An association between the *TM6SF2* E167 K genetic variant and NAFLD was first identified by Kozlitina and colleagues[29] in a GWAS. This genetic variant was found to be highly prevalent in people of European ancestry (7.2%), followed by Hispanic Americans (4.7%) and African Americans (3.4%). This study identified an association

Table 1
Table describing the common genetic polymorphism along with the mean allele frequency (described in 1000 genomics project) and their function

Variant	Gene	Minor Allele Frequency	Effect	Function
rs738409	*PNPLA3*	0.262	p.I148 M	Lipid droplet remodeling
rs58542926	*TM6SF2*	0.07	E167 K	VLDL secretion
rs641738	*MBOAT7*	0.37	Decrease in the protein	Decrease in phosphatidylinositol remodeling
rs780094	*GCKR*	0.30	Loss of function	Regulation of glucose uptake
rs1260326	*GCKR*	0.29	P446 L	Regulation of glucose uptake leading to increased de-novo-lipogenesis
rs72613567	*HSD17B13*	0.40	Loss of function	Lipid droplet remodeling
rs1051338	*LIPA*	0.29	Loss of function	LIPA gene encodes lysosomal acid lipase that breaks down fats
rs2642438	*MARC1*	0.19	p.A165 T	Has antioxidant activity
rs228063	*NCAN*	0.03	Pro92Ser	Hypothesized to control the brain–liver axis.

between the *TM6SF2* E167 K genetic variant and increased hepatic triglyceride content. It has been found that the *TM6SF2* wild allele plays a role in very low density lipoprotein (VLDL) secretion. This missense mutation leads to a decrease in the secretion of VLDL cholesterol, resulting in the accumulation of triglycerides within the liver.[29] Liu and colleagues[30] showed an association between the E167 K variant and hepatic fat and histologic fibrosis stages in a European Caucasian cohort. The effect of the E167 K variant on hepatic steatosis and fibrosis progression was further documented in studies performed in Chinese[31] and Japanese cohorts.[32] Dongiovanni and colleagues[33] were the first to document that the E167 K variant is associated with steatosis, fibrosis, and steatohepatitis. The association of this E167 K variant with HCC in patients with NAFLD is unclear.[34] Liu and colleagues[30] examined this association in patients with NAFLD. They reported a univariate association between the genetic variant and risk of HCC (odds ratio [OR] 1.922, 95% confidence interval [CI] 1.31

Table 2
Effect of genetic polymorphisms on risk of steatosis, NASH and fibrosis

Variant	Gene	Steatosis	NASH	Fibrosis
rs738409	*PNPLA3*	↑	↑	↑
rs58542926	*TM6SF2*	↑	↑	↑
rs641738	*MBOAT7*	↑	↑	↑
rs780094, rs1260326	*GCKR*	↑	↑	↑
rs1051338	*LIPA*	↑	↑[72] (only ↑ in transaminases)	n/a
C282Y/H63D	*HFE*	↑	↑	↑
rs72613567	*HSD17B13*	↑	↓	↓ (tendency toward decreased fibrosis)
rs2642438	*MARC1*	n/a	↓	↓
rs228063	*NCAN*	↑	↑	↑

to 2.81. $P = 6.81 \times 10^{-4}$). However, this association was not significant in multivariate analysis after adjusting for other factors.[30]

The presence of *TM6SF2* has also been studied in the pediatric population. Grandone and colleagues[35] were the first to study the effect of this gene in the pediatric population. Their study of 1010 obese children in Italy found a significant association between this genetic variant and the risk of steatosis and elevated transaminases. These results were further validated by Mancina and colleagues[36] in their study on 423 children/adolescents.

Although associated with deleterious effects on the liver, *TM6SF2* polymorphism is associated with decreased risk of atherosclerosis.[33] The reduced risk of atherosclerosis may be related to decreased VLDL secretion in these patients. Therapeutic strategies for overcoming the effects of this variant on the liver while maintaining its possible beneficial effects on atherosclerotic disease need further investigation.

Studies have also focused on the combined impact of *TM6SF2* and *PNPLA3* on NAFLD and progression. Chen and colleagues studied the additive effect of these variants. They found that the copresence of both mutations is associated with a higher triglyceride and total cholesterol content in hepa 1 to 6 cells.[37] Wang and colleagues[38] also documented that the copresence of both alleles is associated with a higher risk of NAFLD in the Han Chinese population.

A study by Paternostro and colleagues[39] could not show the additive effect of these genes on the risk of developing NASH or fibrosis on histological analysis in patients with biopsy-proven NAFLD. These results contradict the study by Koo and colleagues,[40] who showed that the presence of both these variants together increases the risk of NASH and fibrosis. Krawczyk and colleagues[41] reported the combined effect of these genes on serum aminotransferases but not on histological severity in biopsy-confirmed patients with NAFLD. Given the conflicting data, further research is needed regarding these gene interactions.

Membrane-bound o-acyltransferase domain containing 7

The membrane-bound o-acyltransferase domain containing 7 (*MBOAT7*) gene, located on chromosome 19, encodes a protein that is involved in acyl chain remodeling of phosphatidylinositol (PI) in the Lands cycle.[42,43] This enzyme regulates the amount of free arachidonic acid, which is a potential trigger for inflammation and fibrosis in the liver.[44] The *MBOAT7* gene is highly expressed in the liver and is attached to the ER, mitochondria-associated membranes, and lipid droplets.[45] This gene was first identified in a GWAS in patients with alcohol-related cirrhosis.[46] Subsequent studies on patients with NAFLD revealed an association between *MBOAT7* and NAFLD.[45,47]

It has been reported that the presence of the genetic variant rs641738 leads to decreased levels of MBOAT protein,[45] further leading to a decrease in PI remodeling.[48] It has also been hypothesized that the presence of rs641738 leads to increased sterol regulatory-element binding proteins (SREBP) expression, leading to increased de-novo lipogenesis.[49]

Mancina and colleagues[45] genotyped 3854 participants from the Dallas Heart Study and 1149 European individuals. These investigators found that this gene was associated with increased hepatic fat, liver damage, and fibrosis compared with the patients containing the wild gene. Their study reported that the association was restricted to European-Caucasian individuals. No significant association was found between African Americans and Hispanics. Luukkonen and colleagues[48] also studied 125 patients and reported that the presence of this genetic variant is associated with increased histological severity of NASH and severity of fibrosis. Since then, multiple studies have reported a lack of association between this genetic variant and NAFLD/NASH.[50–52] Given the conflicting data, Teo and colleagues[53] performed a meta-analysis on the *MBOAT7* gene and its effect on the spectrum of NAFLD. They reported that the rs641738 C > T gene was associated with increased hepatic fat content. These results did not differ based on the modality of imaging. No association was found between histological NASH and rs641738. However, a positive association between this gene and ALT levels was reported only in Caucasian adults.[53] The study also found an association between this variant and fibrosis. An association between rs641738 and HCC was also reported in the meta-analysis. This study reported a 30%,40%, and 50% increased risk of NAFLD, advanced fibrosis, and cirrhosis, respectively, in carriers compared with non-carriers.[53]

The 1000 genomes project comprehensively describes common human genetic variants using whole-genome sequencing.[54] The minor allele frequency of the genetic polymorphism in 1000 genomics project 3 was 37.4%. This gene is more prevalent in South Asian patients (56.4%), followed by patients of European descent (44%).[54] A copresence of *PNPLA3, TM6SF2, and MBOAT7* genetic variants has been studied on the risk of NAFLD. In the cohort of 172 patients, the copresence of these genetic variants has been associated with a higher degree of steatosis and histological severity of NASH.[55] Further studies examining the interactions between *MBOAT7* and other genes are warranted.

Glucokinase regulatory gene

Glucokinase regulatory (*GCKR*) gene, located on chromosome 2, codes the glucokinase regulatory protein, which is implicated in regulating glucose homeostasis by controlling the hepatic glucose uptake activity.[56,57] A single nucleotide mutation at position 227 leads to the conversion of the arginine codon to a premature stop codon, resulting in incomplete transcription of the protein.[58] This mutation leads to increased hepatic glucose content, which can further increase hepatic de-novo lipogenesis leading to fatty liver.[59] The rs780094 genetic variant has a mean allele frequency of 0.30.[54]

GWAS have studied the link between the *GCKR* gene and the presence of fatty liver. The study by Speliotes and colleagues[60] indicated that *GCKR* gene variant rs780094 is associated with an increased risk of hepatic steatosis based on CT imaging and histology. Yang and colleagues[61] reported an association between this genetic variant and increased risk of NAFLD in 903 Chinese patients. In 2014, a meta-analysis by Zain and colleagues[62] on five studies reported that this gene was associated with a higher risk of NAFLD (OR 1.25). Since then, multiple studies have examined this gene's role in NAFLD. A study by Petta and colleagues[63] reported that rs780094 is associated with fibrosis in patients with NAFLD. Tan and colleagues[64] reported that the presence of rs780094 predisposes to NAFLD, NASH, and significant fibrosis.

Another genetic polymorphism, rs1260326, has also been identified. A single nucleotide mutation from C > T leads to the coding of leucine instead of proline at position 446 (P446 L). Studies have found an association between rs1260326 and NAFLD. This association was reported by Santoro and colleagues[65] in their study of 446 obese patients. An updated meta-analysis by Li and colleagues[66] reported that the presence of rs780094 and rs1260326 is associated with an increased risk of NAFLD. A study by Hudert and colleagues[67] on 70 patients with biopsy-proven NAFLD reported that the presence of this gene is associated with a higher risk of fibrosis. Tan and colleagues[64] also reported similar findings in their study, revealing that the presence of rs1260326 and rs780094 is associated with the risk of NAFLD, NASH, and significant fibrosis. The rs1260326 SNP is in strong linkage disequilibrium with the rs780094 gene.[68] This strong linkage might explain the association of both these polymorphisms with NAFLD and severity. Pirola and colleagues[69] reported a rare nonsense mutation (rs149847328, p.Arg227Ter) in the *GCKR* gene. This mutation was associated with rapid progression from F0 to F4 within 5 years.

The association of genetic variants in the *GCKR* gene with *PNPLA3* I148 M has been studied. In a study on 455 obese children, Santoro and colleagues[59] reported that genetic variants in the *GCKR* and *PNPLA3* act in conjunction to increase the susceptibility toward fatty liver disease. He reported that the copresence of SNP's explained 39% of the hepatic fat content. A study by Goffredo and colleagues[70] documented that the copresence of *PNPLA3* I148 M, *TM6SF2* variant E167 K, and *GCKR* rs1260326 had an additive effect on the hepatic fat fraction. Further studies exploring these interactions are warranted.

Lipase A, lysosomal acid-type gene

The lipase A, lysosomal acid-type (*LIPA*) gene encodes for the lysosomal acid lipase (LAL) enzyme. This enzyme is responsible for the hydrolysis of cholesterol esters and triglycerides in lysosomes.[71] A common genetic variant rs1051338 involves the replacement of adenine with cytosine in position 46.[72] This leads to a change in the signal peptide, causing decreased transport of the enzyme LAL to the lysosome and increased cytoplasmic degradation. This results in a decrease in LAL protein and enzymatic activity.[72]

Reduction in the levels of LAL has been observed in patients with NAFLD.[73] This impairment of LAL may lead to increased intrahepatic accumulation of lipids.[74] The mechanism by which LAL causes increased hepatic lipid accumulation is still under investigation. However, Ouimet and colleagues[75] reported that reduction in LAL is associated with activation of transcription factors of SREBP, which activates increased lipogenesis.[76]

Pasta and colleagues[71] documented that rs1051338 polymorphism of the *LIPA* gene contributes to a worse form of dyslipidemia and is associated with a higher degree of steatosis in patients with NAFLD. They studied 74 patients and reported that the presence of rs1051338 is associated with an increased risk of developing severe hepatic steatosis. The study also reported higher ALT and AST levels in patients carrying the rs1051338 variant compared with others.[71]

LAL deficiency is an autosomal recessive disorder caused by mutations in the *LIPA* gene. In untreated infants, this disease is fatal.[77] However, in adults, it can lead to hepatomegaly, elevated AST and ALT, liver fibrosis, and cirrhosis.[78,79] A phase 3 trial evaluating the human enzyme replacement therapy for this enzyme deficiency revealed that human enzyme replacement therapy was associated with a significant reduction in the ALT levels.[80] There is limited data on the role of this gene in the pathogenesis of NASH and fibrosis. Further research is needed to understand the effect of this gene on severe forms of NAFLD.

HFE gene

HFE gene encodes the HFE protein, which regulates the production of hepcidin, the central iron regulatory hormone in humans.[81] Heterozygosity for the *HFE* C282Y mutation is associated with an increased risk of fatty liver disease. The two most common variants of the *HFE* gene are C282Y and H63D mutations.[82] C282Y HFE mutation is associated with decreased serum hepcidin and increased parenchymal iron.[83] Iron deposition in the liver can also lead to increased oxidative stress[84–86] and reduced VLDL secretion.[87] Hepatic iron can also result in ER stress,[88] stellate cell activation,[89] and macrophage activation.[90–92] It can also increase cholesterol synthesis.[93]

Nelson and colleagues[94] reported that *HFE* C282Y mutation is associated with advanced hepatic fibrosis in patients with NASH. In a study on 126 patients with NASH, C282Y heterozygous were more likely to have bridging fibrosis or cirrhosis. On the contrary, a study in Poland reported that the presence of these mutations had no association with the risk of fibrosis.[95] It has also been postulated that the pattern of hepatic iron deposition influences histological severity.[96] The literature has documented that iron deposition in the reticuloendothelial system is associated with advanced histological features such as fibrosis, portal inflammation, ballooning of hepatocytes, and definite NASH compared with patients with hepatocellular iron or patients with mixed iron patterns.[96]

Over the years, multiple studies have evaluated the role of *HFE* gene mutation in patients with NAFLD. In 2011, a meta-analysis reported that heterozygosity for the gene mutation is not associated with the presence of NAFLD.[97] This analysis was limited to Caucasians due to the small size of the Non-Caucasian population. An updated meta-analysis in 2018 reported that the presence of C282Y and H63D is associated with an increased risk of developing NAFLD and HCC but not cirrhosis.[98] The study also reported an increased risk of HCC in patients with *HFE* C282Y mutation. An increased risk of developing non-cirrhosis HCC was also reported in patients with *HFE* H63D mutation.

Because of the role of iron deposition in the pathogenesis of NAFLD, studies have focused on the role of phlebotomy as a potential treatment of NAFLD. Initial studies by Valenti and colleagues[99] on 21 patients reported that iron reduction by phlebotomy was associated with improved histological severity in patients with NAFLD and hyperferritinemia. Similar results were reported by Khodadoostan and colleagues[100] in their study of 32 patients with NAFLD. They also reported an improvement in ALT, AST, and ALP levels with phlebotomy sessions and an improvement in the histological severity of NAFLD/NASH. Most studies investigating the role of phlebotomy had a small sample size. Further prospective trials with a large sample size are needed to elucidate the role of phlebotomy as a potential management option in patients with NAFLD/NASH.

Hydroxysteroid 17-beta dehydrogenase 13

Hydroxysteroid 17-beta dehydrogenase 13 (*HSD17B13*) is located on chromosome 4, and its expression is highly restricted to the liver. It is expressed on hepatocytes and located on lipid droplets.[101] *HSD17B13* is thought to be essential in regulating liver lipid droplet biogenesis, growth, and degradation.[101] *HSD17B13* has retinol dehydrogenase activity.[102] Retinol esters, when activated, are known to play a pivotal role in fibrogenesis, which might be the underlying mechanism of worsening histological severity in patients with NAFLD.[103]

GWAS has identified an SNP in the *HSD17B13* gene that is associated with NAFLD; the rs683414 SNP was associated with increased steatosis but decreased inflammation and ballooning in 768 adult Caucasians with biopsy-proven NAFLD and cirrhosis in the general population.[102] rs72613567 is associated with a protective effect against the histological severity of NASH.[104] The patients with this genetic variant have decreased *HSD17B13* protein in the liver.[104] A meta-analysis by Wang and colleagues on liver disease patients reported that the rs72613567 variant protects against cirrhosis and HCC. In their study, the presence of the rs72613567 variant showed a trend toward decreased inflammation and reduced fibrosis in patients with NAFLD.[105]

Because of the potential role of *HSD17B13* in the pathogenesis of NASH, pharmaceutical companies are studying *HSD17B13* as a potential therapeutic target against the progression of NAFLD.[106,107] These studies are in the early phase of their trials, and long-term follow-up will be required before a conclusion can be drawn regarding their benefits and side effects.

Mitochondrial Amidoxime-reducing component 1 enzyme gene

Mitochondrial Amidoxime-reducing component 1 enzyme (*MARC1*) encodes Mitochondrial Amidoxime-reducing Component 1 Enzyme.[108] Emdin and colleagues[109] identified a missense mutation in the gene (*MARC1*p.A165 T), rs262438, which is protective against NAFLD. This work was confirmed by Luukkonen and colleagues,[110] who observed that the rs2642438 variant was associated with a lower prevalence of NASH in a cohort of 369 patients. Patients with the genetic variant had a lower prevalence of lobular inflammation, activity, and fibrosis. However, the prevalence of steatosis and ballooning were comparable between the two groups.

It was previously hypothesized that the genetic variant leads to the loss of alpha helix and altered metal-ion binding ability of the protein. However, Struwe and colleagues[111] studied the crystal structure and found that the alpha helix predicted to be lost is fully intact in the genetic variant. Further research in understanding the mechanisms that confer protection in patients with NAFLD is necessary.

NCAN locus

The *NCAN* locus contains 20 genes and is located on chromosome 19.[112] Neurocan is the protein product of this gene and is primarily expressed in the central nervous tissue.[113] Rs2228063 encodes a nonsynonymous mutation (Pro92Ser), altering the protein structure and function.[114] Although this protein is not directly expressed in the liver, this protein is thought to exert its effect through the brain-liver axis.[114] This gene is also noted to be in strong linkage disequilibrium with the E167 K variant of the TM6SF2 gene, which is associated with the progression of fatty liver disease.[115] Speliotes and colleagues[60] found an association between the rs2228603 and NAFLD. The results were further confirmed by Gorden and colleagues,[114] who observed that the presence of this genetic variant is not only associated with the degree of hepatic steatosis but also with histological features of NASH, such as signs of lobular inflammation and fibrosis.

Other genes

In recent years, there have been multiple other genes that have been studied in association with NAFLD and NASH, some of which are described below

The *APOC3* gene encodes apolipoprotein C-III, which is a VLDL that inhibits lipoprotein lipase and hepatic lipase.[112] Polymorphism in *APOC3* is associated with higher susceptibility to developing NAFLD in the southern Han Chinese population[116]; Valenti and colleagues[115] investigated *APOC3* polymorphisms T-455C and C-482T in European patients with NAFLD and found no protective effects of the *APOC3* wild-type and diagnosis of NASH. The *APOE* gene encodes apolipoprotein E, which is involved in endocytosis and clearance of chylomicron and VLDL particles by the liver.[117] Polymorphism in this gene is associated with an increased risk of NASH.[117] Verrijken and colleagues[118] also investigated another gene variant, rs2854117, and found no significant association. The data regarding genes encoding lipoproteins is mixed, and further research is needed to explore the diagnosis.

Oxidative stress on hepatocytes is instrumental in developing NAFLD and NASH.[119] Various studies have evaluated the effects of genetic variants in mitochondria. One such gene is the superoxide dismutase 2 (SOD2) gene which catalyzes the conversion of superoxide by-products of oxidative phosphorylation to hydrogen peroxide and oxygen.[120] Namikawa and colleagues[121] performed a case-control study and found that the homozygous variant genotype was significantly associated with NASH. Another study performed by Al-Serri and colleagues[122] on a European cohort found that the *SOD2T* variant was associated with advanced fibrosis. Uncoupling protein 3 (*UCP3*) gene encodes a mitochondrial protein primarily expressed in skeletal muscle and is protective against oxidative stress from B oxidation of fatty acids.[120] The glutamate-cysteine ligase catalytic subunit (*GCLC*) gene is involved in the synthesis of glutathione which is well known to counteract oxidative stress.[123] Variants of *GCLC* have been shown to have a significant association with NASH in prior studies.[123]

Cell death-inducing DFFA-like effector Beta (*CIDEB*) is a gene that encodes lipid-droplet protein.[124] It has been postulated that the CIDEB protein is a key driver of liver disease in humans. Studies on human HepG2 or HuH-7 cell lines have shown that silencing of the *CIDEB* gene in oleate-challenged human hepatoma cells prevents the accumulation of lipid droplets.[125] A recent study by Verweij and colleagues reported that the presence of rare coding variants in *CIDEB* is associated with a decreased risk of liver disease across different underlying causes, including NASH. In their analysis, 0.7% of the total population carried the rare predicted loss-of-function variants or missense variants in *CIDEB*, Interestingly, the effect size of the CIDEB gene was deemed to be 2 to 3 times larger than *HSD17B13* splice loss-of-function or predicted loss of function genetic variants.[125] The role of these genetic variants in protection against chronic liver disease needs to be further explored. Therapeutic targets against this gene may be beneficial in the management of obesity, hyperlipidemia, and fatty liver.

The *TMPRSS6* gene encodes transmembrane protease, a cell surface enzyme involved in liver matrix remodeling.[120] This enzyme also plays a role in cleaving a coreceptor necessary for the transcription of hepcidin; therefore, mutations in the gene can affect iron status.[126] Valenti and colleagues documented that the genetic polymorphism was associated with reduced hepatic iron and less severe hepatocyte ballooning. No differences were noted in other histological characteristics of NASH.[127]

The *CLOCK* gene is involved in the regulation of circadian rhythm and metabolism. Its variants have been shown to influence both behavior and obesity.[120] Sookoian and colleagues[128] studied variants of this gene in the Argentinian population and found an association of these variants with NAFLD and overall fibrosis score compared with controls.

Polygenic scores

A powerful application of the identified genetic markers is using polygenic models to calculate the risk of NAFLD and its complications.

Gellert-Kristensen and colleagues studied the combined effect of *PNPLA3, TM6SF2*, and *HSD17B13* variants. He combined them into a risk score from 0 to 6 depending on risk-increasing alleles. An increase in score is associated with an increase in serum ALT levels.[129] In their meta-analysis of Copenhagen studies and UK biobank, they found that a genetic score of 6 was associated with a 12 times higher risk of developing cirrhosis and 29 times higher risk of developing HCC.[130] Bianco and colleagues[131] used the polygenic risk score to predict cancer in patients with and without cirrhosis. They reported that the polygenic score predicted HCC more robustly than single variants. This polygenic score was created by including *PNPLA3, TM6SF2, MBOAT7, and GCKR*, weighted by their effect size on hepatic fat. This study included Europeans, African Americans, Hispanics, and Non-Hispanic Whites in the United States. Thomas and colleagues[132] studied this polygenic risk score in Asian patients. They reported that the polygenic risk score was also associated with the risk of HCC in East Asian patients.

Gao and colleagues[130] studied a polygenic risk score incorporating comorbidities and genetic variants. The examined variables included sex, metabolic syndrome, insulin resistance, serum aspartate transaminase, *PNPLA3* genetic variant, and HSD17B13. They generated a nomogram that had a high area under the curve (AUC) in both internal and external validation cohorts with good calibration. This study was restricted to Asian individuals from China and South Korea. De Vincentis and colleagues[133] reported that a high polygenic risk score-hepatic fat content (PRS-HFC) score is associated with an increased risk of liver injury and severe liver disease. They reported that PRS-HFC improved diagnostic accuracy and positive predictive value in patients with intermediate and high fibrosis scores. Long and colleagues[134] suggested that the addition of ethnicity as a covariate would be helpful in adjusting the ethnicity-specific effects in PRS. Further studies in different ethnic groups will be beneficial in validating the role of PRS in patients with different ethnic backgrounds. Wang and colleagues built a genetic risk score using 11 independent single nucleotide polymorphisms. This 11 SNP-associated genetic risk score showed an increased risk of NAFLD in multi-ethnic populations. The results were further statistically significant in multiple ethnicities (OR ranging from 1.3 in African Americans to 1.52 in Latinos).[135] With the growing knowledge regarding the genetics of NAFLD, the application of genetic risk scores can be beneficial in identifying at-risk individuals.

SUMMARY

Because of the growing prevalence of NAFLD, the role of genetic markers in the progression of this disease needs to be understood. At this time, the management of NAFLD includes lifestyle management and managing the comorbidities related to metabolic syndrome. However, with the growing knowledge of the genetic markers, patients who are at high risk of progression can be identified early. Also, potential therapeutic targets directed against these genetic markers can be studied and will be beneficial in delaying the progression of this disease.

CLINICS CARE POINTS

- In the recent decade, there has been an increase in the understanding of the genetics of NASH- PNPLA3 was the first gene that was identifed as a risk factor for the development of NASH- Since then, multiple additional genes such as TM6SF2, MBOAT7, HSD17B13 have been identified.
- Development and implementation of polygenic scores can be beneficial in predicting the severity of NASH in the coming years.
- Development of therapeutic targets aimed at genetic polymorphics can be explored as a management option in patients with NASH in the future.

DISCLOSURE

The authors declare no relevant or material financial interests that relate to the research described in this article.

REFERENCES

1. Mitra S, De A, Chowdhury A. Epidemiology of non-alcoholic and alcoholic fatty liver diseases. Transl Gastroenterol Hepatol 2020;5:16.

2. Estes C, Razavi H, Loomba R, et al. Modeling the epidemic of nonalcoholic fatty liver disease demonstrates an exponential increase in burden of disease. Hepatology 2018;67(1):123–33.
3. Adams LA, Lymp JF, St Sauver J, et al. The natural history of nonalcoholic fatty liver disease: a population-based cohort study. Gastroenterology 2005;129(1):113–21.
4. Jansen PL. Non-alcoholic steatohepatitis. Eur J Gastroenterol Hepatol 2004; 16(11):1079–85 [published correction appears in Eur J Gastroenterol Hepatol 2005;63(7):241].
5. Nagaoki Y, Hyogo H, Aikata H, et al. Recent trend of clinical features in patients with hepatocellular carcinoma. Hepatol Res 2012;42(4):368–75.
6. Schwimmer JB, Celedon MA, Lavine JE, et al. Heritability of nonalcoholic fatty liver disease. Gastroenterology 2009;136(5):1585–92.
7. Eslam M, George J. Genetic contributions to NAFLD: leveraging shared genetics to uncover systems biology. Nat Rev Gastroenterol Hepatol 2020;17(1):40–52.
8. Sookoian S, Pirola CJ. Genetic predisposition in nonalcoholic fatty liver disease. Clin Mol Hepatol 2017;23(1):1–12.
9. Sillanpää MJ. Overview of techniques to account for confounding due to population stratification and cryptic relatedness in genomic data association analyses. Heredity 2011;106:511–9.
10. Cardon LR, Bell JI. Association study designs for complex diseases. Nat Rev Genet 2001;2(2):91–9.
11. Romeo S, Kozlitina J, Xing C, et al. Genetic variation in PNPLA3 confers susceptibility to nonalcoholic fatty liver disease. Nat Genet 2008;40(12):1461–5.
12. Jenkins CM, Mancuso DJ, Yan W, et al. Identification, cloning, expression, and purification of three novel human calcium-independent phospholipase A2 family members possessing triacylglycerol lipase and acylglycerol transacylase activities. J Biol Chem 2004;279(47):48968–75.
13. Kotronen A, Johansson LE, Johansson LM, et al. A common variant in PNPLA3, which encodes adiponutrin, is associated with liver fat content in humans. Diabetologia 2009;52(6):1056–60.
14. Sookoian S, Castaño GO, Burgueño AL, et al. A nonsynonymous gene variant in the adiponutrin gene is associated with nonalcoholic fatty liver disease severity. J Lipid Res 2009;50(10):2111–6.
15. Dai G, Liu P, Li X, et al. Association between PNPLA3 rs738409 polymorphism and nonalcoholic fatty liver disease (NAFLD) susceptibility and severity: a meta-analysis. Medicine (Baltimore) 2019;98(7):e14324.
16. Rotman Y, Koh C, Zmuda JM, et al. The association of genetic variability in patatin-like phospholipase domain-containing protein 3 (PNPLA3) with histological severity of nonalcoholic fatty liver disease. Hepatology 2010;52(3):894–903.
17. Sookoian S, Pirola CJ. Meta-analysis of the influence of I148M variant of patatin-like phospholipase domain containing 3 gene (PNPLA3) on the susceptibility and histological severity of nonalcoholic fatty liver disease. Hepatology 2011; 53(6):1883–94.
18. Valenti L, Alisi A, Galmozzi E, et al. I148M patatin-like phospholipase domain-containing 3 gene variant and severity of pediatric nonalcoholic fatty liver disease. Hepatology 2010;52(4):1274–80.
19. Larrieta-Carrasco E, León-Mimila P, Villarreal-Molina T, et al. Association of the I148M/PNPLA3 variant with elevated alanine transaminase levels in normal-weight and overweight/obese Mexican children. Gene 2013;520(2):185–8.

20. Krawczyk M, Maier IB, Liebe R, et al. 1392 the common adiponutrin (pnpla3) variant is associated with subclinical liver injury already in young age: analysis of a cohort of paediatric patients. J Hepatol 2013;58:S559–60.
21. Valenti L, Dongiovanni P, Ginanni Corradini S, et al. PNPLA3 I148M variant and hepatocellular carcinoma: a common genetic variant for a rare disease. Dig Liver Dis 2013;45(8):619–24.
22. Trepo E, Guyot E, Ganne-Carrie N, et al. PNPLA3 (rs738409 C>G) is a common risk variant associated with hepatocellular carcinoma in alcoholic cirrhosis. Hepatology 2012;55(4):1307–8.
23. Burza MA, Pirazzi C, Maglio C, et al. PNPLA3 I148M (rs738409) genetic variant is associated with hepatocellular carcinoma in obese individuals. Dig Liver Dis 2012;44(12):1037–41.
24. Marzuillo P, Grandone A, Perrone L, et al. Weight loss allows the dissection of the interaction between abdominal fat and PNPLA3 (adiponutrin) in the liver damage of obese children. J Hepatol 2013;59(5):1143–4.
25. Lindén D, Ahnmark A, Pingitore P, et al. Pnpla3 silencing with antisense oligonucleotides ameliorates nonalcoholic steatohepatitis and fibrosis in Pnpla3 I148M knock-in mice. Mol Metab 2019;22:49–61.
26. BasuRay S, Wang Y, Smagris E, et al. Accumulation of PNPLA3 on lipid droplets is the basis of associated hepatic steatosis. Proc Natl Acad Sci U S A 2019; 116(19):9521–6.
27. Carim-Todd L, Escarceller M, Estivill X, et al. Cloning of the novel gene TM6SF1 reveals conservation of clusters of paralogous genes between human chromosomes 15q24->q26 and 19p13.3->p12. Cytogenet Cell Genet 2000;90(3–4): 255–60.
28. Mahdessian H, Taxiarchis A, Popov S, et al. TM6SF2 is a regulator of liver fat metabolism influencing triglyceride secretion and hepatic lipid droplet content. Proc Natl Acad Sci U S A 2014;111(24):8913–8.
29. Kozlitina J, Smagris E, Stender S, et al. Exome-wide association study identifies a TM6SF2 variant that confers susceptibility to nonalcoholic fatty liver disease. Nat Genet 2014;46(4):352–6.
30. Liu YL, Reeves HL, Burt AD, et al. TM6SF2 rs58542926 influences hepatic fibrosis progression in patients with non-alcoholic fatty liver disease. Nat Commun 2014;5(1):4309.
31. Wong VW, Wong GL, Tse CH, et al. Prevalence of the TM6SF2 variant and nonalcoholic fatty liver disease in Chinese. J Hepatol 2014;61(3):708–9.
32. Akuta N, Kawamura Y, Arase Y, et al. Relationships between genetic variations of PNPLA3, TM6SF2 and histological features of nonalcoholic fatty liver disease in Japan. Gut Liver 2016;10(3):437–45.
33. Dongiovanni P, Petta S, Maglio C, et al. Transmembrane 6 superfamily member 2 gene variant disentangles nonalcoholic steatohepatitis from cardiovascular disease. Hepatology 2015;61(2):506–14.
34. Yang J, Trépo E, Nahon P, et al. PNPLA3 and TM6SF2 variants as risk factors of hepatocellular carcinoma across various etiologies and severity of underlying liver diseases. Int J Cancer 2019;144(3):533–44.
35. Grandone A, Cozzolino D, Marzuillo P, et al. TM6SF2 Glu167Lys polymorphism is associated with low levels of LDL-cholesterol and increased liver injury in obese children. Pediatr Obes 2016;11(2):115–9.
36. Mancina RM, Sentinelli F, Incani M, et al. Transmembrane-6 superfamily member 2 (TM6SF2) E167K variant increases susceptibility to hepatic steatosis in obese children. Dig Liver Dis 2016;48(1):100–1.

37. Chen L, Du S, Lu L, et al. The additive effects of the *TM6SF2 E167K* and *PNPLA3 I148M* polymorphisms on lipid metabolism. Oncotarget 2017;8(43): 74209–16.
38. Wang X, Liu Z, Wang K, et al. Additive effects of the risk alleles of PNPLA3 and TM6SF2 on non-alcoholic fatty liver disease (NAFLD) in a Chinese population. Front Genet 2016;7:140.
39. Paternostro R, Staufer K, Traussnigg S, et al. Combined effects of PNPLA3, TM6SF2 and HSD17B13 variants on severity of biopsy-proven non-alcoholic fatty liver disease. Hepatol Int 2021;15(4):922–33.
40. Koo BK, Joo SK, Kim D, et al. Additive effects of PNPLA3 and TM6SF2 on the histological severity of non-alcoholic fatty liver disease. J Gastroenterol Hepatol 2018;33(6):1277–85.
41. Krawczyk M, Rau M, Schattenberg JM, et al. Combined effects of the PNPLA3 rs738409, TM6SF2 rs58542926, and MBOAT7 rs641738 variants on NAFLD severity: a multicenter biopsy-based study. J Lipid Res 2017;58(1):247–55.
42. Caddeo A, Jamialahmadi O, Solinas G, et al. MBOAT7 is anchored to endomembranes by six transmembrane domains. J Struct Biol 2019;206(3):349–60.
43. Lee HC, Kubo T, Kono N, et al. Depletion of mboa-7, an enzyme that incorporates polyunsaturated fatty acids into phosphatidylinositol (PI), impairs PI 3-phosphate signaling in Caenorhabditis elegans. Genes Cells 2012;17(9): 748–57.
44. Sztolsztener K, Chabowski A, Harasim-Symbor E, et al. Arachidonic acid as an early indicator of inflammation during non-alcoholic fatty liver disease development. Biomolecules 2020;10(8):1133.
45. Mancina RM, Dongiovanni P, Petta S, et al. The MBOAT7-TMC4 variant rs641738 increases risk of nonalcoholic fatty liver disease in individuals of european descent. Gastroenterology 2016;150(5):1219–30.e6.
46. Buch S, Stickel F, Trépo E, et al. A genome-wide association study confirms PNPLA3 and identifies TM6SF2 and MBOAT7 as risk loci for alcohol-related cirrhosis. Nat Genet 2015;47(12):1443–8.
47. Thangapandi VR, Knittelfelder O, Brosch M, et al. Loss of hepatic Mboat7 leads to liver fibrosis. Gut 2020;70(5):940–50.
48. Luukkonen PK, Zhou Y, Hyötyläinen T, et al. The MBOAT7 variant rs641738 alters hepatic phosphatidylinositols and increases severity of non-alcoholic fatty liver disease in humans. J Hepatol 2016;65(6):1263–5.
49. Xia M, Chandrasekaran P, Rong S, et al. Hepatic deletion of Mboat7 (LPIAT1) causes activation of SREBP-1c and fatty liver. J Lipid Res 2021;62:100031.
50. Krawczyk M, Jiménez-Agüero R, Alustiza JM, et al. PNPLA3 p.I148M variant is associated with greater reduction of liver fat content after bariatric surgery. Surg Obes Relat Dis 2016;12(10):1838–46.
51. Kawaguchi T, Shima T, Mizuno M, et al. Risk estimation model for nonalcoholic fatty liver disease in the Japanese using multiple genetic markers. PLoS One 2018;13(1):e0185490. Sookoian SC, ed.
52. Lin YC, Chang PF, Chang MH, et al. Genetic determinants of hepatic steatosis and serum cytokeratin-18 fragment levels in Taiwanese children. Liver Int 2018; 38(7):1300–7.
53. Teo K, Abeysekera KWM, Adams L, et al. rs641738C>T near MBOAT7 is associated with liver fat, ALT and fibrosis in NAFLD: a meta-analysis. J Hepatol 2021; 74(1):20–30.
54. Auton A, Brooks LD, Durbin RM, et al. The 1000 Genomes Project Consortium. A global reference for human genetic variation. Nature 2015;526(7571):68–74.

55. Longo M, Meroni M, Paolini E, et al. TM6SF2/PNPLA3/MBOAT7 loss-of-function genetic variants impact on NAFLD development and progression both in patients and in in vitro models. Cell Mol Gastroenterol Hepatol 2022;13(3):759–88.
56. Warner JP, Leek JP, Intody S, et al. Human glucokinase regulatory protein (GCKR): cDNA and genomic cloning, complete primary structure, and chromosomal localization. Mamm Genome 1995;6(8):532–6.
57. Jonas W, Schürmann A. Genetic and epigenetic factors determining NAFLD risk. Mol Metab 2021;50:101111.
58. Veiga-da-Cunha M, Delplanque J, Gillain A, et al. Mutations in the glucokinase regulatory protein gene in 2p23 in obese French caucasians. Diabetologia 2003;46(5):704–11.
59. Santoro N, Caprio S, Pierpont B, et al. Hepatic de novo lipogenesis in obese youth is modulated by a common variant in the GCKR gene. J Clin Endocrinol Metab 2015;100(8):E1125–32 [published correction appears in J Clin Endocrinol Metab 2020;105(2):].
60. Speliotes EK, Yerges-Armstrong LM, Wu J, et al. Genome-wide association analysis identifies variants associated with nonalcoholic fatty liver disease that have distinct effects on metabolic traits. PLoS Genet 2011;7(3):e1001324.
61. Yang Z, Wen J, Tao X, et al. Genetic variation in the GCKR gene is associated with non-alcoholic fatty liver disease in Chinese people. Mol Biol Rep 2011; 38(2):1145–50.
62. Zain SM, Mohamed Z, Mohamed R. Common variant in the glucokinase regulatory gene rs780094 and risk of nonalcoholic fatty liver disease: a meta-analysis. J Gastroenterol Hepatol 2015;30(1):21–7.
63. Petta S, Miele L, Bugianesi E, et al. Glucokinase regulatory protein gene polymorphism affects liver fibrosis in non-alcoholic fatty liver disease. PLoS One 2014;9(2):e87523.
64. Tan HL, Zain SM, Mohamed R, et al. Association of glucokinase regulatory gene polymorphisms with risk and severity of non-alcoholic fatty liver disease: an interaction study with adiponutrin gene. J Gastroenterol 2014;49(6):1056–64.
65. Santoro N, Zhang CK, Zhao H, et al. Variant in the glucokinase regulatory protein (GCKR) gene is associated with fatty liver in obese children and adolescents. Hepatology 2012;55(3):781–9.
66. Li J, Zhao Y, Zhang H, et al. Contribution of Rs780094 and Rs1260326 polymorphisms in GCKR gene to non-alcoholic fatty liver disease: a meta-analysis involving 26,552 participants. Endocr Metab Immune Disord Drug Targets 2021;21(9):1696–708.
67. Hudert CA, Selinski S, Rudolph B, et al. Genetic determinants of steatosis and fibrosis progression in paediatric non-alcoholic fatty liver disease. Liver Int 2018; 39(3):540–56.
68. Vaxillaire M, Cavalcanti-Proença C, Dechaume A, et al. The common P446L polymorphism in GCKR inversely modulates fasting glucose and triglyceride levels and reduces type 2 diabetes risk in the DESIR prospective general French population. Diabetes 2008;57(8):2253–7.
69. Pirola CJ, Flichman D, Dopazo H, et al. A rare nonsense mutation in the glucokinase regulator gene is associated with a rapidly progressive clinical form of nonalcoholic steatohepatitis. Hepatol Commun 2018;2(9):1030–6.
70. Goffredo M, Caprio S, Feldstein AE, et al. Role of TM6SF2 rs58542926 in the pathogenesis of nonalcoholic pediatric fatty liver disease: a multiethnic study. Hepatology 2016;63(1):117–25.

71. Pasta A, Borro P, Cremonini AL, et al. Effect of a common missense variant in LIPA gene on fatty liver disease and lipid phenotype: new perspectives from a single-center observational study. Pharmacol Res Perspect 2021;9(5):e00820.
72. Morris GE, Braund PS, Moore JS, et al. Coronary artery disease-associated *LIPA* coding variant rs1051338 reduces lysosomal acid lipase levels and activity in lysosomes. Arterioscler Thromb Vasc Biol 2017;37(6):1050–7.
73. Baratta F, Pastori D, Polimeni L, et al. Does lysosomial acid lipase reduction play a role in adult non-alcoholic fatty liver disease? Int J Mol Sci 2015;16(12): 28014–21.
74. Pericleous M, Kelly C, Wang T, et al. Wolman's disease and cholesteryl ester storage disorder: the phenotypic spectrum of lysosomal acid lipase deficiency. Lancet Gastroenterol Hepatol 2017;2(9):670–9.
75. Ouimet M, Franklin V, Mak E, et al. Autophagy regulates cholesterol efflux from macrophage foam cells via lysosomal acid lipase. Cell Metab 2011;13(6): 655–67.
76. Skop V, Cahová M, Papáčková Z, et al. Autophagy-lysosomal pathway is involved in lipid degradation in rat liver. Physiol Res 2012;61(3):287–97.
77. Jones SA, Rojas-Caro S, Quinn AG, et al. Survival in infants treated with sebelipase Alfa for lysosomal acid lipase deficiency: an open-label, multicenter, dose-escalation study. Orphanet J Rare Dis 2017;12(1):25.
78. Grabowski GA, Charnas L, Du H. Lysosomal acid lipase deficiencies: the Wolman disease/cholesteryl ester storage disease spectrum. In: Valle D, Beaudet AL, Vogelstein B, et al, editors. *The online metabolic and molecular bases of inherited disease*. 8th edition. New York: McGraw-Hill; 2012. https://doi.org/10.1036/ommbid.172.
79. Bernstein DL, Hülkova H, Bialer MG, et al. Cholesteryl ester storage disease: review of the findings in 135 reported patients with an underdiagnosed disease. J Hepatol 2013;58(6):1230–43.
80. Burton BK, Balwani M, Feillet F, et al. A phase 3 trial of sebelipase alfa in lysosomal acid lipase deficiency. N Engl J Med 2015;373(11):1010–20.
81. Kowdley KV, Gochanour EM, Sundaram V, et al. Hepcidin signaling in health and disease: ironing out the details. Hepatol Commun 2021;5(5):723–35.
82. Kowdley KV, Brown KE, Ahn J, et al. ACG clinical guideline: hereditary hemochromatosis. Am J Gastroenterol 2019;114(8):1202–18 [published correction appears in Am J Gastroenterol 2019;114(12):1927].
83. Nelson JE, Brunt EM, Kowdley KV. Nonalcoholic steatohepatitis clinical research network. lower serum hepcidin and greater parenchymal iron in nonalcoholic fatty liver disease patients with C282Y HFE mutations. Hepatology 2012;56(5): 1730–40.
84. Fujita N, Miyachi H, Tanaka H, et al. Iron overload is associated with hepatic oxidative damage to DNA in nonalcoholic steatohepatitis. Cancer Epidemiol Biomarkers Prev 2009;18(2):424–32.
85. Nakashima T, Sumida Y, Furutani M, et al. Elevation of serum thioredoxin levels in patients with nonalcoholic steatohepatitis. Hepatol Res 2005;33(2):135–7.
86. Messner DJ, Rhieu BH, Kowdley KV. Iron overload causes oxidative stress and impaired insulin signaling in AML-12 hepatocytes. Dig Dis Sci 2013;58(7): 1899–908.
87. Pan M, Cederbaum AI, Zhang YL, et al. Lipid peroxidation and oxidant stress regulate hepatic apolipoprotein B degradation and VLDL production. J Clin Invest 2004;113(9):1277–87.

88. Tan TC, Crawford DH, Jaskowski LA, et al. Excess iron modulates endoplasmic reticulum stress-associated pathways in a mouse model of alcohol and high-fat diet-induced liver injury. Lab Invest 2013;93(12):1295–312.
89. Rigamonti C, Andorno S, Maduli E, et al. Iron, hepatic stellate cells and fibrosis in chronic hepatitis C. Eur J Clin Invest 2002;32(Suppl 1):28–35.
90. Maliken BD, Nelson JE, Klintworth HM, et al. Hepatic reticuloendothelial system cell iron deposition is associated with increased apoptosis in nonalcoholic fatty liver disease. Hepatology 2013;57(5):1806–13.
91. Chen L, Xiong S, She H, et al. Iron causes interactions of TAK1, p21ras, and phosphatidylinositol 3-kinase in caveolae to activate IkappaB kinase in hepatic macrophages. J Biol Chem 2007;282(8):5582–8.
92. Handa P, Morgan-Stevenson V, Maliken BD, et al. Iron overload results in hepatic oxidative stress, immune cell activation, and hepatocellular ballooning injury, leading to nonalcoholic steatohepatitis in genetically obese mice. Am J Physiol Gastrointest Liver Physiol 2016;310(2):G117–27.
93. Graham RM, Chua AC, Carter KW, et al. Hepatic iron loading in mice increases cholesterol biosynthesis. Hepatology 2010;52(2):462–71.
94. Nelson JE, Bhattacharya R, Lindor KD, et al. HFE C282Y mutations are associated with advanced hepatic fibrosis in Caucasians with nonalcoholic steatohepatitis. Hepatology 2007;46(3):723–9.
95. Raszeja-Wyszomirska J. Nonalcoholic fatty liver disease andHFEgene mutations: a polish study. World J Gastroenterol 2010;16(20):2531.
96. Nelson JE, Wilson L, Brunt EM, et al. Relationship between the pattern of hepatic iron deposition and histological severity in nonalcoholic fatty liver disease. Hepatology 2011;53(2):448–57.
97. Hernaez R, Yeung E, Clark JM, et al. Hemochromatosis gene and nonalcoholic fatty liver disease: a systematic review and meta-analysis. J Hepatol 2011;55(5): 1079–85.
98. Ye Q, Qian BX, Yin WL, et al. Association between the HFE C282Y, H63D polymorphisms and the risks of non-alcoholic fatty liver disease, liver cirrhosis and hepatocellular carcinoma: an updated systematic review and meta-analysis of 5,758 cases and 14,741 controls. PLoS One 2016;11(9):e0163423.
99. Valenti L, Fracanzani AL, Dongiovanni P, et al. A randomized trial of iron depletion in patients with nonalcoholic fatty liver disease and hyperferritinemia. World J Gastroenterol 2014;20(11):3002–10.
100. Khodadoostan M, Zamanidoost M, Shavakhi A, et al. Effects of phlebotomy on liver enzymes and histology of patients with nonalcoholic fatty liver disease. Adv Biomed Res 2017;6:12.
101. Zhang HB, Su W, Xu H, et al. HSD17B13: a potential therapeutic target for NAFLD. Front Mol Biosci 2022;8:824776.
102. Ma Y, Belyaeva OV, Brown PM, et al. 17-beta hydroxysteroid dehydrogenase 13 is a hepatic retinol dehydrogenase associated with histological features of nonalcoholic fatty liver disease. Hepatology 2019;69(4):1504–19.
103. Czuba LC, Wu X, Huang W, et al. Altered vitamin a metabolism in human liver slices corresponds to fibrogenesis. Clin Transl Sci 2021;14(3):976–89.
104. Pirola CJ, Garaycoechea M, Flichman D, et al. Splice variant rs72613567 prevents worst histologic outcomes in patients with nonalcoholic fatty liver disease. J Lipid Res 2019;60(1):176–85.
105. Wang P, Wu CX, Li Y, et al. HSD17B13 rs72613567 protects against liver diseases and histological progression of nonalcoholic fatty liver disease: a

systematic review and meta-analysis. Eur Rev Med Pharmacol Sci 2020;24(17):8997–9007.
106. Availabe at: https://clinicaltrials.gov/ct2/show/NCT04565717 ClinicalTrials.gov: NCT04565717. Accessed February 28, 2023.
107. Availabe at: https://clinicaltrials.gov/ct2/show/NCT04202354 ClinicalTrials.gov: NCT04202354. Accessed February 28, 2023.
108. Havemeyer A, Bittner F, Wollers S, et al. Identification of the missing component in the mitochondrial benzamidoxime prodrug-converting system as a novel molybdenum enzyme. J Biol Chem 2006;281(46):34796–802.
109. Emdin CA, Haas ME, Khera AV, et al. A missense variant in mitochondrial amidoxime reducing component 1 gene and protection against liver disease. PLoS Genet 2020;16(4):e1008629 [published correction appears in PLoS Genet 2021;17(4):e1009503].
110. Luukkonen PK, Juuti A, Sammalkorpi H, et al. MARC1 variant rs2642438 increases hepatic phosphatidylcholines and decreases severity of non-alcoholic fatty liver disease in humans. J Hepatol 2020;73(3):725–6.
111. Struwe MA, Clement B, Scheidig A. Letter to the editor: the clinically relevant MTARC1 p.Ala165Thr variant impacts neither the fold nor active site architecture of the human mARC1 protein. Hepatol Commun 2022;6(11):3277–8 [published online ahead of print, 2022 May 13].
112. Borén J, Packard CJ, Taskinen MR. The roles of ApoC-III on the metabolism of triglyceride-rich lipoproteins in humans. Front Endocrinol 2020;11:474.
113. Rauch U, Feng K, Zhou XH. Neurocan: a brain chondroitin sulfate proteoglycan. Cell Mol Life Sci 2001;58(12–13):1842–56.
114. Gorden A, Yang R, Yerges-Armstrong LM, et al. Genetic variation at NCAN locus is associated with inflammation and fibrosis in non-alcoholic fatty liver disease in morbid obesity. Hum Hered 2013;75(1):34–43.
115. Valenti L, Nobili V, Al-Serri A, et al. The APOC3 T-455C and C-482T promoter region polymorphisms are not associated with the severity of liver damage independently of PNPLA3 I148M genotype in patients with nonalcoholic fatty liver. J Hepatol 2011;55(6):1409–14.
116. Li MR, Zhang SH, Chao K, et al. Apolipoprotein C3 (-455T>C) polymorphism confers susceptibility to nonalcoholic fatty liver disease in the Southern Han Chinese population. World J Gastroenterol 2014;20(38):14010–7.
117. Sazci A, Akpinar G, Aygun C, et al. Association of apolipoprotein E polymorphisms in patients with non-alcoholic steatohepatitis. Dig Dis Sci 2008;53(12):3218–24.
118. Verrijken A, Beckers S, Francque S, et al. A gene variant of PNPLA3, but not of APOC3, is associated with histological parameters of NAFLD in an obese population. Obesity 2013;21(10):2138–45.
119. Ma Y, Lee G, Heo SY, et al. Oxidative stress is a key modulator in the development of nonalcoholic fatty liver disease. Antioxidants (Basel) 2021;11(1):91.
120. Stelzer G, Rosen N, Plaschkes I, et al. The gene cards suite: from gene data mining to disease genome sequence analyses. Curr Protoc Bioinformatics 2016;54:1.
121. Namikawa C, Shu-Ping Z, Vyselaar JR, et al. Polymorphisms of microsomal triglyceride transfer protein gene and manganese superoxide dismutase gene in non-alcoholic steatohepatitis. J Hepatol 2004;40(5):781–6.
122. Al-Serri A, Anstee QM, Valenti L, et al. The SOD2 C47T polymorphism influences NAFLD fibrosis severity: evidence from case-control and intra-familial allele association studies. J Hepatol 2012;56(2):448–54.

123. Oliveira CP, Stefano JT, Cavaleiro AM, et al. Association of polymorphisms of glutamate-cystein ligase and microsomal triglyceride transfer protein genes in non-alcoholic fatty liver disease. J Gastroenterol Hepatol 2010;25(2):357–61.
124. Ye J, Li JZ, Liu Y, et al. Cideb, an ER- and lipid droplet-associated protein, mediates VLDL lipidation and maturation by interacting with apolipoprotein B. Cell Metab 2009;9(2):177–90.
125. Verweij N, Haas ME, Nielsen JB, et al. Germline mutations in *CIDEB* and protection against liver disease. N Engl J Med 2022;387(4):332–44.
126. Silvestri L, Pagani A, Nai A, et al. The serine protease matriptase-2 (TMPRSS6) inhibits hepcidin activation by cleaving membrane hemojuvelin. Cell Metab 2008;8(6):502–11.
127. Valenti L, Rametta R, Dongiovanni P, et al. The A736V TMPRSS6 polymorphism influences hepatic iron overload in nonalcoholic fatty liver disease. PLoS One 2012;7(11):e48804. Targher G, ed.
128. Sookoian S, Castaño G, Gemma C, et al. Common genetic variations in CLOCK transcription factor are associated with nonalcoholic fatty liver disease. World J Gastroenterol 2007;13(31):4242–8.
129. Gellert-Kristensen H, Richardson TG, Davey Smith G, et al. Combined effect of PNPLA3, TM6SF2, and HSD17B13 variants on risk of cirrhosis and hepatocellular carcinoma in the general population. Hepatology 2020;72(3):845–56.
130. Gao F, Zheng KI, Chen SD, et al. Individualized polygenic risk score identifies NASH in the Eastern Asia region: a derivation and validation study. Clin Transl Gastroenterol 2021;12(3):e00321.
131. Bianco C, Jamialahmadi O, Pelusi S, et al. Non-invasive stratification of hepatocellular carcinoma risk in non-alcoholic fatty liver using polygenic risk scores. J Hepatol 2021;74(4):775–82.
132. Thomas CE, Diergaarde B, Kuipers AL, et al. NAFLD polygenic risk score and risk of hepatocellular carcinoma in an East Asian population [published online ahead of print, 2022 May 3]. Hepatol Commun 2022;6(9):2310–21.
133. De Vincentis A, Tavaglione F, Jamialahmadi O, et al. A polygenic risk score to refine risk stratification and prediction for severe liver disease by clinical fibrosis scores. Clin Gastroenterol Hepatol 2022;20(3):658–73.
134. Long J, Bian J, Zhao H. Polygenic risk score: a promising predictor for hepatocellular carcinoma in the population with non-alcoholic fatty liver disease. J Hepatol 2021;74(6):1493–4.
135. Wang J, Conti DV, Bogumil D, et al. Association of genetic risk score with NAFLD in an ethnically diverse cohort. Hepatol Commun 2021;5(10):1689–703.

Role of Liver Biopsy in Clinical Trials and Clinical Management of Nonalcoholic Fatty Liver Disease

Zachary D. Goodman, MD, PhD

KEYWORDS

• Liver biopsy • Histopathology • Nonalcoholic fatty liver disease • Clinical trial

KEY POINTS

- Nonalcoholic fatty liver disease constitutes a spectrum of lesions that can be evaluated and characterized by liver biopsy.
- Nonalcoholic steatohepatitis is the most histologically severe form of nonalcoholic fatty liver disease and a frequent precursor of cirrhosis and its complications.
- There is no approved medical therapy for nonalcoholic steatohepatitis, and consequently numerous clinical trials are in various stages of planning and execution to evaluate new treatments.
- Liver biopsy is useful in assessing the stage of disease and presence or absence of features of nonalcoholic steatohepatitis (NASH), and it is the gold standard for inclusion of subjects in clinical trials.
- The demonstration of regression of fibrosis stage and/or resolution of NASH on liver biopsy are acceptable surrogate clinical trial endpoints for treatment of pre-cirrhotic NASH.

INTRODUCTION

The uses of liver biopsy have evolved over decades as it became a mainstay of clinical practice and investigation in the mid-twentieth century. The principal goal of a liver biopsy is to establish a diagnosis if possible or to generate a differential diagnosis from the recognition of morphologic features characteristic of the various diseases that may affect the liver. Liver diseases can produce several patterns of injury, but when the histologic pattern is supplemented by clinical, radiologic, and laboratory findings in context with, the differential diagnosis will often be limited to a few possibilities, or the correct diagnosis may be obvious. Steatosis (fatty liver) and steatohepatitis constitute one of the most important patterns of liver injury.

The author has nothing to disclose.
Center of Liver Diseases, Inova Fairfax Hospital, 3300 Gallows Road, Falls Church, VA 22042, USA
E-mail address: zachary.goodman@inova.org

Clin Liver Dis 27 (2023) 353–362
https://doi.org/10.1016/j.cld.2023.01.017

liver.theclinics.com

Fatty Liver Disease and Steatohepatitis: Histologic Lesions

Alcoholic liver disease (ALD) and nonalcoholic fatty liver disease (NAFLD) share histologic features and are frequently indistinguishable in the absence of reliable history. However, the frequent clinical indications for liver biopsy differ between patients with ALD, who typically only undergo biopsy when they are severely ill, and patients with NAFLD, who typically have liver biopsy to investigate asymptomatic liver enzyme elevations. Thus, alcoholics tend to have more severe degrees of histologic injury, but the same spectrum of severity may appear in both ALD and NAFLD, at least in adults. NAFLD in children may be similar to the same disease in adults, but it is recognized that most of the children who undergo liver biopsy for suspected fatty liver disease show a different pattern of injury,[1] often termed "pediatric NAFLD," which will not be considered in this review.

Cardinal features include.

1. *Centrilobular (zone 3 of Rappaport acinus) predominance.* Biopsies from individuals with mild or early disease and undistorted hepatic architecture tend to show features of fatty liver disease in tissue around the central veins, which roughly corresponds to the physiologic zone 3 of the hepatic acinus described by Rappaport.[2] With the progression and increasing severity of disease, the hepatic architecture becomes distorted, making it difficult to discern the microscopic anatomical landmarks, but the presence of pathologic features can help identify tissue derived from a centrilobular (zone 3) origin.
2. *Fat.* Steatosis, characterized by triglyceride accumulation in hepatocytes, produces cytoplasmic lipid droplets which appear as vacuoles, usually macrovesicular but sometimes microvesicular or a mixture of small and large vacuoles.
3. *Inflammation.* Spotty lobular inflammation is usually present. Mild cases have a predominance of lymphocytes and macrophages, whereas neutrophils may be present or numerous in more severe cases. Portal inflammation may also be present, especially when there is advanced fibrosis.
4. *Ballooning degeneration ± Mallory–Denk bodies*. Normal hepatocytes maintain a polyhedral shape through a skeleton formed of filaments of keratin types 8 and 18. Damage to the hepatocyte cytoskeleton causes liver cells to swell and become misshapen, whereas the cytoplasm becomes pale and granular or wispy (**Fig. 1**). Damaged keratin filaments and other cellular components can form a Mallory–Denk body, which is a sequestosome, a subcellular structure that can serve as a substrate for degradation by the proteasome. Mallory–Denk bodies are irregular eosinophilic cytoplasmic inclusions that vary considerably in size and shape and may not be seen in every ballooned cell as they may be out of the plane of section.
5. *Fibrosis.* Detected with a Masson trichrome or other connective tissue stain (**Fig. 2**). In the earliest or mildest stage, the fibrous tissue forms a delicate lattice-like network of collagen in the centrilobular areas where the hepatic stellate cells that produce collagen are preferentially located. The fibrosis has a characteristic pericellular–perisinusoidal pattern that surrounds the liver cell plates and outlines the sinusoids, similar to the pattern of fibrosis that occurs in congestive hepatopathy but without features of venous congestion. With disease progression and increasing severity, there is an increase in the pericellular fibrosis and portal–periportal fibrosis with enlargement of portal tracts and eventually bridging fibrosis linking lobular components with vascularized septa. Parenchymal nodules surrounded by fibrous scars are characteristic of cirrhosis, which may similarly be early (incomplete) or advanced.

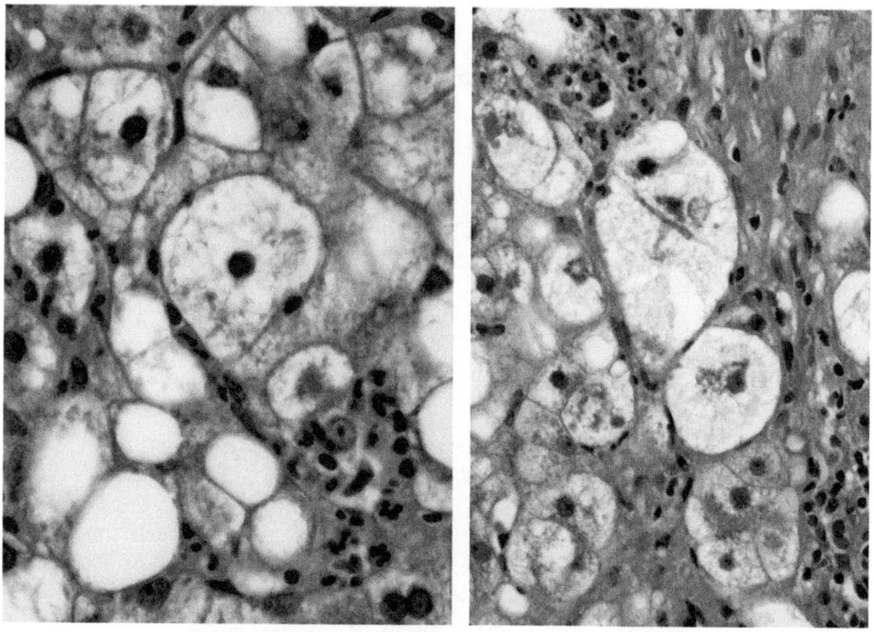

Fig. 1. Ballooning degeneration with Mallory–Denk bodies. Affected hepatocytes are enlarged, misshapen and have pale cytoplasm with irregular eosinophilic inclusions (hematoxylin-eosin X400).

Histologic Classification of Fatty Liver Disease and Steatohepatitis

The concepts and criteria that have become established in NAFLD derived from the similarities to what had been observed in ALD. Thus, ALD was often classified into three entities based on the presence and severity of the features listed above: (1) alcoholic fatty liver characterized by centrilobular injury, fat, and often some inflammation; (2) alcoholic hepatitis when there is also ballooning; and (3) alcoholic cirrhosis, with or without concomitant alcoholic hepatitis when sufficient fibrosis, nodularity, and architectural distortion are present.[3] In NAFLD, the corresponding terms are (1) steatosis (often called "simple steatosis") or nonalcoholic fatty liver (NAFL); (2) nonalcoholic steatohepatitis (NASH); and (3) cirrhosis, with or without active steatohepatitis.

NAFLD activity score. The Pathology Subcommittee of the NIDDK-sponsored NASH Clinical Research Network expanded this simple classification and developed a histologic scoring system intended to assess changes with therapy for use in clinical trials. As with other modern scoring systems in various forms of liver disease, the stage of disease, characterized by progression to end-stage liver failure, was scored separately from disease grade, which was intended to incorporate features likely to have a pathogenetic role in causing the injury leading to disease progression. However, when the grading system was devised and published in 2005, there were no natural history studies to show which features were most important in pathogenesis, so the grading system, which was named the NAFLD activity score (NAS), included features based on reproducibility and usefulness in distinguishing "definite NASH" from "borderline NASH" or "not NASH" based on a review of 32 liver biopsies by nine pathologists and analysis of the data with kappa statistics and logistic regression analysis.[4,5] The final system included four of the five features with the best correlation with a diagnosis of definite NASH (**Table 1**). For this limited sample of 32 biopsies,

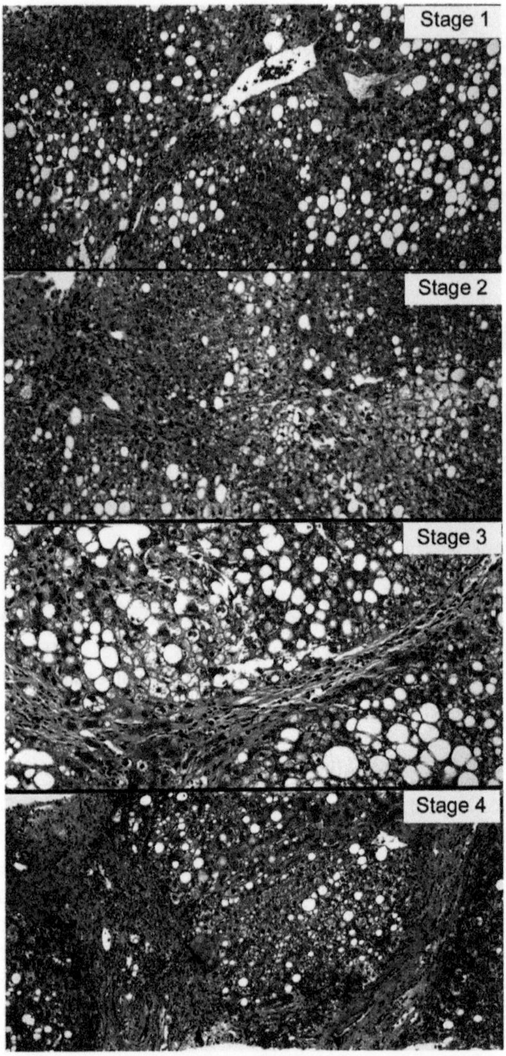

Fig. 2. Stages of fibrosis according to NASH CRN criteria. Collagenous scarring is identified by blue color in trichrome stains. Stage 1: centrilobular perisinusoidal fibrosis; Stage 2: centrilobular and periportal fibrosis; Stage 3: bridging fibrosis; Stage 4: cirrhosis (Masson trichrome X100).

interobserver agreement was nearly perfect (k = 0.81) with a five category staging system for fibrosis and agreement for degree of steatosis was substantial (k = 0.79), but ballooning (k = 0.56) and lobular inflammation (k = 0.45) had only moderate interobserver agreement. Distinction between diagnostic categories (NASH vs borderline NASH vs not NASH) not based on scores but on the pathologists' overall impressions also had substantial agreement (k = 0.61) but was far from perfect. Nevertheless, this was the first such scoring system for NAFLD, and it has come to be the method most often used for evaluating liver biopsies in clinical trials. Subsequent experience refined the number of diagnostic categories to five entities (**Table 2**) that have been incorporated into practice guidelines and reporting recommendations.[6,7]

Table 1
Grading and staging with nonalcoholic fatty liver disease activity score and nonalcoholic steatohepatitis CRN fibrosis stage

Feature (Interobserver Kappa[a])	Score	Kappa (2005)[4]	Kappa (2019)[5]
Steatosis		0.79	0.77
<5%	0		
5%–33%	1		
33%–66%	2		
>66%	3		
Lobular inflammation		0.45	0.46
None	0		
<2 foci per 200X field	1		
2–4 foci per 200X field	2		
>4 foci per 200X field	3		
Ballooning (kappa = 0.56)		0.56	0.54
None	0		
Few ballooned cells	1		
Many cells/prominent ballooning	2		
NAS (steatosis + lobular inflammation + ballooning) 0–8			
Fibrosis (kappa = 0.84)	Stage	0.84	0.75
None	0		
Perisinusoidal or periportal	1		
Mild centrilobular (zone 3) perisinusoidal	1A		
Moderate centrilobular (zone 3) perisinusoidal	1B		
Portal/periportal	1C		
Perisinusoidal and portal/periportal	2		
Bridging fibrosis	3		
Cirrhosis	4		
Diagnostic categories (kappa = 0.61)		0.61	0.66
NASH			
Possible/borderline NASH			
Not NASH			

[a] Kappa statistic interpretation for interobserver agreement: 1.0: Perfect agreement, 0.81–1.0: Almost perfect agreement, 0.61–0.80: Substantial agreement, 0.41–0.60: Moderate agreement, 0.21–0.40: Fair agreement, 0–0.20: Slight agreement, 0.0: Chance agreement.

Biopsy sampling, interobserver variability, and placebo effect. A major drawback to any system that relies on needle biopsy tissue examination is the inevitable possibility of sampling variability. It is widely cited that a needle biopsy represents only 1/50,000 of the liver,[8] which is approximately correct for a 1 cm long needle core from a 16 g needle weighing about 10 mg. It is also widely recognized that pathologic features are unevenly distributed in chronic liver disease, both within an individual case and in a population with a specific diagnosis. In most diseases, the members of a population with that diagnosis will have a spectrum of severity, so that an accurate assessment requires a specimen large enough to show pathologic changes that may be missed in small biopsies from subjects at the mild end of the spectrum, whereas conversely those with severe disease are more readily recognized with small biopsies.

Table 2
Diagnostic categories for nonalcoholic fatty liver disease as used by nonalcoholic steatohepatitis CRN[4,5]

Category	Definition	Fibrosis
Not NAFLD	<5% steatosis	None or any amount up to cirrhosis
NAFL, not NASH	≥5% steatosis ± lobular and portal inflammation	None or any amount up to cirrhosis
Borderline steatohepatitis	Most, but not all criteria for steatohepatitis present	None or any amount up to cirrhosis
Zone 3	+ accentuation in zone 3	
Zone 1	+ accentuation in zone 1	
Definite steatohepatitis	All criteria present (steatosis, Ballooning, lobular inflammation)	None or any amount up to cirrhosis

Thus, sampling variability produces mostly one-sided errors and in general, "the smaller the biopsy, the milder the disease".[9] The same is probably true for NAFLD, but most studies have been relatively small case series, and some have found significant discrepancies between paired biopsies of the same liver,[8] whereas others have found negligible differences.[10] Nevertheless, studies of sampling variability in chronic hepatitis C concluded that 2 cm long biopsies taken with a 16-gauge biopsy needle and containing at least 11 portal tracts were sufficiently accurate for most clinical and investigational purposes, and this recommendation was incorporated into the AASLD Liver Biopsy Practice Guideline.[11] Interobserver and intraobserver variability is also a constant source of potentially discrepant results, as evidenced by the kappa statistics in the previous section, and furthermore even after years of use, repeat of the experiment showed the same degree of interobserver variability (see **Table 1**), which must be considered in clinical trial design and interpretation. Indeed, it has been suggested that the so-called "placebo effect" of fibrosis regression in a proportion of subjects in randomized clinical trials is actually due predominantly to sampling variability and not to true improvement.[12]

Natural History

As noted previously, the NAS and NASH Clinical Research Network (CRN) fibrosis stages were proposed as a method for grading and staging of NAFLD before there was evidence of the relative importance of the pathologic features in the natural history of the disease and its subtypes. Subsequent long-term natural history studies have found that in subjects with biopsy-proven NAFLD, cardiovascular disease rather than liver disease was the most common cause of death (38% to 43%) followed by extrahepatic malignancy (18% to 23%), both similar to control populations.[13,14] Liver-related deaths or transplantation due to cirrhosis complications or hepatocellular carcinoma were the third most common cause (9%) and were largely confined to those with cirrhosis (stage 4) or less often bridging fibrosis (stage 3). A large meta-analysis of 1495 subjects that included these along with other three series found only occasional liver-related deaths among subjects with stages 1 and 2 on initial biopsy.[15] Nevertheless, multivariate analysis consistently identifies advanced fibrosis stage as the strongest and only independent predictor of liver-related outcomes. Other histologic features, including the components of NAS and portal inflammation, correlate with fibrosis stage, and the analysis of serial biopsies has demonstrated that changes in stage also correlate with changes in many of the features.[5] A causal relationship with hepatocellular injury and inflammation driving progression of fibrosis seems likely but difficult to prove.

Liver Biopsy Use in Clinical Trials

For regulatory agency approval, a new treatment or form of therapy must be shown to be safe and effective for a specific clinical application. Studies to evaluate the safety and efficacy of pharmacologic agents for treatment of NAFLD are typically double-blind randomized placebo-controlled clinical trials. Patients recruited for participation in a trial undergo evaluation for a list of inclusion and exclusion criteria, and only those who conform to the inclusion criteria without the presence of any exclusion criteria are allowed to be enrolled and randomized. Findings on liver biopsy performed within a certain time before randomization (usually 6 months or a year) are among the criteria, but as liver biopsy is an invasive procedure, biopsies are typically reserved for those who have satisfied all other criteria. If a biopsy had already been performed within the screening timeframe, then it would be used as the baseline evaluation. If not, then a new biopsy would be required.

Histologic inclusion criteria are specified in trial protocols, usually after consultation with the regulatory agencies. Following Food and Drug Administration (FDA) guidance,[16–18] most trials now limit enrollment to subjects with definite NASH with full complement of diagnostic features as defined by the NASH CRN and with NAS of 4 or greater. To meet this requirement, the biopsies are usually reviewed by a central pathologist, and the most recent recommendation is for a pathology adjudication committee of at least two pathologists to agree on the precise score. Subjects whose biopsies have no fibrosis or CRN stage 1 with minimal risk of liver-related clinical outcomes are excluded, and pre-cirrhotic and cirrhotic stages of the disease are usually enrolled in separate but parallel trials. For trials of treatment of NASH with pre-cirrhotic fibrosis, the biopsies must have CRN stage 2 or 3 but not cirrhosis. For NASH cirrhosis, there must be nodules surrounded by fibrotic septa, but the cirrhosis may be early (or incomplete) or it may be established. Patients with advanced cirrhosis may also be enrolled, although the risk of decompensation may make them ineligible. As steatosis may decrease to less than 5% after cirrhosis has developed, some trials allow enrollment of a limited number of subjects with compatible clinical features, but not necessarily all the histologic features of NASH.

Liver biopsies in clinical trials may also be used as a measure of efficacy by demonstrating histologic improvement. Efficacy in a randomized controlled trial typically is determined by comparison of a treatment group with a randomly assigned placebo control group. The treatment is considered efficacious if the treated group has significantly better measures of clinical outcomes than placebo in the terms of how the patients feel, function, or survive. Surrogate outcomes, such as changes in liver biopsies or other laboratory tests or indirect measures, may be substituted when they have been shown to accurately predict clinical outcomes. Use of liver biopsy as an outcome requires a suitable baseline biopsy and one or more follow-up biopsy to determine whether the therapeutic intervention under study produces histologic benefit. Early trials were hampered by the rudimentary state of knowledge about relationships between histologic features and natural history so the definition of benefit has evolved. The NAS was developed for use as a tool to assess changes in histology, and it has usually been incorporated into the evaluations, although its role has changed with advances in understanding the natural history of fatty liver disease. As trials for treatment of chronic viral hepatitis often defined histologic improvement as a 2-point decrease in the Histology Activity Index with no worsening of fibrosis stage, a similar 2-point decrease in NAS with no increase in fibrosis stage was sometimes used in NASH trials.[19] More complex definitions of response could also be used; for example, in the PIVENS trial, improvement was defined as a decrease in the ballooning score by one or more point associated with a decrease in NAS by either 2 points or to a NAS $\leq$3 with no increase in fibrosis stage.[20] In the course of the early NASH trials, it was observed that some subjects in both the placebo and active treatment groups had follow-up biopsies that were no longer diagnostic of definite NASH, usually because of absence of ballooning. Thus, "NASH resolution" has been introduced as a possible endpoint, sometimes defined as overall histopathological assessment and sometimes defined in terms of NAS as a score of 0 for ballooning with $\leq$1 for inflammation and any degree of steatosis.[21,22] Sampling variability undoubtedly accounts for some loss of ballooning, so a placebo control group is essential for comparison and statistical analysis to show that the histologic change is attributable to the therapeutic intervention. With recognition of the importance of fibrosis stage in the natural history, "improvement in fibrosis" defined as a decrease in the NASH CRN four-stage scale by one or more stages was also introduced as a potential endpoint.

FDA GUIDANCE ON ENDPOINTS IN NONALCOHOLIC STEATOHEPATITIS CLINICAL TRIALS

In 2018 and 2019, the FDA published Guidance for Industry with recommendations for the development of drugs for the treatment of NASH followed by a summary of current thinking from the Division of Hepatology and Nutrition in 2021[16–18] that suggests different goals and endpoints for cirrhotic versus noncirrhotic NASH.

For cirrhotic stage NASH, the FDA guidance recommends only clinical outcomes as endpoints to support marketing applications. Liver biopsy is recommended to assure the correct diagnosis of NASH and to confirm cirrhosis at baseline, but currently in the opinion of the agency, there is insufficient evidence to support the use of histologic improvement or other laboratory test as a surrogate endpoint reasonably likely to predict clinical benefit. Even regression of cirrhosis to pre-cirrhotic bridging fibrosis is not accepted as a surrogate endpoint as it has not been shown convincingly to predict improved survival or reduction in other adverse clinical events.

For pre-cirrhotic NASH with moderate or bridging fibrosis (NASH CRN stages 2 and 3), FDA guidance allows surrogate histopathologic endpoints as discussed in the previous section[16–18] to be considered in the context of safety, clinical need, and magnitude of change in the decision to grant accelerated approval of marketing a new therapy. In this context, three options were suggested as sufficient evidence of efficacy.

A. The resolution of steatohepatitis with no worsening of fibrosis stage.
B. Improvement in fibrosis stage with no worsening of steatohepatitis in any of the three components of NAS.
C. Both A and B.

If conditional approval is granted based on surrogate endpoints, the sponsor is then obligated to conduct sufficiently long and adequately powered post-marketing phase 4 trials to verify clinical benefit by showing superiority of the drug to placebo in such things as progression to cirrhosis, mortality, hepatic decompensation and other such events. However, as no form of pharmacologic therapy has received regulatory approval for the treatment of NASH or fatty liver disease, either through the traditional approval pathway or through accelerated approval based on surrogate endpoints, this remains a theoretical possibility rather than a proven strategy.

LIVER BIOPSY IN CLINICAL MANAGEMENT OF NONALCOHOLIC FATTY LIVER DISEASE

Outside the context of a clinical trial, liver biopsy is of limited use in fatty liver disease. The biopsy may be useful in establishing the diagnosis and excluding alternative forms of liver disease, and it may help in assessing disease severity and prognosis, but there is no indication for therapeutic guidance in routine management of the individual patient. Lifestyle modification consisting of diet, exercise, and weight loss can be recommended to nearly anyone with fatty liver disease, but there are no pharmacologic agents or bariatric surgical procedures that have received regulatory approval or recommendation by the AASLD practice guideline.[11] Nevertheless, when there is strong clinical suspicion of active disease with or without advanced fibrosis, liver biopsy findings may be helpful in encouraging lifestyle changes and adherence to regimens for management of diabetes and other comorbidities. A liver biopsy may also reveal coexisting but unsuspected autoimmune, biliary tract, granulomatous or vascular disease. In addition, the assessment of fibrosis remains an important predictor of prognosis.

SUMMARY

NAFLD and nonalcoholic steatohepatitis constitute a spectrum of histologic lesions characterized by varying degrees of hepatocellular injury and fat accumulation with inflammation and scarring. In clinical trials, liver biopsies are performed and evaluated to confirm the diagnosis of nonalcoholic steatohepatitis and to assess fibrosis stage for subject enrollment. In trials for treatment of pre-cirrhotic NASH, liver biopsies can be used to evaluate the surrogate endpoints of NASH resolution and fibrosis improvement.

REFERENCES

1. Schwimmer JB, Behling C, Newbury R, et al. Histopathology of pediatric nonalcoholic fatty liver disease. Hepatology 2005;42:641–9.
2. Rappaport AM. The structural and functional unit in the human liver (liver acinus). Anat Rec 1954;119:11–27.
3. Alcoholic liver disease: morphological manifestations. Review by an international group. Lancet 1981;1(8222):707–11.
4. Kleiner DE, Brunt EM, Van Natta M, et al. Design and validation of a histological scoring system for nonalcoholic fatty liver disease. Hepatology 2005;41:1313–21.
5. Kleiner DE, Brunt EM, Wilson LA, et al. Association of histologic disease activity with progression of nonalcoholic fatty liver disease. JAMA Netw Open 2019;2(10): e1912565.
6. Chalasani N, Younossi Z, Lavine JE, et al. The diagnosis and management of nonalcoholic fatty liver disease: practice guidance from the American Association for the Study of Liver Diseases. Hepatology 2018;67:328–57.
7. Brunt EM, Kleiner DE, Carpenter DH, et al. American association for the study of liver diseases NASH task force. NAFLD: reporting histologic findings in clinical practice. Hepatology 2021;73:2028–38.
8. Ratziu V, Charlotte F, Heurtier A, et al. Sampling variability of liver biopsy in nonalcoholic fatty liver disease. Gastroenterology 2005;128:1898–906.
9. Colloredo G, Guido M, Sonzogni A, et al. Impact of liver biopsy size on histological evaluation of chronic viral hepatitis: the smaller the sample, the milder the disease. J Hepatol 2003;39:239–44.

10. Larson SP, Bowers SP, Palekar NA, et al. Histopathologic variability between the right and left lobes of the liver in morbidly obese patients undergoing Roux-en-Y bypass. Clin Gastroenterol Hepatol 2007;5:1329–32.
11. Rockey DC, Caldwell SH, Goodman ZD, et al. American association for the study of liver diseases. Liver biopsy. Hepatology 2009;49:1017–44.
12. Rowe IA, Parker R. The placebo response in randomized trials in nonalcoholic steatohepatitis simply explained. Clin Gastroenterol Hepatol 2022 Mar;20(3):e564–72.
13. Angulo P, Kleiner DE, Dam-Larsen S, et al. Liver fibrosis, but no other histologic features, is associated with long-term outcomes of patients with nonalcoholic fatty liver disease. Gastroenterology 2015;149:389–97.e10.
14. Ekstedt M, Hagstrom H, Nasr P, et al. Fibrosis stage is the strongest predictor for disease-specific mortality in NAFLD after up to 33 years of follow-up. Hepatology 2015;61:1547–54.
15. Dulai PS, Singh S, Patel J, et al. Increased risk of mortality by fibrosis stage in nonalcoholic fatty liver disease: systematic review and meta-analysis. Hepatology 2017;65:1557–65.
16. U.S. Department of Health and Human Services, Food and drug administration, center for drug evaluation and research. Noncirrhotic nonalcoholic steatohepatitis with liver fibrosis: developing drugs for treatment draft guidance for industry, Available at: https://www.fda.gov/media/119044/download, 2018. Accessed December 29, 2022.
17. U.S. Department of Health and Human Services, Food and Drug Administration, Center for Drug Evaluation and Research. Nonalcoholic Steatohepatitis with Compensated Cirrhosis: Developing Drugs for Treatment: Guidance for Industry. 2019, Available at:https://www.fda.gov/media/127738/download. Accessed December 29, 2022.
18. Anania FA, Dimick-Santos L, Mehta R, et al. Nonalcoholic steatohepatitis: current thinking from the division of hepatology and nutrition at the food and drug administration. Hepatology 2021;73:2023–7.
19. Neuschwander-Tetri BA, Loomba R, Sanyal AJ, et al. Farnesoid X nuclear receptor ligand obeticholic acid for non-cirrhotic, non-alcoholic steatohepatitis (FLINT): a multicentre, randomised, placebo-controlled trial. Lancet 2015;385:956–65.
20. Sanyal AJ, Chalasani N, Kowdley KV, et al. Pioglitazone, vitamin E, or placebo for nonalcoholic steatohepatitis. N Engl J Med 2010;362:1675–85.
21. Sanyal AJ, Brunt EM, Kleiner DE, et al. Endpoints and clinical trial design for nonalcoholic steatohepatitis. Hepatology 2011;54(1):344–53.
22. Cheung A, Neuschwander-Tetri BA, Kleiner DE, et al. Liver forum case definitions working group. defining improvement in nonalcoholic steatohepatitis for treatment trial endpoints: recommendations from the liver forum. Hepatology 2019; 70(5):1841–55.

Roles of Radiological Tests in Clinical Trials and the Clinical Management of Nonalcoholic Fatty Liver Disease

Winston Dunn, MD[a,*], Laurent Castera, MD[b,c],
Rohit Loomba, MD[d]

KEYWORDS

• Fibrosis • Liver biopsy • NAFLD • NASH • Ultrasound

KEY POINTS

- The CAP performs well in detecting fatty liver for NAFLD diagnosis but is unable to differentiate between hepatic steatosis grades and cannot be relied on to track longitudinal changes.
- MRI-PDFF is a better technique for evaluating longitudinal changes and is currently used as a primary endpoint in trials investigating antisteatotic properties of therapeutic agents.
- When assessing liver fibrosis to determine the need for referral to hepatology specialists from primary care, the probability of detecting liver fibrosis using radiological testing is low.
- The probability of detecting liver fibrosis using radiological testing techniques is high when performed at referral centers for the purposes of clinical trial prescreening, and reasonable imaging strategies include the combination of FIB-4 and VCTE, the FAST Score, MAST, and MEFIB.

INTRODUCTION

Nonalcoholic fatty liver disease (NAFLD) is one of the most common causes of chronic liver disease worldwide.[1] The presence of fatty liver can be diagnosed by various imaging modalities or liver biopsy. Ultrasound remains the most widely used first-line tool despite its well-known limitations (low sensitivity and operator dependence). An

[a] Division of Gastroenterology and Hepatology, Department of Medicine, University of Kansas Medical Center, 3901 Rainbow Boulevard, Kansas City, KS 66160, USA; [b] Université de Paris, UMR1149 (CRI), INSERM, Paris, France; [c] Service d'Hépatologie, Assistance Publique-Hôpitaux de Paris (AP-HP), Hôpital Beaujon, Clichy, France; [d] Division of Gastroenterology and Hepatology, Department of Medicine, NAFLD Research Center, University of California San Diego, La Jolla, CA, USA
* Corresponding author.
E-mail address: wdunn2@kumc.edu

Clin Liver Dis 27 (2023) 363–372
https://doi.org/10.1016/j.cld.2023.01.020

NAFLD diagnosis requires the exclusion of excessive alcohol use, prosteatotic medications, and concurrent liver diseases. NAFLD can be classified with or without significant fibrosis and with or without substantial nonalcoholic steatohepatitis (NASH). Fibrosis is the only predictor of all-cause and liver-related mortality,[2] even after adjustment for NASH.[3,4] However, patients with NAFLD with NASH may experience more rapid fibrosis progression than patients with NAFLD without NASH[5]; therefore, clinical trial typically targets patients with NASH and stage 2 fibrosis or greater, coined as "at-risk NASH."

Although NAFLD affects a quarter of the global and US populations,[1] only 5.9% and 1.6% of the population are considered at risk for disease progression due to the presence of NASH and stages 2 and 3 fibrosis or greater, respectively.[6] Liver biopsy is the current reference standard for confirming NASH and fibrosis stage. However, the associated costs and invasive nature of liver biopsy make this procedure impractical for use in large-scale, population-based studies.[7]

Radiological tests able to assess the stage of disease and the risk of disease progression in patients with NAFLD have been proposed for both the clinical management of NAFLD and the enrichment of candidates for clinical trials. Radiological tests include ultrasound-based tests such as vibration-controlled transient elastography (VCTE; FibroScan, Echosens, Paris, France) allowing controlled attenuation parameter (CAP) and liver stiffness measurements and magnetic resonance–based tests such as MRI-proton density fat fraction (MRI-PDFF) and magnetic resonance elastography (MRE).[8] Radiological tests can address the following: (1) quantifying liver fat for NAFLD diagnosis; (2) assessing liver fibrosis stage; and (3) evaluating longitudinal changes over time. Liver fibrosis needs to be assessed during clinical trial prescreening, as most clinical trials target populations with stage 2 fibrosis or greater, with or without an NAS of 4. Liver fibrosis is also assessed when determining whether a patient should be referred to hepatology specialists from primary care, which is recommended for patients with stage 3 fibrosis or greater or who are identified as being at risk for a liver-related outcome.

QUANTIFYING LIVER FAT FOR NONALCOHOLIC FATTY LIVER DISEASE DIAGNOSIS

Ultrasound-Based Tests

CAP, which quantifies the loss of ultrasound signal as it penetrates the liver, can be used to diagnose steatosis. Although CAP is accurate for diagnosing the presence of steatosis, it is not adequately sensitive to differentiate among different histological grades.[9,10] In a prospective study[10] of bariatric surgery patients undergoing liver biopsy comparing the diagnostic performances of CAP with MRI-PDFF, CAP had an area under the receiver operating characteristic curve (AUROC) value of 0.83 for the diagnosis of steatosis greater than 5%, but the AUROC value decreased to 0.79 and 0.73 for the diagnosis of steatosis greater than 33% and greater than 66%, respectively. In addition, CAP was outperformed by MRI-PDFF. Given the CAP's poor performance in quantifying steatosis, it may not be adequate for detecting dynamic changes in steatosis in the context of monitoring progression in clinical care or clinical trials.

The optimal cutoff value for diagnosing NAFLD varies depending on the patient population and the probe being used.[11] Two types of probes, M and XL, are available, and the device automatically recommends the use of an XL probe if the skin to liver capsule distance is greater than 25 mm. The optimal cutoff value when using the XL probe may be 10 dB/m higher than when using the M probe.[12] An individual patient data meta-analysis[13] including data for 2346 patients and using XL probe indicated that CAP results can be influenced by cause, diabetes, and body mass index. In studies of patients with NAFLD, optimal CAP cutoff values at 288 dB/m[14] and 306 dB/m[15] were proposed when using MRI-PDFF and liver biopsy as references, respectively. Finally, in the absence of consensual cutoffs, recent European Association for the Study of the Liver (EASL) guidelines[16] stated that, given their sensitivity greater than 90%, values greater than 275 dB/m could be used to diagnose NAFLD.

Magnetic Resonance–Based Tests

As MRI-PDFF is the most accurate noninvasive method to quantify steatosis,[17] it has been used in many clinical trials.[18] MR spectroscopy (MRS) is another highly accurate method for measuring steatosis[19] but is limited by costs, instrument availability, and analytical algorithms. Although the findings derived from MRI-PDFF and MRS correlate closely in clinical trials,[20] a cross-sectional study suggested that MRI-PDFF may be more accurate than MRS.

Evaluating Longitudinal Changes Over Time

Currently, MRI-PDFF is the only technique able to evaluate change in steatosis grade over time, with a reasonable AUROC of 0.70. The ability of MRI-PDFF to detect a greater than or equal to 2-point improvement in NAS or NASH resolution and the ability of MRE to measure fibrosis improvements remain suboptimal, and liver biopsies continue to be necessary to assess improvements in phase 3 clinical trials. However, the reference standard that MRI-PDFF is being compared with is liver biopsy, which is characterized by significant variability that may adversely affect the relative performance of MRI-PDFF. MRI-PDFF is currently allowed for the assessment of primary endpoints in phase 2 clinical trials when evaluating agents believed to have a strong antisteatotic effect.

In a study of selonsertib,[21] 54 patients underwent paired liver biopsies and MRE assessments performed at baseline and at week 24. Fibrosis improvement ($\geq$1-stage reduction) was noted in 18 (33%) liver biopsy samples. The AUROC value for the ability of MRE to detect fibrosis improvement was 0.62, and the optimal threshold was a relative change of 0%. Among 65 patients with paired liver biopsies and MRI-PDFF assessments performed at baseline and at week 24, steatosis improvement ($\geq$1-grade reduction) was noted in 18 (28%) liver biopsy samples. The AUROC value for the ability of MRI-PDFF to predict steatosis improvement was 0.70, and the optimal threshold was a relative change of 0%. In a secondary analysis of the FLINT trial,[22] paired MRI-PDFF and liver biopsies from 78 patients were compared to determine the ability of MRI-PDFF to detect a histologically determined 2-point improvement in NAS without fibrosis worsening. MRI-PDFF had an AUROC value of 0.60, using a relative improvement of 30% as the optimal cutoff value. Alternatively,[23] MRI-PDFF was able to identify a 1-grade reduction in steatosis with an AUROC value of 0.81 and a 1-grade worsening in steatosis with an AUROC value of 0.81.

In a meta-analysis of 7 clinical trials, including 346 subjects,[24] MRI-PDFF responders (relative decline of $\geq$30% in liver fat) were significantly more likely than nonresponders to have a greater than or equal to 2-point improvement in NAS (51% vs 14%, pooled odds ratio [OR]: 6.98) and NASH resolution (41% vs 7%, pooled OR: 5.45).

MRI-PDFF interexamination repeatability has been estimated with a standard deviation (SD) of less than 0.5%. A longitudinal hepatic change of greater than 1.8% in MRI-PDFF, which is twice the maximum aggregate (SD), represents real change rather than measurement imprecision.[25] The reduction in AUROC values observed in longitudinal studies compared with cross-sectional studies may be associated with the use of liver biopsies as the reference and the degree of variability observed in biopsy results. In the colesevelam study,[20] an increase in hepatic steatosis compared with placebo after 24 weeks was detected by MRI-PDFF but not by liver biopsy. In 50 patients with data for longitudinal liver biopsies,[26] MRI-PDFF, MRS-PDFF, liver enzyme, and weight measurements, patients who displayed a greater than 1% increase or decrease in PDFF showed parallel increases in body weights and liver enzymes that could not be confirmed by histology. Both studies suggest that MRI-PDFF may be more sensitive than liver biopsy for determining changes in liver fat content.

ASSESSING LIVER FIBROSIS OR FIBROTIC NONALCOHOLIC STEATOHEPATITIS IN THE CONTEXT OF CLINICAL TRIAL PRESCREENING

Ultrasound-Based Tests

Advanced fibrosis

A meta-analysis of 37 primary studies including 5735 patients[27] showed that VCTE had AUROC values of 0.85 and 0.90 for diagnosing advanced stage 3 fibrosis or greater and cirrhosis. Youden index identified optimal cutoff values of 9.1 kPa for stage 3 fibrosis or greater and 10.4 kPa for cirrhosis. NASH-specific studies from NASH Clinical Research Network[9] and other pooled analysis[28] showed that VCTE had AUROC values of 0.83 to 0.84 for diagnosing advanced fibrosis and 0.84 to 0.93 for diagnosing cirrhosis. Youden index identified optimal cutoff values of 8.6 to 8.8 kPa for advanced fibrosis and 11.8 to 13.1 kPa for cirrhosis.

Many studies have explored the use of a dual-cutoff strategy with VCTE for the diagnosis of advanced fibrosis. Advanced fibrosis can be ruled out by lower cutoff values and ruled in by higher cutoff values, although patients between the 2 cutoff values will continue to require a liver biopsy to confirm fibrosis. In a meta-analysis,[27] dual cutoff values of 7.4 and 12.1 kPa were able to achieve 90% sensitivity and specificity. Using a single cutoff value of 9.1 kPa resulted in the misclassification of 22% of patients, whereas the use of dual values resulted in the misclassification of 10% of patients and the classification of 31% of patients as indeterminate.

Combining simple, noninvasive blood tests with VCTE, either simultaneously or sequentially, can improve screening accuracy. For example, various strategies have been developed for combining paired cutoff values for both the fibrosis-4 (FIB-4) and VCTE.[27,29] In this large meta-analysis in 5737 patients with NAFLD, the sequential combination of FIB-4 cutoffs (<1.3; ≥ 2.67) followed by VCTE cutoffs (<8.0; ≥ 10.0 kPa) to rule-in or rule-out advanced fibrosis had sensitivity and specificity (95% CI) of 66% (63–68) and 86% (84–87), with 33% needing a biopsy to establish a final diagnosis.

The rate at which patients are classified as indeterminate or misclassified depends on the prevalence of advanced fibrosis. In screening for the STELLAR[30] study, for which the prevalence of advanced fibrosis was as high as 70% to 80%, a simultaneous strategy may be preferred, as it lowers the misclassification rate from 20% to 5% at the cost of indeterminate rate.

Fibrotic nonalcoholic steatohepatitis

The FibroScan-aspartate aminotransferase (FAST) score (Echosens, Paris, France) has been proposed to select eligible candidates for clinical trials, that is, patients with fibrotic NASH (stage ≥ 2 fibrosis with NAS ≥ 4).[31] It combines CAP, liver stiffness, and aspartate transaminase levels and can be calculated on a free app. It ranges from 0 to 1, with rule-out and rule-in cutoffs of 0.35 (90% sensitivity) and 0.67 (90% specificity). Its AUROC was 0.80 in the training cohort and 0.85 in the validation cohort.[27] Further independent validation[32] of the FAST score shows that this score is highly[33,34] reproducible and unaffected by differences in ultrasound equipment or probes. Limitation of the FAST score is its low positive predictive value.

Magnetic Resonance Elastography–Based Tests

Advanced fibrosis

MRE has excellent accuracy with AUROC of 0.93 for the diagnosis of advanced fibrosis (stage 3 and 4).[35] Several head-to-head comparison studies have shown that MRE outperformed VCTE in detection of fibrosis stages.[36,37] However, use of MRE in clinical practice is hampered by cost and limited availability. Thus MRE is more suited for clinical trials.[16]

MRE combined with the FIB-4 (MEFIB) was developed as a 2-step screening algorithm for clinical trial assessment at the University of California San Diego. The endpoint was stage 2 fibrosis or greater in patients with NAFLD. MRE has an AUROC value of 0.93, and FIB-4 has an AUROC value of 0.78 for the detection of fibrosis. The sequential application of the FIB-4 and MRE was proposed, in which patients with FIB-4 scores greater than or equal to 1.6 receive MRE screening at a referral center. A high positive predictive value of 95% was established for the combination of MRE greater than or equal to 3.3 kPa and FIB-4 greater than or equal to 1.6, and these patients were classified as excellent candidates for screening liver biopsies.[38]

The MEFIB strategy has been shown to be superior to FAST score[39,40] for diagnosing stage 2 fibrosis or greater alone, although FAST was originally designed to diagnose stage 2 or greater with NAS greater than or equal to 4.

Fibrotic nonalcoholic steatohepatitis

The MAST score, an MRI-serum-based score, has been recently proposed for diagnosing fibrotic NASH.[41] It combines MRI-PDFF, liver stiffness using MRE, and aspartate transaminase levels. It ranges from 0 to 1, with rule-out and rule-in cutoffs of 0.165 (90% sensitivity) and 0.242 (90% specificity). Its AUROC was 0.93 in the validation cohort, and it outperformed FAST score. When compared head-to-head with FAST and MEFIB in a US and a Japanese cohort,[40] MAST was outperformed by MEFIB in the US cohort but not in the Japanese cohort. Further studies are needed to clarify how to best use these tests in practice.

ASSESSING LIVER FIBROSIS IN THE CONTEXT OF A DECISION TREE FOR REFERRAL TO HEPATOLOGY SPECIALISTS FROM PRIMARY CARE

Ultrasound-Based Tests

Despite the high prevalence of NAFLD in primary care (25%), only a small minority (<5%) of patients with NAFLD will develop advanced liver fibrosis. The challenge is to identify these patients, who are at the greatest risk of developing complications and need to be referred to liver clinics for specialized management.[42] Sequential algorithms using FIB-4 as the first-line test, followed, if positive (>1.3), by VCTE are the best strategy to define pathways for patients at risk of NAFLD from primary care to liver clinics.

Such strategy was implemented in patients with type 2 diabetes (T2D) seen in primary care setting in East England.[43] FIB-4 was automatically calculated, and VCTE was ordered when the FIB-4 was greater than 1.3. Referral for secondary care was implemented for VCTE greater than 8 kPa. This approach resulted in 12.4% of patients requiring VCTE, 6.4% of patients being referred, and 4.3% of patients being diagnosed with advanced fibrosis. The advanced fibrosis detection rate increased by 7-fold upon referral; however, half of patients diagnosed with advanced fibrosis presented with normal liver function tests at the time of referral.

The prognostic value of the combined FIB-4 and VCTE strategy was evaluated in a cohort study in France.[44] Patients with FIB-4 less than 1.3 or FIB-4 greater than 1.3 and VCTE less than 8 kPa are at very low risk of experiencing a liver-related event.

The study recommended retesting within 3 years among patients without T2D and within 2 years in patients with T2D.

The cost-effectiveness of the FIB-4 and VCTE combination strategy has also been compared with other combination strategies.[45] The FIB-4 and VCTE combination was able to identify patients with cirrhosis with the lowest cost per person and highest diagnostic accuracy of all examined methods, followed by MEFIB.

The sequential FIB-4 and VCTE testing approach has been recommended initially by the EASL,[16] followed by American Association of Clinical Endocrinology (AACE) and American Association for the Study of Liver Disease (AASLD).[46] All these associations propose the performance of an initial screening using the FIB-4. The EASL suggests screening patients with metabolic cofactors without specifically defining which patients to apply the FIB-4 greater than 1.30 criterion for. The AACE and AASLD broadly define the high-risk NAFLD group as those with prediabetes, T2D, obesity, more than 2 cardiometabolic risk factors, steatosis on imaging, or elevated liver enzymes. VCTE is proposed for patients with FIB-4 ranging from 1.3 to 2.67. The EASL guidelines favor VCTE for patients with FIB-4 greater than 1.3, whereas the AACE and AASLD guidelines favor referral to a hepatology specialist without further testing when FIB-4 greater than 2.67.

SUMMARY

Radiological testing is now routinely used for clinical trial prescreening, diagnosis, and treatment and to determine which primary care patients should be referred to hepatology specialists. The CAP performs well in detecting fatty liver for NAFLD diagnosis but is unable to differentiate between hepatic steatosis grades and cannot be relied on to track longitudinal changes. MRI-PDFF is a better technique for evaluating longitudinal changes and is currently used as a primary endpoint in trials investigating antisteatotic properties of therapeutic agents. The probability of detecting liver fibrosis using radiological testing techniques is high when performed at referral centers for the purposes of clinical trial prescreening, and reasonable imaging strategies include the combination of FIB-4 and VCTE, the FAST Score, MAST, and MEFIB. When assessing liver fibrosis to determine the need for referral to hepatology specialists from primary care, the probability of detecting liver fibrosis using radiological testing is low. The strategy currently recommended by the EASL, AACE, and AASLD is the sequential application of FIB-4 and VCTE, based on availability of resources and local imaging capabilities.

CLINICS CARE POINTS

- The CAP performs well in detecting fatty liver for NAFLD diagnosis but is unable to differentiate between hepatic steatosis grades and cannot be relied on to track longitudinal changes.
- MRI-PDFF is a better technique for evaluating longitudinal changes and is currently used as a primary endpoint in trials investigating antisteatotic properties of therapeutic agents.
- When assessing liver fibrosis to determine the need for referral to hepatology specialists from primary care, the probability of detecting liver fibrosis using radiological testing is low.
- The probability of detecting liver fibrosis using radiological testing techniques is high when performed at referral centers for the purposes of clinical trial prescreening, and reasonable imaging strategies include the combination of FIB-4 and VCTE, the FAST Score, MAST, and MEFIB.

CONFLICT OF INTEREST

R. Loomba serves as a consultant to Aardvark Therapeutics, Altimmune, Anylam/Regeneron, Amgen, Arrowhead Pharmaceuticals, AstraZeneca, Bristol-Myer Squibb, CohBar, Eli Lilly, Galmed, Gilead, Glympse bio, Hightide, Inipharma, Intercept, Inventiva, Ionis, Janssen Inc., Madrigal, Metacrine, Inc., NGM Biopharmaceuticals, Novartis, Novo Nordisk, Merck, Pfizer, Sagimet, Theratechnologies, 89 bio, Terns Pharmaceuticals, and Viking Therapeutics. In addition, his institutions received research grants from Arrowhead Pharmaceuticals, Astrazeneca, Boehringer-Ingelheim, Bristol-Myers Squibb, Eli Lilly, Galectin Therapeutics, Galmed Pharmaceuticals, Gilead, Intercept, Hanmi, Intercept, Inventiva, Ionis, Janssen, Madrigal Pharmaceuticals, Merck, NGM Biopharmaceuticals, Novo Nordisk, Merck, Pfizer, Sonic Incytes, and Terns Pharmaceuticals. Cofounder of LipoNexus Inc. L. Castera has served as a consultant for Alexion, Echosens, Gilead, Intercept, MSD, Novo Nordisk, Pfizer, and Sagimet and has received lectures fees from Echosens, Gilead, Intercept, and Novo Nordisk.

FUNDING STATEMENT

R. Loomba receives funding support from NCATS (5UL1TR001442), United States, NIDDK (U01DK061734, U01DK130190, R01DK106419, R01DK121378, R01DK124318, P30DK120515), United States, and NHLBI (P01HL147835), United States. W. Dunn receives funding support from NIDDK 1K23DK10929401A1 and Gilead NASH Models of Care ISR Program.

REFERENCES

1. Younossi ZM, Koenig AB, Abdelatif D, et al. Global epidemiology of nonalcoholic fatty liver disease-Meta-analytic assessment of prevalence, incidence, and outcomes. Hepatology 2016;64:73–84.
2. Sanyal AJ, Van Natta ML, Clark J, et al. Prospective study of outcomes in adults with nonalcoholic fatty liver disease. N Engl J Med 2021;385:1559–69.
3. Taylor RS, Taylor RJ, Bayliss S, et al. Association between fibrosis stage and outcomes of patients with nonalcoholic fatty liver disease: a systematic review and meta-analysis. Gastroenterology 2020;158:1611–1625 e12.
4. Angulo P, Kleiner DE, Dam-Larsen S, et al. Liver fibrosis, but no other histologic features, is associated with long-term outcomes of patients with nonalcoholic fatty liver disease. Gastroenterology 2015;149:389–397 e10.
5. Kleiner DE, Brunt EM, Wilson LA, et al. Association of histologic disease activity with progression of nonalcoholic fatty liver disease. JAMA Netw Open 2019;2: e1912565.
6. Kim D, Kim WR, Kim HJ, et al. Association between noninvasive fibrosis markers and mortality among adults with nonalcoholic fatty liver disease in the United States. Hepatology 2013;57:1357–65.
7. Anstee QM, Castera L, Loomba R. Impact of non-invasive biomarkers on hepatology practice: past, present and future. J Hepatol 2022;76:1362–78.
8. Castera L, Friedrich-Rust M, Loomba R. Noninvasive assessment of liver disease in patients with nonalcoholic fatty liver disease. Gastroenterology 2019;156: 1264–1281 e4.
9. Siddiqui MS, Vuppalanchi R, Van Natta ML, et al. Vibration-controlled transient elastography to assess fibrosis and steatosis in patients with nonalcoholic fatty liver disease. Clin Gastroenterol Hepatol 2019;17:156–163 e2.

10. Garteiser P, Castera L, Coupaye M, et al. Prospective comparison of transient elastography, MRI and serum scores for grading steatosis and detecting non-alcoholic steatohepatitis in bariatric surgery candidates. JHEP Rep 2021;3: 100381.
11. Karlas T, Petroff D, Sasso M, et al. Individual patient data meta-analysis of controlled attenuation parameter (CAP) technology for assessing steatosis. J Hepatol 2017;66:1022–30.
12. Caussy C, Brissot J, Singh S, et al. Prospective, same-day, direct comparison of controlled attenuation parameter with the M vs the XL probe in patients with nonalcoholic fatty liver disease, using magnetic resonance imaging-proton density fat fraction as the standard. Clin Gastroenterol Hepatol 2020;18: 1842–1850 e6.
13. Petroff D, Blank V, Newsome PN, et al. Assessment of hepatic steatosis by controlled attenuation parameter using the M and XL probes: an individual patient data meta-analysis. Lancet Gastroenterol Hepatol 2021;6:185–98.
14. Caussy C, Alquiraish MH, Nguyen P, et al. Optimal threshold of controlled attenuation parameter with MRI-PDFF as the gold standard for the detection of hepatic steatosis. Hepatology 2018;67:1348–59.
15. Eddowes PJ, Sasso M, Allison M, et al. Accuracy of fibroscan controlled attenuation parameter and liver stiffness measurement in assessing steatosis and fibrosis in patients with nonalcoholic fatty liver disease. Gastroenterology 2019; 156:1717–30.
16. European Association for the Study of the Liver. Electronic address eee, Clinical practice guideline P, Chair, et al. EASL clinical practice guidelines on non-invasive tests for evaluation of liver disease severity and prognosis - 2021 update. J Hepatol 2021;75:659–89.
17. Gu J, Liu S, Du S, et al. Diagnostic value of MRI-PDFF for hepatic steatosis in patients with non-alcoholic fatty liver disease: a meta-analysis. Eur Radiol 2019; 29:3564–73.
18. Kramer H, Pickhardt PJ, Kliewer MA, et al. Accuracy of liver fat quantification with advanced CT, MRI, and ultrasound techniques: prospective comparison with MR spectroscopy. AJR Am J Roentgenol 2017;208:92–100.
19. Hannah WN Jr, Harrison SA. Noninvasive imaging methods to determine severity of nonalcoholic fatty liver disease and nonalcoholic steatohepatitis. Hepatology 2016;64:2234–43.
20. Le TA, Chen J, Changchien C, et al. Effect of colesevelam on liver fat quantified by magnetic resonance in nonalcoholic steatohepatitis: a randomized controlled trial. Hepatology 2012;56:922–32.
21. Jayakumar S, Middleton MS, Lawitz EJ, et al. Longitudinal correlations between MRE, MRI-PDFF, and liver histology in patients with non-alcoholic steatohepatitis: analysis of data from a phase II trial of selonsertib. J Hepatol 2019;70:133–41.
22. Loomba R, Neuschwander-Tetri BA, Sanyal A, et al. Multicenter validation of association between decline in MRI-PDFF and histologic response in NASH. Hepatology 2020;72:1219–29.
23. Middleton MS, Heba ER, Hooker CA, et al. Agreement between magnetic resonance imaging proton density fat fraction measurements and pathologist-assigned steatosis grades of liver biopsies from adults with nonalcoholic steatohepatitis. Gastroenterology 2017;153:753–61.
24. Stine JG, Munaganuru N, Barnard A, et al. Change in MRI-PDFF and histologic response in patients with nonalcoholic steatohepatitis: a systematic review and meta-analysis. Clin Gastroenterol Hepatol 2021;19:2274–2283 e5.

25. Tyagi A, Yeganeh O, Levin Y, et al. Intra- and inter-examination repeatability of magnetic resonance spectroscopy, magnitude-based MRI, and complex-based MRI for estimation of hepatic proton density fat fraction in overweight and obese children and adults. Abdom Imaging 2015;40:3070–7.
26. Noureddin M, Lam J, Peterson MR, et al. Utility of magnetic resonance imaging versus histology for quantifying changes in liver fat in nonalcoholic fatty liver disease trials. Hepatology 2013;58:1930–40.
27. Selvaraj EA, Mozes FE, Jayaswal ANA, et al. Diagnostic accuracy of elastography and magnetic resonance imaging in patients with NAFLD: a systematic review and meta-analysis. J Hepatol 2021;75:770–85.
28. Hsu C, Caussy C, Imajo K, et al. Magnetic resonance vs transient elastography analysis of patients with nonalcoholic fatty liver disease: a systematic review and pooled analysis of individual participants. Clin Gastroenterol Hepatol 2019; 17:630–637 e8.
29. Mozes FE, Lee JA, Selvaraj EA, et al. Diagnostic accuracy of non-invasive tests for advanced fibrosis in patients with NAFLD: an individual patient data meta-analysis. Gut 2022;71:1006–19.
30. Anstee QM, Lawitz EJ, Alkhouri N, et al. Noninvasive tests accurately identify advanced fibrosis due to NASH: baseline data from the STELLAR trials. Hepatology 2019;70:1521–30.
31. Newsome PN, Sasso M, Deeks JJ, et al. FibroScan-AST (FAST) score for the non-invasive identification of patients with non-alcoholic steatohepatitis with significant activity and fibrosis: a prospective derivation and global validation study. Lancet Gastroenterol Hepatol 2020;5:362–73.
32. Woreta TA, Van Natta ML, Lazo M, et al. Validation of the accuracy of the FAST score for detecting patients with at-risk nonalcoholic steatohepatitis (NASH) in a North American cohort and comparison to other non-invasive algorithms. PLoS One 2022;17:e0266859.
33. Oeda S, Takahashi H, Imajo K, et al. Diagnostic accuracy of FibroScan-AST score to identify non-alcoholic steatohepatitis with significant activity and fibrosis in Japanese patients with non-alcoholic fatty liver disease: comparison between M and XL probes. Hepatol Res 2020;50:831–9.
34. Hirooka M, Koizumi Y, Yano R, et al. Validation of the FibroScan-aspartate aminotransferase score by vibration-controlled transient and B-mode ultrasound elastography. Hepatol Res 2021;51:652–61.
35. Loomba R, Wolfson T, Ang B, et al. Magnetic resonance elastography predicts advanced fibrosis in patients with nonalcoholic fatty liver disease: a prospective study. Hepatology 2014;60:1920–8.
36. Park CC, Nguyen P, Hernandez C, et al. Magnetic resonance elastography vs transient elastography in detection of fibrosis and noninvasive measurement of steatosis in patients with biopsy-proven nonalcoholic fatty liver disease. Gastroenterology 2017;152:598–607 e2.
37. Imajo K, Kessoku T, Honda Y, et al. Magnetic resonance imaging more accurately classifies steatosis and fibrosis in patients with nonalcoholic fatty liver disease than transient elastography. Gastroenterology 2016;150:626–637 e7.
38. Jung J, Loomba RR, Imajo K, et al. MRE combined with FIB-4 (MEFIB) index in detection of candidates for pharmacological treatment of NASH-related fibrosis. Gut 2021;70:1946–53.
39. Tamaki N, Imajo K, Sharpton S, et al. Magnetic resonance elastography plus Fibrosis-4 versus FibroScan-aspartate aminotransferase in detection of

candidates for pharmacological treatment of NASH-related fibrosis. Hepatology 2022;75:661–72.
40. Kim BK, Tamaki N, Imajo K, et al. Head to head comparison between MEFIB, MAST, and FAST for detecting stage 2 fibrosis or higher among patients with NAFLD. J Hepatol 2022;77(6):1482–90.
41. Noureddin M, Truong E, Gornbein JA, et al. MRI-based (MAST) score accurately identifies patients with NASH and significant fibrosis. J Hepatol 2022;76:781–7.
42. Castera L, Boursier J. Noninvasive algorithms for the case finding of "at-risk" patients with NAFLD. Semin Liver Dis 2022;42(3):313–26.
43. Mansour D, Grapes A, Herscovitz M, et al. Embedding assessment of liver fibrosis into routine diabetic review in primary care. JHEP Rep 2021;3:100293.
44. Boursier J, Hagstrom H, Ekstedt M, et al. Non-invasive tests accurately stratify patients with NAFLD based on their risk of liver-related events. J Hepatol 2022;76:1013–20.
45. Vilar-Gomez E, Lou Z, Kong N, et al. Cost effectiveness of different strategies for detecting cirrhosis in patients with nonalcoholic fatty liver disease based on United States health care system. Clin Gastroenterol Hepatol 2020;18:2305–2314 e12.
46. Cusi K, Isaacs S, Barb D, et al. American association of clinical endocrinology clinical practice guideline for the diagnosis and management of nonalcoholic fatty liver disease in primary care and endocrinology clinical settings: co-sponsored by the american association for the study of liver diseases (AASLD). Endocr Pract 2022;28:528–62.

Noninvasive Tests Used in Risk Stratification of Patients with Nonalcoholic Fatty Liver Disease

Linda Henry, PhD[a,b,c,d], Katherine Elizabeth Eberly, MD[a,c], Dipam Shah, MD[a,c], Ameeta Kumar, MD[a,c], Zobair M. Younossi, MD, MPH[a,b,c,*]

KEYWORDS

• Fibrosis • Liver disease • Nonalcoholic fatty liver disease • Noninvasive test • Fib-4 • VCTE CAP • MRI-PDFF • ELF • MRE

KEY POINTS

- NAFLD is increasing expotentially in parallel to the obesity and T2 diabetes epidemics.
- The lack of non-invasive tests have hindered knowing the true prevalence of NAFLD.
- The presence of fibrosis is the most significant predictor of mortality in those with NAFLD so patients with NAFLD and fibrosis stage 2 or greater are considered to have "high risk" NAFLD.
- There are now several non-invasive tests that recommended to identify patients with NAFLD and those with high risk NAFLD.
- The current risk stratifying non-invasive tests to be used in primary care and endocrinology include the use of ultrasound, MRI-PDFF or VCTE Cap scores to identify steatosis. Fib-4 < or >/= 1.3 is used to risk stratify patients as to who should remain with their primary care or endocrinologist (FIB-4 <1.3) for management of their NAFLD and cariometabolic risk factors and those who need further testing and should be referred to a specialist (Fib -4 >/= 1.3).

[a] Inova Medicine, Inova Health System, 3300 Gallows Road, Falls Church, VA 22042, USA; [b] Liver and Obesity Research Program, Inova Health System, 3300 Gallows Road, Falls Church, VA 22042, USA; [c] Department of Medicine, Center for Liver Diseases, Inova Fairfax Medical Campus, 3300 Gallows Road, Falls Church, VA 22042, USA; [d] Center for Outcomes Research in Liver Diseases, 2411 I Street, Northwest Washington, DC 20037, USA
* Corresponding author. Beatty Liver and Obesity Research Program, Claude Moore Health Education and Research Building, 3300 Gallows Road, Falls Church, VA 22042.
E-mail address: Zobair.Younossi@inova.org

Clin Liver Dis 27 (2023) 373–395
https://doi.org/10.1016/j.cld.2023.01.022
liver.theclinics.com

INTRODUCTION

The most current estimate suggests that in 2019, 38% of the world's adult population had nonalcoholic fatty liver disease (NAFLD).[1] NAFLD is a complex liver disease that occurs as a result of multiple risk factors including metabolic comorbidities (eg, insulin resistance, obesity, type 2 diabetes mellitus [T2D], hypertension, dyslipidemia), genetic predisposition (eg, PNPLA3 I148M), environmental factors (eg, lack of access to healthy food), gut dysbiosis, and dysregulation of bile acids.[2–5] The most potentially progressive form of NAFLD, nonalcoholic steatohepatitis (NASH), affects about 5% of the general population.[1] It is estimated that 10% to 15% of patients with NASH can potentially progress to advanced fibrosis, cirrhosis, hepatocellular carcinoma, liver transplantation, and death.[6–8] In addition to these clinical outcomes, NAFLD and NASH are associated with impairment of health-related quality of life, loss of work productivity, and tremendous economic burden.[9–19] Therefore, it has become increasingly important to efficiently identify patients with NAFLD who are at risk for progression, manage their cardiometabolic risks as well as provide them with future NASH-specific drug regimens. In this context, the most important clinical predictors of adverse outcomes among those with NAFLD are the presence of T2D and other components of metabolic syndrome.[6,20] Furthermore, presence of significant hepatic fibrosis on histology (≥stage 2 fibrosis) has been consistently shown to be the most important independent predictor of mortality among patients with NAFLD.[21–24]

Although histologic stage of fibrosis has been historically determined by liver biopsy, there has been intense efforts to develop and validate noninvasive methods to estimate stage of fibrosis and predict long-term outcomes.[25] In addition, because most of the patients with NAFLD are usually first seen in primary care or endocrinology practices, the need for simple, noninvasive tests (NITs) that can accurately and efficiently determine which patients have NAFLD and are at risk for progressive liver disease are urgently needed.[26] Once identified, these patients at high risk can then be referred to gastrohepatology for evaluation and managed by a multispecialty team.[26] Despite great strides in the past decade in the field of NITs for NAFLD, their utilization in clinical practice and the disease awareness about NAFLD remain low.[27–29]

The following section briefly describes the currently available NITS with an algorithm to assist practitioners on how to implement the use of these NITs in clinical practice.

From Histology to Noninvasive Tests Used for Assessment of Hepatic Steatosis, Fibrosis, and Activity

The diagnosis of NAFLD is based on the presence of steatosis in which at least 5% of the hepatocytes are fat filled in the absence of excessive alcohol use (men >3 drinks/day; women >1.5 drinks/day), other steatogenic liver conditions, viral hepatitis, and exposure to steatogenic medications.[30,31] In this context, there are also 3 histologically determined components of disease that can be used for diagnosis,[25] which include hepatic steatosis, hepatic fibrosis, and histologic activity of steatohepatitis.[25] Because (as previously discussed) the most important histologic predictor of long-term outcome is stage of fibrosis,[21–24] emphasis has been placed on the development of noninvasive biomarkers and algorithms to determine stage of fibrosis.[21–24,26,27,32,33] The following paragraphs will describe in more detail different modalities assessing hepatic steatosis, fibrosis, and activity in NAFLD that have been recently developed.

Hepatic steatosis: the most efficient method to assess hepatic steatosis rely on imaging modalities. These modalities include ultrasound, controlled attenuation parameter (CAP) of vibration-controlled elastography (VCTE), and MRI-proton density fat fraction (MRI-PDFF).[34,35] Although other noninvasive algorithms such as fatty liver index (FLI) and hepatic steatosis index (HSI) are good indices for establishing hepatic steatosis, they have mostly been used in research studies rather than clinical practice.[26,36] These specific modalities for assessment of hepatic steatosis are discussed in subsequent paragraphs.

Hepatic fibrosis: in addition to hepatic fat, estimation of hepatic fibrosis can be made by radiologic modalities using estimation of liver stiffness with VCTE, shear wave elastography (SWE), and acoustic radiation force impulse (ARFI) or magnetic resonance elastography (MRE).[37] The areas under the curve results are similar for fibrosis stages F1 to F3 for VCTE liver stiffness measure (VCTE-LSM), 2-dimensional SWE (2DSWE), and MRE, but MRE has been shown to have the best results for finding cirrhosis.[38–40] This finding is especially important for those with a small intercostal space (eg, women), as MRE has been shown to be easier to perform in patients with narrow intercostal space. MRE also allows for the measurement of larger liver area, avoiding sampling variability caused by the heterogeneity of advanced fibrosis.[38–40] In addition, there may be limitations based on test availability and the need for skilled staff as well as higher costs. Therefore, in many cases, these tests are reserved to be used as second-line or third-line tests that can assist in risk stratification and subsequent clinical management.[35,38]

In addition to these radiologic NITs, blood biomarkers test can estimate stage of fibrosis. These biomarkers use direct or indirect markers of hepatic injury, inflammation, fibrogenesis, or extracellular matrix remodeling.[41,42] The most commonly used serum fibrosis NIT is enhanced liver fibrosis (ELF) score.[37] A number of other simple tests have also been developed and validated to estimate stage of fibrosis (FIB-4, NAFLD fibrosis score [NFS], and so on). Of these, FIB-4 has been extensively used in algorithms for risk stratification in clinical practice.[37] In fact, given that most patients with NAFLD may be diagnosed by their primary care or endocrinology physicians, the professional liver disease societies recommend the use of FIB-4 (<1.3) and NFS (<-1.45), due to their high negative predictive values (NPV, $\geq$ 90%) to determine the presence or absence of the risk for advanced fibrosis or cirrhosis, which means these markers can be used to exclude patients who may be at high risk of liver-related morbidity or mortality.[30,43–46]

Histologic activity scores: historically, NAFLD activity score (NAS) was developed to assess histologic activity of steatohepatitis. The NAS was designed and validated by the Pathology Committee of the NASH Clinical Research Network to describe the spectrum of lesions found with NAFLD and as an assessment method for clinical trials.[33,47] The NAS is composed of 4 components considered to be imperative for the determination of disease activity and are graded on a scale. The following are the NAS components with their assigned scores where higher NASs relate to fibrosis progression rather than a change in the liver disease (ie, an increase in an NAS correlates with fibrosis progression and a decrease correlates with fibrosis improvement: steatosis [0–3], lobular inflammation [0–2], hepatocellular ballooning [0–2], and fibrosis [0–4]).[33]

Given that NAS requires a liver biopsy, a number of NITs estimating histologic disease activity have been developed, which include FibroScan-aspartate aminotransferase (FAST) score and MRI-aspartate aminotransferase (MAST) score.[48–50] The FAST score is a new combination test using both FibroScan and liver enzymes (AST) and is described in more detail later as is the MAST score, another combination test.[48,49] However, an important feature of both the FAST and MAST scores is that they do not require a liver biopsy. The combination of an imaging modality and a liver enzyme obtained from a simple blood draw has the ability to identify patients with NASH (NAS >4) and fibrosis with a F2 or greater stage.[48,49]

In addition to these radiologic modalities, NIS4 was recently developed using patients from several NASH clinical trials and is composed of 4 biomarkers commonly associated with NASH, which include miR-34a-5p, alpha-2 macroglobulin, YKL-40, and glycated hemoglobin. In addition, the NIS4 score does not seem to be influenced by age, sex, body mass index (BMI), or aminotransferase levels. A score less than 0.36 was established as a rule out high-risk NASH cut-off score with a sensitivity of 82%, a specificity of 63%, and a NPV of 78%. A NIS4 score of greater than 0.63 was identified as a rule in cut-off for high-risk NASH with a sensitivity of 51%, a specificity of 87%, and a positive predictive value (PPV) of 79.2%.[51]

The role of these radiologic and serum biomarkers of steatohepatitis activity in clinical practice is still being determined but is described in more detail in the following sections with a description of a proposed algorithm of how these diagnostic modalities can be used in clinical practice.

Specific Imaging and Noninvasive Modalities for Assessment of Hepatic Steatosis

Ultrasound

Historically, the most commonly used radiologic NIT to assess hepatic steatosis has been ultrasound (US). In fact, in many cases, NAFLD has been diagnosed incidentally in patients who were undergoing US testing for other purposes (**Table 1**).[62] US is easily obtained in a clinical practice with immediate results being available. However, in NAFLD, US is less accurate when there is mild steatosis, which cannot be detected by this modality. Also, US is dependent on a skilled operator and may not be as accurate in those with obesity.[55,57,63–65] In a meta-analysis of studies including 4720 patients comparing US with liver histology, US was sensitive for the detection of moderate-to-severe steatosis (approximating to steatosis in >33% of hepatocytes) with a sensitivity of 84.8% (95% confidence interval [CI] 79.5–88.9) and specificity of 93.6% (95% CI 87.2–97.0) but did not reliably detect steatosis of less than 20%.[55] Therefore, US is considered a qualitative rather than a quantitative diagnostic tool for establishing fatty liver but remains the most common method for NAFLD diagnosis.

Vibration-controlled transient elastography–controlled attenuation parameter

In the past decade, CAP has been increasingly used to determine the presence of hepatic steatosis. CAP is obtained with the use of one-dimensional transient elastography (TE) FibroScan (Echosens, Paris France), which measures the ultrasonic attenuation of the echo wave. One study reported the areas under receiver operating characteristic curve (AUROC) for estimation of steatosis grades greater than or equal to S1, S2, and S3 were 0.97, 0.86, and 0.75, respectively, suggesting that the optimal CAP cutoffs for estimation of steatosis grades greater than or equal to S1, S2, and S3 were 263 dB/m, 281 dB/m, and 283 dB/m, respectively.[66] When examined by obesity status, among the nonobese patients, the AUROC for estimation of steatosis grades greater than or equal to S1 and S2 were 0.99 and 0.99, respectively. Among the obese patients, the AUROC for steatosis grades greater than or equal to S1, S2, and S3 were 0.92, 0.64, and 0.58, respectively.[66] Others have suggested that CAP values greater than or equal to285 dB/m provided a sensitivity of 80% and specificity of 77% for determining the presence of liver steatosis greater than or equal to5%, whereas others have found that the different cutoffs produced AUROCs that varied between 0.88 and 0.70 for detection of steatosis.[67] A most recent study found that although CAP is very good for the detection of mild hepatic steatosis, CAP cannot grade steatosis in patients with NAFLD adequately, and its accuracy can be impaired by high BMI, sex, age, and high levels of AST.[67] Therefore, further work is needed to

Table 1
Noninvasive tests for steatosis

Test	Cutoffs	AUROC	Sensitivity (%)	Specificity (%)	PPV (%)	NPV (%)	LR−	LR+	Reference #
Simple Biomarkers									
HSI	>41.6	0.81	61	83	99	10	9.2	—	Lee et al,[52] 2010
HSI	>43.0	0.65	59	68	71	56	1.8	—	Lee et al,[52] 2010
FLI	>60	0.83	76	87	99	15	5.7	—	Bedogni et al,[53] 2006
FLI	>82	0.65	59	69	71	56	1.9	—	Bedogni et al,[53] 2006
USFLI	≥30 (rule in)	0.80	62	88	—	—	0.43	5.2	Ruhl & Everhart,[54] 2015
USFLI	<10 (rule out)	0.80	86	48	—	—	0.28	1.7	Ruhl & Everhart,[54] 2015
Imagining									
Ultrasound	>33% hepatic steatosis	—	84	94	—	—	—	—	Fishbein et al,[55] 2005
CAP	236	0.88	62	91	99	67	—	—	Myers et al,[56] 2012
	270	0.73	78	81	73	75	—	—	Myers et al,[56] 2012
	283	—	76	79	87	64	—	—	Myers et al,[56] 2012
	302	0.70	64	74	76	94	—	—	Myers et al,[56] 2012
CT Scan	>0% steatosis	—	46	94	—	—	—	—	[57–60]
	>5% steatosis	—	50	94	—	—	—	—	[57–60]
	>30% steatosis	—	91	97	—	—	—	—	[57–60]
MRI-PDFF (≥1)	5.2	0.98	90	93	89.2	51.9	—	—	Myers et al,[56] 2012
MRI-PDFF (≥2)	11.3	0.90	79	84	85	78	—	—	Myers et al,[56] 2012
MRI-PDFF (≥3)	17.1	0.790	74	81	63	95	—	—	Myers et al,[56] 2012
Ultrasound >33% hepatic steatosis	—	—	84	94	—	—	—	—	Brunt et al,[61] 2019

Abbreviations: CT, computed tomography; USFLI, United States fatty liver index.

validate the correct threshold scores as well as comparison of CAP with other radiologic modalities. None the less, CAP may be most useful as a second test in those whose first test places them in an indeterminate zone or are suspected of having mild steatosis.[68,69]

Magnetic resonance imaging-derived proton density fat fraction

MRI-PDFF is a quantitative imaging biomarker for hepatic steatosis.[70] The MRI itself is a method to quantify the relative amount of water and fat signal arising from the tissue. PDFF is defined as the ratio of the density of mobile protons from triglycerides and the total density of protons from mobile triglycerides and mobile water. It is expressed as an absolute percentage (%) and ranges from 0% to –100%. Within the liver, hepatic steatosis via PDFF is displayed as the percentage of cells containing intracellular droplets of fat.[38,39] Severe steatosis (grade 3) is defined as an MRI-PDFF of greater than or equal to 17.1%. In this context, MRI-PDFF may be the most accurate method to assess hepatic steatosis in NAFLD.[38,39]

Magnetic resonance spectroscopy

Magnetic resonance spectroscopy (MRS) is similar to MRI-PDFF but displays a reading that requires expertise to interpret, and the analysis must be performed off-line with specialized software.[70] Both MRI modalities address confounding factors and are not affected by scanner field strength, patient factors (age, sex, BMI, cause of liver disease), and concomitant liver abnormalities (iron overload and necroinflammation).[70] Despite these advantages, MR-based technologies are limited due to access and costs.[70]

Computed tomography scan

Computed tomography (CT) may be useful to detect and quantify moderate-to-severe hepatic steatosis but its utility is limited, particularly at low fat concentrations, which is most relevant for clinical practice. In addition, CT scans expose patients to radiation, which makes this therapy less attractive, especially as alternative noninvasive imaging methods such as MRI are available.[57–60]

Simple Biomarkers for Detecting Nonalcoholic Fatty Liver Disease

Fatty liver index

The FLI is based on BMI, waist circumference, triglycerides, and gamma glutamyl transferase (GGT). The FLI has an accuracy of 0.84 (95% CI 0.81–0.87) for detecting fatty liver. A FLI score of less than 30 (sensitivity of 87%; negative likelihood ratio = 0.2) has been found to have good NPV, whereas an FLI greater than or equal to 60 can be used to rule in hepatic steatosis (specificity = 86%; positive likelihood ratio = 4.3).[53] The following is the formula used to calculate FLI:

FLI = (e 0.953*loge (triglycerides) + 0.139*BMI + 0.718*loge (ggt) +0.053*waist circumference–15.745)/(1 + e 0.953*loge (triglycerides) + 0.139*BMI + 0.718*loge (ggt) + 0.053*waist circumference–15.745) * 100.

United States fatty liver index

The United States FLI (USFLI) is an improved version of FLI designed specifically for the multiethnic US population. It is also a biochemical model that predicts the presence of fatty liver based on age, race/ethnicity, waist circumference, GGT activity, fasting insulin, and fasting glucose and is defined as follows:

US FLI = (e–0.8073*non-Hispanic black + 0.3458*Mexican American + 0.0093*age + 0.6151*loge(GGT) + 0.0249*waist circumference + 1.1792*loge(insulin) + 0.8242*loge(glucose)–14.7812)/(1 + e–0.8073*non-Hispanic black + 0.3458*Mexican

American + 0.0093*age + 0.6151*loge(GGT) + 0.0249*waist circumference + 1.17 92*loge(insulin) + 0.8242*loge(glucose) – 14.7812) * 100.

This model has been previously validated with an AUROC of 0.80 (95% CI 0.77–0.83) for the detection of fatty liver in subjects with values greater than or equal to 30.[53,54]

Hepatic steatosis index

The HSI was developed in a study using Korean population. The derivation of the HSI is based on gender, the presence or absence of diabetes mellitus as well as the alanine transaminase (ALT) and aspartate transaminase (AST) ratio and BMI.[52] Therefore, the HSI calculation formula is 8 x(ALT/AST ratio)+BMI (+2, if female; +2, if diabetes mellitus). HSI has an AUROC of 0.812 (95% CI, 0.801–0.824) for detecting fatty liver. At values of less than 30.0 or greater than 36.0, HSI ruled out NAFLD with a sensitivity of 92.5% (95% CI, 91.4–93.5) and a negative likelihood ratio of 0.186 (95% CI, 0.163–0.213), and at a value of greater than 36.0, HSI could detect NAFLD with a specificity of 92.4% (95% CI, 91.3–93.4) and a positive likelihood ratio of 6.069 (95% CI, 5.284–6.970).[71] Studies providing external validation of HSI in different population are needed.

Specific Imaging and Noninvasive Modalities for Assessment of Hepatic Fibrosis

As previous discussed, liver biopsy and histologic assessments have been the gold standard for diagnosing NASH and staging of fibrosis.[25] Nevertheless, liver biopsy is not without its limitations, risks, and costs, making it impractical for use when stratifying patients in a general clinical practice (**Table 2**).[72–75] On the other hand, liver biopsy remains an important diagnostic tool especially to exclude other causes of liver disease that may be superimposed on NAFLD.[76]

Vibration-controlled elastography liver stiffness measure for estimating hepatic fibrosis

VCTE-LSM is obtained using FibroScan (Echosens, Paris France).[34,77,78] This test is an US-based method in which a probe generates a low-frequency, acoustic shear wave that travels through the liver. The velocity of the waves captured correlates with the amount of liver stiffness. The higher the value, the greater the degree of liver stiffness/fibrosis. LSM values range from 1.5 to 75 kPa. LSM values of 8 to 12 kPa (median LSM 8.6 kPa has a sensitivity of 66% and specificity of 80%) are considered to represent an intermediate risk of advanced fibrosis (F3–F4), whereas those with a greater than or equal to 12 kPa are considered to be at high risk for advanced fibrosis.[34,78] However, one limitation of VCTE is that it can have a high failure rate ranging between 5% and 27%, especially in the presence of obesity. The use of a specified probe (M or XL) can reduce the error rate to less than 10%. In addition, it is recommended that VCTE is performed at least 3 hours after a meal to reduce error.[79–81]

Magnetic resonance imaging and elastography

As noted earlier, this technology decomposes the signals obtained from the liver and addresses confounding factors such as scanner field strength, patient factors (age, sex, BMI, cause of liver disease), and concomitant liver abnormalities (iron overload and necroinflammation).[70,82–84] The role of routine MRI in clinical practice for assessment of NAFLD is very limited.[82,83] On the other hand, the role of MR technology MRE for assessment of liver stiffness in NAFLD is quite promising.[82–84]

MRE is an MRI-based method for quantitatively imaging tissue stiffness and is available from several manufacturers of MRI scanners as an option that includes special hardware and software. Quantitative stiffness images (elastograms) of the liver can be obtained rapidly during breath-hold acquisitions and can therefore be readily

Table 2
Noninvasive tests for fibrosis

Test	Cutoffs	AUROCs	Sensitivity	Specificity	PPV	NPV	LR−	LR+	Comments
Simple Biomarkers									
FIB-4	1.30	0.86	85	65	36	95	.36	2.32	46
	2.67	0.86	39	95	67	84	.03	7.85	46
	3.25	0.86	26	98	75	85	—	—	46
APRI	1	0.67	27	89	37	84	—	—	46
BARD	2–4	0.77	89	44	27	96	—	—	46
NFS	<−1.455	0.81	82	77	56	93	0.23	3.56	99,100
NFS	>0.676	0.81	51	98	90	85	0.50	25.97	99,100
AST/ALT ratio	> 0.8	0.83	74	78	44	93	—	—	43
NIS4 (rule out)	<0.36	—	82	63	—	78	—	—	54
NIS4 (rule in)	>0.63	—	51	87	—	92	—	—	54
Imaging									
MRE ≥ 1	2.5 kPa	0.80	75	86	99	85	—	—	61
MRE ≥ 2	3.4 kPa	0.89	87	85	88	84	—	—	61
MRE ≥ 3	4.8 kPa	0.89	75	87	75	81	—	—	61
MRE ≥ 4	6.7 kPa	0.97	91	95	59	99	—	—	61
TE ≥ 1	7.0 kPa	0.78	62	100	100	87	—	—	61
TE ≥ 2	11.0 kPa	0.82	65	89	88	66	—	—	61
TE ≥ 3	11.4 kPa	0.88	86	84	75	92	—	—	61
TE ≥ 4	14.0 kPa	0.92	100	76	73	100	—	—	61
2DSWE	7.1 kPa		94	52	—	—	—	—	92
	9.2 kPa		93	81	—	—	—	—	92
	11.3 kPa		75	88	—	—	—	—	92
ARFI ≥ F2	0.95	0.77	90	36	—	—	—	—	93
	1.32	0.77	56	91	—	—	—	—	93

ARFI ≥ F3	1.15	0.84	90	63	—	—	—	—	93
	1.53	0.84	59	90	—	—	—	—	93
ARFI F4	1.3	0.84	90	67	—	—	—	—	93
	2.04	0.84	44	90	—	—	—	—	93
Combination									
ELF	7.7	0.85	93	34	7	99	—	—	109,110
ELF	9.8	0.85	65	86	20	98	—	—	109,110
ELF	10.51	0.85	51	93	26	97	—	—	109,110
ELF	11.3	0.85	36	96	34	97	—	—	109,110
FibroMeter (F ≥ 2)	0.30	0.94	79	96	—	—	—	—	107
FibroTest F ≥ 2	.30	0.81	77	77	—	—	—	—	107
FibroTest F ≥ 3	.70	0.83	15	98	—	—	—	—	107
MAST	0.165	0.93	72	90	29	98	—	—	51
MAST	0.242	0.93	75	90	50	97	—	—	51
FAST	0.35–0.67	0.85	89	64	—	94	—	—	50
FAST	>0.67	0.85	92	49	—	69	—	—	50

Abbreviations: APRI, AST to platelet ratio; BARD, BMI, AST/ALT ratio, Diabetes; ELF, enhanced liver function; FAST, fibroscan +AST; FIB-4, fibrosis 4 score; MAST, MRE + AST; MRE, magnetic resonance elastography.

included in conventional liver MRI protocols.[82–84] Fibrosis stages 0 to 4 (F0–F4) defined using MRE values based on a previous meta-analysis are as follows: (F0 <2.61 kPa; F1, 2.61–2.96 kPa; F2 = 2.97–3.61kPa; F3 = 3.62–4.68 kPa; F4 = 4.69 kPa).[56,84]

Two-dimensional shear wave elastography

2D-SWE is integrated into a conventional US imaging machine and can measure liver stiffness during a routine ultrasound scan with results returned in real time where elasticity is displayed on a color map.[85,86] Furthermore, although several confounders (age, BMI, and severe steatosis) regarding the diagnostic accuracy of serum fibrosis markers or TE have been reported, in a recent study, the AUROCs remained greater than 0.80% regardless of the presence of these confounders. Researchers in one study reported the sensitivity and specificity of 2D-SWE for the optimal cutoffs of 7.15 for fibrosis stage less than 2 (93.8% and 52%), 9.15 for fibrosis stage 2 to 3 (93.1% and 80.9%), and 11.0 for fibrosis stage 3 to 4 (75.3% and 85.8%), respectively.[86] As such, 2DSWE may be a viable alternative to regular US for finding high-risk patients when performed by very experienced sonographers or radiologists after the patient has fasted for at least 2 hours.

Acoustic radiation force impulse

ARFI is an ultrasound-based diagnostic technique that uses nonexternal compression to generate short-duration acoustic radiation forces (<1 ms) at a specified area of interest. The generated wave scan provides both qualitative or quantitative wave velocity value responses that correspond to liver stiffness.[87] ARFI has been shown to provide similar accuracy as transient elastography in diagnosing significant fibrosis or cirrhosis. It is also a potential viable option for offices that do not have access to TE equipment, as AFRI does not require separate equipment and has good interoperator reliability while producing very good displays of anatomical structures and measurements, which are not hindered by age, sex, or BMI (https://www.siemens-healthineers.com/en-us/ultrasound/arfi-elastography). In a comparison study with liver biopsy, ARFI returned AUROCs between 0.77 and 0.84 for fibrosis level F2, F3, and cirrhosis.[87]

Simple Biomarkers for Fibrosis

There are several simple NITs (BMI, AST, ALT, and Diabetes (BARD); AST to platelet ratio [APRI]; FIB-4; NFS) used in clinical practice. These NITs incorporate "indirect" markers of liver fibrosis such as aminotransaminases accompanied with clinical parameters (age, sex, presence of insulin resistance/T2DM, and andromorphic assessments). A recent meta-analysis confirmed that the current advocated published cutoffs to determine the presence of significant or advanced fibrosis are appropriate. Specifically, the investigators determined that the summary sensitivities and specificities of BARD score (threshold of 2) for advanced fibrosis was 0.76 and 0.61, whereas an APRI threshold of 1.0 and 1.5 provided sensitivities and specificities of 18.3% and 96.1% for advanced fibrosis. An FIB-4 threshold of 2.67 and 3.25 provided sensitivities and specificitiess for advanced fibrosis of 26.6% and 96.5% and 31.8% and 96.0%, respectively. For the NFS threshold of −1.455, the summary sensitivities and specificities for advanced fibrosis were 0.72 and 0.70.[88] Based on their analysis, the investigators suggested that the NFS and FIB-4 offer the best diagnostic performance for detecting advanced fibrosis. In fact, the use of the indirect biomarker FIB-4 is suggested for use in primary care and endocrinology practices as a screening tool for fibrosis and in determining whether a patient will need a specialist referral.[26,37,88–90] However, the following section provides further details about these NITS.

Fibrosis-4

The FIB-4 is an algorithm based on age, levels of platelets, AST, and ALT to indicate the presence or absence of advanced fibrosis (fibrosis stage 3–4). Using FIB-4 threshold values of less than 1.3 and greater than 2.67 for the absence and presence of advanced fibrosis, respectively, a liver biopsy may be avoided in 78% of patients with NAFLD, and as such, these values were used in this study.[90] However, it is important to note that because both the NFS and FIB-4 use age as one criterion in their model calculation, it is suggested that for those aged 65 years and older, an FIB-4 score of greater than 2.0 be used as the initial cutoff rather than greater than 1.3 and an NFS score greater than 0.12.[90] Furthermore, the FIB-4 has not been shown to be accurate for those younger than 35 years again because of age. However, given the slow progressive nature of this disease, at this time, screening for fibrosis in the younger group is not as pressing although, if the current trajectory of disease continues, the younger age group will warrant further NIT exploration.[8,91,92]

Nonalcoholic fatty liver disease fibrosis score

The NFS uses age, platelets, AST and ALT ratio, albumin levels, BMI, and impaired fasting glucose/diabetes. In patients with NAFLD applying a low cut-off score of less than −1.455 excluded advanced fibrosis with high accuracy, whereas applying a high cut-off score of greater than 0.675 diagnosed the presence of advanced fibrosis with high accuracy (AUROC of 0.88 and 0.82 in the estimation and validation groups). By applying the low cut-off score (−1.455), advanced fibrosis could be excluded with high accuracy (NPV of 93% and 88% in the estimation and validation groups, respectively). By applying the high cut-off score (0.676), the presence of advanced fibrosis could be diagnosed with high accuracy (PPV of 90% and 82% in the estimation and validation groups, respectively). Using the NFS may avoid liver biopsy in 75%.[88,93] The following is the formula for the NFS score:

NAFLD fibrosis score (NFS) = 1.675 + 0.037 X age (years) +0.094 X BMI (kg/m2) +1.13 X IFG/diabetes (yes = 1, no = 0) +0.99 X AST/ALT ratio–0.013 X platelet (109/L) −0.66 X albumin (g/dL).

Aspartate aminotransferase to platelet ratio

The AST:platelet ratio index uses AST's upper limit of normal and platelet count to determine the presence of advanced fibrosis and cirrhosis.[90,94] The higher the fibrosis stage, the lower the AST levels and platelet counts, which returned high sensitivity and specificity as well as good positive and negative predictability. The APRI formula is as follows: AST level (/ULN)/Platelet counts (109/L) x 100.[94]

HEPAmet. The HEPAmet score was developed using data from the HEPAmet registry in Spain and validated in a cohort of patients from France, Italy, China, and Cuba.[95] A HEPAmet score of less than 0.12 is considered to be low risk for advanced fibrosis, whereas a score of 0.12 to 00.47 indicates intermediate risk, and a score greater than 0.47 is at high risk for advanced fibrosis with good sensitivity, specificity, as well as good negative and positive predictability.[95]

The final biochemical model is 1/(1 + e [5.390–0:986 x Age [45_64 years of age]-1.719 x Age [>65 years of age] + 0.875x Male sex −0.896 x AST [35–69 IU/L]-2.126 x AST [>70 IU/L]- 0.027x Albumin [4–4:49 g = dL]- 0.897 x Albumin [<4 g = dL]- 0.899 x HOMA [2–3:99 with no Diabetes Mellitus]- 1.497 x HOMA [>4 with no Diabetes Mellitus]-2.184 x[Diabetes Mellitus – 0.882x platelets x 1:000/uL [155_219] – 2.233 x platelets x 1.000/uL = mL [<155]).

BARD score

The BARD score is composed of BMI (B), AST/ALT ratio (AAR), and Diabetes (D).[96] The formula is BARD score = AAR≥ 0.8 (2 points), BMI≥ 28 (1 point), presence of diabetes (1 point) for a total score of 4; however, a score of 2 to 4 was found to be indicative of advanced fibrosis; therefore, a BARD score greater than or equal to 2 is considered a positive BARD score. When comparing NAFLD alone plus NASH with fibrosis stages 0 to 2 to NASH with fibrosis stages 3 to 4, AUROC for the use of the BARD score was found to be 0.81. The PPV and NPV were 43% and 96%, respectively, in the development cohort, whereas in the validation cohort, the AUC was 0.78 with a PPV and an NPV of 27% and 97%, respectively. A positive BARD score was associated with an odds ratio of 17 (CI 9.2–31.9) for detecting stage 3 to 4 fibrosis. However, the BARD score seems to be more accurate at predicting advanced fibrosis in nondiabetics compared with diabetic patients most likely because of the higher weight given to AAR. Nonetheless, as noted by the BARD developers, an easily remembered simple application of the score is that patients with NAFLD with an AAR greater than or equal to 0.8 or those who are both obese and have diabetes are at enough risk to warrant further evaluation but a negative score (BARD <2) in one with NAFLD by imaging also warrants further evaluation.[96]

Complex Serum Biomarker of Fibrosis

In addition, there are complex biomarkers, which include the FibroTest, FibroMeter, ELF, and type IV collagen 7S, N-terminal propeptide of type 3 collagen (Pro-C3), that are reliant on the direct markers of fibrogenesis and fibrinolysis such as serum tissue metalloproteinases and hyaluronic acid.[97] Of all these tests, ELF is the more robust test that has recently received regulatory approval for risk stratification of patients with NAFLD.

Enhanced liver function score

The ELF panel consists of plasma levels of 3 matrix turnover proteins (hyaluronic acid, TIMP-1, and procollagen III, N-terminal propeptide [PIIINP]) and has an AUROC of 0.90 with 80% sensitivity and 90% specificity for detecting advanced fibrosis.[98–107] The ELF score also has 3 distinct cut-off values that can be readily used in practice without an indeterminate zone. These zones for advanced fibrosis are low risk with an ELF score of less than 9.8, midrisk with an ELF score greater than or equal to 9.8 and less than 11.3, and higher risk with an ELF score greater than or equal to 11.3.[100–107] The ELF score is the preferred test in the NICE (UK) guideline for determining the presence of high-risk NAFLD.[108] It is also part of American Association of Clinical Endocrinology clinical practice guidelines where ELF is recommended to be used as the second-line test for patients who fall into the indeterminate zone with the use of FIB-4 or to confirm the likelihood of the presence of significant or advanced fibrosis.[109] As such, ELF has also been the only test that is considered a prognostic test (what is likely to happen) with independently validated 9.8 and 11.3 cutoffs where a unit increase in ELF score is associated with a doubling of risk.[100,101] A recent study determined that patients with NASH with an ELF score greater than or equal to 11.3 have 2.5 to 2.8 increased risk of experiencing a liver-related event.[102,103] The use of the ELF score has also been predictive of patient-reported outcomes.[110] However, the ELF's high sensitivity (0.73) and specificity (0.80, AUC:0.83) are only apparent in a setting in where there is a very high prevalence (>50%) of fibrosis.[107] The following is the ELF formula: ELF score*† = 2.278 + 0.851 ln (CHA) + 0.751 ln (CPIIINP) + 0.394 ln (CTIMP-1).[100–107]

PRO-C3

The accumulation of excess extracellular matrix (ECM) leads to liver fibrosis progression and the release of PRO-C3, which reflects the formation and degradation of ECM.[111–116] In a study that included 431 patients with biopsy-proven NAFLD, the AUROC of PRO-C3 for detecting advanced fibrosis was 0.81 to 0.83 with a diagnostic accuracy similar to FIB-4 and NFS.[115] To improve the diagnostic accuracy, a new scoring system, ADAPT score, was created with the addition of age, presence of diabetes, and platelet counts to PRO-C3.[114] When ADAPT was used, the AUROC for advanced fibrosis improved to 0.86 to 0.87.[114] Another study that included 517 patients with biopsy-proven NAFLD demonstrated that the diagnostic accuracy of ADAPT for advanced fibrosis was higher than other noninvasive markers such as FIB-4.[115] Because ELF, type IV collagen 7S, or PRO-C3 reflect fibrogenesis, it may be useful for determining treatment response or longitudinal changes in liver fibrosis. However, validation studies are relatively small compared with FIB-4 or NFS, and further data are needed. Furthermore, both tests can be affected by the presence of other fibrotic diseases.[116]

FibroTest

The FibroTest is a biomarker test that uses the results of 6 blood serum tests (alpha-2-macroglobulin, haptoglobin, apolipoprotein A1, GGT, total bilirubin, and ALT) to generate a score that is correlated with the degree of liver damage.[99] However, a recent meta-analysis determined that the FibroTest returned the best value for patients with cirrhosis (AUC = 0.92) and moderate values for those with significant and advanced fibrosis (AUC = 0.77).[100]

FibroMeter

The FibroMeter is a patented (Echosens, Paris France) formula that includes the parameters prothrombin index, AST, ALT, Urea, GGT, alpha-2-macroglobulin, and platelets. A recent meta-analysis found that FibroMeter itself had an AUC of 0.82 in determining the presence of F3 or greater; with the addition of VCTE, the AUC increased to 0.94. However, given the various versions of the FibroMeter, further head-to-head test of its performance among patients with NAFLD is recommended.[100]

Combination Tests for Assessment of Fibrosis and Steatohepatitis

There are also several tests such as the FAST, MAST, and MEFIB score that combine imagining and biomarkers to determine those with "at-risk" NASH. The FAST score is the use of fibroscan to diagnose NAFLD and fibrosis along with the serum biomarker AST. The MAST score is the use of MRI-PDFF or MRE to diagnose NASH and fibrosis along with the AST level. The MEFIB is a combination of MRE and the FIB-4 score. The MEFIB index is considered to be positive with a MRE score greater than or equal to 3.3kPa and FIB-4 greater than or equal to 1.6. A recent meta-analysis of individual patient data found that a positive MEFIB index was highly associated with hepatic decompensation, whereas a negative MEFIB had high NPV for hepatic decompensation at 5 years.[117,118]

FibroScan-aspartate aminotransferase score

The FAST score is a simple algorithm that combines LSM and CAP obtained from the FibroScan device along with AST.[48] The FAST score cutoffs of 0.35 (sensitivity of 90%) and 0.67 (specificity of 90%) are used to assess for significant fibrosis (F2) where an FAST score of 0.67 indicates having significant fibrosis. FAST score cutoffs of 0.38 (sensitivity of 91%) and 0.76 (specificity of 92%) can be used to assess for fibrosis stage 3. However, a score between 0.35 and 0.67 is considered to be in the grey zone where one cannot rule in or rule out significant fibrosis, but at the present time, as this test was developed for use in specialty practices, consideration for biopsy and eligibility for trials or treatment can be further evaluated.[48]

The formula for the FAST score is as follows:

$$\text{FAST} = e{-}1{\cdot}65 + 1{\cdot}07 \times \ln(\text{LSM}){+}2{\cdot}66{*}10\text{-}8 \times \text{CAP3-}63{\cdot}3 \times \text{AST-}11{+}e{-}1{\cdot}65 + 1{\cdot}07 \times \ln(\text{LSM}){+}2{\cdot}66{*}10\text{-}8 \times \text{CAP3-}$$

Magnetic resonance imaging-aspartate aminotransferase score

The MAST score is composed of MRI results with AST results.[49] In the validation cohorts, the MAST score produced a 90% specificity for a cutoff of 0.242, which corresponded to a sensitivity of 75.0%, PPV of 50.0% and NPV of 96.5%. At a 90% sensitivity cutoff of 0.165, a specificity of 72.2%, PPV of 29.4%, and NPV of 98.1% were obtained. Compared with NFS and FIB-4, the MAST score resulted in fewer patients having indeterminate scores and an overall higher AUC. Compared with FAST, MAST exhibited a higher AUC and overall better discrimination.[49]

Combination of fibrosis-4 and enhanced liver fibrosis score and fibrosis-4 and magnetic resosnance elastography

Another important study of patients with NAFLD who underwent FIB-4 followed by ELF established 2 different thresholds (rule out advanced fibrosis: ELF score of $\geq$7.2 with a FIB-4 score $\geq$ 0.74, NPV of 95.1, sensitivity of 92.5%; rule in advanced fibrosis: ELF score$\geq$ 9.8 with a FIB-4 score $\geq$ 2.9, PPV 95.0%, specificity 99.7%) that can be used to rule in advanced fibrosis. This study suggests that by implanting different cutoffs for these 2 tests clinical care pathways can be established to risk stratify patients with NAFLD.[105]

Finally, MRE and FIB-4 (MEFIB) score has recently been studied, which is a combination of imagining and biomarkers to determine those with "at-risk" NASH. The clinical utility and large-scale external validation studies of this combination and others are still pending so at this time, one combination test cannot be recommended over others.[117,119]

Algorithm in Practice to Identify High-Risk Nonalcoholic Fatty Liver Disease

Although a number of the current NITs have excellent NPV for excluding advanced fibrosis, they have poor PPV to identify those with significant fibrosis who should be identified in clinical practice and linked to care. In this context, a number of algorithms have suggested sequential risk stratification to help identify patients who are at risk for progressive liver disease.[27,109,118,120,121]

One approach to identify patients with high-risk NAFLD is depicted in **Fig. 1**. In this context, Fib-4 is the suggested first-line test to exclude those patients who are unlikely to have advanced fibrosis. In fact, patients with FIB-4 score of less than 1.3 is recommended to stay under the care of their primary care or endocrinology care practices for management of cardiometabolic risks. In contrast, patients with FIB-4 greater than or equal to 1.3 should be considered for further evaluation or a referral to a specialist. The next step in the evaluation depends on test availability and the associated costs. In general, the second line testing with ELF or VCTE-LSM should be performed to determine the risk for significant or advanced fibrosis. These test results will then define the next steps as well as the appropriate management (see **Fig. 1**). For those patients whose tests are contradictory, another test such as MRE may be considered. Finally, on a case-by-case basis, liver biopsy may be needed in rare circumstances, especially if another superimposed liver pathology is suspected.

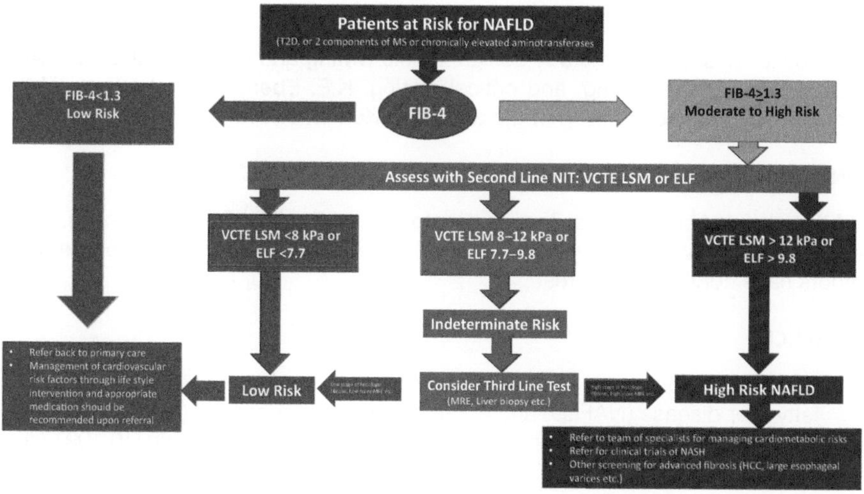

Fig. 1. Risk Stratification of Patients with NAFLD. (Modified Younossi Z et al APT 2022, Younossi Z et al AJG 2020, Cusi K et al Endocr Pract. 2022.)

SUMMARY

As the prevalence of NAFLD and NASH continue to increase, the necessity for identifying and linking the high-risk patients to appropriate care in a timely fashion is becoming imperative. Currently, a number of reasonably well-validated noninvasive tests for estimated hepatic fibrosis and steatosis are available. To assist the front-line health care providers (primary care physicians and endocrinologists), several algorithms incorporating a practical and easy-to-use noninvasive test in a stepwise fashion have been developed. As we increase awareness about NAFLD, it is critical to provide tools and algorithms to enhance the identification of high-risk NAFLD and linkage to appropriate care using multidisciplinary care pathways.

CLINICS CARE POINTS

- Patients with diabetes or 2 or more metabolic comorbidities in the absence of excessive alcohol intake, viral hepatitis and other steatotic causes of liver disease should be suspected of having NAFLD.
- Ultrasound, MRI-PDFF or VCTECAP can be used to determine the presence of steatosis.
- Fib-4 < 1.3 indicates that a patients is at low risk of having fibrosis and should continued to be managed in their primary care or endocrinology office.
- Patients with a FIB-4 score >/= 1.3 should undergo further testing with VCTE LSM and or ELF score and referred to a specialist.
- All non-invasive tests still have limitations so these recommedations will evolve over time as more study is completed.

FUNDING SUPPORT

None.

AUTHOR CONTRIBUTIONS

Z.M. Younossi: supervisor, study design, article writing and critical editing. L. Henry: study design, article writing, and critical editing. K.E. Eberly: critical editing of the article. D. Shah: critical editing of the article. A. Kumar: critical editing of the article.

CONFLICTS OF INTEREST

Z.M. Younossi: Abbott, Astra Zeneca, Bristol-Myers Squibb, Gilead Sciences, Intercept, Madridgal, Merck, NovoNordisk, and Siemens Healthineers. None of the other authors have conflicts of interest.

REFERENCES

1. Younossi Z., Golabi P., Paik J., et al., The global epidemiology of nonalcoholic fatty liver disease (NAFLD) and non-alcoholic steatohepatitis (NASH): a systematic review [published online January 3, 2023]. *Hepatology.* doi:10.1097/HEP.0000000000000004.
2. Romeo S, Kozlitina J, Xing C, et al. Genetic variation in PNPLA3 confers susceptibility to nonalcoholic fatty liver disease. Nat Genet 2008;40(12):1461–5.
3. Leung C, Rivera L, Furness JB, et al. The role of the gut microbiota in NAFLD. Nat Rev Gastroenterol Hepatol 2016;13(7):412–25.
4. Chávez-Talavera O, Haas J, Grzych G, et al. Bile acid alterations in nonalcoholic fatty liver disease, obesity, insulin resistance and type 2 diabetes: what do the human studies tell? Curr Opin Lipidol 2019;30(3):244–54.
5. Loomba R, Friedman SL, Shulman GI. Mechanisms and disease consequences of nonalcoholic fatty liver disease. Cell 2021;184(10):2537–64.
6. Anstee QM, Targher G, Day CP. Progression of NAFLD to diabetes mellitus, cardiovascular disease or cirrhosis [Internet]. Nat Rev Gastroenterol Hepatol 2013;10:330–44.
7. Nyberg LM, Cheetham TC, Patton HM, et al. The natural history of NAFLD, a community-based study at a large health care delivery system in the United States. Hepatol Commun 2020;5(1):83–96.
8. Allen AM, Therneau TM, Ahmed OT, et al. Clinical course of non-alcoholic fatty liver disease and the implications for clinical trial design. J Hepatol 2022;77(5):1237–45.
9. Younossi ZM, Stepanova M, Lawitz EJ, et al. Patients with nonalcoholic steatohepatitis experience severe impairment of health-related quality of life. Am J Gastroenterol 2019;114(10):1636–41.
10. Younossi ZM, Stepanova M, Anstee QM, et al. Reduced patient-reported outcome scores associate with level of fibrosis in patients with nonalcoholic steatohepatitis. Clin Gastroenterol Hepatol 2019;17(12):2552–60.e10.
11. Younossi ZM, Yilmaz Y, Yu ML, et al. Clinical and patient-reported outcomes from patients with nonalcoholic fatty liver disease across the world: data from the global non-alcoholic steatohepatitis (NASH)/ non-alcoholic fatty liver disease (NAFLD) registry. Clin Gastroenterol Hepatol 2022;20(10):2296–306.e6.
12. Younossi ZM, Wong VW, Anstee QM, et al. Fatigue and pruritus in patients with advanced fibrosis due to nonalcoholic steatohepatitis: the impact on patient-reported outcomes. Hepatol Commun 2020;4(11):1637–50.
13. Younossi ZM, Tampi R, Priyadarshini M, et al. Burden of illness and economic model for patients with nonalcoholic steatohepatitis in the United States. Hepatology 2019;69(2):564–72.

14. Younossi ZM, Tampi RP, Racila A, et al. Economic and Clinical burden of nonalcoholic steatohepatitis in patients with type 2 diabetes in the U.S. Diabetes Care 2020;43(2):283–9.
15. Tampi RP, Wong VW, Wong GL, et al. Modelling the economic and clinical burden of nonalcoholic steatohepatitis in East Asia: data from Hong Kong. Hepatol Res 2020;50(9):1024–31.
16. Sayiner M, Arshad T, Golabi P, et al. Extrahepatic manifestations and healthcare expenditures of nonalcoholic fatty liver disease in the Medicare population. Hepatol Int 2020;14(4):556–66.
17. Younossi ZM, Blissett D, Blissett R, et al. The economic and clinical burden of nonalcoholic fatty liver disease in the United States and Europe. Hepatology 2016;64(5):1577–86.
18. Nguyen AL, Park H, Nguyen P, et al. Rising inpatient encounters and economic burden for patients with nonalcoholic fatty liver disease in the USA. Dig Dis Sci 2019;64(3):698–707.
19. Younossi Z.M., Paik J.M., Henry L., et al., The Growing Economic and Clinical Burden of Nonalcoholic Steatohepatitis (NASH) in the United States, J Clin Exp Hepatol, 2022, Available at: https://www.sciencedirect.com/science/article/abs/pii/S0973688322005321#:~:text=NASH%20cases%20in%20the%20U.S,(13.46%25%20to%2013.05%25).
20. Golabi P, Otgonsuren M, Suen W, et al. Predictors of inpatient mortality and resource utilization for the elderly patients with chronic hepatitis C (CH-C) in the United States. Medicine (Baltim) 2016;95(3):e2482.
21. Dulai PS, Singh S, Patel J, et al. Increased risk of mortality by fibrosis stage in nonalcoholic fatty liver disease: systematic review and meta-analysis. Hepatology 2017;65(5):1557–65.
22. Taylor RS, Taylor RJ, Bayliss S, et al. Association between fibrosis stage and outcomes of patients with nonalcoholic fatty liver disease: a systematic review and meta-analysis. Gastroenterology 2020;158(6):1611–25.e12.
23. Hagström H, Nasr P, Ekstedt M, et al. Fibrosis stage but not NASH predicts mortality and time to development of severe liver disease in biopsy-proven NAFLD. J Hepatol 2017;67(6):1265–73.
24. Younossi ZM, Stepanova M, Rafiq N, et al. Nonalcoholic steatofibrosis independently predicts mortality in nonalcoholic fatty liver disease. Hepatol Commun 2017;1(5):421–8.
25. Goodman ZD. Chapter 7 Hepatic Histopathology. Schiff ER, Maddrey WC, Sorrell MF, editors. First published: 31 October 2011. https://doi.org/10.1002/9781119950509.
26. Younossi ZM, Corey KE, Alkhouri N, et al. Clinical assessment for high-risk patients with non-alcoholic fatty liver disease in primary care and diabetology practices [Internet]. Aliment Pharmacol Ther 2020;52:513–26.
27. Ekstedt M, Hagström H, Nasr P, et al. Fibrosis stage is the strongest predictor for disease-specific mortality in NAFLD after up to 33 years of follow-up [Internet]. Hepatology 2015;61:1547–54.
28. Angulo P, Kleiner DE, Dam-Larsen S, et al. Liver fibrosis, but no other histologic features, is associated with long-term outcomes of patients with nonalcoholic fatty liver disease [Internet]. Gastroenterology 2015;149:389–97.e10.
29. Singh A, Dhaliwal AS, Singh S, et al. Awareness of nonalcoholic fatty liver disease is increasing but remains very low in a representative US cohort. Dig Dis Sci 2020;65(4):978–86.

30. Chalasani N, Younossi Z, Lavine JE, et al. The diagnosis and management of nonalcoholic fatty liver disease: practice guidance from the American Association for the Study of Liver Diseases. Hepatology 2018;67:328–57.
31. NHANES guidelines for alcohol use, 2023. Available at: https://www.nice.org.uk/guidance/ng49/resources/nonalcoholic-fatty-liver-disease-nafld-assessment-and-management-pdf-1837461227461. Accessed Febuary 17, 2023.
32. Tsochatzis EA, Newsome PN. Non-alcoholic fatty liver disease and the interface between primary and secondary care. Lancet Gastroenterol Hepatol 2018;3:509–17.
33. Kleiner DE, Brunt EM, Van Natta M, et al, Nonalcoholic Steatohepatitis Clinical Research Network. Design and validation of a histological scoring system for nonalcoholic fatty liver disease. Hepatology 2005;41(6):1313–21.
34. Castera L, Friedrich-Rust M, Loomba R. Noninvasive assessment of liver disease in patients with nonalcoholic fatty liver disease. Gastroenterology 2019;156(5):1264–81.e4.
35. Piazzolla VA, Mangia A. Noninvasive diagnostics of NAFLD and NASH. Cells 2020;9(4):1005.
36. Sourianarayanane A, McCullough AJ. Accuracy of steatosis and fibrosis NAFLD scores in relation to vibration controlled transient elastography: an NHANES analysis. Clin Res Hepatol Gastroenterol 2022;46(7):101997.
37. Younossi Z, Alkhouri N, Cusi K, et al. A practical use of noninvasive tests in clinical practice to identify high-risk patients with nonalcoholic steatohepatitis. Aliment Pharmacol Ther 2023;57(3):304–12.
38. Park CC, Nguyen P, Hernandez C, et al. Magnetic resonance elastography vs transient elastography in detection of fibrosis and noninvasive measurement of steatosis in patients with biopsy-proven nonalcoholic fatty liver disease. Gastroenterology 2017;152(3):598–607.e2.
39. Imajo K, Honda Y, Kobayashi T, et al. Direct comparison of US and MR elastography for staging liver fibrosis in patients with nonalcoholic fatty liver disease. Clin Gastroenterol Hepatol 2022;20(4):908–17.e11.
40. Hines CD, Bley TA, Lindstrom MJ, et al. Repeatability of magnetic resonance elastography for quantification of hepatic stiffness. J Magn Reson Imaging 2010;31:725–31.
41. Anstee QM, Castera L, Loomba R. Impact of non-invasive biomarkers on hepatology practice: past, present and future. J Hepatol 2022;76(6):1362–78.
42. Sandrin L, Fourquet B, Hasquenoph JM, et al. Transient elastography: a new noninvasive method for assessment of hepatic fibrosis. Ultrasound Med Biol 2003;29:1705–13.
43. Xiao G, Zhu S, Xiao X, et al. Comparison of laboratory tests, ultrasound, or magnetic resonance elastography to detect fibrosis in patients with nonalcoholic fatty liver disease:a meta-analysis. Hepatology 2017;66:1486–501.
44. Sumida Y, Yoneda M, Hyogo H, et al. Validation of the FIB4 index in a Japanese nonalcoholic fatty liver disease population. BMC Gastroenterol 2012;12:2.
45. Castellana M, Donghia R, Guerra V, et al. Fibrosis-4 index vs nonalcoholic fatty liver disease fibrosis score in identifying advanced fibrosis in subjects with nonalcoholic fatty liver disease: a meta-analysis. Am J Gastroenterol 2021;116:1833–41.
46. Tokushige K, Ikejima K, Ono M, et al. Evidence-based clinical practice guidelines for nonalcoholic fatty liver disease/nonalcoholic steatohepatitis 2020. J Gastroenterol 2021;56:951–63.

47. Pai RK, Jairath V, Hogan M, et al. Reliability of histologic assessment for NAFLD and development of an expanded NAFLD activity score. Hepatology 2022; 76(4):1150–63.
48. Newsome PN, Sasso M, Deeks JJ, et al. FAST) score for the non-invasive identification of patients with non-alcoholic steatohepatitis with significant activity and fibrosis: a prospective derivation and global validation study. Lancet Gastroenterol Hepatol 2020;5(4):362–73 [Erratum in: Lancet Gastroenterol Hepatol. 2020 Apr;5(4):e3. PMID: 32027858; PMCID: PMC7066580.
49. Noureddin M, Truong E, Gornbein JA, et al. MRI-based (MAST) score accurately identifies patients with NASH and significant fibrosis. J Hepatol 2022;76(4): 781–7.
50. Kleiner DE, Brunt EM, Wilson LA, et al. Association of histologic disease activity with progression of nonalcoholic fatty liver disease. JAMA Netw Open 2019;2: e1912565.
51. Harrison SA, Ratziu V, Boursier J, et al. A blood-based biomarker panel (NIS4) for non-invasive diagnosis of non-alcoholic steatohepatitis and liver fibrosis: a prospective derivation and global validation study. Lancet Gastroenterol Hepatol 2020;5(11):970–85.
52. Lee JH, Kim D, Kim HJ, et al. Hepatic steatosis index: a simple screening tool reflecting nonalcoholic fatty liver disease. Dig Liver Dis 2010;42:503–8.
53. Bedogni G, Bellentani S, Miglioli L, et al. The Fatty Liver Index: a simpleand accurate predictor of hepaticsteatosis in the general population. BMC Gastroenterol 2006;6:33.
54. Ruhl CE, Everhart JE. Fatty liver indices in the multiethnic United States national health and nutrition examination survey. Aliment Pharmacol Ther 2015;41:65–76.
55. Fishbein M, Castro F, Cheruku S, et al. Hepatic MRI for fat quantitation: its relationship to fat morphology, diagnosis, and ultrasound. J Clin Gastroenterol 2005; 39(7):619–25.
56. Myers RP, Pollett A, Kirsch R, et al. Controlled Attenuation Parameter (CAP): a noninvasive method for the detection of hepatic steatosis based on transient elastography. Liver Int 2012;32(6):902–10.
57. Saadeh S, Younossi ZM, Remer EM, et al. The utility of radiological imaging in nonalcoholic fatty liver disease. Gastroenterology 2002;123(3):745–50.
58. Limanond P, Raman SS, Lassman C, et al. Macrovesicular hepatic steatosis in living related liver donors: correlation between CT and histologic findings. Radiology 2004;230(1):276–80.
59. Fazel R, Krumholz HM, Wang Y, et al. Exposure to low-dose ionizing radiation from medical imaging procedures. N Engl J Med 2009;361(9):849–57.
60. Birnbaum BA, Hindman N, Lee J, et al. Multi-detector row CT attenuation measurements: assessment of intra- and interscanner variability with an anthropomorphic body CT phantom. Radiology 2007;242(1):109–19.
61. Brunt EM, Kleiner DE, Wilson LA, et al, Nonalcoholic Steatohepatitis Clinical Research Network. Improvements in histologic features and diagnosis associated with improvement in fibrosis in nonalcoholic steatohepati-tis: results from the Nonalcoholic Steatohepatitis Clinical Research Network Treatment Trials. Hepatology 2019;70:522–31.
62. de Moura Almeida A, Cotrim HP, Barbosa DBV, et al. Fatty liver disease in severe obese patients: diagnostic value of abdominal ultrasound. World J Gastroenterol 2008;14:1415–8.

63. Bril F, Ortiz-Lopez C, Lomonaco R, et al. Clinical value of liver ultrasound for the diagnosis of nonalcoholicfatty liver disease in overweight and obese patients. Liver Internat 2015;35:2139–46.
64. Hernaez R, Lazo M, Bonekamp S, et al. Diagnostic accuracy and reliability of ultrasonography for the detection of fatty liver: a meta-analysis. Hepatology 2011;54(3):1082–90.
65. Imajo K, Kessoku T, Honda Y, et al. Magnetic resonance imaging more accurately classifies steatosis and fibrosis in patients with nonalcoholic fatty liver disease than transient elastography. Gastroenterology 2016;150(3):626–37.e7.
66. Petroff D, Blank V, Newsome PN, et al. Assessment of hepatic steatosis by controlled attenuation parameter using the M and XL probes: an individual patient data meta-analysis. The Lancet Gastroenterology & Hepatology 2021; 6(3):185–98.
67. Pu K, Wang Y, Bai S, et al. Diagnostic accuracy of controlled attenuation parameter (CAP) as a non-invasive test for steatosis in suspected non-alcoholic fatty liver disease: a systematic review and meta-analysis. BMC Gastroenterol 2019;19:51. https://doi.org/10.1186/s12876-019-0961-9.
68. Le MH, Cheung R, Nguyen MH. Transient elastography and serum-based tests for diagnosis of fatty liver and advanced fibrosis in a community cohort- a cross sectional analysis. Dig Dis 2022. https://doi.org/10.1159/000526503. Epub ahead of print. PMID: 35973400.
69. Caussy C, Reeder SB, Sirlin CB, et al. Noninvasive, quantitative assessment of liver fat by MRI-PDFF as an endpoint in NASH trials. Hepatology 2018. https://doi.org/10.1002/hep.29797.
70. Reeder SB, Cruite I, Hamilton G, et al. Quantitative assessment of liver fat with magnetic resonance imaging and spectroscopy. J Magn Reson Imaging 2011; 34(4):729–49.
71. Zaitoun AM, Al Mardini H, Awad S, et al. Quantitative assessment of fibrosis and steatosis in liver biopsies from patients with chronic hepatitis C. J Clin Pathol 2001;54(6):461–5.
72. Maharaj B, Maharaj RJ, Leary WP, et al. Sampling variability and its influence on the diagnostic yield of percutaneous needle biopsy of the liver. Lancet 1986; 1(8480):523–5.
73. Younossi ZM, Gramlich T, Liu YC, et al. Nonalcoholic fatty liver disease; Assessment of variability in pathologic interpretations. Mod Pathol 1998;11:560–5.
74. Matteoni CA, Younossi ZM, Gramlich T, et al. Nonalcoholic fatty liver disease: a spectrum of clinical and pathological severity. Gastroenterology 1999;116: 1413–9.
75. Kleiner DE, Makhlouf HR. Histology of nonalcoholic fatty liver disease and nonalcoholic steatohepatitis in adults and children. Clin Liver Dis 2016;20:293–312.
76. Younossi ZM, Stepanova M, Rafiq N, et al. Pathologic criteria for nonalcoholic steatohepatitis: interprotocol agreement and ability to predict liver-related mortality. Hepatology 2011;53:1874–82.
77. Eddowes PJ, Sasso M, Allison M. Accuracy of FibroScan controlled attenuation parameter and liver stiffness measurement in assessing steatosis and fibrosis in patients with nonalcoholic fatty liver disease. Gastroenterology 2019;156: 1717–30 [PubMed: 30689971].
78. Siddiqui MS, Vuppalanchi R, Van Natta ML, et al, NASH Clinical Research Network. Vibration-controlled transient elastography to assess fibrosis and steatosis in patients with nonalcoholic fatty liver disease. Clin Gastroenterol Hepatol 2019;17(1):156–63.e2.

79. Wong GL, Chan HL, Choi PC, et al. Association between anthropometric parameters and measurements of liver stiffness by transient elastography. Clin Gastroenterol Hepatol 2013;11:295–302. e1-e3 [PubMed: 23022698].
80. Friedrich-Rust M, Hadji-Hosseini H, Kriener S, et al. Transient elastography with a new probe for obese patients for non-invasive staging of non-alcoholic steatohepatitis. Eur Radiol 2010;20:2390–6 [PubMed: 20526777].
81. Vuppalanchi R, Siddiqui MS, Van Natta ML, et al. Performance characteristics of vibration-controlled transient elastography for evaluation of nonalcoholic fatty liver disease. Hepatology 2018;67:134–44 [PubMed: 28859228].
82. Noureddin M, Lam J, Peterson MR, et al. Utility of magnetic resonance imaging versus histology for quantifying changes in liver fat in nonalcoholic fatty liver disease trials. Hepatology 2013;58:1930–40.
83. Carrión JA, Navasa M, Forns X. MR elastography to assess liver fibrosis. Radiology 2008;247:591.
84. Hsu C, Caussy C, Imajo K, et al. Magnetic resonance vs transient elastography analysis of patients with nonalcoholic fatty liver disease: a systematic review and pooled analysis of individual participants. Clin Gastroenterol Hepatol 2019; 17(4):630–7.e8.
85. Kakegawa T, Sugimoto K, Kuroda H, et al, GITHY Liver Study Group. Diagnostic accuracy of two-dimensional shear wave elastography for liver fibrosis: a multicenter prospective study. Clin Gastroenterol Hepatol 2022;20(6):e1478–82.
86. Herrmann E, de Lédinghen V, Cassinotto C, et al. Assessment of biopsy-proven liver fibrosis by two-dimensional shear wave elastography: an individual patient data-based meta-analysis. Hepatology 2018;67(1):260–72.
87. Cassinotto C, Boursier J, de Lédinghen V, et al. Liver stiffness in nonalcoholic fatty liver disease: a comparison of supersonic shear imaging, FibroScan, and ARFI with liver biopsy. Hepatology 2016;63(6):1817–27.
88. Lissen E, Clumeck N, Sola R, et al. Development of a simple noninvasive index to predict significant fibrosis in patients with HIV/HCV coinfection. Hepatology 2006;43:1317–25.
89. Sun W, Cui H, Li N, et al. Comparison of FIB-4 index, NAFLD fibrosis score and BARD score for prediction of advanced fibrosis in adult patients with nonalcoholic fatty liver disease: a meta-analysis study. Hepatol Res 2016 Aug; 46(9):862–70.
90. McPherson S, Hardy T, Dufour JF, et al. Age as a confounding factor for the accurate non-invasive diagnosis of advanced NAFLD fibrosis. Am J Gastroenterol 2017;112(5):740–51.
91. Paik JM, Kabbara K, Eberly KE, et al. Global burden of NAFLD and chronic liver disease among adolescents and young adults. Hepatology 2022;75(5): 1204–17.
92. Arshad T, Paik JM, Biswas R, et al. Nonalcoholic fatty liver disease prevalence trends among adolescents and young adults in the United States, 2007-2016. Hepatol Commun 2021;5(10):1676–88.
93. Angulo P, Hui JM, Marchesini G, et al. The NAFLD fibrosis score: a noninvasive system that identifies liver fibrosis in patients with NAFLD. Hepatology 2007;45: 846–54.
94. Wai CT, Greenson JK, Fontana RJ, et al. A simple noninvasive index can predict both significant fibrosis and cirrhosis in patients with chronic hepatitis C. Hepatology 2003;38:518–26.
95. Ampuero J, Pais R, Aller R, et al, HEPAmet Registry. Development and validation of hepamet fibrosis scoring system-a simple, noninvasive test to identify

patients with nonalcoholic fatty liver disease with advanced fibrosis. Clin Gastroenterol Hepatol 2020;18(1):216–25.e5.
96. Harrison SA, Oliver D, Arnold HL, et al. Development and validation of a simple NAFLD clinical scoring system for identifying patients without advanced disease. Gut 2008;57:1441–7.
97. Alkhouri N, McCullough AJ. Noninvasive diagnosis of NASH and liver fibrosis within the spectrum of NAFLD. Gastroenterol Hepatol 2012;8(10):661–8.
98. Staufer K, Halilbasic E, Spindelboeck W, et al. Evaluation and comparison of six noninvasive tests for prediction of significant or advanced fibrosis in nonalcoholic fatty liver disease. United European Gastroenterol J 2019;7(8):1113–23.
99. Van Dijk AM, Vali Y, Mak AL, et al. Systematic review with meta-analyses: diagnostic accuracy of fibrometer tests in patients with non-alcoholic fatty liver disease. J Clin Med 2021;10(13):2910.
100. Sharma C, Cococcia S, Ellis N, et al. Systematic review: accuracy of the enhanced liver fibrosis test for diagnosing advanced liver fibrosis and cirrhosis. J Gastroenterol Hepatol 2021;36(7):1788–802.
101. Sanyal AJ, Harrison SA, Ratziu V, et al. The natural history of advanced fibrosis due to nonalcoholic steatohepatitis: data from the simtuzumab trials. Hepatology 2019;70(6):1913–27.
102. Miele L, De Michele T, Marrone G, et al. Enhanced liver fibrosis test as a reliable tool for assessing fibrosis in nonalcoholic fatty liver disease in a clinical setting. Int J Biol Markers 2017;32(4):e397–402. PMID: 28862712. Miele L, et al. Int J Biol Markers. 2017; 32(4): e397-e402.
103. Irvine KM, Wockner LF, Shanker M, et al. The Enhanced liver fibrosis score is associated with clinical outcomes and disease progression in patients with chronic liver disease. Liver Int 2016 Mar;36(3):370–7. https://doi.org/10.1111/liv.12896. Epub 2015 Aug 28. PMID: 26104018.Irvine KM, et al. Liver Int. 2016;36:370-377.
104. Dellavance A, Fernandes F, Shimabokuro N, et al. Enhanced liver fibrosis (ELF) score: analytical performance and distribution range in a large cohort of blood donors. Clin Chim Acta 2016;461:151–5.
105. Younossi ZM, Felix S, Jeffers T, et al. Performance of the enhanced liver fibrosis test to estimate advanced fibrosis among patients with nonalcoholic fatty liver disease. JAMA Netw Open 2021;4:e2123923 [PubMed: 34529067].
106. Inadomi C, Takahashi H, Ogawa Y, et al. Accuracy of the Enhanced Liver Fibrosis test, and combination of the Enhanced Liver Fibrosis and non-invasive tests for the diagnosis of advanced liver fibrosis in patients with non-alcoholic fatty liver disease. Hepatol Res 2020;50:682–92 [PubMed: 32090397].
107. Vali Y, Lee J, Boursier J, et al. Enhanced liver fibrosis test for the non-invasive diagnosis of fibrosis in patients with NAFLD: a systematic review and meta-analysis. J Hepatol 2020;73:252–62 [PubMed: 32275982].
108. NICE guideline NG49. Available at: https://www.nice.org.uk/guidance/ng49/resources/nonalcoholic-fatty-liver-disease-nafld-assessment-and-management-pdf-1837461227461.
109. Cusi K, Isaacs S, Barb D, et al. American association of clinical endocrinology clinical practice guideline for the diagnosis and management of nonalcoholic fatty liver disease in primary care and endocrinology clinical settings: co-sponsored by the american association for the study of liver diseases (AASLD). Endocr Pract 2022;28(5):528–62.
110. Younossi ZM, Anstee QM, Wai-Sun Wong V, et al. The association of histologic and noninvasive tests with adverse clinical and patient-reported outcomes in

patients with advanced fibrosis due to nonalcoholic steatohepatitis. Gastroenterology 2021;160(5):1608–19.e13.

111. Arpino V, Brock M, Gill SE. The role of TIMPs in regulation of extracellular matrix proteolysis. Matrix Biol 2015;44-46:247–54.
112. Rosenberg WM, Voelker M, Thiel R, et al. Serum markers detect the presence of liver fibrosis: a cohort study. Gastroenterology 2004;127:1704–13.
113. Mak AL, Lee J, van Dijk AM, et al. Systematic review with meta-analysis: diagnostic accuracy of pro-C3 for hepatic fibrosis in patients with non-alcoholic fatty liver disease. Biomedicines 2021;9(12):1920.
114. Daniels SJ, Leeming DJ, Eslam M, et al. ADAPT: an algorithm incorporating PRO-C3 accurately identifies patients with NAFLD and advanced fibrosis. Hepatology 2019;69(3):1075–86.
115. Nielsen MJ, Leeming DJ, Goodman Z, et al. Comparison of ADAPT, FIB-4 and APRI as non-invasive predictors of liver fibrosis and NASH within the CENTAUR screening population. J Hepatol 2021;75:1292–300.
116. Erhardtsen E, Rasmussen DGK, Frederiksen P, et al. Determining a healthy reference range and factors potentially influencing PRO-C3 - a biomarker of liver fibrosis. JHEP Rep 2021;3(4):100317.
117. Ajmera V, Nguyen K, Tamaki N, et al. Prognostic utility of magnetic resonance elastography and MEFIB index in predicting liver-related outcomes and mortality in individuals at risk of and with nonalcoholic fatty liver disease. Therap Adv Gastroenterol 2022;15. 17562848221093869.
118. Long MT, Noureddin M, Lim JK. AGA clinical practice update: diagnosis and management of nonalcoholic fatty liver disease in lean individuals: expert review. Gastroenterology 2022;163(3):764–74.e1.
119. Ajmera V, Kim BK, Yang K, et al. Liver stiffness on magnetic resonance elastography and the MEFIB index and liver-related outcomes in nonalcoholic fatty liver disease: a systematic review and meta-analysis of individual participants. Gastroenterology 2022. S0016-5085(22)00735-1.
120. Srivastava A, Gailer R, Tanwar S, et al. Prospective evaluation of a primary care referral pathway for patients with non-alcoholic fatty liver disease. J Hepatol 2019;71(2):371–8.
121. Kanwal F, Shubrook JH, Adams LA, et al. Clinical care pathway for the risk stratification and management of patients with nonalcoholic fatty liver disease. Gastroenterology 2021;161(5):1657–69.

Current Treatment Options, Including Diet, Exercise, and Medications: The Impact on Histology

Mazen Noureddin, MD, MHSc[a,b], Manal F. Abdelmalek, MD, MPH[c,*]

KEYWORDS

- Nonalcoholic fatty liver disease • Nonalcoholic steatohepatitis
- Life-style modification • Fibrosis • Metabolic syndrome

KEY POINTS

- Current treatments of NAFLD/ NASH target the effective treatment of metabolic drivers and/or co-morbidities such as insulin resistance, obesity and diabetes mellitus.
- Multidisciplinary teams and approach to managing patients with NAFLD/NASH may optimize success with behavioral and life-style modification.
- Alcohol use, even in small amounts, should be avoided in patients with NASH and fibrosis due to risk of accelerating fibrosis progression.
- Although there are currently no FDA approved drugs for the treatment of NAFLD/NASH, treatment of obesity and/or diabetes with approved therapies for these indication may improve NAFLD/NASH.

INTRODUCTION

Fibrosis in the presence of steatohepatitis is the primary predictor of disease progression and negative clinical outcomes.[1–3] Although fibrosis of the primary determinant of adverse outcomes, patients with nonalcoholic steatohepatitis (NASH) and significant hepatic fibrosis (fibrosis stage $\geq$ F2) have a higher risk for liver-related morbidity and mortality.[4] When energy excess exceeds metabolic needs and disposal capacity, the increase in dietary carbohydrates and saturated fat consumption the formation accumulation of intrahepatic fat[5–8] resulting in the development of insulin resistance, which is nearly universal in patients with nonalcoholic fatty liver disease (NAFLD). Given the strong association between NAFLD and metabolic comorbidities, current treatment(s)

[a] Sherrie and Alan Conover Center for Liver Disease and Transplantation, Houston Methodist Hospital, Houston, TX, USA; [b] Houston Research Institute and Houston Liver Institute, Houston, TX, USA; [c] Division of Gastroenterology & Hepatology, Department of Medicine, Mayo Clinic, Rochester, MN, USA
* Corresponding author. Mayo Clinic Rochester, 200 1st Street, SW, Rochester, MN 55905.
E-mail address: abdelmalek.manal@mayo.edu

Clin Liver Dis 27 (2023) 397–412
https://doi.org/10.1016/j.cld.2023.01.008
1089-3261/23/

target improvement in insulin resistance, whether it be through lifestyle modification or the use of available pharmacotherapies to optimize metabolic drivers and/or consequences of metabolic stress. Promotion of healthy lifestyle, weight loss, and aggressive treatment of comorbid conditions such as type 2 diabetes mellitus (T2DM), dyslipidemia, and hypertension have the potential to improve liver histology and potentially alter the natural history for disease progression.

MULTIDISCIPLINARY LIFESTYLE INTERVENTION IN NONALCOHOLIC STEATOHEPATITIS

The lack of pharmacologic interventions for NASH makes lifestyle measures exceedingly important. Long-term adoption of these measures; however, is challenging. Improve dietary composition independent of weight loss may improve NASH. Weight loss of 5-10% of the initial body weight and moderate increases in physical activity can also improve the histologic features of NAFLD/NASH.

Lifestyle modification with a healthy diet and routine physical activity is the foundation of treatment not only for NAFLD but also for its associated metabolic comorbidities and improved cardiometabolic health.[9] Although long-term goals of lifestyle modification are difficult to achieve and sustain, a multidisciplinary team and approach provides the best chance for success in achieving weight loss goals and reducing the liver and cardiovascular morbidity and mortality in patients with NAFLD.[10]

Weight Loss

Weight loss is the foundation for the treatment of NAFLD/NASH in patients with overweight or obese status. Even modest amounts of weight loss can be impactful, especially for those with milder diseases. Weight loss of 3% to 5% improves insulin resistance, hepatic steatosis, and steatohepatitis. Greater degrees of weight loss have the potential to further improve liver injury. Thresholds of weight loss that exceed 10% may resolve steatohepatitis and improve hepatic fibrosis.[11–15] Although majority of patients may be able to achieve modest degrees of weight loss, few patients (≤10%) achieve effective weight loss despite structured interventions at 1 year, and fewer than half of these maintain the weight loss 5 years after intervention.[11,16] The challenge of sustaining weight loss highlights the need for ongoing nutrition support through multidisciplinary care and consideration of pharmacotherapy as a complement to lifestyle modification.

Sustained weight loss improves peripheral sensitivity and reduces adipose tissue stress,[17] which can reduce the drive for liver injury in NASH. Psychological barriers and eating disorders can impede the implementation of a successful dietary and exercise plan. Therefore, the engagement of behavioral specialists, health psychologists, dieticians, and/or nutritionists may be an in-variable resource for select patients to optimize success.[18,19]

Impact of Exercise

Exercise independent of weight loss has a beneficial effect on NAFLD and should be tailored to the patient's preferences and physical abilities.[20–24] Regular moderate exercise at least five times a week for a total of 150 min per week or an increase in physical activity by more than 60 min per week can prevent her improve NAFLD.[9,22,25,26] More vigorous exercise is needed for the resolution of NASH with even higher intensity exercise shown to reduce hepatic fibrosis.[27]

Studies combining diet with increases in physical activity consistently show reduction in liver fat proportional to the intensity of the intervention.[28–31] Patients should be encouraged to adapt optimal intensity exercise, tailored to their personal preferences and enjoyment such that long-term maintenance of lifestyle modification can be achieved.[22,23,26] Even in those patients with NASH-related advanced hepatic fibrosis or cirrhosis, regular physical activity has been shown to reduce portal pressure,[32] improve frailty, sarcopenia, and quality of life.[33] Other approaches (ie, participation in structured life-style intervention programs and/or enrollment in clinical trials for the treatment of NAFLD/NASH) may increase the potential for adherence.

ROLE OF MACRONUTRIENT COMPOSITION

Changes in dietary composition (eg, low carbohydrate vs low-fat diet, intermittent fasting, Mediterranean diet, etc.) and different intensities of caloric restriction appear comparable and their ability to improve NAFLD and NASH.[34] A Mediterranean diet is often recommended for patients with NAFLD/NASH based on its demonstrable reduction and liver fat[35,36] while also lending cardiovascular benefits.[37] Intermittent calorie restriction (the 5:2 diet) and a low-carb high-fat diet (LCHF) were assessed in terms of their effect on the reduction of hepatic steatosis. Both diets led to a decrease in hepatic steatosis (on imaging) and weight loss compared with the standard of care.[38] Another recent study compared the effect of the LCHF diet on T2DM and NAFLD compared with a high-carbohydrate, low-fat (HCLF) diet. Within the trial duration (6 months), LCHF diet had greater improvements in hemoglobin A_{1c} (mean difference in change, −6.1) and more weight loss (mean difference in change, −3.8 kg). Nevertheless, they did not differ in their effect on liver histology.[39] Red meat processed red, poultry and cholesterol have been associated with NAFLD, whereas fibers had the inverse relationship.[40] These associations were stronger between red meat and cholesterol and NAFLD with cirrhosis compared with those without cirrhosis (*P* heterogeneity $\leq$0.014). To promote long-term adherence and compliance, dietary interventions and modification should be tailored to the patient's culture on personal preferences.

Impact of Fructose Consumption

A diet containing excess calories in the form of refined carbohydrates, sugar-sweetened beverages, and excess saturated fats (Western diet) is associated with obesity and NAFLD.[41–43] excess fructose consumption is associated with increased risk for NAFLD acquisition[44,45] and progression.[46] Excess fructose consumption ($\geq$7 drinks per week) has been associated with hepatic fibrosis, independent of calorie intake, in a dose dependent manner[46]

Coffee Consumption

Coffee consumption, potentially due to polyphenol and independent of caffeine content, may lend a benefit for NAFLD/NASH. Drinking at least three cups of coffee per day has been shown epidemiologic studies and meta-analyses to decrease the risk of NAFLD and hepatic fibrosis.[47–50]

Role of Alcohol Consumption

Alcohol intake, even in small quantities, can serve as a cofactor for fatty liver disease acquisition and progression. Alcohol use should be quantified in patients with risk factors for NAFLD.[51] Although earlier epidemiologic studies suggested a protective effect of mild alcohol consumption on the development of NAFLD,[52] subsequent studies have shown that moderate alcohol use was associated with persistent hepatic steatosis, elevated liver aminotransferases, and lower thirds of NASH resolution compared with patients who did not consume alcohol.[53] Moderate alcohol (21 to 39 g [women] and 31 to 59 g [men] per day) use increases the probability of advanced fibrosis,[54] particularly in patients with obesity or T2DM, indicating potential synergistic effects of insulin resistance and alcohol on liver disease progression. Obesity and alcohol use synergistically increase the risk of liver injury, cirrhosis, hepatocellular carcinoma, and death from liver disease.[55–57] Heavy alcohol consumption accelerates fibrosis progression and should be avoided in all patients with NAFLD/NASH.[51]

REPURPOSED MEDICATIONS FOR NONALCOHOLIC FATTY LIVER DISEASE/ STEATOHEPATITIS

Although there are currently no US Food and Drug Administration (FDA)-approved drugs for the treatment of NASH at any disease stage, medications approved for commonly associated comorbidities such as T2DM and obesity have been shown to reduce liver enzymes, steatosis, and histology features of steatohepatitis. Therefore, early intervention with medications approved for treatment of complications of metabolic syndrome may be considered in patients with NAFLD/NASH (**Table 1**).

Vitamin E

In the Pioglitazone versus Vitamin E versus Placebo for the Treatment of Non-Diabetic Patients with Nonalcoholic Steatohepatitis (PIVENS) study, a randomized double-blind placebo-controlled multicenter trial of pioglitazone versus vitamin E (rrr α-tocopherol, the natural form of vitamin E) 800 IU daily for 96 weeks, treatment with vitamin E improved the histologic features of steatohepatitis ($\geq$2 point reduction in NAFLD Activity Score [NAS]) compared with placebo.[58] A subsequent meta-analysis supported these findings showing that vitamin E improved serum aminotransferases, hepatic steatosis, necroinflammatory, and hepatocellular ballooning on liver histology.[59,60] A reduction in serum alanine aminotransferase to $\leq$ 40 U/L and by $\geq$ 30% of baseline value after initiation of vitamin E is associated with improvement in histological parameters.[61] Although vitamin E has not been shown to lend a meaningful reduction in hepatic fibrosis, a retrospective, single-center study of 236 patients with NASH and advanced fibrosis showed that vitamin E use was associated with

Table 1
Repurposed drugs which may improve nonalcoholic steatohepatitis

Drug	Population	Duration	Primary End Point
Therapies recommended for NASH by International Societies			
Vitamin E [rrr α-tocopherol]	NASH without cirrhosis	96 weeks	Improvement in NAS by two points. Met by Vitamin E 800 IU
Pioglitazone	NASH without cirrhosis Pre-diabetes and diabetes	18 months	Improvement in NAS by two points. Met by Pioglitazone 45 mg
Therapies obesity or metabolic syndrome that has initial efficacy evidence in NASH			
Liraglutide	NASH without cirrhosis	48 weeks	Resolution of NASH with no worsening in fibrosis. Met by liraglutide 1.8 mg daily
Semaglutide	NASH with fibrosis stage 1 to stage 3	72 weeks	Resolution of NASH with no worsening in fibrosis. Met by semaglutide 0.4 mg daily

lower rates of hepatic decompensation (37% vs 62%, $p = 0.04$) and higher transplant-free survival (78% vs 49%, $p < 0.01$).[62] Vitamin E reduced morbidity and mortality independent of underlying diabetes status. However, concerns regarding the bleeding risks of high-dose vitamin E, specifically risk for hemorrhagic stroke and prostate cancer has been raised, although this observation has not yet been confirmed by prospective studies.[63,64] The potential risks of high dose (eg, 800 IU daily) long-term use of vitamin E should be discussed with patients prior to initiation.

Thiazolidinediones

Thiazolidinediones (TZDs) are ligands for peroxisome proliferator-activated receptor (PPAR) γ approved for the treatment of T2DM.[65] Treatment with pioglitazone in patients with NASH, both with and without prediabetes or diabetes, improved insulin resistance, serum lipids, glycemic control, and histologic features of steatohepatitis[58,66–68] In the PIVENS trial, pioglitazone treatment did not meet the *a priori* primary endpoint of a $\geq$ 2-point reduction NAFLD activity score (NAS) without worsening of fibrosis, although 47% had NASH resolution compared with 21% of participants receiving placebo ($P < 0.001$).[58] Subsequently, in an 18-month study of patients with either prediabetes or T2DM and NASH, pioglitazone treatment led to NASH resolution and a trend toward fibrosis improvement.[69]

A meta-analysis showed that pioglitazone was better in achieving NASH resolution as well as fibrosis improvement than placebo.[70] Pioglitazone use is associated with potential side effects including weight gain, bone loss in postmenopausal women, the debated risks of heart failure, and those with preexisting cardiac dysfunction and bladder cancer.[71–73] Although pioglitazone may improve NASH and lend secondary prevention of macrovascular events in patients with T2DM[74–76] its use in clinical practice has been overtaken by newer insulin-sensitizing agents (Sodium glucose cotransporter-2 inhibitors [SGLT-2] inhibitors and glucagon-like peptide 1 [GLP-1] receptor agonists) with more pronounces effects on weight loss and cardiovascular mortality.[75,77,78]

Glucagon-Like Peptide-1 Receptor Agonists

GLP-1 receptor agonist or currently approved by the FDA for the indication of obesity and diabetes for both adults and children.[79–83] The biological effects of GLP-1 receptor agonists on glycemic control, lipids, weight loss, as well as improved cardiovascular outcomes[78,84] makes them an attractive therapeutic option for the treatment of NASH.[85] In a phase 2 double-blinded, randomized, placebo-controlled phase 2 trial of liraglutide (1.8 mg subcutaneously daily) compared with placebo for patients with biopsy-proven NASH, liraglutide improved steatosis, resolved steatohepatitis and reduced fibrosis progression compared with placebo.[86]

In an adequately powered Phase 2b RCT of daily subcutaneous semaglutide, 320 patients with NASH (F1-3) were randomized to 0.1, 0.2, or 0.4 mg or placebo daily for 72 weeks (primary endpoint, resolution of NASH without worsening fibrosis).[87] NASH resolution was dose dependent and occurred in 59% in the treatment group versus 17% in the placebo group ($p < 0.001$).[87] despite the evidence of improvement in NASH, there was no significant reduction in fibrosis over 72 weeks of treatment; however, semaglutide appeared to lend protection against fibrosis progression compared with placebo. Likewise, tirzepatide, a novel, first-in-class, dual-glucose-dependent insulininotropic polypeptide (GIP)/GLP-1 receptor agonist,[88] has been shown to be safe and effective for the treatment of obesity and diabetes.[89,90]

In a study of patients with NAFLD randomly assigned to treatment with tirzepatide 5 mg ($n = 71$); tirzepatide 10 mg ($n = 79$); tirzepatide 15 mg ($n = 72$); and insulin degludec ($n = 74$), the absolute reduction in liver fat content at week 52 was significantly greater for the pooled tirzepatide 10 mg and 15 mg groups (−8.09%, SE 0.57) versus the insulin degludec group (−3.38%, 0.83). The estimated treatment difference versus insulin degludec was −4.71% (95% CI −6.72 to −2.70; $p < 0.0001$). Tirzepatide also showed a significant reduction in visceral and subcutaneous adipose tissue volumes compared with insulin degludec in patients with T2DM.[91] In a phase 3 double-blind, randomized, controlled trial, tirzepatide showed weight loss up to 20.9% (95% CI, −21.8 to −19.9) with doses up to 15-mg once weekly compared with 3.1% (95% CI, −4.3 to −1.9) with placebo ($P < 0.001$).[92] This degree of weight loss was associated with an absolute reduction of the liver fat content of 8.1% suggesting a potential benefit of GIP/GLP1 receptor agonists in patients with NASH.

Tirzepatide, a recently approved GLP1/ GIP receptor agonist (RA) shows weight loss as high as 20.9% compared with 3.1% in the placebo group, and an absolute reduction in liver fat content of 8.1%, suggesting a possible benefit in NASH.[92] Both semaglutide and tirzepatide may be considered for the treatment of obesity and diabetes in patients with NASH. A large phase 3 clinical study of semaglutide (*ClinicalTrials.gov Identifier:* NCT04822181) and phase 2 study of tirzepatide (*ClinicalTrials.gov Identifier*: NCT04166773) are currently underway.

Sodium glucose cotransporter-2 inhibitors

SGLT-2i are glucose-lowering agents that improve glucose control by target renal glucose resorption from the globular filtrate while promoting weight loss and lowering serum uric acid levels.[93] SGLT-2is are approved for the treatment of diabetes mellitus, induce modest degrees of weight loss, and have cardiorenal protective benefits.[94] The protective role of SGLT-2i against NAFLD progression also seems to be mediated by effects beyond those on body weight. Indeed, it has been shown that SGLT-2i treatment improves IR and ameliorates the intracellular free fatty acids (FFA), total cholesterol (TC), and triglycerides (TG) accumulation by reducing the expression of genes involved in *de novo* lipogenesis, FA uptake, and hepatic TG secretion, whereas it also promotes the expression of key regulatory genes of fatty acid β-oxidation.[95–98] SGLT-2is induce 2% to 3% weight loss and have cardiorenal protective benefits.[94,99–101]

Although the role of SGLT-2i in the treatment of NAFLD/NASH is limited by a small sample size and lack of histologic outcomes, current data suggest that SGLT-2i improve metabolic risk factor and liver fat content in patients with NAFLD/NASH.[102–105] Despite the limitations in available data regarding the therapeutic efficacy of SGLT-2is on NAFLD/NASH, their use for the treatment of diabetes may lend consideration for their inclusion in treatment alternatives to improving glycemic control and optimizing the cardiometabolic risk factors known to be associated with NAFLD/NASH.[106]

Available agents without evidence of histological benefits in Nonalcoholic steatohepatitis

Although metformin has been tentatively used in the treatment of insulin resistance and T2DM, there is no compelling evidence that metformin improves the histology of NAFLD and NASH in adults or children.[107–111] ursodeoxycholic acid has hepatic effects related to changes in the bile acid pool, immune modulation, and potential cytoprotection. Ursodeoxycholic acid has shown antifibrotic effects in primary biliary cholangitis and has been studied for the treatment of NASH. Although initial studies suggested the benefit of NASH,[112–114] subsequent large, randomized placebo-controlled trials failed to show any histologic benefit.[115,116]

Dipeptidyl peptidase 4 (DPP-4) inhibitors are used with diet and exercise to control high blood sugar in adults with T2DM. Sitagliptin inhibits the pro-fibrotic and pro-inflammatory changes in a high-fat-induced NAFLD model[117] and may improve non-invasive markers of fibrosis in humans.[118,119] Although safe in a patient with T2DM and NAFLD,[120] in a randomized, double-blind, placebo-controlled studies, sitagliptin has not been shown to be effective in improving liver fat and liver fibrosis in patients with NAFLD.[121–123] However, Other drugs that have been shown to improve serum lipids (ie, n-3 polyunsaturated fatty acids, fish oil, ethyl-eicosapentaenoic acid, ezetimibe and fenofibrate), these drugs were not shown to have liver-specific benefits in a patient with NAFLD/NASH.[124–127] A recent meta-analysis of six studies (two randomized controlled and four single-arm trials) involving 273 participants with NAFLD and NASH suggested that ezetimibe attenuated serum aminotransferase, hepatic steatosis, and hepatocyte ballooning; however, did not improve hepatic inflammation or fibrosis.[128] The effect of silymarin (milk thistle) in patients with NAFLD/NASH remains inconclusive. A recent meta-analysis of eight randomized controlled trials of silymarin compared with placebo, suggested that silymarin was effective in reducing aminotransferases, irrespective of weight loss.

In the meta-analysis, eight randomized clinical trials were included to evaluate the role of silymarin in the treatment of NAFLD/NASH. Silymarin treatment led to a statistically significant greater reduction in the levels of transaminases compared with the placebo, irrespective of weight loss. In phase 2 randomized controlled trials, silymarin was safe and well tolerated but did not improve the histologic features of NASH.[129,130]

Role of Statins in Patients with Nonalcoholic Fatty Liver Disease/Steatohepatitis

Patients with NAFLD are twice as likely to have dyslipidemia[131] and atherogenic lipid subtraction[132,133] compared with those without NAFLD. As patients have progressed to cirrhosis, they continue to remain at increased risk for cardiovascular disease[134–136]; therefore, management of dyslipidemia NAFLD should include the use of moderate to high-intensity statins as first-line therapy based on lipid risk levels and atherosclerotic cardiovascular disease (ASCVD) risk scores. Statins are safe in patients with NAFLD across the disease spectrum and lead to demonstrable reduction in cardiovascular morbidity and mortality.[29,137–139] Unfortunately, statin therapy remains underutilized in clinical practice despite extensive data showing safety, even among patients with cirrhosis.[140–143] Recent data from large cohort studies suggest that statins may have beneficial effects on decreasing the future risk for hepatocellular cancer and hepatic decompensation.[137]

SUMMARY

Although liver-directed pharmacology therapy for the treatment of NAFLD/NASH does not currently exist, treatment options inclusive of dietary modification, increased physical activity, and effectively managing complications of metabolic syndrome including obesity, diabetes, and/or dyslipidemia have the potential to improve the histologic feature of NASH. Efficacy data are available to support the use of pioglitazone and vitamin E in NASH and data are emerging regarding the role of GLP-1 receptor agonists, GLP-1/GIP dual agonists, and SGLT-2i for the treatment of NASH. Pending approved pharmacologic therapies for NASH, providers must strive to earnestly optimize metabolic risk factors contributing to NAFLD/NASH disease acquisition and progression in hopes that such interventions will improve not only cardiometabolic risk but also the associated hepatic manifestation of metabolic syndrome.

CLINICS CARE POINTS

- In patients with NASH, the goal of treatment is to reverse steatohepatitis and fibrosis, or at least halt fibrosis progression by directing early interevention at reversing the unfavorable metabolic profile.
- Successful interevention favors a multidisciplinary team including primary care, nutrition/dietician, behavioral therapists, endocrinologists and gastroenterologist/hepatologist in a patient tailored approach.
- When considering treatment for diabetes, preference should be lent to those therapies (ie. pioglitazone, liraglutide, and semaglutide) with reported histologic improvement in patients with NASH.

REFERENCES

1. Taylor RS, Taylor RJ, Bayliss S, et al. Association between fibrosis stage and outcomes of patients with nonalcoholic fatty liver disease: a systematic review and meta-analysis. Gastroenterology 2020;158:1611–25, e1612.
2. Dulai PS, Singh S, Patel J, et al. Increased risk of mortality by fibrosis stage in nonalcoholic fatty liver disease: systematic review and meta-analysis. Hepatology 2017;65:1557–65.
3. Simon TG, Roelstraete B, Khalili H, et al. Mortality in biopsy-confirmed nonalcoholic fatty liver disease: results from a nationwide cohort. Gut 2021;70:1375–82.
4. Hagstrom H, Nasr P, Ekstedt M, et al. Fibrosis stage but not NASH predicts mortality and time to development of severe liver disease in biopsy-proven NAFLD. J Hepatol 2017;67:1265–73.
5. Donnelly KL, Smith CI, Schwarzenberg SJ, et al. Sources of fatty acids stored in liver and secreted via lipoproteins in patients with nonalcoholic fatty liver disease. J Clin Invest 2005;115:1343–51.
6. Sanders FWB, Acharjee A, Walker C, et al. Hepatic steatosis risk is partly driven by increased de novo lipogenesis following carbohydrate consumption. Genome Biol 2018;19:79.
7. Luukkonen PK, Sädevirta S, Zhou Y, et al. Saturated fat is more metabolically harmful for the human liver than unsaturated fat or simple sugars. Diabetes Care 2018;41:1732–9.
8. Berná G, Romero-Gomez M. The role of nutrition in non-alcoholic fatty liver disease: pathophysiology and management. Liver Int 2020;40:102–8.
9. Semmler G, Datz C, Reiberger T, et al. Diet and exercise in NAFLD/NASH: beyond the obvious. Liver Int 2021;41:2249–68.
10. Duell PB, Welty FK, Miller M, et al. Nonalcoholic fatty liver disease and cardiovascular risk: a scientific statement from the American heart association. Arterioscler Thromb Vasc Biol 2022;42:e168–85.
11. Vilar-Gomez E, Martinez-Perez Y, Calzadilla-Bertot L, et al. Weight loss through lifestyle modification significantly reduces features of nonalcoholic steatohepatitis. Gastroenterology 2015;149:367–78, e365; [quiz: e314-365].
12. Patel NS, Doycheva I, Peterson MR, et al. Effect of weight loss on magnetic resonance imaging estimation of liver fat and volume in patients with nonalcoholic steatohepatitis. Clin Gastroenterol Hepatol 2015;13:561–568 e561.
13. Patel NS, Hooker J, Gonzalez M, et al. Weight loss decreases magnetic resonance elastography estimated liver stiffness in nonalcoholic fatty liver disease. Clin Gastroenterol Hepatol 2017;15:463–4.

14. Long MT, Noureddin M, Lim JK. AGA clinical practice update: diagnosis and management of nonalcoholic fatty liver disease in lean individuals: expert review. Gastroenterology 2022;163:764–74.
15. Koutoukidis DA, Astbury NM, Tudor KE, et al. Association of weight loss interventions with changes in biomarkers of nonalcoholic fatty liver disease: a systematic review and meta-analysis. JAMA Intern Med 2019;179:1262–71.
16. Malespin MH, Barritt ASt, Watkins SE, et al. Weight loss and weight regain in usual clinical practice: results from the TARGET-NASH observational cohort. Clin Gastroenterol Hepatol 2022;20:2393–2395 e2394.
17. Kahn CR, Wang G, Lee KY. Altered adipose tissue and adipocyte function in the pathogenesis of metabolic syndrome. J Clin Investig 2019;129:3990–4000.
18. Stewart KE, Haller DL, Sargeant C, et al. Readiness for behaviour change in non-alcoholic fatty liver disease: implications for multidisciplinary care models. Liver Int 2015;35:936–43.
19. Thoma C, Day CP, Trenell MI. Lifestyle interventions for the treatment of non-alcoholic fatty liver disease in adults: a systematic review. J Hepatol 2012;56: 255–66.
20. Hainer V, Toplak H, Stich V. Fat or fit: what is more important? Diabetes Care 2009;32(Suppl 2):S392–7.
21. Sargeant JA, Aithal GP, Takamura T, et al. The influence of adiposity and acute exercise on circulating hepatokines in normal-weight and overweight/obese men. Appl Physiol Nutr Metab 2018;43:482–90.
22. Sung KC, Ryu S, Lee JY, et al. Effect of exercise on the development of new fatty liver and the resolution of existing fatty liver. J Hepatol 2016;65:791–7.
23. Bae JC, Suh S, Park SE, et al. Regular exercise is associated with a reduction in the risk of NAFLD and decreased liver enzymes in individuals with NAFLD independent of obesity in Korean adults. PLoS One 2012;7:e46819.
24. Careau V, Halsey LG, Pontzer H, et al. Energy compensation and adiposity in humans. Curr Biol 2021;31:4659–4666 e4652.
25. St George A, Bauman A, Johnston A, et al. Independent effects of physical activity in patients with nonalcoholic fatty liver disease. Hepatology 2009;50:68–76.
26. Johnson NA, Sachinwalla T, Walton DW, et al. Aerobic exercise training reduces hepatic and visceral lipids in obese individuals without weight loss. Hepatology 2009;50:1105–12.
27. Kistler KD, Brunt EM, Clark JM, et al. Physical activity recommendations, exercise intensity, and histological severity of nonalcoholic fatty liver disease. Am J Gastroenterol 2011;106:460–8 [quiz: 469].
28. Abdelbasset WK, Tantawy SA, Kamel DM, et al. A randomized controlled trial on the effectiveness of 8-week high-intensity interval exercise on intrahepatic triglycerides, visceral lipids, and health-related quality of life in diabetic obese patients with nonalcoholic fatty liver disease. Medicine (Baltim) 2019;98:e14918.
29. Bril F, Portillo Sanchez P, Lomonaco R, et al. Liver safety of statins in prediabetes or T2DM and nonalcoholic steatohepatitis: post hoc analysis of a randomized trial. Journal of Clinical Endocrinology & Metabolism 2017;102:2950–61.
30. van Kleef LA, Hofman A, Voortman T, et al. Objectively measured physical activity is inversely associated with nonalcoholic fatty liver disease: the rotterdam study. Am J Gastroenterol 2022;117:311–8.
31. Tsunoda K, Kitano N, Kai Y, et al. Dose-response relationships of accelerometer-measured sedentary behaviour and physical activity with non-alcoholic fatty liver disease. Aliment Pharmacol Ther 2021;54:1330–9.

32. Berzigotti A, Albillos A, Villanueva C, et al. Effects of an intensive lifestyle intervention program on portal hypertension in patients with cirrhosis and obesity: the SportDiet study. Hepatology 2017;65:1293–305.
33. Williams FR, Berzigotti A, Lord JM, et al. Review article: impact of exercise on physical frailty in patients with chronic liver disease. Aliment Pharmacol Ther 2019;50:988–1000.
34. Properzi C, O'Sullivan TA, Sherriff JL, et al. Ad libitum mediterranean and low-fat diets both significantly reduce hepatic steatosis: a randomized controlled trial. Hepatology 2018;68:1741–54.
35. Kawaguchi T, Charlton M, Kawaguchi A, et al. Effects of mediterranean diet in patients with nonalcoholic fatty liver disease: a systematic review, meta-analysis, and meta-regression analysis of randomized controlled trials. Semin Liver Dis 2021;41:225–34.
36. Haigh L, Kirk C, El Gendy K, et al. The effectiveness and acceptability of Mediterranean diet and calorie restriction in non-alcoholic fatty liver disease (NAFLD): a systematic review and meta-analysis. Clin Nutr 2022;41:1913–31.
37. Kouvari M, Boutari C, Chrysohoou C, et al. Mediterranean diet is inversely associated with steatosis and fibrosis and decreases ten-year diabetes and cardiovascular risk in NAFLD subjects: results from the ATTICA prospective cohort study. Clin Nutr 2021;40:3314–24.
38. Holmer M, Lindqvist C, Petersson S, et al. Treatment of NAFLD with intermittent calorie restriction or low-carb high-fat diet - a randomised controlled trial. JHEP Rep 2021;3:100256.
39. Hansen CD, Gram-Kampmann EM, Hansen JK, et al. Effect of calorie-unrestricted low-carbohydrate, high-fat diet versus high-carbohydrate, low-fat diet on type 2 diabetes and nonalcoholic fatty liver disease : a randomized controlled trial. Ann Intern Med 2023;176(1):10–21.
40. Noureddin M, Zelber-Sagi S, Wilkens LR, et al. Diet associations with nonalcoholic fatty liver disease in an ethnically diverse population: the multiethnic cohort. Hepatology 2020;71:1940–52.
41. Yasutake K, Nakamuta M, Shima Y, et al. Nutritional investigation of non-obese patients with non-alcoholic fatty liver disease: the significance of dietary cholesterol. Scand J Gastroenterol 2009;44:471–7.
42. Meng G, Zhang B, Yu F, et al. Soft drinks consumption is associated with nonalcoholic fatty liver disease independent of metabolic syndrome in Chinese population. Eur J Nutr 2018;57:2113–21.
43. Vilar-Gomez E, Nephew LD, Vuppalanchi R, et al. High-quality diet, physical activity, and college education are associated with low risk of NAFLD among the US population. Hepatology 2022;75:1491–506.
44. Ouyang X, Cirillo P, Sautin Y, et al. Fructose consumption as a risk factor for non-alcoholic fatty liver disease. J Hepatol 2008;48:993–9.
45. Jensen T, Abdelmalek MF, Sullivan S, et al. Fructose and sugar: a major mediator of non-alcoholic fatty liver disease. J Hepatol 2018;68:1063–75.
46. Abdelmalek MF, Suzuki A, Guy C, et al. Increased fructose consumption is associated with fibrosis severity in patients with nonalcoholic fatty liver disease. Hepatology 2010;51:1961–71.
47. Chen YP, Lu FB, Hu YB, et al. A systematic review and a dose-response meta-analysis of coffee dose and nonalcoholic fatty liver disease. Clin Nutr 2019;38:2552–7.
48. Saab S, Mallam D, Cox GA 2nd, et al. Impact of coffee on liver diseases: a systematic review. Liver Int 2014;34:495–504.

49. Wijarnpreecha K, Thongprayoon C, Ungprasert P. Coffee consumption and risk of nonalcoholic fatty liver disease: a systematic review and meta-analysis. Eur J Gastroenterol Hepatol 2017;29:e8–12.
50. Setiawan VW, Porcel J, Wei P, et al. Coffee drinking and alcoholic and nonalcoholic fatty liver diseases and viral hepatitis in the multiethnic cohort. Clin Gastroenterol Hepatol 2017;15:1305–7.
51. Blomdahl J, Nasr P, Ekstedt M, et al. Moderate alcohol consumption is associated with advanced fibrosis in non-alcoholic fatty liver disease and shows a synergistic effect with type 2 diabetes mellitus. Metabolism 2021;115:154439.
52. Dunn W, Sanyal AJ, Brunt EM, et al. Modest alcohol consumption is associated with decreased prevalence of steatohepatitis in patients with non-alcoholic fatty liver disease (NAFLD). J Hepatol 2012;57:384–91.
53. Ajmera V, Belt P, Wilson LA, et al. Among patients with nonalcoholic fatty liver disease, modest alcohol use is associated with less improvement in histologic steatosis and steatohepatitis. Clin Gastroenterol Hepatol 2018;16:1511–20.
54. Chang Y, Ryu S, Kim Y, et al. Low levels of alcohol consumption, obesity, and development of fatty liver with and without evidence of advanced fibrosis. Hepatology 2020;71:861–73.
55. Loomba R, Yang HI, Su J, et al. Synergism between obesity and alcohol in increasing the risk of hepatocellular carcinoma: a prospective cohort study. Am J Epidemiol 2013;177:333–42.
56. Loomba R, Bettencourt R, Barrett-Connor E. Synergistic association between alcohol intake and body mass index with serum alanine and aspartate aminotransferase levels in older adults: the Rancho Bernardo Study. Aliment Pharmacol Ther 2009;30:1137–49.
57. Hart CL, Morrison DS, Batty GD, et al. Effect of body mass index and alcohol consumption on liver disease: analysis of data from two prospective cohort studies. BMJ 2010;340:c1240.
58. Sanyal AJ, Chalasani N, Kowdley KV, et al. Pioglitazone, vitamin E, or placebo for nonalcoholic steatohepatitis. N Engl J Med 2010;362:1675–85.
59. Sato K, Gosho M, Yamamoto T, et al. Vitamin E has a beneficial effect on nonalcoholic fatty liver disease: a meta-analysis of randomized controlled trials. Nutrition 2015;31:923–30.
60. Xu R, Tao A, Zhang S, et al. Association between vitamin E and non-alcoholic steatohepatitis: a meta-analysis. Int J Clin Exp Med 2015;8:3924–34.
61. Hoofnagle JH, Van Natta ML, Kleiner DE, et al. Vitamin E and changes in serum alanine aminotransferase levels in patients with non-alcoholic steatohepatitis. Aliment Pharmacol Ther 2013;38:134–43.
62. Vilar-Gomez E, Vuppalanchi R, Gawrieh S, et al. Vitamin E improves transplant-free survival and hepatic decompensation among patients with nonalcoholic steatohepatitis and advanced fibrosis. Hepatology 2020;71:495–509.
63. Gaziano JM, Sesso HD, Christen WG, et al. Multivitamins in the prevention of cancer in men: the Physicians' Health Study II randomized controlled trial. JAMA 2012;308:1871–80.
64. Neuhouser ML, Barnett MJ, Kristal AR, et al. Dietary supplement use and prostate cancer risk in the Carotene and Retinol Efficacy Trial. Cancer Epidemiol Biomarkers Prev 2009;18:2202–6.
65. Upadhyay J, Polyzos SA, Perakakis N, et al. Pharmacotherapy of type 2 diabetes: an update. Metabolism 2018;78:13–42.

66. Aithal GP, Thomas JA, Kaye PV, et al. Randomized, placebo-controlled trial of pioglitazone in nondiabetic subjects with nonalcoholic steatohepatitis. Gastroenterology 2008;135:1176–84.
67. Belfort R, Harrison SA, Brown K, et al. A placebo-controlled trial of pioglitazone in subjects with nonalcoholic steatohepatitis. N Engl J Med 2006;355:2297–307.
68. Cusi K. Pioglitazone for the treatment of NASH in patients with prediabetes or type 2 diabetes mellitus. Gut 2018;67:1371.
69. Cusi K, Orsak B, Bril F, et al. Long-term pioglitazone treatment for patients with nonalcoholic steatohepatitis and prediabetes or type 2 diabetes mellitus: a randomized trial. Ann Intern Med 2016;165:305–15.
70. Majzoub AM, Nayfeh T, Barnard A, et al. Systematic review with network meta-analysis: comparative efficacy of pharmacologic therapies for fibrosis improvement and resolution of NASH. Aliment Pharmacol Ther 2021;54:880–9.
71. Tang H, Shi W, Fu S, et al. Pioglitazone and bladder cancer risk: a systematic review and meta-analysis. Cancer Med 2018;7:1070–80.
72. Yau H, Rivera K, Lomonaco R, et al. The future of thiazolidinedione therapy in the management of type 2 diabetes mellitus. Curr Diab Rep 2013;13:329–41.
73. Viscoli CM, Inzucchi SE, Young LH, et al. Pioglitazone and risk for bone fracture: safety data from a randomized clinical trial. J Clin Endocrinol Metab 2017;102:914–22.
74. Dormandy JA, Charbonnel B, Eckland DJ, et al. Secondary prevention of macrovascular events in patients with type 2 diabetes in the PROactive Study (PROspective pioglitAzone Clinical Trial in macroVascular Events): a randomised controlled trial. Lancet 2005;366:1279–89.
75. Nissen SE, Nicholls SJ, Wolski K, et al. Comparison of pioglitazone vs glimepiride on progression of coronary atherosclerosis in patients with type 2 diabetes: the PERISCOPE randomized controlled trial. JAMA 2008;299:1561–73.
76. Kernan WN, Viscoli CM, Furie KL, et al. Pioglitazone after ischemic stroke or transient ischemic attack. N Engl J Med 2016;374:1321–31.
77. Zinman B, Wanner C, Lachin JM, et al. Empagliflozin, cardiovascular outcomes, and mortality in type 2 diabetes. N Engl J Med 2015;373:2117–28.
78. Marso SP, Bain SC, Consoli A, et al. Semaglutide and cardiovascular outcomes in patients with type 2 diabetes. N Engl J Med 2016;375:1834–44.
79. Bacha F. FDA approval of GLP-1 receptor agonist (liraglutide) for use in children. Lancet Child Adolesc Health 2019;3:595–7.
80. Chadda KR, Cheng TS, Ong KK. GLP-1 agonists for obesity and type 2 diabetes in children: systematic review and meta-analysis. Obes Rev 2021;22:e13177.
81. Thondam SK, Cuthbertson DJ, Aditya BS, et al. A glucagon-like peptide-1 (GLP-1) receptor agonist in the treatment for hypothalamic obesity complicated by type 2 diabetes mellitus. Clin Endocrinol 2012;77:635–7.
82. Wilding JPH, Batterham RL, Calanna S, et al. Once-weekly semaglutide in adults with overweight or obesity. N Engl J Med 2021;384:989–1002.
83. Rubino DM, Greenway FL, Khalid U, et al. Effect of weekly subcutaneous semaglutide vs daily liraglutide on body weight in adults with overweight or obesity without diabetes: the STEP 8 Randomized clinical trial. JAMA 2022;327:138–50.
84. Nikolic D, Patti AM, Giglio RV, et al. Liraglutide improved cardiometabolic parameters more in obese than in non-obese patients with type 2 diabetes: a real-world 18-month prospective study. Diabetes Ther 2022;13:453–64.
85. Barritt ASt, Marshman E, Noureddin M. Review article: role of glucagon-like peptide-1 receptor agonists in non-alcoholic steatohepatitis, obesity and diabetes-what hepatologists need to know. Aliment Pharmacol Ther 2022;55:944–59.

86. Armstrong MJ, Gaunt P, Aithal GP, et al. Liraglutide safety and efficacy in patients with non-alcoholic steatohepatitis (LEAN): a multicentre, double-blind, randomised, placebo-controlled phase 2 study. Lancet 2016;387:679–90.
87. Newsome PN, Buchholtz K, Cusi K, et al. A placebo-controlled trial of subcutaneous semaglutide in nonalcoholic steatohepatitis. N Engl J Med 2021;384: 1113–24.
88. Tall Bull S, Nuffer W, Trujillo JM. Tirzepatide: a novel, first-in-class, dual GIP/GLP-1 receptor agonist. J Diabetes Complications 2022;36:108332.
89. Venniyoor A. Tirzepatide once weekly for the treatment of obesity. N Engl J Med 2022;387:1433–4.
90. Permana H, Yanto TA, Hariyanto TI. Efficacy and safety of tirzepatide as novel treatment for type 2 diabetes: a systematic review and meta-analysis of randomized clinical trials. Diabetes Metab Syndr 2022;16:102640.
91. Gastaldelli A, Cusi K, Fernandez Lando L, et al. Effect of tirzepatide versus insulin degludec on liver fat content and abdominal adipose tissue in people with type 2 diabetes (SURPASS-3 MRI): a substudy of the randomised, open-label, parallel-group, phase 3 SURPASS-3 trial. Lancet Diabetes Endocrinol 2022; 10:393–406.
92. Jastreboff AM, Aronne LJ, Ahmad NN, et al. Tirzepatide once weekly for the treatment of obesity. N Engl J Med 2022;387:205–16.
93. Tahrani AA, Barnett AH, Bailey CJ. SGLT inhibitors in management of diabetes. Lancet Diabetes Endocrinol 2013;1:140–51.
94. Alkabbani W, Gamble JM. Profile of ipragliflozin, an oral SGLT-2 inhibitor for the treatment of type 2 diabetes: the evidence to date. Drug Des Devel Ther 2021; 15:3057–69.
95. Luo J, Sun P, Wang Y, et al. Dapagliflozin attenuates steatosis in livers of high-fat diet-induced mice and oleic acid-treated L02 cells via regulating AMPK/mTOR pathway. Eur J Pharmacol 2021;907:174304.
96. Nasiri-Ansari N, Nikolopoulou C, Papoutsi K, et al. Empagliflozin attenuates non-alcoholic fatty liver disease (NAFLD) in high fat diet fed ApoE((-/-)) mice by activating autophagy and reducing ER stress and apoptosis. Int J Mol Sci 2021; 22(2):818.
97. Lee JY, Lee M, Lee JY, et al. Ipragliflozin, an SGLT2 inhibitor, ameliorates high-fat diet-induced metabolic changes by upregulating energy expenditure through activation of the AMPK/SIRT1 pathway. Diabetes Metab J 2021;45: 921–32.
98. Petito-da-Silva TI, Souza-Mello V, Barbosa-da-Silva S. Empaglifozin mitigates NAFLD in high-fat-fed mice by alleviating insulin resistance, lipogenesis and ER stress. Mol Cell Endocrinol 2019;498:110539.
99. Hodrea J, Saeed A, Molnar A, et al. SGLT2 inhibitor dapagliflozin prevents atherosclerotic and cardiac complications in experimental type 1 diabetes. PLoS One 2022;17:e0263285.
100. Yabiku K, Nakamoto K, Tsubakimoto M. Effects of sodium-glucose cotransporter 2 inhibition on glucose metabolism, liver function, ascites, and hemodynamics in a mouse model of nonalcoholic steatohepatitis and type 2 diabetes. J Diabetes Res 2020;2020:1682904.
101. Fawzy AM, Rivera-Caravaca JM, Underhill P, et al. Incident heart failure, arrhythmias and cardiovascular outcomes with sodium-glucose cotransporter 2 (SGLT2) inhibitor use in patients with diabetes: insights from a global federated electronic medical record database. Diabetes Obes Metab 2022.

102. Cusi K, Bril F, Barb D, et al. Effect of canagliflozin treatment on hepatic triglyceride content and glucose metabolism in patients with type 2 diabetes. Diabetes Obes Metab 2019;21:812–21.
103. Latva-Rasku A, Honka MJ, Kullberg J, et al. The SGLT2 inhibitor dapagliflozin reduces liver fat but does not affect tissue insulin sensitivity: a randomized, double-blind, placebo-controlled study with 8-week treatment in type 2 diabetes patients. Diabetes Care 2019;42:931–7.
104. Kahl S, Gancheva S, Strassburger K, et al. Empagliflozin effectively lowers liver fat content in well-controlled type 2 diabetes: a randomized, double-blind, phase 4, placebo-controlled trial. Diabetes Care 2020;43:298–305.
105. Eriksson JW, Lundkvist P, Jansson PA, et al. Effects of dapagliflozin and n-3 carboxylic acids on non-alcoholic fatty liver disease in people with type 2 diabetes: a double-blind randomised placebo-controlled study. Diabetologia 2018;61:1923–34.
106. Cusi K. Time to include nonalcoholic steatohepatitis in the management of patients with type 2 diabetes. Diabetes Care 2020;43:275–9.
107. Lavine JE, Schwimmer JB, Van Natta ML, et al. Effect of vitamin E or metformin for treatment of nonalcoholic fatty liver disease in children and adolescents: the TONIC randomized controlled trial. JAMA 2011;305:1659–68.
108. Loomba R, Lutchman G, Kleiner DE, et al. Clinical trial: pilot study of metformin for the treatment of non-alcoholic steatohepatitis. Aliment Pharmacol Ther 2009;29:172–82.
109. Nair S, Diehl AM, Wiseman M, et al. Metformin in the treatment of non-alcoholic steatohepatitis: a pilot open label trial. Aliment Pharmacol Ther 2004;20:23–8.
110. Schwimmer JB, Middleton MS, Deutsch R, et al. A phase 2 clinical trial of metformin as a treatment for non-diabetic paediatric non-alcoholic steatohepatitis. Aliment Pharmacol Ther 2005;21:871–9.
111. Shields WW, Thompson KE, Grice GA, et al. The effect of metformin and standard therapy versus standard therapy alone in nondiabetic patients with insulin resistance and nonalcoholic steatohepatitis (NASH): a pilot trial. Therap Adv Gastroenterol 2009;2:157–63.
112. Dufour JF, Oneta CM, Gonvers JJ, et al. Randomized placebo-controlled trial of ursodeoxycholic acid with vitamin e in nonalcoholic steatohepatitis. Clin Gastroenterol Hepatol 2006;4:1537–43.
113. Laurin J, Lindor KD, Crippin JS, et al. Ursodeoxycholic acid or clofibrate in the treatment of non-alcohol-induced steatohepatitis: a pilot study. Hepatology 1996;23:1464–7.
114. Ratziu V. Treatment of NASH with ursodeoxycholic acid: pro. Clin Res Hepatol Gastroenterol 2012;36(Suppl 1):S41–5.
115. Leuschner UF, Lindenthal B, Herrmann G, et al. High-dose ursodeoxycholic acid therapy for nonalcoholic steatohepatitis: a double-blind, randomized, placebo-controlled trial. Hepatology 2010;52:472–9.
116. Lindor KD, Kowdley KV, Heathcote EJ, et al. Ursodeoxycholic acid for treatment of nonalcoholic steatohepatitis: results of a randomized trial. Hepatology 2004;39:770–8.
117. Ren J, Wang X, Yee C, et al. Sitagliptin is more effective than gliclazide in preventing pro-fibrotic and pro-inflammatory changes in a rodent model of diet-induced non-alcoholic fatty liver disease. Molecules 2022;27.
118. Zhou ST, Cui W, Kong L, et al. Efficacy of sitagliptin on nonalcoholic fatty liver disease in high-fat-diet-fed diabetic mice. Curr Med Sci 2022;42:513–9.

119. Doustmohammadian A, Nezhadisalami A, Safarnezhad Tameshke F, et al. A randomized triple-blind controlled clinical trial evaluation of sitagliptin in the treatment of patients with non-alcoholic fatty liver diseases without diabetes. Front Med 2022;9:937554.
120. Fukuhara T, Hyogo H, Ochi H, et al. Efficacy and safety of sitagliptin for the treatment of nonalcoholic fatty liver disease with type 2 diabetes mellitus. Hepato-Gastroenterology 2014;61:323–8.
121. Cui J, Philo L, Nguyen P, et al. Sitagliptin vs. placebo for non-alcoholic fatty liver disease: a randomized controlled trial. J Hepatol 2016;65:369–76.
122. Zhang Y, Cai T, Zhao J, et al. Effects and safety of sitagliptin in non-alcoholic fatty liver disease: a systematic review and meta-analysis. Horm Metab Res 2020;52:517–26.
123. Wang X, Zhao B, Sun H, et al. Effects of sitagliptin on intrahepatic lipid content in patients with non-alcoholic fatty liver disease. Front Endocrinol 2022;13:866189.
124. Argo CK, Patrie JT, Lackner C, et al. Effects of n-3 fish oil on metabolic and histological parameters in NASH: a double-blind, randomized, placebo-controlled trial. J Hepatol 2015;62:190–7.
125. Sanyal AJ, Abdelmalek MF, Suzuki A, et al. No significant effects of ethyl-eicosapentanoic acid on histologic features of nonalcoholic steatohepatitis in a phase 2 trial. Gastroenterology 2014;147:377–384 e371.
126. Loomba R, Sirlin CB, Ang B, et al. Ezetimibe for the treatment of nonalcoholic steatohepatitis: assessment by novel magnetic resonance imaging and magnetic resonance elastography in a randomized trial (MOZART trial). Hepatology 2015;61:1239–50.
127. Fernandez-Miranda C, Perez-Carreras M, Colina F, et al. A pilot trial of fenofibrate for the treatment of non-alcoholic fatty liver disease. Dig Liver Dis 2008; 40:200–5.
128. Nakade Y, Murotani K, Inoue T, et al. Ezetimibe for the treatment of non-alcoholic fatty liver disease: a meta-analysis. Hepatol Res 2017;47:1417–28.
129. Navarro VJ, Belle SH, D'Amato M, et al. Silymarin in non-cirrhotics with non-alcoholic steatohepatitis: a randomized, double-blind, placebo controlled trial. PLoS One 2019;14:e0221683.
130. Wah Kheong C, Nik Mustapha NR, Mahadeva S. A randomized trial of silymarin for the treatment of nonalcoholic steatohepatitis. Clin Gastroenterol Hepatol 2017;15:1940–1949 e1948.
131. Mantovani A, Byrne CD, Bonora E, et al. Nonalcoholic fatty liver disease and risk of incident type 2 diabetes: a meta-analysis. Diabetes Care 2018;41:372–82.
132. Siddiqui MS, Fuchs M, Idowu MO, et al. Severity of nonalcoholic fatty liver disease and progression to cirrhosis are associated with atherogenic lipoprotein profile. Clin Gastroenterol Hepatol 2015;13:1000–8.
133. Patel S, Siddiqui MB, Roman JH, et al. Association between lipoprotein particles and atherosclerotic events in nonalcoholic fatty liver disease. Clin Gastroenterol Hepatol 2021;19:2202–4.
134. Corey KE, Wilson LA, Altinbas A, et al. Relationship between resolution of non-alcoholic steatohepatitis and changes in lipoprotein sub-fractions: a post-hoc analysis of the PIVENS trial. Aliment Pharmacol Ther 2019;49:1205–13.
135. Corey KE, Vuppalanchi R, Wilson LA, et al. NASH resolution is associated with improvements in HDL and triglyceride levels but not improvement in LDL or non-HDL-C levels. Aliment Pharmacol Ther 2015;41:301–9.

136. Harrison SA, Bashir MR, Guy CD, et al. Resmetirom (MGL-3196) for the treatment of non-alcoholic steatohepatitis: a multicentre, randomised, double-blind, placebo-controlled, phase 2 trial. Lancet 2019;394:2012–24.
137. Kaplan DE, Serper MA, Mehta R, et al. Effects of hypercholesterolemia and statin exposure on survival in a large national cohort of patients with cirrhosis. Gastroenterology 2019;156:1693–706.
138. Ekstedt M, Franzen LE, Mathiesen UL, et al. Statins in non-alcoholic fatty liver disease and chronically elevated liver enzymes: a histopathological follow-up study. J Hepatol 2007;47:135–41.
139. Abdallah M, Brown L, Provenza J, et al. Safety and efficacy of dyslipidemia treatment in NAFLD Patients: a Meta-analysis of randomized controlled trials. Ann Hepatol 2022. https://doi.org/10.1016/j.aohep.2022.100738:100738.
140. Bays H, Cohen DE, Chalasani N, et al. An assessment by the statin liver safety task force: 2014 update. Journal of Clinical Lipidology 2014;8:S47–57.
141. Blais P, Lin M, Kramer JR, et al. Statins are underutilized in patients with nonalcoholic fatty liver disease and dyslipidemia. Dig Dis Sci 2016;61:1714–20.
142. Patel SS, Guzman LA, Lin F-P, et al. Utilization of aspirin and statin in management of coronary artery disease in patients with cirrhosis undergoing liver transplant evaluation. Liver Transplant 2018;24:872–80.
143. Athyros VG, Tziomalos K, Gossios TD, et al. Safety and efficacy of long-term statin treatment for cardiovascular events in patients with coronary heart disease and abnormal liver tests in the Greek Atorvastatin and Coronary Heart Disease Evaluation (GREACE) Study: a post-hoc analysis. Lancet 2010;376:1916–22.

The Role Bariatric Surgery and Endobariatric Therapies in Nonalcoholic Steatohepatitis

Aaron Yeoh, MD[a], Robert Wong, MD, MS[a,b],
Ashwani K. Singal, MD, MS[c,d,e,*]

KEYWORDS

- Bariatric surgery • Endoscopic bariatric and metabolic therapies
- Bariatric endoscopy • Nonalcoholic fatty liver disease • Nonalcoholic steatohepatitis

KEY POINTS

- Nonalcoholic fatty liver disease (NAFLD) is the most common cause of chronic liver disease worldwide, and second leading etiology for liver transplantation.
- Currently, there are no approved medical therapies, and weight loss through lifestyle modifications remains mainstay of therapy.
- Bariatric surgery is the most effective therapy for weight loss and improves liver histology.

INTRODUCTION

Nonalcoholic fatty liver disease (NAFLD) is rapidly increasing in its magnitude, mirroring the global increase in the prevalence of obesity. The prevalence of NAFLD is approximately 25% worldwide and in the United States.[1,2] Approximately 25% of patients with NAFLD progress to nonalcoholic steatohepatitis (NASH), with increased risks of cirrhosis and hepatocellular carcinoma.[1] A reduction in body weight and lifestyle intervention with diet and exercise remains the first line for patients with NAFLD.[3] In one study, 10% weight loss over 52 weeks resolved NASH in 90%, and even a 5% weight loss resolved NASH resolution in 26% of patients.[4] However, only 10% of individuals in this study could lose 10% weight loss, highlighting difficulties in achieving weight loss with lifestyle intervention alone.[4] Currently, there are no approved pharmacologic therapies for NAFLD.[5]

[a] Division of Gastroenterology and Hepatology, Stanford University School of Medicine, Palo Alto, CA, USA; [b] Gastroenterology Section, Veterans Affairs Palo Alto Healthcare System, Palo Alto, CA, USA; [c] University of South Dakota Sanford School of Medicine; [d] Avera Medical Group Liver Disease and Transplant Institute, Avera McKennan University Hospital, Clinical Research Affairs Avera Transplant Institute, 1315 South Cliff Avenue, Sioux Falls, SD 57105, USA; [e] VA Medical Center, Sioux Falls, SD, USA
* Corresponding author. Avera Medical Group Liver Disease and Transplant Institute.
E-mail address: ashwanisingal.com@gmail.com

Clin Liver Dis 27 (2023) 413–427
https://doi.org/10.1016/j.cld.2023.01.009 liver.theclinics.com
1089-3261/23/

Bariatric surgery (BS) is approved for individuals who have failed lifestyle intervention and have either class III obesity (body mass index [BMI] ≥ 40 mg/kg^2) or class II obesity (BMI ≥ 35 mg/kg^2) with an obesity-related comorbidity. Over the last decade, endoscopic bariatric and metabolic therapies (EBMT) have emerged as novel therapies for the treatment of obesity and diabetes mellitus. There is increasing evidence that both BS and EBMT improve serologic, radiographic, and histologic profiles in patients with NASH. This review aimed to summarize the current evidence of BS and EBMT in NASH.

BARIATRIC SURGERY

BS includes procedures with restrictive or restrictive with malabsorptive effects. Restrictive surgeries like sleeve gastrectomy (SG) and adjustable gastric banding (AGB) decrease caloric intake by reducing the stomach size. Restrictive with malabsorption surgeries like Roux-en-Y Gastric Bypass (RYGB) and Biliopancreatic Diversion with Duodenal Switch have an additional effect of bypassing the proximal small bowel, resulting in hormonal effects that improve insulin resistance.[6] Restrictive procedures can be revised to RYGB or Bilio-Pancreatic Diversion-Duodenal Switch (BPD-DS) if desired weight loss is not achieved.

Several studies examining the role of BS in NASH have shown improvement in liver histology, in those with advanced fibrosis.[7] In a study on 340 laparoscopic BS (42% no steatosis, 44% mild NASH, and 14% advanced fibrosis), overall complication rate was 13%, similar in the three groups.[8] Overall complication rate was 13% with no significant difference in complications observed between the three groups.[8]

Various BS procedures have been in practice since the 1950s and the field has rapidly evolved, over the last decade. Between 2011 and 2019, the use of AGB has decreased and increased for SG and RYGB.[9] Of all BS in 2019, SG contributed 61.4%, RYGB in 32.4 (15.4% revisions), and AGB in 1.1% only.[9] In this review, we focus on the role of RYGB and SG in patients with NASH (**Table 1**).

Roux-en-Y Gastric Bypass Surgery

Since the first reported RYGB in 1995 on 91 patients with NAFLD,[10] several observational studies have examined the benefit of RYGB in patients with NASH. In a meta-analysis of 15 studies (10 RYGB) with 766 paired liver biopsies, pooled proportion of patients with either improvement of steatosis, steatohepatitis, and fibrosis was 91.6% (95% CI 82.4 to 97.5), 81.3% (95% CI 61.9% to 94.9%), and 65.5% (95% CI 38.2 to 88.1), respectively.[11] The limitations of this meta-analysis were variations across studies on type of biopsy performed, histopathology grading systems, and type of BS. A more recent meta-analysis included 32 studies (25 RYGB) with 3093 paired liver biopsy specimens, mean steatosis resolution was in 80% (95% CI 66 to 91), lobular inflammation in 57% (95% CI 29 to 83), ballooning degeneration in 80% (95% CI 65 to 91), and fibrosis in 51% (95% 39 to 63) of patients.[12]

Several studies have investigated long-term outcomes after RYGB in NASH. In a small prospective study on nine patients with NASH, RYGB was associated with improvement in hepatic steatosis, inflammation, and ballooning in 55%, 100%, and 88.8%, respectively, after a mean of 55 months.[13] In another study of 1236 obese patients (86% NAFLD), BS (55% RYGB, 45% AGB) reported histology data on liver biopsies taken at 0 (n = 1201), 1 (n = 578), and 5 years (n = 413).[14] Mean ± standard deviation (SD) NAFLD activity score (NAS) decreased from 2.0 ± 1.5 to 0.7 ± 1.0 at year 1 and this benefit was sustained for 5 years.[14]

Table 1
Summary of bariatric surgeries and endoscopic bariatric metabolic therapies

Procedure Name	Mechanism	Pros	Cons	Reversible	Company	FDA Approved
Bariatric surgery						
Roux-en-Y Gastric Bypass Surgery	Restrictive with malabsorption	Most effective procedure for weight loss and reversal of diabetes mellitus.	Post-operative complications like dumping syndrome, nutritional deficiencies, and alcohol use.	No	N.A.	Yes
Surgical Sleeve Gastrectomy	Restrictive	Durable weight loss with lower surgical risk and post-operative complications compared with RYGB.	Smaller weight loss and effect on insulin resistance. Risk for anastomotic leak and potential worsening of gastroesophageal reflux.	No	N.A.	Yes
Endoscopic bariatric metabolic therapies (gastric devices)						
Intragastric balloon	Restrictive	Relatively simple endoscopic procedure, good safety profile.	Nausea and GI distress frequent. Weight regain common after balloon removal	Yes	Multiple approved devices	Yes
Aspiration Therapy	Restrictive (ingested food aspiration)	Relatively simple endoscopic procedure. Durable weight control device.	Requires frequent emptying after each meal. Potentially unpleasant for patients.	Yes	Aspire Bariatrics	Yes
Endoscopic Sleeve Gastroplasty	Restrictive	Durable weight loss. Good procedure for patients refusing	Less weight loss compared with bariatric surgery.	No	Apollo Endo-surgery	Yes

(*continued on next page*)

Table 1
(*continued*)

Procedure Name	Mechanism	Pros	Cons	Reversible	Company	FDA Approved
		surgical options. Faster recovery than bariatric surgery.	Requires advanced endoscopic training.			
Primary Obesity Surgery Endo-luminal (POSE)	Restrictive	Durable weight loss.	Less weight loss compared with bariatric surgery. Requires advanced endoscopic training.	No	USGI Medical	Yes
Endoscopic bariatric metabolic therapies (small bowel devices)						
Endo-barrier	Malabsorption	Targeted therapy for patients who are unfit or unwilling to undergo surgery. Minimal side effects.	Requires endoscopic expertise and fluoroscopy. Temporary effect for 12 mos.	Yes	GI Dynamics	No
Duodenal Mucosa Resurfacing	Malabsorption	Targeted therapy for patients unfit or unwilling to undergo surgery. Minimal side effects.	Requires endoscopic expertise and fluoroscopy. Unclear duration of benefit.	No	Fractyl Health	No

Sleeve Gastrectomy

SG is a common BS, with its benefits shown in patients with NASH.[15] For example, in one study on 84 patients with NAFLD diagnosed on ultrasound and receiving SG, 56% showed NAFLD resolution after a median follow-up of 3.3 years.[16] In another study on 72 patients, liver elastography measurement (LSM) on fibroscan improved from 7.5 ± 5.0 kPa before surgery to 5.6 ± 2.5 kPa at 6 months of follow-up.[17] In the same study, hepatic steatosis as measured by controlled attenuation parameter improved from 309.2 ± 68.7 dB/M to 217.4 ± 56.4 dB/M.[17] In a recent study, SG in 174 patients with NAFLD (46% with advanced fibrosis) showed a mean change in NAFLD fibrosis score of 0.46 (±1.02), -0.55 (±0.98) and -0.55 (±1.12) at 6, 12, and 24 months, respectively.[18] In yet another study on 79 patients with NAFLD (NASH in 63%) in Japan, NASH resolved in 25 of 28 patients with a follow-up at 12 months.[19] In another similar study on 94 patients (83 NASH), the mean NAFLD activity score decreased from 5.20 to 2.63 at 1-year follow-up.[20] Interestingly, only 1 of 26 patients with F3 fibrosis did not show fibrosis improvement at 12 months.[20]

Roux-en-Y Gastric Bypass versus Sleeve Gastrectomy for Nonalcoholic Fatty Liver Disease

Several studies have compared the efficacy of RYGB with SG in patients with NAFLD. For example, in a study from India on 134 patients (88 NAFLD and 45 NASH) undergoing BS, of 30 patients (20 SG and 10 RYGB) with paired biopsy at a mean follow-up of 7.1 months, 9 showed resolution and 11 improvement of NASH, with no differences comparing SG versus RYGB.[21] In a similar study on 40 patients (16 RYGB and 24 SG), there was a larger reduction in steatosis at 12 months with RYGB versus SG (−0.91 versus −0.33, $p = 0.007$), but no difference on NAFLD activity score −3.0 versus −2.25, $p = 0.24$.[22] In a meta-analysis of 20 studies comparing RYGB versus SG in patients with NASH, mean changes in NAFLD activity score and NAFLD fibrosis score tended to be larger in RYGB: −2.8 versus −2.3 and −1.0 versus −0.7, respectively, $p > 0.05$ for both.[23] In a clinical trial on 100 individuals with diabetes mellitus randomized 1:1 to SG or RYGB, changes in hepatic steatosis (MRI proton density fat fraction) declined −19.7%, in SG and −21.5% in the RYGB group, $p > 0.05$. None of the patients had significant fibrosis (enhanced liver fibrosis score), with 94% in SG and 100% in the RYGB at 1 year after BS.[24]

Our careful literature review suggests that BS may be considered for patients with NASH. However, currently this is not recommended to treat NASH and this diagnosis by itself is not an approved indication for BS.[25] Further, there is also inadequate evidence to confirm the superiority of RYGB or SG. The decision to choose one over another must consider an informed decision between the surgeon and patient explaining the pros and cons of each of these procedures (see **Table 1**). Further, limitations of BS should be recognized especially weight regain, recurrence of NAFLD, nutritional deficiencies after RYGB, and risk or worsening of alcohol use disorder.[7,26,27] Long-term prospective studies are needed to examine weight trajectory and recurrence of NASH among subjects receiving BS.

MECHANISMS OF WEIGHT LOSS AND IMPROVED METABOLIC PROFILE AFTER BARIATRIC SURGERY

Weight loss following BS occurs via the direct effects of reduced caloric intake and the indirect effects of RYGB on the gastrointestinal physiology. Ghrelin produced in the gastric fundus is the primary hormone to stimulate appetite.[28] Whereas ghrelin secretion is increased following lifestyle-mediated weight loss, its levels fall following BS.[28]

This may in part help explain the sustained weight loss after BS compared with typical weight regain with lifestyle modification, where increasing ghrelin levels "push back", making sustained weight loss difficult.

Improvement in metabolic profile and NASH following BS is due to increased hepatic insulin sensitivity and reduced peripheral insulin resistance due to gradual weight loss.[29] The rapid transit of digested nutrients to the distal small bowel following BS stimulates small intestinal cells which secrete glucagon-like peptide-1 (GLP-1) and peptide YY which have multiple endocrine effects including an increase in insulin sensitivity and modulation of ghrelin and leptin, which result in a decrease in appetite.[30] GLP-1 also has direct effects on the liver with activation of PPAR-γ genes, enhancing hepatic fat oxidation, lipid export, and insulin sensitivity.[31] GLP-1 also attenuates hepatic expression of TNF-alpha and interleukins 6 and 1, which improves hepatic inflammation and slows the progression of NASH.[28,31]

Changes in the gut microbiome and bile acids also play a role in improving the metabolic profile and NASH. There are more than 40 trillion microorganisms and at least 1000 bacterial species in the gastrointestinal tract of humans.[32] Individuals with obesity have dysbiosis with lower gut microbiome diversity and a reduction in the phyla *Bifidobacterium* with an increase in the phyla *Firmicutes*.[33] Microbiome dysbiosis increases gut permeability and worsens bacterial translocation, increased production and absorption of fatty acids, and changes in immune function.[34] Taken together, these lead to the worsening of hepatic inflammation and NASH. Following BS, levels of *Firmicutes* decrease with an increase in the phyla of other bacteria.[34] Bile acids and restoration of primary to secondary bile acids play a modulatory role in energy homeostasis, glucose and lipid metabolism, and inflammatory pathways, primarily through binding the Takeda G receptor 5 (TGR5) and farnesoid X receptor (FXR).[33,35] Although there are many plausible explanations linking the microbiome and bile acids, further studies are needed to better understand the precise mechanisms that drive benefits in NASH histology following BS.

ENDOSCOPIC BARIATRIC AND METABOLIC THERAPIES

Over the last few years, EBMT has emerged as an effective and safe option to treat obesity. Endoscopic therapies can be intragastric devices (balloons, endoscopic sleeve gastroplasty [ESG], and aspiration therapy) that restrict food intake or small bowel devices (Endo-barrier and duodenal mucosal resurfacing [DMR]) targeting metabolic profile and insulin resistance (see **Table 1**). In a meta-analysis of 18 studies on 863 patients with NAFLD, the use of restrictive EBMT was associated with a reduction in liver fibrosis with a standardized mean difference (SMD) of 0.7 (95% CI 0.1, 1.3; $p = 0.02$).[36] There was also a significant improvement in hepatic steatosis (SMD: −1.0, 95% CI −1.2 to −0.8) and NAFLD activity score (−2.5, 95% CI −3.5 to −1.5).[36]

Gastric Endoscopic Bariatric and Metabolic Therapies

Intragastric balloon

Intragastric balloons (IGBs) are space-occupying devices filled with saline or gas and designed to reduce gastric volume, promote early satiety, and slow gastric emptying (**Fig. 1**A). IGB was US Food and Drug Administration (FDA) approved in 1985 but was withdrawn from the market in 1992, as it did not lead to the substantial weight change.[37] Since then, several IGB devices have become available, and are now in common use worldwide. Three IGBs are currently FDA approved in the United States: Obera (Apollo Endo-surgery), Reshape Duo (Reshape Medical), and Obalon (Obalon

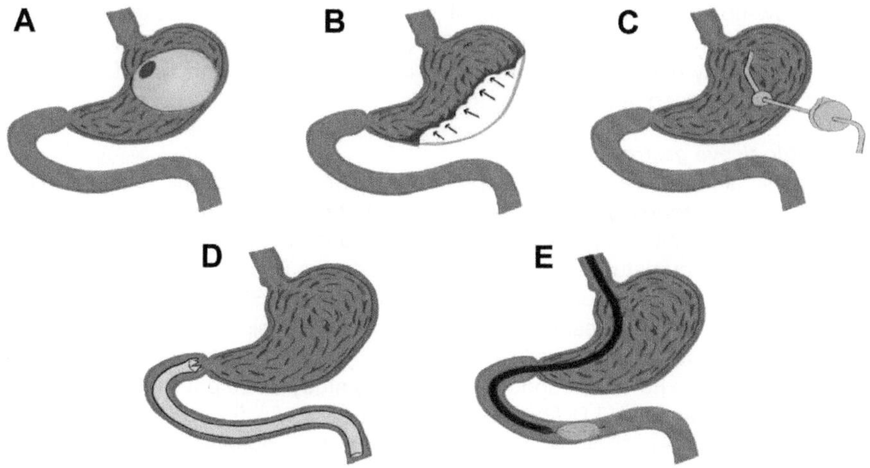

Fig. 1. Schematic representation of EBMT: (*A*) *Intragastric Balloon*: Obera single balloon seen in gastric body, (*B*) *Endoscopic Sleeve Gastroplasty*: Full-thickness bites with suturing device causing apposition of tissue along greater curvature, (*C*) *Aspiration Therapy*: Percutaneous gastrostomy tube with connection to external device for drainage of partially digested food, (*D*) *Endo-barrier:* 60 cm plastic liner anchored in duodenal bulb allowing chyme to bypass duodenum, (*E*) *Duodenal Mucosa Resurfacing*: Ablation of 10 cm of duodenum mucosa with hydrothermal balloon.

Therapeutics). The typical volume of an IGB is 500 – 700 mL and balloons are removed approximately after 6 months of placement.

Most studies of IGB have focused on weight loss and have looked only at indirect markers of NASH including alanine aminotransferase (ALT), AST, and gamma-glutamyl transpeptidase (GGT). An early observational study on 93 obese patients showed that IGB placement was associated with a greater reduction in ALT and GGT from baseline among NAFLD versus those without hepatic steatosis on ultrasound with 30 versus 23 IU/L and 28 versus 20 IU/L, respectively; $p < 0.01$ for both.[38] In a prospective study, proportion of patients with severe hepatic steatosis on ultrasound reduced to 4% at 6 months from 52% before IGB was placed.[39] In another study on 26 patients, liver stiffness and hepatic steatosis were reduced at 6 months after IGB placement versus baseline value (13.3 ± 3.2 kPa vs 11.3 ± 2.8 kPa) and (355 dB/m, 95% CI 298–400 vs 296, 95% CI 255–352 dB/m), $P < 0.01$ for both analyses.[40] Serial IGB placement (at least two 6-month IGB) have also been shown to gradually improve markers of NASH with the greatest improvement within the first 6 months.[41] In a pilot randomized controlled study on 18 patients with biopsy-confirmed NASH, IGB with lifestyle changes versus sham IGB with lifestyle changes reduced NAFLD activity score (2 ± 0.75 vs 4 ± 2.25; $p < 0.03$) at 6 months.[42] There was no change in median lobular inflammation, hepatocellular ballooning, or fibrosis scores in either group.[42]

In a meta-analysis of nine studies, use of IGB ($N = 442$) showed improved steatosis in 79.2%, reduction in liver volume on CT scan, and improvement in NAFLD activity score.[43] Common adverse events were nausea and vomiting. There were no serious adverse events or patient mortality.[43] Although overall the IGB is safe and effective, IGB placement requires expertise and training, which limits availability in every endoscopic center at a national level. Weight regain is also common following IGB removal. In a retrospective study of 65 patients who underwent IGB from 2009 to 2016 with a mean follow-up at 3.3 years, only 39% of patients were satisfied with the procedure and 89% went on to regain weight or undergo another bariatric procedure.[44] Thus, although IGB may have a role in prompting initial weight loss and NAFLD improvement, it is not an adequate long-term therapy.

Endoscopic sleeve gastroplasty

ESG, a minimally invasive endoscopic procedure mimics the anatomic changes of SG (**Fig. 1**B). An endoscopic suturing device is used to take full-thickness suture bites of the gastric wall and cause apposition of the anterior and posterior walls of the stomach along the greater curvature. The most common device is OverStitch (Apollo Endosurgery). In a study on 118 adults with obesity and NAFLD, ESG reduced hepatic steatosis index by 4 points per year ($p < 0.001$), and NAFLD fibrosis score by 0.3 points per year ($p = 0.034$) at 2 years of follow-up.[45] Notably, 20% of patients improved liver fibrosis from F3-4 to F0-2.[45] In another prospective study on 26 patients with NAFLD, ESG improved mean NAFLD fibrosis score from 0.23 to −0.20 at 6 and −0.55 at 12 months of follow-up.[46] No major adverse events were observed.[46] The results of an ongoing randomized controlled trial comparing SG to ESG in NASH patients with obesity (NCT04060368) will hopefully provide evidence-based data for clinicians to choose one procedure over the other in routine practice.[47]

Another novel therapy is the Primary Obesity Surgery Endo-luminal (POSE) procedure, which uses full-thickness plication of the gastric body with endoscopically deployed anchors. In a prospective multicenter study on 44 patients, POSE procedure was associated with weight loss of 15.7%, 12 units lowering in ALT, and −0.5 kPa liver stiffness measurement at 12 months.[48] However, these results did not reach statistical significance.[48]

Both ESG and POSE may provide durable results unlike IGB, which are only in place for 6 months on average. Although ESG and POSE require additional training, they may have a role for individuals who would benefit from durable restrictive gastric changes but are unwilling or are too sick to undergo BS.

Aspiration therapy

Aspiration Therapy is a simple FDA-approved EBMT (**Fig. 1**C), and can be used for a long period along with lifestyle intervention. The device consists of a percutaneous endoscopic gastrostomy tube port connected with an external device, that allows for the drainage of approximately 30% of ingested calories following a meal.[49] In a meta-analysis of five studies on 590 patients receiving aspiration therapy, mean reductions in AST and ALT were 2.7 and 7.5 units, respectively, with an improvement in metabolic syndrome at 1 year follow-up.[49]

Small bowel endoscopic bariatric and metabolic therapies

These therapies replicate the hormonal effect seen with restrictive and malabsorptive BS, with improved metabolic profile and even complete resolution of diabetes mellitus.[50] However, these therapies currently are not FDA-approved for routine use in clinical practice.

Endo-barrier

One alternative to surgical small bowel bypass is the Endo-barrier (GI Dynamics), an endo-luminal duodenal-jejunal bypass liner (**Fig. 1**D).[51] The device is a 60-cm impermeable liner that is implanted endoscopically under fluoroscopic guidance and affixed to the duodenal bulb with anchors. The liner allows for digested gastric contents to bypass absorption in the duodenum and be delivered into the jejunum. In a study on 20 patients with obesity and diabetes mellitus receiving Endo-barrier therapy, the median (IQR) liver stiffness on fibroscan reduced from 10.4 to 5.3 kPa, $p < 0.01$ at 12 months.[52] Hepatic steatosis also improved with median controlled attenuation parameter decreasing from 343 to 317 dB/m, $p < 0.05$.[52] In a meta-analysis of 10 studies on 211 subjects, hemoglobin A1C and weight decreased by 0.9% and 5.1 kg, respectively.[53]

Duodenal mucosal resurfacing

DMR is an endoscopic procedure designed to ablate duodenal mucosa and improve insulin resistance-associated conditions such as diabetes mellitus and metabolic syndrome. The procedure is performed with the Revita system (Fractyl Laboratories) which uses a hydrothermal catheter under fluoroscopic guidance to ablate approximately 10 cm of mucosa in the duodenum distal to the ampulla of Vater. In the first prospective trial of DMR (Revita 1), 37 subjects underwent DMR, and 27 of these followed for 24 months.[54] There was a durable improvement in HbA1c by 1.4% (SD = 0.8), with a reduction in ALT of 16.6 U/L (SD = 14.2) and AST of 9.6 (SD = 5.1).[54] In a second study (Revita 2) in Europe and Brazil, a total of 109 patients were randomized to undergo DMR vs sham procedure.[55] Metabolic parameters were measured including hepatic steatosis quantified by MRI proton density fat fraction. Overall, there was a nonsignificant reduction in fat quantification at 6 months in the DMR versus sham group (−5.4 vs −2.2%, $p = 0.035$).[55]

BARIATRIC SURGERY IN PATIENTS WITH CIRRHOSIS

Compensated Cirrhosis

The data on the safety of BS procedures in patients with cirrhosis are limited. In a systematic review of 15 studies, BS resulted in 60.4% excess weight loss with remission of NAFLD in 58% of patients. However, the BS procedure was complicated in 19.2%, with 2.67 higher odds of complications in patients with cirrhosis. Patient mortality rates were 0.9% for compensated cirrhosis and 18.2% for decompensated cirrhosis.[56] The outcome of BS in cirrhosis is proportional to center experience, with a reduced risk of complications, especially at centers with more than 50 cases per year.[57] Patients with decompensated cirrhosis and those with compensated cirrhosis at a higher surgical risk should be excluded. Several scoring systems can be used to estimate surgical risks such as Child-Pugh-Turcotte (CTP), Model for End-Stage Liver Disease (MELD), and University of Pennsylvania Veterans Affairs Cohort (UPenn VOCAL) scores.[58–60]

Patients Awaiting Liver Transplantation

Obesity is known to impact surgical outcomes with a higher risk of complications and longer hospitalization.[61] Hence, class III obesity is considered a relative contraindication for transplantation at several centers.[62] Patients need to lose weight to a level so that they become eligible for transplantation. In a retrospective study on 32 LT candidates (median MELD score 12 and BMI 45), with class III obesity but well-controlled cirrhosis complications receiving SG, there was no mortality and only one patient developed a major complication of the gastric leak that was successfully managed conservatively. Median weight loss at 6 months was 22 kg (excess weight loss of 33.4%), making 28 candidates eligible for LT.[63] Similar results have been reported in another study with the use of BS including SG and RYGB.[63]

Considering the risk of performing SG in patients with uncontrolled complications of cirrhosis and those with high MELD scores who cannot wait for BMI to reach eligibility level, the Mayo clinic in MN developed a program in 2006 on simultaneous SG performed at LT for candidates who are unable to achieve a BMI <35 before LT with lifestyle intervention. In a prospective study of 35 patients enrolled, of 7 patients requiring

LT and SG, there were no deaths and only one patient developed a major complication of suture leak that was managed conservatively.[64] Recently, the same group reported long-term outcomes in 13 of 29 patients who completed ≥3 years of follow-up. Compared with 36 patients becoming LT eligible with lifestyle intervention, those receiving LT and SG were more likely to maintain >10% weight loss (100% vs 29.4%) and a higher total weight loss (34.8 ± 17.3 vs 3.9 ± 13.3%) at ≥3 years, $P < 0.001$ for both. LT recipients with simultaneous SG also had better control of metabolic syndrome and NAFLD.[65]

Liver Transplant Recipients

Although the advent of effective immune-suppression regimens has improved patient and graft survival, obesity, metabolic syndrome, and NAFLD are the most important long-term issues among transplant recipients. Data on BS among LT recipients are limited, with RYGB in 7 patients[66] and SG in 37 patients (33 by laparoscopic) from four different reports.[67–70] However, there is high morbidity with major complications in nine patients within the first 30 days, mostly related to wound dehiscence or anastomotic leak. In a study of 303 patients, a matched cohort of 48 patients (12 previous LT) showed that non-LT patients had higher major complication rate (25 vs 3%, $P = 0.043$), shorter hospital stay (1.7 vs 3.1 d, $P < 0.001$), and higher excess weight loss (54 vs 45%, $P < 0.001$). Technical feasibility and control of metabolic conditions was similar in the two groups. There were no perioperative deaths in either group.[70] SG is preferred over RYGB, as it will not impair the absorption of immune-suppression medications and maintains anatomy allowing biliary/pancreatic intervention if needed. The treatment needs to be personalized with pre-LT SG for those with low biologic MELD and well-controlled complications of cirrhosis.

SUMMARY

Lifestyle modification with diet and exercise is currently the mainstay of treatment of NASH. However, it is difficult to achieve and more importantly sustain the lost weight. BS is an alternative option for NAFLD patients with severe obesity or with moderate obesity with an associated comorbidity. EBMT are emerging options and may be considered for patients who are poor surgical candidates and when weight loss is desired for a short period of time such as helping patients to meet a cut-off on BMI for LT eligibility.

Although data are emerging on BS in patients with cirrhosis, well-designed prospective studies are needed in this population. Prospective studies are also needed to guide on the appropriate timing of SG during pre-, peri-, or post-LT period. It also remains to be seen whether patients who become eligible for LT with lifestyle intervention should be offered SG to improve their long-term outcomes and control of metabolic abnormalities. Finally, randomized controlled trials are needed to evaluate if BS and EBMT may be appropriate to be considered irrespective of BMI for the treatment of patients with NASH.

In summary, while considering an intervention for managing obesity in patients with NASH, a close collaborative multidisciplinary approach with the patient, hepatologist, and surgeon is critical. The aim is to provide maximum benefit with the least amount of risk to the patient. Main factors to consider in decision-making in routine clinical practice include disease stage and liver function, advantages and disadvantages of BS or EBMT procedure, the desired goal of short-term or long-term weight loss, FDA approval of the procedure, and most importantly the local expertise while approaching a given patient with NAFLD (see **Table 1**).

CLINICS CARE POINTS

- Lifestyle modification with diet and exercise is currently the mainstay of treatment for NASH and there are no FDA approved pharmacotherapies.
- It is difficult to achieve the required weight loss of 7-10% from baseline, and more importantly challenging to sustain the lost weight.
- A diagnosis of NAFLD or NASH by itself is not an approved indication for bariatric surgery.
- A close collaboration in a multidisciplinary team with hepatologist, surgeon, dietitian, and endocrinologist is required for managing metabolic syndrome in patients with NAFLD.
- Prospective studies are needed to develop guidance on the timing of bariatric surgery during pre-, peri-, or post-transplant period among NASH patients waiting or receiving liver transplantation.

DISCLOSURE

A. Yeoh reports no conflict of interest. R. Wong reports outside the submitted work research grants (to his institution) from Gilead Sciences and Exact Sciences. He also reports consulting for Gilead Sciences, United States and Salix Pharmaceuticals. He reports personal fees unrelated to the submitted work from Chronic Liver Disease Foundation and ACG for educational initiatives. He has received research funding support from ACG, AASLD, NIAAA, and NIMHD, United States outside the submitted work. A.K. Singal reports outside the submitted work personal fees from Gilead, Medscape Gastroenterology, Chronic Liver Disease Foundation, Up-to-Date, and ACG; non-financial support from AASLD, United States and American Porphyria Foundation, United States; and grants from NIAAA and NIDDK, United States outside the submitted work.

REFERENCES

1. Younossi ZM, Koenig AB, Abdelatif D, et al. Global epidemiology of nonalcoholic fatty liver disease-Meta-analytic assessment of prevalence, incidence, and outcomes. Hepatology 2016;64(1):73–84.
2. Vernon G, Baranova A, Younossi ZM. Systematic review: the epidemiology and natural history of non-alcoholic fatty liver disease and non-alcoholic steatohepatitis in adults. Aliment Pharmacol Ther 2011;34(3):274–85.
3. Romero-Gomez M, Zelber-Sagi S, Trenell M. Treatment of NAFLD with diet, physical activity and exercise. J Hepatol 2017;67(4):829–46.
4. Vilar-Gomez E, Martinez-Perez Y, Calzadilla-Bertot L, et al. Weight loss through lifestyle modification significantly reduces features of nonalcoholic steatohepatitis. Gastroenterology 2015;149(2):367–378 e365 [quiz: e314-365].
5. Sanyal AJ, Chalasani N, Kowdley KV, et al. Pioglitazone, vitamin E, or placebo for nonalcoholic steatohepatitis. N Engl J Med 2010;362(18):1675–85.
6. Affinati AH, Esfandiari NH, Oral EA, et al. Bariatric surgery in the treatment of type 2 diabetes. Curr Diab Rep 2019;19(12):156.
7. Chauhan M, Singh K, Thuluvath PJ. Bariatric surgery in NAFLD. Dig Dis Sci 2022; 67(2):408–22.
8. Weingarten TN, Swain JM, Kendrick ML, et al. Nonalcoholic steatohepatitis (NASH) does not increase complications after laparoscopic bariatric surgery. Obes Surg 2011;21(11):1714–20.

9. Umehara T. Nonalcoholic fatty liver disease with elevated alanine aminotransferase levels is negatively associated with bone mineral density: Cross-sectional study in U.S. adults. PLoS One 2018;13(6):e0197900.
10. Silverman EM, Sapala JA, Appelman HD. Regression of hepatic steatosis in morbidly obese persons after gastric bypass. Am J Clin Pathol 1995;104(1): 23–31.
11. Mummadi RR, Kasturi KS, Chennareddygari S, et al. Effect of bariatric surgery on nonalcoholic fatty liver disease: systematic review and meta-analysis. Clin Gastroenterol Hepatol 2008;6(12):1396–402.
12. Lee Y, Doumouras AG, Yu J, et al. Complete resolution of nonalcoholic fatty liver disease after bariatric surgery: a systematic review and meta-analysis. Clin Gastroenterol Hepatol 2019;17(6):1040–1060 e1011.
13. Schneck AS, Anty R, Patouraux S, et al. Roux-En Y gastric bypass results in long-term remission of hepatocyte apoptosis and hepatic histological features of non-alcoholic steatohepatitis. Front Physiol 2016;7:344.
14. Caiazzo R, Lassailly G, Leteurtre E, et al. Roux-en-Y gastric bypass versus adjustable gastric banding to reduce nonalcoholic fatty liver disease: a 5-year controlled longitudinal study. Ann Surg 2014;260(5):893–8 [discussion: 898-899].
15. Iannelli A, Treacy P, Sebastianelli L, et al. Perioperative complications of sleeve gastrectomy: review of the literature. J Minim Access Surg 2019;15(1):1–7.
16. Algooneh A, Almazeedi S, Al-Sabah S, et al. Non-alcoholic fatty liver disease resolution following sleeve gastrectomy. Surg Endosc 2016;30(5):1983–7.
17. Batman B, Altun H, Simsek B, et al. The effect of laparoscopic sleeve gastrectomy on nonalcoholic fatty liver disease. Surg Laparosc Endosc Percutan Tech 2019;29(6):548–9.
18. Koh ZJ, Salgaonkar HP, Lee WJJ, et al. Improvement in non-alcoholic fatty liver disease score correlates with weight loss in obese patients undergoing laparoscopic sleeve gastrectomy: a two-centre study from an asian cohort. Obes Surg 2019;29(3):862–8.
19. Nikai H, Ishida K, Umemura A, et al. Effects of laparoscopic sleeve gastrectomy on non-alcoholic steatohepatitis and liver fibrosis in Japanese patients with severe obesity. Obes Surg 2020;30(7):2579–87.
20. Salman MA, Salman AA, Abdelsalam A, et al. Laparoscopic sleeve gastrectomy on the horizon as a promising treatment modality for NAFLD. Obes Surg 2020; 30(1):87–95.
21. Praveen Raj P, Gomes RM, Kumar S, et al. The effect of surgically induced weight loss on nonalcoholic fatty liver disease in morbidly obese Indians: "NASHOST" prospective observational trial. Surg Obes Relat Dis 2015;11(6):1315–22.
22. Pedersen JS, Rygg MO, Serizawa RR, et al. Effects of roux-en-Y gastric bypass and sleeve gastrectomy on non-alcoholic fatty liver disease: a 12-month follow-up study with paired liver biopsies. J Clin Med 2021;10(17):1–12.
23. Baldwin D, Chennakesavalu M, Gangemi A. Systematic review and meta-analysis of Roux-en-Y gastric bypass against laparoscopic sleeve gastrectomy for amelioration of NAFLD using four criteria. Surg Obes Relat Dis 2019;15(12):2123–30.
24. Seeberg KA, Borgeraas H, Hofso D, et al. Gastric bypass versus sleeve gastrectomy in type 2 diabetes: effects on hepatic steatosis and fibrosis : a randomized controlled trial. Ann Intern Med 2022;175(1):74–83.
25. Chalasani N, Younossi Z, Lavine JE, et al. The diagnosis and management of nonalcoholic fatty liver disease: practice guidance from the American Association for the Study of Liver Diseases. Hepatology 2018;67(1):328–57.

26. Jimenez LS, Mendonca Chaim FH, Mendonca Chaim FD, et al. Impact of weight regain on the evolution of non-alcoholic fatty liver disease after roux-en-Y gastric bypass: a 3-year follow-up. Obes Surg 2018;28(10):3131–5.
27. Yarra P, Dunn W, Younossi Z, et al. Association of previous gastric bypass surgery and patient outcomes in alcohol-associated cirrhosis hospitalizations. Dig Dis Sci 2022.
28. Seymour KA, Abdelmalek MF. The role of bariatric surgery in the management of nonalcoholic steatohepatitis. Curr Opin Gastroenterol 2021;37(3):208–15.
29. Laursen TL, Hagemann CA, Wei C, et al. Bariatric surgery in patients with non-alcoholic fatty liver disease - from pathophysiology to clinical effects. World J Hepatol 2019;11(2):138–49.
30. Beckman LM, Beckman TR, Earthman CP. Changes in gastrointestinal hormones and leptin after Roux-en-Y gastric bypass procedure: a review. J Am Diet Assoc 2010;110(4):571–84.
31. Kim YO, Schuppan D. When GLP-1 hits the liver: a novel approach for insulin resistance and NASH. Am J Physiol Gastrointest Liver Physiol 2012;302(8): G759–61.
32. Sender R, Fuchs S, Milo R. Are we really vastly outnumbered? Revisiting the ratio of bacterial to host cells in humans. Cell 2016;164(3):337–40.
33. Talavera-Urquijo E, Beisani M, Balibrea JM, et al. Is bariatric surgery resolving NAFLD via microbiota-mediated bile acid ratio reversal? A comprehensive review. Surg Obes Relat Dis 2020;16(9):1361–9.
34. Leung C, Rivera L, Furness JB, et al. The role of the gut microbiota in NAFLD. Nat Rev Gastroenterol Hepatol 2016;13(7):412–25.
35. Yuan L, Bambha K. Bile acid receptors and nonalcoholic fatty liver disease. World J Hepatol 2015;7(28):2811–8.
36. Jirapinyo P, McCarty TR, Dolan RD, et al. Effect of endoscopic bariatric and metabolic therapies on nonalcoholic fatty liver disease: a systematic review and meta-analysis. Clin Gastroenterol Hepatol 2022;20(3):511–24.e511.
37. Lari E, Burhamah W, Lari A, et al. Intra-gastric balloons - the past, present and future. Ann Med Surg (Lond). 2021;63:102138.
38. Ricci G, Bersani G, Rossi A, et al. Bariatric therapy with intragastric balloon improves liver dysfunction and insulin resistance in obese patients. Obes Surg 2008;18(11):1438–42.
39. Forlano R, Ippolito AM, Iacobellis A, et al. Effect of the BioEnterics intragastric balloon on weight, insulin resistance, and liver steatosis in obese patients. Gastrointest Endosc 2010;71(6):927–33.
40. Salomone F, Currenti W, Magrì G, et al. Effects of intragastric balloon in patients with nonalcoholic fatty liver disease and advanced fibrosis. Liver Int 2021;41(9): 2112–6.
41. Nguyen V, Li J, Gan J, et al. Outcomes following serial intragastric balloon therapy for obesity and nonalcoholic fatty liver disease in a single centre. Can J Gastroenterol Hepatol 2017;2017:4697194.
42. Lee YM, Low HC, Lim LG, et al. Intragastric balloon significantly improves nonalcoholic fatty liver disease activity score in obese patients with nonalcoholic steatohepatitis: a pilot study. Gastrointest Endosc 2012;76(4):756–60.
43. Chandan S, Mohan BP, Khan SR, et al. Efficacy and safety of intragastric balloon (IGB) in non-alcoholic fatty liver disease (NAFLD): a comprehensive review and meta-analysis. Obes Surg 2021;31(3):1271–9.

44. Haddad AE, Rammal MO, Soweid A, et al. Intragastric balloon treatment of obesity: long-term results and patient satisfaction. Turk J Gastroenterol 2019; 30(5):461–6.
45. Hajifathalian K, Mehta A, Ang B, et al. Improvement in insulin resistance and estimated hepatic steatosis and fibrosis after endoscopic sleeve gastroplasty. Gastrointest Endosc 2021;93(5):1110–8.
46. Jagtap N, Kalapala R, Katakwar A, et al. Endoscopic sleeve gastroplasty - minimally invasive treatment for non-alcoholic fatty liver disease and obesity. Indian J Gastroenterol 2021;40(6):572–9.
47. Lavín-Alconero L, Fernández-Lanas T, Iruzubieta-Coz P, et al. Efficacy and safety of endoscopic sleeve gastroplasty versus laparoscopic sleeve gastrectomy in obese subjects with Non-Alcoholic SteatoHepatitis (NASH): study protocol for a randomized controlled trial (TESLA-NASH study). Trials 2021;22(1):756.
48. Lopez Nava G, Arau RT, Asokkumar R, et al. Prospective multicenter study of the primary obesity surgery endoluminal (POSE 2.0) procedure for treatment of obesity. Clin Gastroenterol Hepatol 2022.
49. Jirapinyo P, de Moura DTH, Horton LC, et al. Effect of aspiration therapy on obesity-related comorbidities: systematic review and meta-analysis. Clin Endosc 2020;53(6):686–97.
50. Cohen RV, Shikora S, Petry T, et al. The diabetes surgery summit II guidelines: a disease-based clinical recommendation. Obes Surg 2016;26(8):1989–91.
51. Ruban A, Ashrafian H, Teare JP. The endobarrier: duodenal-jejunal bypass liner for diabetes and weight loss. Gastroenterol Res Pract 2018;2018:7823182.
52. Gollisch KS, Lindhorst A, Raddatz D. EndoBarrier gastrointestinal liner in type 2 diabetic patients improves liver fibrosis as assessed by liver elastography. Exp Clin Endocrinol Diabetes 2017;125(2):116–21.
53. Rohde U, Hedback N, Gluud LL, et al. Effect of the EndoBarrier Gastrointestinal Liner on obesity and type 2 diabetes: a systematic review and meta-analysis. Diabetes Obes Metab 2016;18(3):300–5.
54. van Baar ACG, Deviere J, Hopkins D, et al. Durable metabolic improvements 2 years after duodenal mucosal resurfacing (DMR) in patients with type 2 diabetes (REVITA-1 Study). Diabetes Res Clin Pract 2022;184:109194.
55. Mingrone G, van Baar AC, Deviere J, et al. Safety and efficacy of hydrothermal duodenal mucosal resurfacing in patients with type 2 diabetes: the randomised, double-blind, sham-controlled, multicentre REVITA-2 feasibility trial. Gut 2022; 71(2):254–64.
56. Bai J, Jia Z, Chen Y, et al. Bariatric surgery is effective and safe for obese patients with compensated cirrhosis: a systematic review and meta-analysis. World J Surg 2022;46(5):1122–33.
57. Are VS, Knapp SM, Banerjee A, et al. Improving outcomes of bariatric surgery in patients with cirrhosis in the United States: a nationwide assessment. Am J Gastroenterol 2020;115(11):1849–56.
58. Child CG, Turcotte JG. Surgery and portal hypertension. Major Probl Clin Surg 1964;1:1–85.
59. Teh SH, Nagorney DM, Stevens SR, et al. Risk factors for mortality after surgery in patients with cirrhosis. Gastroenterology 2007;132(4):1261–9.
60. Mahmud N, Fricker Z, Hubbard RA, et al. Risk prediction models for post-operative mortality in patients with cirrhosis. Hepatology 2021;73(1):204–18.
61. Schaeffer DF, Yoshida EM, Buczkowski AK, et al. Surgical morbidity in severely obese liver transplant recipients - a single Canadian Centre Experience. Ann Hepatol 2009;8(1):38–40.

62. Thapar M, Bonkovsky HL. Indications for liver transplant and AASLD guidelines. Hepatology 2015;61(1):408.
63. Sharpton SR, Terrault NA, Posselt AM. Outcomes of sleeve gastrectomy in obese liver transplant candidates. Liver Transpl 2019;25(4):538–44.
64. Heimbach JK, Watt KD, Poterucha JJ, et al. Combined liver transplantation and gastric sleeve resection for patients with medically complicated obesity and end-stage liver disease. Am J Transplant 2013;13(2):363–8.
65. Zamora-Valdes D, Watt KD, Kellogg TA, et al. Long-term outcomes of patients undergoing simultaneous liver transplantation and sleeve gastrectomy. Hepatology 2018;68(2):485–95.
66. Al-Nowaylati AR, Al-Haddad BJ, Dorman RB, et al. Gastric bypass after liver transplantation. Liver Transpl 2013;19(12):1324–9.
67. Lin MY, Tavakol MM, Sarin A, et al. Safety and feasibility of sleeve gastrectomy in morbidly obese patients following liver transplantation. Surg Endosc 2013;27(1):81–5.
68. Khoraki J, Katz MG, Funk LM, et al. Feasibility and outcomes of laparoscopic sleeve gastrectomy after solid organ transplantation. Surg Obes Relat Dis 2016;12(1):75–83.
69. Osseis M, Lazzati A, Salloum C, et al. Sleeve gastrectomy after liver transplantation: feasibility and outcomes. Obes Surg 2018;28(1):242–8.
70. Tsamalaidze L, Stauffer JA, Arasi LC, et al. Laparoscopic sleeve gastrectomy for morbid obesity in patients after orthotopic liver transplant: a matched case-control study. Obes Surg 2018;28(2):444–50.

Future Treatment Options and Regimens for Nonalcoholic Fatty Liver Disease

Sven Francque, MD, PhD[a,b,c,d,e,*], Vlad Ratziu, MD, PhD[f,g,h,*]

KEYWORDS

• Pharmacological treatment • NASH resolution • Fibrosis regression • Endpoints

KEY POINTS

- Assessing treatment efficacy in noncirrhotic nonalcoholic steatohepatitis currently relies on surrogate endpoints likely to predict clinically meaningful benefit.
- The failure of several drugs to hit their endpoints in phase 3 is in part reflective of the complex pathophysiology of the disease and the need to target the main drivers.
- Drugs that have a substantial impact on the metabolic drivers of the disease show promise but need further confirmation.
- Targeting several intrahepatic and extrahepatic key pathways simultaneously is probably required to achieve success in most patients.
- New compounds and innovative approaches are likely to change the therapeutic landscape in the near future.

INTRODUCTION

Although the progress in the field of nonalcoholic steatohepatitis (NASH) pharmacological treatment seems less spectacular compared with some other liver diseases, it has been significant and probably even decisive for future developments. A myriad of pathogenic studies aimed at identifying druggable targets (**Fig. 1**). The availability of candidate pharmacological agents and the flurry of NASH trials have provided the impetus for drug regulatory agencies to define a regulatory framework for drug

[a] Department of Gastroenterology and Hepatology, Antwerp University Hospital, Antwerp, Belgium; [b] Laboratory of Experimental Medicine and Paediatrics (LEMP), Faculty of Medicine and Health Sciences, University of Antwerp, Antwerp, Belgium; [c] InflaMed Centre of Excellence, University of Antwerp, Antwerp, Belgium; [d] Translational Sciences in Inflammation and Immunology, University of Antwerp, Antwerp, Belgium; [e] European Reference Network on Hepatological Diseases (ERN RARE-LIVER), Antwerp University Hospital, Drie Eikenstraat 665, Edegem B-2650, Belgium; [f] Sorbonne Université, Paris, France; [g] Institute of Cardiometabolism and Nutrition, Assistance Publique-Hôpitaux De Paris, Hôpital Pitié-Salpêtrière, 47-83 Boulevard de l'Hôpital, Paris Cedex 13 75651, France; [h] INSERM UMRS 1138 CRC, Paris, France
* Corresponding authors.
E-mail addresses: sven.francque@uza.be (S.F.); vlad.ratziu@inserm.fr (V.R.)

Clin Liver Dis 27 (2023) 429–449
https://doi.org/10.1016/j.cld.2023.01.010
liver.theclinics.com

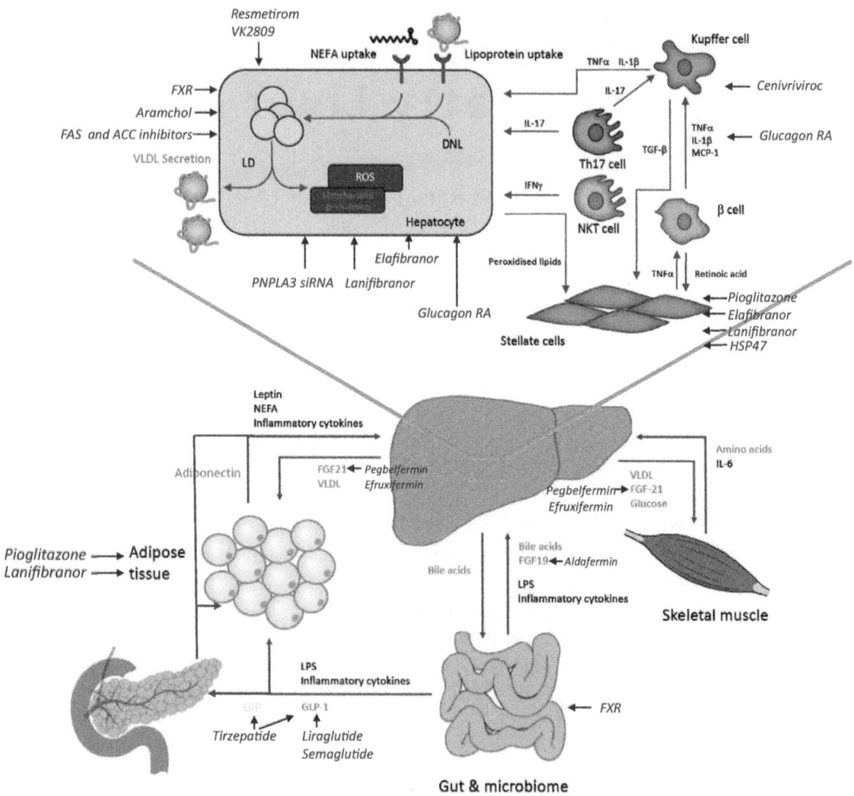

Fig. 1. Therapeutic targets in the complex pathophysiology of NASH. NASH is the result of a complex interplay of metabolic, inflammatory, and fibrogenic processes. Within the liver, hepatocytes and several of its intracellular organelles, most notably mitochondria, play an important role, alongside the stellate cells and several resident and infiltrating immune cells of different populations. NASH furthermore results from and affects an important crosstalk between the liver, the adipose tissue, the gut (including the gut microbiome), the muscle, and the pancreas. The cardiovascular system is also involved (not depicted, see[120]). Drugs that have been tested in NASH or that are under development have differential targets whether hepatic or extrahepatic. ACC, acetyl-CoA carboxylase; DNL, de novo lipogenesis; FAS, fatty acid synthase; FGF19, fibroblast growth factor 1; FGF21, fibroblast growth factor 21; FXR, farnesoid receptor X; GIP, glucose-dependent insulinotropic polypeptide; GLP-1, glucagon-like peptide 1; IFNγ, interferon gamma; IL1-β, interleukin 1 beta; IL-6, interleukin 6; IL-17, interleukin 17; LD, lipid droplets; LPS, lipopolysaccharide; MCP-1, monocyte chemoattractant protein 1; NEFA, nonesterified fatty acids; NKT cell, natural killer T cell; PNPLA3, patatin-like phospholipase domain-containing protein 3; RA, receptor agonist; ROS, reactive oxygen species; siRNA, small interfering RNA; Th17, T helper 17 cell; TGFβ, tumor growth factor beta; TNFα, tumor necrosis factor alpha; VLDL, very-low-density lipoproteins. (Figure adapted from[117] [courtesy J. Haas] and [121].)

approval in NASH.[1] The recognition of fibrotic NASH as a serious and life-threatening condition has justified an accelerated approval pathway[2]; this allows a drug to be given conditional approval, while awaiting the evidence of clinical benefit required for definitive approval. The rationale is to ensure faster patient access to potentially useful drugs in an area of unmet clinical need. Surrogate endpoints for conditional approval have been clearly defined: regression of fibrosis or resolution of NASH. These histological changes are achievable within a 12- to 18-month timeframe[3,4] and are therefore feasible within a trial context. Whether meeting these surrogate endpoints will result in clinical benefit has been questioned because no prospective demonstration is available yet; however, their use is currently supported by regulatory agencies.[2] Numerous retrospective studies have shown that fibrosis stage is associated with liver-related mortality and liver-related events,[5] and fibrosis stage reversal can even benefit patients with cirrhosis.[6] An important observation is that steatohepatitis itself increases the risk of liver-related events more than steatosis alone, even in the absence of fibrosis.[7] Moreover, changes in steatohepatitis status[8] (and, more widely speaking, in activity grade[9]) are positively associated with changes in fibrosis.[8,10] Thus, the chosen surrogates seem appropriate because they are achievable and have prognostic value. There are, however, caveats. Requiring complete NASH resolution could be unnecessarily strict, given the aforementioned relationship between changes in activity and changes in fibrosis. More importantly, documenting the disappearance of steatohepatitis, as defined by the absence of ballooned hepatocytes, can be very challenging, as even expert pathologists have difficulty agreeing on hepatocyte ballooning.[11] Finally, there are differences between European and American regulatory agencies regarding which combination of surrogate histological endpoints are acceptable.[12]

Clinical benefit required for definitive approval is typically tested in large long-term outcome trials[13] and is defined by mortality, liver transplantation, the occurrence of cirrhotic complications but also progression to compensated cirrhosis (defined clinically or histologically). In trials of midterm duration (typically 5 years) progression to cirrhosis is expected to be the most frequently occurring event. Although these outcomes have been repeatedly outlined by the regulatory agencies, the final decision relies not only on efficacy parameters but also on a complex assessment of the risk-benefit balance in the wider context of competing comorbidities in patients with NASH; this seems particularly relevant given that the chronic nature of the illness requires long-term therapy.

Recent Progress in Pharmacological Treatment

Over the past 15 years, many compounds have been explored for their utility in the treatment of NASH. A substantial number of trials have failed to meet prespecified primary endpoints. For some pathways, pharmacological intervention does seem to hold promise, and some new targets and approaches are currently explored.[14]

Farnesoid X Receptor Agonists

The farnesoid X receptor (FXR) plays an important role in bile acid metabolism but also on several metabolic, inflammatory, and fibrogenic pathways. FXR is present in the liver and the intestine, with some differences in effect according to the site.[15] Bile acids are the natural ligands of FXR. Ursodeoxycholic acid (UDCA) has no FXR agonistic effect, but the modified bile acid, obeticholic acid (OCA), is a potent FXR agonist currently licensed for the treatment of primary biliary cholangitis. In patients with NASH, the phase 2b Farnesoid X Receptor Ligand Obeticholic Acid in NASH Treatment (FLINT) study[16] demonstrated improvement of histological activity of steatohepatitis as defined by a greater than or equal to 2 points reduction in NAS (a composite score of steatosis, hepatocyte ballooning, and lobular inflammation) but also a beneficial effect on fibrosis without, however, a significant effect on resolution of NASH. Importantly, OCA has been the first (and to date the only one) to subsequently confirm the beneficial effects on fibrosis regression in the phase 3, REGENERATE trial (interim analysis on histological endpoints) after 18 months of treatment.[4] Nine hundred thirty-one patients with stage F2-F3 fibrosis were included in the primary analysis of this 3-arm trial. The fibrosis improvement endpoint was achieved by 12% of patients in the placebo group, 18% in the OCA 10 mg group (P = .045), and 23% in the OCA 25 mg group (P = .0002). These results were confirmed on a subsequent reading by different pathologists, including on several patients. NASH resolution is probably achievable given the effect of OCA on hepatocyte ballooning and lobular inflammation, although this endpoint was not formally met. Despite the efficacy on approvable surrogate endpoints, OCA is still not approved at the time of this writing, possibly because of a risk-benefit ratio that is still being assessed. OCA induces indeed several side effects such as dose-related pruritus, an increase in low-density lipoprotein (LDL) cholesterol (manageable with statin therapy) and biliary stones with cholecystitis. A black box warning has been issued due to several fatal cases mostly occurring following off-label prescriptions in patients with decompensated cirrhosis (Child-Pugh B or C) due to cholestatic diseases.

Several other bile acid FXR agonists are investigated, nor-UDCA being the most advanced (currently in phase 2) and promising. Non–bile acid FXR agonists are also actively developed with the prospect of reducing the unwanted side effects of OCA as a consequence of a lack of their enterohepatic cycle or due to different hepatic versus intestinal tropism or optimized pharmacokinetics. Compounds such as EDP-305[17] or MET-409[18] have confirmed a reduction in steatosis and biochemical efficacy but also pruritus as a dose-limiting, class effect, with, however, increases in LDL of a lesser magnitude.[19] Data from a 16-week trial of vonafexor, another nonsteroidal FXR agonist, suggested additional renal benefits to be further confirmed in larger trials.[20] Unfortunately, the only histological data available with a second-generation FXR agonist, a year-long trial of tropifexor, did not demonstrate efficacy when evaluated by traditional pathology, although assessment by digital pathology indicated patterns of fibrosis regression.[21] Tropifexor has been tested in a combination therapy with cenicriviroc and showed no benefit in favor of the combination,[22,23] although it is unclear whether this is due to the lack of efficacy of cenicriviroc.[24,25]

Fibroblast Growth Factors

As part of the FXR pathway, fibroblast growth factor (FGF) 19 is released by the intestinal cells on FXR stimulation, reaches the liver via the portal vein, and exerts its actions on bile acid metabolism via the FGF receptor 4 (FGFR4)/β-klotho (KLB) complex. FGFR4 is mainly expressed in the liver that confers a liver-targeted action of FGF19. FGF19 regulates hepatic bile acid synthesis by decreasing the expression of the rate-limiting enzyme (cholesterol 7 alpha-hydroxylase [CYP7A1]) of bile acid synthesis (which is also directly regulated by FXR).[26] FGF19 also affects lipid and glucose metabolism. However, by signaling via the IL-6/STAT3 pathway, FGF19 can drive tumorigenesis.[27]

NGM282 or aldafermin is an engineered FGF19 analogue that lacks the effect on the STAT3 pathway and hence most likely lacks the tumorigenic effect of FGF19. It demonstrated a significant reduction in liver fat content in a study including 82 patients with NASH.[28] A 24-week treatment in patients with F2-F3 fibrosis failed to reach the endpoint of fibrosis regression,[29]despite powerful suppression of toxic hydrophobic bile acids.[30] The drug is still under investigation in F4 patients (EudraCT Number: 2019–002341–38, NCT04210245).

FGF21 is another member of the FGF19 subfamily, also acting as a hormone. It is a so-called hepatokine, a peptide hormone mainly produced by the liver (but also by multiple other organs, including the pancreas; circulating levels are, however, mainly determined by the hepatic production) regulating sugar intake, glucose homeostasis, and energy expenditure. It also needs the KLB coreceptor and acts mainly through the FGFR1c, which is mainly coexpressed with KLB in the central nervous system and adipocytes.[26] Interestingly, in view of the peroxisome proliferator–activated receptor (PPAR) drugs in the pipeline, its expression in the liver is regulated by PPARα. Animal data suggest enhanced NASH and associated metabolic derangements induced by FGF21 deficiency and improvement on FGF21 administration.[31] Interestingly, obese humans have increased circulating FGF21 levels, suggesting cellular FGF21 resistance.[32]

Recent data demonstrated a beneficial effect on liver fat content of Pegbelfermin, an injectable pegylated analogue of human FGF21, along with a reduction in biomarkers of liver injury and fibrosis. Phase 2b studies with histological endpoints at week 24 were, however, negative possibly due to a waning of the effect (tachyphylaxis) after the first few months of therapy.[33] Efruxifermin, a human FGF21 with 3 mutations fused to an immunoglobulin G1 Fc domain, showed strong antisteatogenic effects in an early study.[34] Recently released results from a 24-week study demonstrated significant improvements in NASH resolution and fibrosis regression over placebo.[35] A small uncontrolled study of pegozafermin, another pegylated FGF21, has shown NASH resolution or fibrosis reduction in 47% of patients after 20 weeks of therapy with a strong antisteatogenic and biochemical response including improvement of lipid parameters. These promising compounds are to be further tested in longer, phase 2b trials.

Peroxisome Proliferator–Activated Receptor Agonists

PPARs were first described as members of the steroid hormone receptor superfamily of ligand-activated transcription factors causing proliferation of peroxisomes. Peroxisomes play an important role in fatty acid catabolism and in the pentose pathway and hence in energy metabolism. They also play a role in the reduction of reactive oxygen species.[36] However, the actions of the PPAR target pathways involve several other cell organelles, most notably mitochondria. The pleiotropic actions of PPARs ultimately makes them critical regulators of not only fatty acid metabolism[37] but also glucose metabolism, inflammation, and fibrogenesis.[37,38]

Three PPAR isotypes have been identified (α, β/δ, and γ),[39,40] the expression and actions of which differ according to isotype, organ, and intraorgan cell type, resulting in a complex system of nuclear receptor–mediated interorgan crosstalk.[41] The main ligands for PPARs are fatty acids and their metabolites.

Despite preclinical rationale,[42] clinical data on PPARα single agonists are scarce. Fenofibrate reduces lipid levels by activating PPARα, which is highly expressed in the liver, but has no effect on insulin sensitivity[43] or hepatic steatosis.[44] Pemafibrate, which also showed benefits in preclinical nonalcoholic fatty liver disease (NAFLD) models and in patients with diabetes and dyslipidemia, also failed to reduce liver fat content.[45]

Thiazolidinediones (TZD) are PPARγ agonists that improve insulin resistance (IR) by direct effects on adipose tissue.[46] PPARγ activation in humans is associated with a broad spectrum of metabolic effects in great part derived from restoring adipose tissue biology[47,48] and a decrease in chronic systemic inflammation,[49,50] changes that are strongly associated with improvement in liver histology in patients with NASH.[51] In patients with prediabetes or type 2 diabetes (T2DM), pioglitazone 45 mg daily for 6 months improved NASH with a trend toward improvement in fibrosis compared with placebo.[52] A subsequent 18-month randomized controlled trial (RCT) in 101 patients with biopsy-proven NASH[53] confirmed these results. More recently, in an RCT of 105 patients with T2DM, pioglitazone plus vitamin E improved steatosis, hepatocyte ballooning, and inflammation.[54] The effect of pioglitazone on liver fibrosis is still unclear, as the landmark 2-year, PIVENS trial did not show an effect on fibrosis, instead all other histological parameters of steatohepatitis improved.[48]

The dual PPARα/γ agonist saroglitazar has beneficial effects in experimental models of NASH[55] and significantly decreases alanine transaminase levels and improves the cardiometabolic profile of subjects with biopsy-proven NASH.[56] A randomized, double-blind, phase 2 trial showed a significant effect on liver fat content after 16 weeks of treatment.[57] A study with histological endpoints is ongoing (NCT05011305).

The selective PPARβ/δ agonist seladelpar (MBX-8025) improves insulin sensitivity and steatohepatitis in mouse models of NAFLD[58] but its development in human NAFLD has been abandoned.

In rodent models of NASH and/or liver fibrosis, the dual PPARα/δ agonist elafibranor reduced liver fibrosis progression.[59] In the phase 2b GOLDEN 505 study of 274 noncirrhotic patients with biopsy-proven NASH, elafibranor 120 mg daily, was superior to placebo (20% vs 11%; $P = .018$) in patients with higher baseline NAFLD activity score (NAS $\geq$ 4).[60] Furthermore, a secondary post hoc analysis based on a revised definition for the resolution of NASH (with disappearance of ballooning and disappearance of lobular inflammation or persistence of mild lobular inflammation [score of 0 or 1], without worsening in liver fibrosis [progression by $\geq$ 1 stage]) was met with the 120 mg daily dose in the intention-to-treat population (19% vs 12%, $P = .045$).[60] Also, patients who improved NASH also improved fibrosis. However, the phase 3 RESOLVE-IT trial (NCT02704403)[61] did not confirm a significant benefit of elafibranor over placebo in inducing NASH resolution.[62]

The concept of combining PPARα, -β/δ, and -γ activation may represent a novel and potentially more efficacious therapeutic approach compared with single or dual agonists by targeting the large array of disturbances that contribute to the development and progression of NASH.[63,64] Lanifibranor (IVA337) is an indole sulfonamide PPAR agonist that activates all 3 subtypes α, β/δ, and γ, giving it the potential to address all the key features of NASH,[63] namely inflammation, steatosis, ballooning, and fibrosis.[65] In in vitro and in vivo preclinical studies, lanifibranor prevented and induced the regression of preexisting fibrotic damage in the liver and other organs without the classic effects on body weight, fluid retention, and heart weight increase reported with TZDs. Lanifibranor also improved metabolic features relevant to NASH.[63] A 24-week treatment with 800 or 1200 mg once daily showed dose-dependent significant effects on both resolution of NASH without worsening of fibrosis (45% for 1200 mg vs 19% on placebo, $P < .001$) and regression of fibrosis without worsening of NASH (42% vs 24%, $P = .011$) as well as on the composite endpoint of NASH resolution and fibrosis stage improvement (31% vs 7%, $P < .001$) with a good safety and tolerability profile.[66] The compound is now being tested in a large phase 3 study (EudraCT Number: 2020–004986–38, NCT04849728).

Incretins and Other Metabolic Hormones

Another approach is related to incretins and other hormones that are mainly known to handle body energy homeostasis and hence regulate glucose and lipid metabolism in the main involved organs. Glucagon-like peptide 1(GLP-1) is mainly secreted by intestinal L cells (mainly located in the ileum and colon) after exposure to nutrients. It stimulates insulin secretion by pancreatic β cells and inhibits glucagon secretion, hence contributing to the control of postprandial glycaemia. GLP-1 also affects on satiety by action on the central nervous system and by slowing gastric emptying and intestinal transit. It also has a positive impact on beta-cell health and proliferation.[67]

Treatment with GLP-1 receptor agonist have shown considerable benefit in the treatment of diabetes and obesity and conferring long-term cardiovascular protection. Several studies have assessed their utility for the treatment of NASH. Data with histological endpoints come from a small 1-year trial with liraglutide and a larger 18-month trial with semaglutide.[3,68] Both studies show, besides improvements in body weight, glycemic control, and lipid profile, an improvement in liver histology in terms of features of steatohepatitis. Semaglutide at a daily dose of 0.4 mg subcutaneously resulted in a placebo-subtracted effect size of 42% for NASH resolution with no worsening of fibrosis, confirming previous observations with liraglutide.

Looking at the global picture of fibrosis improvers, stabilizers, or worseners, the overall picture suggests nevertheless a beneficial effect on fibrosis with numerically less fibrosis worseners and more improvers in semaglutide-treated versus placebo-treated patients, but without reaching the endpoint of 1-stage regression of fibrosis without worsening of NASH despite 18 months of treatment and a strong effect on steatohepatitis.[3]

An important question is hence to understand the drivers of improvement. As no GLP-1 receptors are present in the liver, it is likely that the observed results are attributable to the improvement of the metabolic milieu and hence indirect actions of the drug. Whether longer treatment will result in more pronounced effects on fibrosis remains to be demonstrated. Side effects are mainly gastrointestinal. The drug is currently in the phase 3 ESSENCE trial (EudraCT 2019–004594–44, NTC U1111-1244–3678).

Dual agonists are currently being tested associating an effect on glucagon, glucose-dependent insulinotropic polypeptide (GIP), or FGF21 receptors in addition to GLP1 receptors. Some of these drugs have shown particularly strong weight loss effects.[69] BI 456906 is a dual agonist of GLP-1 and glucagon (GCG) receptors. Of note, glucagon secretion as such is inhibited by GLP-1. The endocrine action of glucagon increases fatty acid disposal through beta-oxidation (and, possibly, energy expenditure) and can hence reduce body weight. The dual compound is hence expected to result in a more pronounced body weight compared with the individual molecules, which might also translate into a more pronounced improvement in liver histology. Furthermore, in contrast to GLP-1, glucagon receptors are present in the liver and GCG receptors might directly increase the fatty acid oxidation in the liver, potentially reducing the lipotoxicity. Glucagon also affects bile acid metabolism, inflammation, and immune cell activation.[70] Such partially direct intrahepatic effects might theoretically further enhance efficacy. The phase 2 trial is ongoing (EudraCT 2020–002723–11; NCT04771273).

Another neuroendocrine peptide hormone under study is amylin, which is cosecreted with insulin by pancreatic β cells in response to food intake and which affects several postprandial processes, for example, delays gastric emptying and suppresses of glucagon secretion.[71] Besides its glucoregulatory properties, amylin has binding sites in areas of the brain known to be involved in the regulation of energy homeostasis. Long-acting analogues are currently studied in combination therapies, more specifically with semaglutide (EudraCT 2020–003566–39; NTC NNC0174–0833).

Emerging data suggest that the gut-derived nutrient-induced incretin GIP operates at the interface of metabolism and inflammation. GIP is released after a meal by the K cells in the duodenum and ileum and, similar to GLP-1, increases pancreatic insulin secretion in a glucose-dependent manner. It also affects satiety and energy expenditure. GIP has, however, many other actions, mainly on different types of immune cells and hence influences immune cell metabolism, with direct and indirect effects on adipose tissue depots and energy expenditure, as well as the liver.[72,73] Tirzepatide is a GLP1-GIP dual agonist currently studied in NASH with histological endpoints, after positive results on biomarkers in patients with T2D with markers indicative of the presence of NASH (EudraCT 2019–001550–26; NCT04166773).[74] A triple GLP-1/GIP/glucagon receptor agonist is even in development.[75]

De Novo Lipogenesis

De novo lipogenesis (DNL) is an important source of liver fat in the context of NAFLD. Aramchol, a fatty-acid/bile acid conjugate, is an inhibitor of hepatic stearoyl-CoA desaturase-1, a key enzyme in hepatic lipogenesis that converts saturated fatty acids into monounsaturated fatty acids. Aramchol has direct effects on both hepatocytes and hepatic stellate cells, in the latter associated with increased PPARγ expression and reduced expression of profibrotic genes.[76]

In a 52-week phase 2b study comparing 2 doses of Aramchol with placebo, besides numerically reducing liver fat as measured by MR spectroscopy, Aramchol, 600 mg, resulted in a numerically higher rate of NASH resolution without worsening of fibrosis compared with placebo (16.7 vs 5%, $P = .051$), an analysis restricted to patients with both baseline and end-of-treatment liver biopsy available.[77] Based on these results and the good safety and tolerability profile, the compound is now in phase 3 (EudraCT 2019–002073–56, NCT04104321).

Acetyl-CoA carboxylase (ACC) catalyzes the first step in DNL and modulates mitochondrial fatty acid oxidation. Increased hepatic DNL flux and reduced fatty acid oxidation are hypothesized to contribute to steatosis. Some proinflammatory cells also show increased dependency on DNL, suggesting that ACC may regulate aspects of the inflammatory response in NASH.[78] Firsocostat is a liver-targeted ACC inhibitor that was tested alone or in several combinations in patients with advanced fibrosis for 48 weeks. Albeit no statistical differences were observed compared with placebo, the combination of firsocostat with an FXR agonist had numerically a higher rate of fibrosis regression and also improved several features of steatohepatitis.[79] ACC inhibition typically results in hypertriglyceridemia, which can be mitigated by fibrates or DGAT2 inhibitors.[80] Several ACC1/2 inhibitors and combination therapies are under investigation.[81] Fatty acid synthase is a downstream target of lipogenesis that has been successfully modulated by a small molecule inhibitor, TVB-2640, with strong antisteatogenic and biochemical efficacy in an early phase NASH trial.[82]

Thyromimetics

Thyroid hormones increase energy expenditure and have catabolic properties, acting via the thyroid hormone receptor (THR), a nuclear receptor with different isoforms. In the liver, known effects of thyroid receptor activation on lipid metabolism include increased cholesterol metabolism via expression of the enzyme CYP7A1 and reduced DNL through suppressed expression of hepatic sterol regulatory element-binding protein-1.[83] An intrahepatic hypothyroidism is present in NASH and potentially contributes to its pathophysiology. This intrahepatocytic hypothyroidism is potentially attributable to alterations in hepatic deiodinase expression because of repair-related Hedgehog activation.[84] The incidence of clinical and subclinical hypothyroidism has also been reported to be higher in patients with NAFLD or NASH relative to age-matched controls.[85,86]

The THR agonist resmetirom (MGL-3196) has a selectivity for the TRH-β1 receptor (it is around 28 times more selective than triiodothyronine for THR-β vs THR-α) that is mainly expressed in the liver and the kidney, and therefore, resmetirom most likely lacks some potentially important side effects of thyroid agonism, among others, on bone metabolism. Furthermore, this orally active compound is liver directed and is highly protein bound (>99%), with poor tissue penetration outside the liver.[87] In phase 2, resmetirom significantly reduced liver fat content after 12 weeks of treatment, with concomitant beneficial effects on liver enzymes and markers of liver inflammation, apoptosis, and fibrosis. Paired liver biopsies were obtained in 107 patients in the same trial after 36 weeks of treatment. NASH resolution without fibrosis worsening was significantly more frequent in the resmetirom arm compared with placebo, if patients with greater than 9.5% of weight loss (which only occurred in the placebo group) were excluded from the analysis, or when only MRI-PDFF responders were considered. No fibrosis improvement was detected histologically. There was no effect on body weight and glycemic control, but there was a significant improvement in atherogenic lipids (a decrease in triglycerides and LDL cholesterol, Lipoprotein (a), apolipoprotein [Apo]-B, and Apo-C3). There was no impact on bone mineral density. The compound is now further explored in several phase 3 trials (NCT04951219, NCT04197479, NCT03900429).[88]

Another compound with liver-specific thyromimetic properties is VK2809. VK2809 is a THR β-selective agent using a proprietary prodrug technology that confers lower systemic and tissue distribution relative to thyroid hormone and other thyromimetic drug classes. First-pass extraction of VK2809 in the liver, coupled with liver-specific activation to VK2809A and limited distribution of VK2809A to extrahepatic tissues, should confer a high degree of liver selectivity to the pharmacological effects of this agent. Currently, a phase 2 study with histological endpoints (as secondary endpoints) is ongoing (NCT04173065).[89]

Genetic Targets

Interfering with gene expression by small interfering RNAs (siRNA) is increasingly applied to treat disease. RNA interference is a naturally occurring cellular mechanism for regulation of gene expression: siRNA binds to its complementary messenger RNA (mRNA) sequence, which leads to mRNA cleavage and subsequent suppression of the synthesis and levels of the target protein.[90]

Hydroxysteroid 17β dehydrogenase 13 (HSD17B13) is a member of the 17β hydroxysteroid dehydrogenase (HSD) family, consisting of 14 structurally related enzymes implicated in steroid and fatty acid metabolism.[91] HDS17B13 is primarily expressed in the liver and is a lipid droplet enzyme with retinol dehydrogenase properties. It is highly expressed in patients with NAFLD compared with healthy controls, and variants of the *HSD17B13* gene have recently been associated with reduced hepatic injury, fibrosis, and inflammation among patients with NASH. The most common of these variants results in a truncated version of HSD17B13 protein that is catalytically defective and less stable, suggesting that the wild-type protein is associated with the development of NASH and its loss of function is protective against NASH and adverse outcomes among NASH patients.[92,93] ALN-HSD is an siRNA directly reducing hepatic *HSD17B13* expression, thereby mimicking the genetic loss of HSD17B13 function, which is expected to result in reduction of the hepatic injury in NASH. It is specifically designed for delivery into hepatocytes through conjugation of a carbohydrate ligand to the siRNA, resulting in uptake of siRNA via the asialoglycoprotein receptor after subcutaneous administration and is in early phase of development (NCT04565717). Results from an early trial have demonstrated a 90% inhibition of the expression of HSD17B13 mRNA.[94]

Another target of this approach is heat shock protein 47 (HSP47). HSP47 is a necessary component of the collagen deposition mechanism in myofibroblasts. By acting as an intracellular chaperone of early collagen precursors for type I to type V collagens, HSP47 facilitates collagen formation, prevents collagen degradation, and ensures proper triple-helix formation of procollagen in the endoplasmic reticulum. Although HSP47 is not the initiating factor in the pathologic accumulation of extracellular collagen matrix, several experimental models have shown that HSP47 is required to produce high-quality collagen and that its intracellular levels increase with increased demand for collagen synthesis.[95,96] BMS-986263 is a lipid nanoparticle formulation that incorporates 6 lipid components and a retinoid-conjugated targeting agent (di-retinamide-PEG-di-retinamide [DPD]). The DPD moiety is present on the external surface of the nanoparticle and enables targeting and uptake by hepatic stellate cells via receptors for retinol-binding protein. The lipid nanoparticles contain a siRNA designed to suppress *HSP47* expression. The resultant decreased intracellular level of HSP47 should lead to a decrease in the formation of stable collagen and is hypothesized to result in decreased liver fibrosis. The compound has been tested in patients with hepatitis-C–related advanced fibrosis* and is currently studied in patients with NASH cirrhosis (NCT 04267393).[97]

The isoleucine-to-methionine substitution at position 148 (I148M) (rs738409C > G encoding for PNPLA3 I148M) in the patatin-like phospholipase domain-containing protein 3 (PNPLA3) is strongly associated with NAFLD and its severity and in particular also with the risk of hepatocellular carcinoma (HCC). Homozygosity for the common variant seems to confer a 10-fold increased risk of HCC in NAFLD.[98–100] The I148M PNPLA3 mutation has, however, also been shown to be of importance in other liver diseases.[101] The wild-type PNPLA3 protein has triglyceride and retinyl esters hydrolase activity. The 148M substitution induces a loss of function in this enzymatic activity, which results in an entrapment of triglycerides and retinyl esters in lipid droplets of hepatocytes and hepatic stellate cells.[102] The latter then induces liver damage. The mechanism is related to the accumulation of mutated 148M on lipid droplets, where it escapes proteasomal degradation and inhibits the activity of other lipases.[103] In mice fed an NASH-inducing diet, treatment with antisense oligonucleotide directed against PNPLA3 leads to improvements in steatosis. Furthermore, in mice carrying the human I148M mutant, antisense oligonucleotide treatment improves inflammation and fibrosis.[104] The aim is hence to reduce the overexpression of the I148M variant. Therefore, AZD2693, a compound with an siRNA lowering the mRNA expression of PNPLA3, is currently explored in patients who are homozygotes for the 148M risk allele.

Antifibrotic Drugs

As mentioned, fibrosis is an important target for therapy. Despite NASH being the driver of disease progression, fibrosis is the strongest predictor of liver-related outcomes as well as overall mortality.[105] Liver-related events also drive morbidity and mortality in patients with advanced fibrosis.[106] These patients do not decompensate and die from fibrosis *per se*, but fibrosis progression to cirrhosis results in the development of portal hypertension and hepatic insufficiency, which will drive cirrhosis decompensation. Fibrosis regression or even preventing fibrosis progression is therefore a rational objective, although to what extent this will translate in improved outcomes need to be studied.

Unfortunately, several drugs failed to demonstrate robust fibrosis regression, remarkably, all of them with a plausible antifibrotic mode of action. Cenicriviroc is a dual CCR2 and CCR5 antagonist. CCR2 and CCR5 play an important role in macrophage recruitment and polarization and have been implicated in NASH pathogenesis. Despite this rational mode of action, cenicriviroc did not show an effect on NASH resolution,[17] and the significant benefit of cenicriviroc over placebo in terms of regression of fibrosis after 1 year of treatment[24] was unfortunately not confirmed with additional duration[25] or in a subsequent phase 3 trial. Simtuzumab is a lysyl oxidase homolog 2 antibody interfering with collagen cross-linking and is an example of a pure antifibrotic approach. Yet simtuzumab failed in 2 large NASH trials.[107] Selonsertib is an inhibitor of apoptosis signal-regulating kinase 1, which is involved in response to various cellular stresses. It was tested in a small, 6-month trial, alone or in combination with simtuzumab, and demonstrated a higher proportion of fibrosis regression versus the comparator[108] but without an effect on steatohepatitis, aminotransferases, or metabolic features. Unsurprisingly, the phase 3 trials failed to confirm a significant benefit in terms of fibrosis regression.[109]

WHAT EXPLAINS SO MANY FAILURES?

Several factors need to be considered to find an explanation for this high number of failures.[110] First, the trial endpoints being determined by histological reading, robust pathological assessment is crucial. Unfortunately, even the most experienced pathologists cannot eliminate the significant intra- and interobserver variability, let alone imprecisions or subjectivity in the definition or grading/staging of histological lesions.[11,111] However, a recent subanalysis of the semaglutide phase 2b trial analyzing histological changes by digital pathology yielded the same conclusions as the primary analysis. Although digital pathology does have a higher sensitivity to detect changes for different histological parameters, whether changes that are not detectable through conventional pathology are relevant for clinical outcomes remains to be determined. Another issue with the liver biopsy is sampling variability. Assessing a larger size biopsy or assessing several sections instead of a single slide can improve, although not completely mitigate, this issue but runs into serious feasibility issues in clinical trials. It should, however, be acknowledged that the noninvasive serum and imaging markers have been proposed as alternatives to the liver biopsy but these noninvasive diagnoses also have substantial variability.[112,113] Replacing an imperfect reference standard by another imperfect reference standard will not solve the issue. The limitations of the biopsy hence do not explain the whole picture.

Two other elements need to be considered. First, the definition of the endpoint only considers patients who show improvement in their fibrosis stage. However, halting disease progression might be as valuable, and absence of progression should also result in less progression to cirrhosis and hence liver-related events.[114] The placebo-subtracted effect size of OCA for fibrosis regression was 15% (in the per protocol analysis), whereas 8% less patients progressed compared with placebo, and thereby the overall antifibrotic benefit was higher than anticipated from fibrosis regression only.[4] Lanifibranor showed a comparable picture, with 14% and 5% placebo-subtracted effect size for regression and reduced progression of fibrosis, respectively.[66] The greater than or equal to 1-stage improvement in fibrosis is a high barrier endpoint. Despite numerical differences, semaglutide did not reach this endpoint, but here too fibrosis progression was slower on drug than on placebo, suggesting an overall beneficial impact on fibrosis.[115]

A second element brings back the concept of NASH as the driver of disease progression. Paired biopsy studies have shown that changes in fibrosis and disease activity occur in parallel.[9] One may therefore question if in order to obtain fibrosis regression it is not necessary to reduce disease activity. NASH resolution was the strongest predictor of fibrosis regression in a recent post-hoc analysis of NASH CRN trials,[8] and a subanalysis of the elafibranor phase 2 GOLDEN trial showed correlation between changes in disease activity and fibrosis.[116] Lanifibranor not only induced fibrosis regression but also significantly induced NASH resolution, and OCA significantly improved ballooning and inflammation.[4,66] As mentioned, the strong effect of semaglutide on NASH resolution also was accompanied by a signal of beneficially affecting fibrosis evolution over time.[115] By contrast, cenicriviroc showed no effect on steatohepatitis[25] and had a questionable impact on fibrosis. Also, other compounds without an effect on steatohepatitis (eg, simtuzumab and selonsertib) failed to show an effect on fibrosis.[109] It is therefore likely that drugs that act only on mechanisms of fibrosis but that have no or insufficient effect on the upstream processes of metabolic dysfunction, cell damage, and inflammation may not achieve long-lasting fibrosis regression (**Fig. 2**).

Another legitimate question is whether compounds with a narrow mode of action tackling single pathways (eg, key enzymatic steps in de novo lipogenesis, blockage of a specific chemokine receptor subtype) might fail given the complexity of disease pathophysiology[117] and the existence of many other "rescue" or redundant pathways. Of course, combination therapies seem very appealing, despite having their own numerous challenges.

THE FUTURE OF NONALCOHOLIC STEATOHEPATITIS THERAPEUTICS

Given the complexity of its pathogenesis, there is great interest in the development of combination therapies targeting different aspects of NASH. Several elements will, however, need to be considered.

Antidiabetic drugs such as GLP-1 receptor agonists and sodium-glucose cotransporter-2 (SGLT2) inhibitors have proved efficacy in preventing cardiovascular or nephrological outcomes and are likely to be the background therapy for many diabetic patients with NASH in the near future. Although there are no data on hepatic histological benefit of SGLT2 inhibitors, GLP1 receptor agonists or dual or triple agonists are

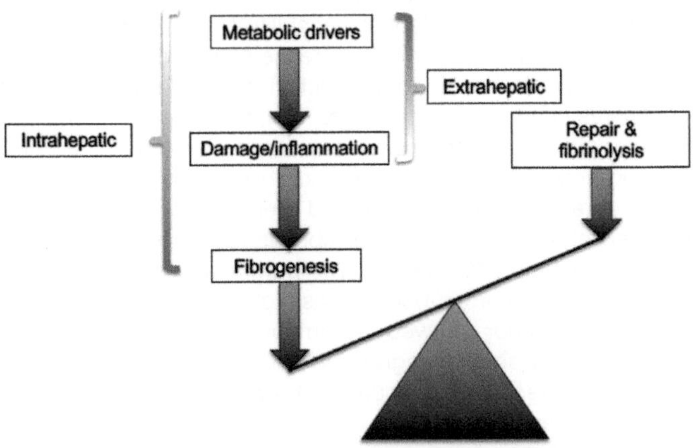

Fig. 2. Progression of disease in nonalcoholic steatohepatitis (NASH). Progression occurs when profibrogenic mechanisms are not sufficiently counteracted by repair mechanisms. Fibrosis is driven by processes of cell damage and inflammation, mostly initiated by lipotoxicity associated with adipose tissue dysfunction and insulin resistance. Thus, hepatic fibrosis is the end-stage adaptive response to injury. This makes the fibrogenic process difficult to control by a putative antifibrotic drug only, if upstream driving pathways are not being controlled. Ideally pleiotropic drugs or combinations thereof should act at several levels of this pathogenic sequence. (*Adapted from* Ref.[122])

actively tested for NASH. If the histological efficacy seen in early trials is confirmed, most diabetic NASH patients will be treated with these drugs, and compounds specifically developed for NASH and not for diabetes or weight loss will have to prove additional efficacy in order to be adopted. Combination strategies will have to consider specific approaches, such as induction and maintenance strategies versus intermittent cycled therapy versus sequential therapies depending on the potency and tolerability of future agents.

Also, given the biological complexity and clinical heterogeneity of NASH and its comorbidities, identification of the precise drivers of disease would support the development of targeted therapeutics. Understanding how precision or individualized medicine should be conducted will require studies on large numbers of well phenotyped and genotyped patients. The use of polygenic risk scores to identify individuals with specific risk characteristics and pathways of liver injury will be pivotal for successful implementation of personalized medicine approaches. Recent data from the Million Veterans Program[118] support this concept but currently do not go beyond providing insights on the development of fatty liver.[119] It will be crucial to integrate genomic, phenomic, and transcriptomic data to advance the field toward specifically targeted therapeutics that will benefit the largest number of patients with NASH.

DISCLOSURE

S. Francque holds a senior clinical investigator fellowship from the Research Foundation Flanders (FWO) (1802154N). His institution has received grants from Astellas, Falk Pharma, Genfit, Gilead Sciences, GlympsBio, Janssens Pharmaceutica, Inventiva, Merck Sharp & Dome, Pfizer, and Roche. S. Francque has acted as consultant for Abbvie, Actelion, Aelin Therapeutics, Aligos Therapeutics, Allergan, Astellas, Astra Zeneca, Bayer, Boehringer Ingelheim, Bristol-Meyers Squibb, CSL Behring, Coherus, Echosens, Eisai, Enyo, Galapagos, Galmed, Genetech, Genfit, Gilead Sciences, Intercept, Inventiva, Janssens Pharmaceutica, Julius Clinical, Madrigal, Medimmune, Merck Sharp & Dome, NGM Bio, Novartis, Novo Nordisk, Promethera, and Roche. S. Francque has been lecturer for Abbvie, Allergan, Bayer, Eisai, Genfit, Gilead Sciences, Janssens Cilag, Intercept, Inventiva, Merck Sharp & Dome, Novo Nordisk, and Promethera. V. Ratziu has acted as consultant for Boehringer Ingelheim, Bristol-Myers-Squibb, Enyo, Intercept Pharmaceuticals, Madrigal, Novo Nordisk, Pfizer, Poxel, and Terns. His institution received research grants from Gilead Sciences and Intercept Pharmaceuticals.

REFERENCES

1. Sanyal AJ, Friedman SL, Mccullough AJ, et al. Challenges and opportunities in drug and biomarker development for nonalcoholic steatohepatitis: findings and recommendations from an American association for the study of liver diseases-U.S. Food and drug administration joint workshop. Hepatology 2015;61(4):1392–405.
2. Anania FA, Dimick-Santos L, Mehta R, et al. Nonalcoholic steatohepatitis: current thinking from the division of hepatology and nutrition at the food and drug administration. Hepatology 2021;73(5):2023–7.
3. Newsome PN, Buchholtz K, Cusi K, et al. A placebo-controlled trial of subcutaneous semaglutide in nonalcoholic steatohepatitis. N Engl J Med 2021;384(12):1113–24.

4. Younossi ZM, Ratziu V, Loomba R, et al. Obeticholic acid for the treatment of non-alcoholic steatohepatitis: interim analysis from a multicentre, randomised, placebo-controlled phase 3 trial. Lancet 2019;394(10215):2184–96.
5. Taylor RS, Taylor RJ, Bayliss S, et al. Association between fibrosis stage and outcomes of patients with nonalcoholic fatty liver disease: a systematic review and meta-analysis. Gastroenterology 2020;158(6). https://doi.org/10.1053/j.gastro.2020.01.043.
6. Sanyal AJ, Anstee QM, Trauner M, et al. Cirrhosis regression is associated with improved clinical outcomes in patients with nonalcoholic steatohepatitis. Hepatology 2022;75(5):1235–46.
7. Simon TG, Roelstraete B, Khalili H, et al. Mortality in biopsy-confirmed nonalcoholic fatty liver disease: results from a nationwide cohort. Gut 2021;70(7):1375–82.
8. Brunt EM, Kleiner DE, Wilson LA, et al, Nonalcoholic Steatohepatitis Clinical Research Network. Improvements in histologic features and diagnosis associated with improvement in fibrosis in nonalcoholic steatohepatitis: results from the nonalcoholic steatohepatitis clinical research network treatment trials. Hepatology 2019;70(2):522–31.
9. Kleiner DE, Brunt EM, Wilson LA, et al. Association of histologic disease activity with progression of nonalcoholic fatty liver disease. JAMA Netw Open 2019;2(10). e1912565.
10. Ratziu V, Francque S, Harrison SH. Improvement in NASH histological activity highly correlates with fibrosis regression. Hepatology 2016;64(LB21).
11. Brunt EM, Clouston AD, Goodman Z, et al. Complexity of ballooned hepatocyte feature recognition: defining a training atlas for artificial intelligence-based imaging in NAFLD. J Hepatol 2022;76(5):1030–41.
12. Loomba R, Ratziu V, Harrison SA. NASH clinical trial design international working group. Expert panel review to compare FDA and EMA guidance on drug development and endpoints in nonalcoholic steatohepatitis. Gastroenterology 2022;162(3):680–8.
13. Ratziu V, Sanyal AJ, Loomba R, et al. REGENERATE: design of a pivotal, randomised, phase 3 study evaluating the safety and efficacy of obeticholic acid in patients with fibrosis due to nonalcoholic steatohepatitis. Contemp Clin Trials 2019;84. 105803.
14. Ratziu V, Francque S, Sanyal A. Breakthroughs in therapies for NASH and remaining challenges. J Hepatol 2022;76(6):1263–78.
15. Chávez-Talavera O, Tailleux A, Lefebvre P, et al. Bile acid control of metabolism and inflammation in obesity, type 2 diabetes, dyslipidemia, and nonalcoholic fatty liver disease. Gastroenterology 2017;152(7):1679–94.e3.
16. Neuschwander-Tetri BA, Loomba R, Sanyal AJ, et al. Farnesoid X nuclear receptor ligand obeticholic acid for non-cirrhotic, non-alcoholic steatohepatitis (FLINT): a multicentre, randomised, placebo-controlled trial. Lancet 2015;385(9972):956–65.
17. Ratziu V, Rinella ME, Neuschwander-Tetri BA, et al. EDP-305 in patients with NASH: a phase II double-blind placebo-controlled dose-ranging study. J Hepatol 2022;76(3):506–17.
18. Harrison SA, Bashir MR, Lee KJ, et al. A structurally optimized FXR agonist, MET409, reduced liver fat content over 12 weeks in patients with nonalcoholic steatohepatitis. J Hepatol 2021;75(1):25–33.

19. Patel K, Harrison SA, Elkhashab M, et al. Cilofexor, a nonsteroidal FXR agonist, in patients with noncirrhotic NASH: a phase 2 randomized controlled trial. Hepatology 2020;72(1):58–71.
20. Ratziu V, Harrison SA, Loustaud-Ratti V, et al. Hepatic and renal improvements with FXR agonist vonafexor in individuals with suspected fibrotic NASH. J Hepatol 2022. https://doi.org/10.1016/j.jhep.2022.10.023. S0168-8278(22) 03160-9.
21. Naoumov N v, Brees D, Loeffler J, et al. Digital pathology with artificial intelligence analyses provides greater insights into treatment-induced fibrosis regression in NASH. J Hepatol 2022;77(5):1399–409.
22. Pedrosa M, Seyedkazemi S, Francque S, et al. A randomized, double-blind, multicenter, phase 2b study to evaluate the safety and efficacy of a combination of tropifexor and cenicriviroc in patients with nonalcoholic steatohepatitis and liver fibrosis: study design of the TANDEM trial. Contemp Clin Trials 2020;88. 105889.
23. Anstee Quentin M, Lucas Kathryn Jean, Francque Sven M, et al. Safety and efficacy of Tropifexor plus Cenicriviroc combination therapy in adult patients with fibrotic NASH: 48 week results from the phase 2b tandem study. Hepatology 2021;74(1 suppl):142.
24. Friedman SL, Ratziu V, Harrison SA, et al. A randomized, placebo-controlled trial of cenicriviroc for treatment of nonalcoholic steatohepatitis with fibrosis. Hepatology 2018;67(5):1754–67.
25. Ratziu V, Sanyal A, Harrison SA, et al. Cenicriviroc treatment for adults with nonalcoholic steatohepatitis and fibrosis: final analysis of the phase 2b CENTAUR study. Hepatology 2020;72(3):892–905.
26. Henriksson E, Andersen B. FGF19 and FGF21 for the treatment of NASH-two sides of the same coin? Differential and overlapping effects of FGF19 and FGF21 from mice to human. Front Endocrinol 2020;11. 601349.
27. Zhao H, Lv F, Liang G, et al. FGF19 promotes epithelial-mesenchymal transition in hepatocellular carcinoma cells by modulating the GSK3β/β- catenin signaling cascade via FGFR4 activation. Oncotarget 2016;7(12):13575–86.
28. Harrison SA, Rinella ME, Abdelmalek MF, et al. NGM282 for treatment of nonalcoholic steatohepatitis: a multicentre, randomised, double-blind, placebo-controlled, phase 2 trial. Lancet 2018;391(10126):1174–85.
29. Harrison SA, Neff G, Guy CD, et al. Efficacy and safety of aldafermin, an engineered FGF19 analog, in a randomized, double-blind, placebo-controlled trial of patients with nonalcoholic steatohepatitis. Gastroenterology 2021;160(1). https://doi.org/10.1053/j.gastro.2020.08.004.
30. Sanyal AJ, Ling L, Beuers U, et al. Potent suppression of hydrophobic bile acids by aldafermin, an FGF19 analogue, across metabolic and cholestatic liver diseases. JHEP Rep 2021;3(3). 100255.
31. Rusli F, Deelen J, Andriyani E, et al. Fibroblast growth factor 21 reflects liver fat accumulation and dysregulation of signalling pathways in the liver of C57BL/6J mice. Sci Rep 2016;6. 30484.
32. Dushay J, Chui PC, Gopalakrishnan GS, et al. Increased fibroblast growth factor 21 in obesity and nonalcoholic fatty liver disease. Gastroenterology 2010; 139(2):456–63.
33. Loomba Rohit, J Sanyal Arun, Nakajima Atsushi, et al. LO5: efficacy and safety of PEGBELFERMIN in patients with nonalcoholic steatohepatitis and stage 3 fibrosis: results from the phase 2b, randomized, double-blind, placebocontrolled falcon 1 study. JHEP 2022;74(1 suppl).

34. Harrison SA, Ruane PJ, Freilich BL, et al. Efruxifermin in non-alcoholic steatohepatitis: a randomized, double-blind, placebo-controlled, phase 2a trial. Nat Med 2021;27(7):1262–71.
35. Harrison SA, Frias JP, Neff GW, et al. Efruxifermin (EFX) in nonalcoholic steatohepatitis with fibrosis: results from a randomized, double-blind, placebo-controlled, phase 2b trial (HARMONY). Hepatology 2022;76(Suppl. 1):LB5.
36. Wanders RJA, Waterham HR. Biochemistry of mammalian peroxisomes revisited. Annu Rev Biochem 2006;75:295–332.
37. Dreyer C, Krey G, Keller H, et al. Control of the peroxisomal beta-oxidation pathway by a novel family of nuclear hormone receptors. Cell 1992;68(5):879–87.
38. Samuel VT, Shulman GI. Nonalcoholic fatty liver disease as a nexus of metabolic and hepatic diseases. Cell Metab 2018;27(1):22–41.
39. Michalik L, Auwerx J, Berger JP, et al. International union of pharmacology. LXI. Peroxisome proliferator-activated receptors. Pharmacol Rev 2006;58(4):726–41.
40. Fajas L, Auboeuf D, Raspé E, et al. The organization, promoter analysis, and expression of the human PPARgamma gene. J Biol Chem 1997;272(30):18779–89.
41. Tailleux A, Wouters K, Staels B. Roles of PPARs in NAFLD: potential therapeutic targets. Biochim Biophys Acta 2012;1821(5):809–18.
42. Larter CZ, Yeh MM, van Rooyen DM, et al. Peroxisome proliferator-activated receptor-α agonist, Wy 14,643, improves metabolic indices, steatosis and ballooning in diabetic mice with non-alcoholic steatohepatitis. J Gastroenterol Hepatol 2012;27(2):341–50.
43. Belfort R, Berria R, Cornell J, et al. Fenofibrate reduces systemic inflammation markers independent of its effects on lipid and glucose metabolism in patients with the metabolic syndrome. J Clin Endocrinol Metab 2010;95(2):829–36.
44. Fabbrini E, Mohammed BS, Korenblat KM, et al. Effect of fenofibrate and niacin on intrahepatic triglyceride content, very low-density lipoprotein kinetics, and insulin action in obese subjects with nonalcoholic fatty liver disease. J Clin Endocrinol Metab 2010;95(6):2727–35.
45. Nakajima A, Eguchi Y, Yoneda M, et al. Randomised clinical trial: Pemafibrate, a novel selective peroxisome proliferator-activated receptor α modulator (SPPARMα), versus placebo in patients with non-alcoholic fatty liver disease. Aliment Pharmacol Ther 2021;54(10):1263–77.
46. Gastaldelli A, Harrison SA, Belfort-Aguilar R, et al. Importance of changes in adipose tissue insulin resistance to histological response during thiazolidinedione treatment of patients with nonalcoholic steatohepatitis. Hepatology 2009;50(4):1087–93.
47. Cusi K. Role of obesity and lipotoxicity in the development of nonalcoholic steatohepatitis: pathophysiology and clinical implications. Gastroenterology 2012;142(4):711–25.e6.
48. Maeda N, Takahashi M, Funahashi T, et al. PPARgamma ligands increase expression and plasma concentrations of adiponectin, an adipose-derived protein. Diabetes 2001;50(9):2094–9.
49. Soccio RE, Chen ER, Lazar MA. Thiazolidinediones and the promise of insulin sensitization in type 2 diabetes. Cell Metabol 2014;20(4):573–91.
50. Ma X, Wang D, Zhao W, et al. Deciphering the roles of PPARγ in adipocytes via dynamic change of transcription complex. Front Endocrinol 2018;9:473.
51. Gastaldelli A, Harrison S, Belfort-Aguiar R, et al. Pioglitazone in the treatment of NASH: the role of adiponectin. Aliment Pharmacol Ther 2010;32(6):769–75.

52. Belfort R, Harrison SA, Brown K, et al. A placebo-controlled trial of pioglitazone in subjects with nonalcoholic steatohepatitis. N Engl J Med 2006;355(22): 2297–307.
53. Cusi K, Orsak B, Bril F, et al. Long-term pioglitazone treatment for patients with nonalcoholic steatohepatitis and prediabetes or type 2 diabetes mellitus a randomized trial. Ann Intern Med 2016;165(5):305–15.
54. Bril F. Role of oral vitamin E for the treatment of nonalcoholic steatohepatitis (NASH) in patients with type 2 diabetes: a randomized controlled trial. Diabetes Care 2019;42(8):1481–8.
55. Jain MR, Giri SR, Bhoi B, et al. Dual PPARα/γ agonist saroglitazar improves liver histopathology and biochemistry in experimental NASH models. Liver Int 2018; 38(6):1084–94.
56. Kaul U, Parmar D, Manjunath K, et al. New dual peroxisome proliferator activated receptor agonist—saroglitazar in diabetic dyslipidemia and non-alcoholic fatty liver disease: integrated analysis of the real world evidence. Cardiovasc Diabetol 2019;18(1):80.
57. Gawrieh S, Noureddin M, Loo N, et al. Saroglitazar, a PPAR-α/γ agonist, for treatment of NAFLD: a randomized controlled double-blind phase 2 trial. Hepatology 2021;74(4):1809–24.
58. Haczeyni F, Wang H, Barn V, et al. The selective peroxisome proliferator-activated receptor-delta agonist seladelpar reverses nonalcoholic steatohepatitis pathology by abrogating lipotoxicity in diabetic obese mice. Hepatol Commun 2017; 1(7):663–74.
59. Staels B, Rubenstrunk A, Noel B, et al. Hepatoprotective effects of the dual peroxisome proliferator-activated receptor alpha/delta agonist, GFT505, in rodent models of nonalcoholic fatty liver disease/nonalcoholic steatohepatitis. Hepatology 2013;58(6):1941–52.
60. Ratziu V, Harrison SA, Francque S, et al. Elafibranor, an agonist of the peroxisome Proliferator−Activated Receptor−α and −δ, induces resolution of nonalcoholic steatohepatitis without fibrosis worsening. Gastroenterology 2016; 150(5):1147–59.e5.
61. Phase 3 study to evaluate the efficacy and safety of elafibranor versus placebo in patients with nonalcoholic steatohepatitis (NASH). Available at: https://ClinicalTrials.gov/show/NCT02704403. Accessed February 17, 2022.
62. Harrison Stephen A, Ratziu Vlad, Dufour Jean-François, et al. The dual PPARα/δ agonist elafibranor did not achieve resolution of NASH without worsening of fibrosis in adult patients with non-alcoholic steatohepatitis and significant fibrosis. Hepatology 2020;72(1 suppl). LP 23.
63. Wettstein G, Luccarini JM, Poekes L, et al. The new-generation pan-peroxisome proliferator-activated receptor agonist IVA337 protects the liver from metabolic disorders and fibrosis. Hepatol Commun 2017;1(6):524–37.
64. Lefere S, Puengel T, Hundertmark J, et al. Differential effects of selective- and pan-PPAR agonists on experimental steatohepatitis and hepatic macrophages. J Hepatol 2020;73(4):757–70.
65. Boubia B, Poupardin O, Barth M, et al. Design, synthesis, and evaluation of a novel series of indole sulfonamide peroxisome proliferator activated receptor (PPAR) α/γ/δ triple activators: discovery of lanifibranor, a new antifibrotic clinical candidate. J Med Chem 2018;61(6):2246–65.
66. Francque SM, Bedossa P, Ratziu V, et al. A randomized, controlled trial of the pan-PPAR agonist lanifibranor in NASH. N Engl J Med 2021;385(17). https://doi.org/10.1056/NEJMoa2036205.

67. Drucker DJ. Mechanisms of action and therapeutic application of glucagon-like peptide-1. Cell Metabol 2018;27(4):740–56.
68. Armstrong MJ, Gaunt P, Aithal GP, et al. Liraglutide safety and efficacy in patients with non-alcoholic steatohepatitis (LEAN): a multicentre, double-blind, randomised, placebo-controlled phase 2 study. Lancet 2016;387(10019): 679–90.
69. Frías JP, Davies MJ, Rosenstock J, et al. Tirzepatide versus semaglutide once weekly in patients with type 2 diabetes. N Engl J Med 2021;385(6):503–15.
70. Habegger KM, Heppner KM, Geary N, et al. The metabolic actions of glucagon revisited. Nat Rev Endocrinol 2010;6(12):689–97.
71. Mack C, Wilson J, Athanacio J, et al. Pharmacological actions of the peptide hormone amylin in the long-term regulation of food intake, food preference, and body weight. Am J Physiol Regul Integr Comp Physiol 2007;293(5): R1855–63.
72. Mantelmacher FD, Zvibel I, Cohen K, et al. GIP regulates inflammation and body weight by restraining myeloid-cell-derived S100A8/A9. Nat Metab 2019;1(1): 58–69.
73. Efimova I, Steinberg I, Zvibel I, et al. GIPR signaling in immune cells maintains metabolically beneficial type 2 immune responses in the white fat from obese mice. Front Immunol 2021;12. 643144.
74. Hartman ML, Sanyal AJ, Loomba R, et al. Effects of novel dual GIP and GLP-1 receptor agonist Tirzepatide on biomarkers of nonalcoholic steatohepatitis in patients with type 2 diabetes. Diabetes Care 2020;43(6):1352–5.
75. Starling S. A new GLP1, GIP and glucagon receptor triagonist. Nat Rev Endocrinol 2022;18(3):135.
76. Iruarrizaga-Lejarreta M, Varela-Rey M, Fernández-Ramos D, et al. Role of Aramchol in steatohepatitis and fibrosis in mice. Hepatol Commun 2017;1(9): 911–27.
77. Ratziu V, de Guevara L, Safadi R, et al. Aramchol in patients with nonalcoholic steatohepatitis: a randomized, double-blind, placebo-controlled phase 2b trial. Nat Med 2021;27(10):1825–35.
78. Matsumoto M, Yashiro H, Ogino H, et al. Acetyl-CoA carboxylase 1 and 2 inhibition ameliorates steatosis and hepatic fibrosis in a MC4R knockout murine model of nonalcoholic steatohepatitis. PLoS One 2020;15(1). e0228212.
79. Loomba R, Noureddin M, Kowdley K v, et al. Combination therapies including cilofexor and firsocostat for bridging fibrosis and cirrhosis attributable to NASH. Hepatology 2021;73(2):625–43.
80. Lawitz EJ, Bhandari BR, Ruane PJ, et al. Fenofibrate mitigates hypertriglyceridemia in nonalcoholic steatohepatitis patients treated with cilofexor/firsocostat. Clin Gastroenterol Hepatol 2022;21(1):143–52.e3.
81. Zhang XJ, Cai J, Li H. Targeting ACC for NASH resolution. Trends Mol Med 2022;28(1):5–7.
82. Loomba R, Mohseni R, Lucas KJ, et al. TVB-2640 (FASN inhibitor) for the treatment of nonalcoholic steatohepatitis: FASCINATE-1, a randomized, placebo-controlled phase 2a trial. Gastroenterology 2021;161(5):1475–86.
83. Ritter MJ, Amano I, Hollenberg AN. Thyroid hormone signaling and the liver. Hepatology 2020;72(2):742–52.
84. Bohinc BN, Michelotti G, Xie G, et al. Repair-related activation of hedgehog signaling in stromal cells promotes intrahepatic hypothyroidism. Endocrinology 2014;155(11):4591–601.

85. Sinha RA, Bruinstroop E, Singh BK, et al. Nonalcoholic fatty liver disease and hypercholesterolemia: roles of thyroid hormones, metabolites, and agonists. Thyroid 2019;29(9):1173–91.
86. Labenz C, Kostev K, Armandi A, et al. Impact of thyroid disorders on the incidence of non-alcoholic fatty liver disease in Germany. United European Gastroenterol J 2021;9(7):829–36.
87. Kelly MJ, Pietranico-Cole S, Larigan JD, et al. Discovery of 2-[3,5-dichloro-4-(5-isopropyl-6-oxo-1,6-dihydropyridazin-3-yloxy)phenyl]-3,5-dioxo-2,3,4,5-tetrahydro[1,2,4]triazine-6-carbonitrile (MGL-3196), a Highly Selective Thyroid Hormone Receptor β agonist in clinical trials for the treatment of dyslipidemia. J Med Chem 2014;57(10):3912–23.
88. Harrison SA, Bashir MR, Guy CD, et al. Resmetirom (MGL-3196) for the treatment of non-alcoholic steatohepatitis: a multicentre, randomised, double-blind, placebo-controlled, phase 2 trial. Lancet 2019;394(10213):2012–24.
89. Zhou J, Waskowicz LR, Lim A, et al. A liver-specific thyromimetic, VK2809, decreases hepatosteatosis in glycogen storage disease type ia. Thyroid 2019; 29(8):1158–67.
90. Elbashir SM, Martinez J, Patkaniowska A, et al. Functional anatomy of siRNAs for mediating efficient RNAi in Drosophila melanogaster embryo lysate. EMBO J 2001;20(23):6877–88.
91. Marchais-Oberwinkler S, Henn C, Möller G, et al. 17β-Hydroxysteroid dehydrogenases (17β-HSDs) as therapeutic targets: protein structures, functions, and recent progress in inhibitor development. J Steroid Biochem Mol Biol 2011; 125(1–2):66–82.
92. Luukkonen PK, Tukiainen T, Juuti A, et al. Hydroxysteroid 17-β dehydrogenase 13 variant increases phospholipids and protects against fibrosis in nonalcoholic fatty liver disease. JCI Insight 2020;5(5). https://doi.org/10.1172/jci.insight.132158.
93. Ma Y, Belyaeva O v, Brown PM, et al. 17-Beta hydroxysteroid dehydrogenase 13 is a hepatic retinol dehydrogenase associated with histological features of nonalcoholic fatty liver disease. Hepatology 2019;69(4):1504–19.
94. Yuen MF. HSD17B13. J Hepatol 2022.
95. Sauk JJ, Smith T, Norris K, et al. Hsp47 and the translation-translocation machinery cooperate in the production of alpha 1(I) chains of type I procollagen. J Biol Chem 1994;269(6):3941–6.
96. Hagiwara S, Iwasaka H, Matsumoto S, et al. An antisense oligonucleotide to HSP47 inhibits paraquat-induced pulmonary fibrosis in rats. Toxicology 2007; 236(3):199–207.
97. Lawitz EJ, Shevell DE, Tirucherai GS, et al. BMS-986263 in patients with advanced hepatic fibrosis: 36-week results from a randomized, placebo-controlled phase 2 trial. Hepatology 2022;75(4):912–23.
98. Dongiovanni P, Donati B, Fares R, et al. PNPLA3 I148M polymorphism and progressive liver disease. World J Gastroenterol 2013;19(41):6969–78.
99. Anstee QM, Darlay R, Cockell S, et al. Genome-wide association study of non-alcoholic fatty liver and steatohepatitis in a histologically characterised cohort. J Hepatol 2020;73(3):505–15.
100. Liu YL, Patman GL, Leathart JBS, et al. Carriage of the PNPLA3 rs738409 C >G polymorphism confers an increased risk of non-alcoholic fatty liver disease associated hepatocellular carcinoma. J Hepatol 2014;61(1):75–81.

101. Trépo E, Caruso S, Yang J, et al. Common genetic variation in alcohol-related hepatocellular carcinoma: a case-control genome-wide association study. Lancet Oncol 2022;23(1):161–71.
102. Pingitore P, Pirazzi C, Mancina RM, et al. Recombinant PNPLA3 protein shows triglyceride hydrolase activity and its I148M mutation results in loss of function. Biochim Biophys Acta 2014;1841(4):574–80.
103. BasuRay S, Smagris E, Cohen JC, et al. The PNPLA3 variant associated with fatty liver disease (I148M) accumulates on lipid droplets by evading ubiquitylation. Hepatology 2017;66(4):1111–24.
104. Lindén D, Ahnmark A, Pingitore P, et al. Pnpla3 silencing with antisense oligonucleotides ameliorates nonalcoholic steatohepatitis and fibrosis in Pnpla3 I148M knock-in mice. Mol Metabol 2019;22:49–61.
105. Dulai PS, Singh S, Patel J, et al. Increased risk of mortality by fibrosis stage in nonalcoholic fatty liver disease: systematic review and meta-analysis. Hepatology 2017;65(5):1557–65.
106. Sanyal AJ, van Natta ML, Clark J, et al. Prospective study of outcomes in adults with nonalcoholic fatty liver disease. N Engl J Med 2021;385(17):1559–69.
107. Harrison SA, Abdelmalek MF, Caldwell S, et al. Simtuzumab is ineffective for patients with bridging fibrosis or compensated cirrhosis caused by nonalcoholic steatohepatitis. Gastroenterology 2018;155(4):1140–53.
108. Loomba R, Lawitz E, Mantry PS, et al. The ASK1 inhibitor selonsertib in patients with nonalcoholic steatohepatitis: a randomized, phase 2 trial. Hepatology 2018;67(2):549–59.
109. Harrison SA, Wong VWS, Okanoue T, et al. Selonsertib for patients with bridging fibrosis or compensated cirrhosis due to NASH: results from randomized phase III STELLAR trials. J Hepatol 2020;73(1):26–39.
110. Ratziu V, Friedman SL. Why do so many NASH trials fail? Gastroenterology 2020. https://doi.org/10.1053/j.gastro.2020.05.046. S0016-5085(20)30680-6.
111. Davison BA, Harrison SA, Cotter G, et al. Suboptimal reliability of liver biopsy evaluation has implications for randomized clinical trials. J Hepatol 2020;73(6):1322–32.
112. Chow JCL, Wong GLH, Chan AWH, et al. Repeating measurements by transient elastography in non-alcoholic fatty liver disease patients with high liver stiffness. J Gastroenterol Hepatol 2019;34(1):241–8.
113. Ruhl CE, Everhart JE. Diurnal variation in serum alanine aminotransferase activity in the US population. J Clin Gastroenterol 2013;47(2):165–73.
114. Ratziu V. A critical review of endpoints for non-cirrhotic NASH therapeutic trials. J Hepatol 2018;68(2):353–61.
115. Newsome PN, Sejling AS, Sanyal AJ. Semaglutide or placebo for nonalcoholic steatohepatitis. Reply. *N Engl J Med.* 2021;385(2):e6.
116. Ratziu V, Harrison S, Francque S, et al. A post-hoc analysis of the Golden505 trial demonstrates histological and cardiometabolic efficacy of elafibranor 120 mg in patients with moderate or severe NASH that are eligible for pharmacotherapy. JHEP 2016;150(5):1147–59.e5.
117. Haas JT, Francque S, Staels B. Pathophysiology and mechanisms of nonalcoholic fatty liver disease. Annu Rev Physiol 2016;78:181–205.
118. Gaziano JM, Concato J, Brophy M, et al. Million Veteran Program: a mega-biobank to study genetic influences on health and disease. J Clin Epidemiol 2016;70:214–23.

119. Vujkovic M, Ramdas S, Lorenz KM. A genome-wide association study for nonalcoholic fatty liver disease identifies novel genetic loci and trait-relevant candidate genes in the Million Veteran Program. medRxiv 2021.
120. Hampson SJ. Nursing interventions for the first three postpartum months. J Obstet Gynecol Neonatal Nurs 1989;18(2):116–22.
121. Francque S, Vonghia L. Pharmacological treatment for non-alcoholic fatty liver disease. Adv Ther 2019;36(5):1052–74.
122. Francque SM, Marchesini G, Kautz A, et al. Non-alcoholic fatty liver disease: a patient guideline. JHEP Rep 2021;3(5). 100322.

Special Population

Lean Nonalcoholic Fatty Liver Disease

Ajay Duseja, MD, DM, FAASLD, FACG, FAMS, FSGEI, FISG, FINASL, Master-ISG[a,*],
Arka De, MD, DM[a], Vincent Wong, MD[b,c]

KEYWORDS

- Nonalcoholic fatty liver disease • Nonalcoholic steatohepatitis • Body mass index • Waist circumference • Obesity • Overweight • Liver fibrosis

KEY POINTS

- The prevalence of nonalcoholic fatty liver disease (NAFLD) in lean individuals is around 10%.
- In general, lean patients with NAFLD have milder liver disease but data on long-term outcomes are conflicting.
- Patients who are lean but have severe liver disease should be assessed thoroughly for other liver diseases or secondary causes of fatty liver.
- Noninvasive tests such as simple fibrosis scores and vibration-controlled transient elastography work well in the lean population.
- Lifestyle intervention is effective in reversing NAFLD in lean patients but a lesser degree of weight reduction is needed for the beneficial effects.

INTRODUCTION

Nonalcoholic fatty liver disease (NAFLD) affects at least 25% of the global adult population and is one of the leading causes of cirrhosis and hepatocellular carcinoma (HCC) in western countries.[1] It is strongly associated with obesity and the metabolic syndrome. In fact, NAFLD is considered the hepatic manifestation of the metabolic syndrome. Adipose tissue is also the main source of lipids to the liver. The toxic lipid species in turn cause hepatic inflammation, tissue injury, and fibrosis.

Despite the tight link between obesity and NAFLD, it is clear from multiple epidemiologic studies that a significant proportion of patients with NAFLD have relatively normal body mass index (BMI). This condition is often coined as "lean" or "nonobese"

[a] Department of Hepatology, Post Graduate Institute of Medical Education and Research, Chandigarh, India; [b] Department of Medicine and Therapeutics, Medical Data Analytics Center, The Chinese University of Hong Kong, Hong Kong; [c] State Key Laboratory of Digestive Disease, Institute of Digestive Disease, The Chinese University of Hong Kong, Hong Kong
* Corresponding author. Department of Hepatology, Post Graduate Institute of Medical Education and Research Chandigarh, India - 160012.
E-mail address: ajayduseja@yahoo.co.in

Clin Liver Dis 27 (2023) 451–469
https://doi.org/10.1016/j.cld.2023.01.011 liver.theclinics.com
1089-3261/23/

NAFLD.[2] In a way, this reflects the spectrum of NAFLD across different degrees of adiposity. Other components of the metabolic syndrome also contribute to the development of NAFLD with substantial individual variability in the relative importance of various metabolic factors. Furthermore, BMI is an imperfect marker of adiposity. It is important to recognize that a normal BMI does not always indicate metabolic health.

In this article, we discuss the definitions of obesity and review the epidemiology of NAFLD in the general population and lean individuals. We also describe the pathogenesis, clinical features, and outcomes of NAFLD in lean individuals. Based on this knowledge, we highlight key issues in the assessment and treatment of this special population.

DEFINING ADIPOSITY IN LEAN NONALCOHOLIC FATTY LIVER DISEASE

In simple terms, adiposity refers to excess body fat and is largely a consequence of net positive energy balance.[3] It is important to note that in the NAFLD literature, BMI alone has been used for defining "lean" (BMI <25 kg/m^2 in Western populations and <23 kg/m^2 in Asians) and "nonobese" (BMI <30 kg/m^2 in Western populations and <25 kg/m^2 in Asians).[4,5] However, BMI is a poor surrogate of adiposity. Indeed, an individual with a muscular physique and a high fat-free mass may well have a high BMI despite body fat percentage being within normal limits.[6] Further, BMI does not provide any information on the distribution of body fat, which is important for clinical outcomes.

According to the adipose tissue expandability hypothesis, adipose tissue has a restricted capacity to accumulate new fat stores, and when this capacity is exhausted, fat deposits in ectopic sites such as the liver.[3] Most of the evidence suggests that subcutaneous adipose tissue (SAT), which is expandable and plastic is the primary site for the initial fat storage. On the contrary, visceral adipose tissue (VAT) is associated with increased lipolysis, insulin resistance, and proinflammatory and fibrogenic mediators and may be more important in governing the risk of NAFLD.[7,8] Further, SAT itself is not a homogeneous entity from a metabolic standpoint and is subject to different epigenetic regulation depending on its location in the upper body (abdominal subcutaneous fat) or lower body (gluteofemoral fat).Gluteofemoral fat shows a hyperplastic response to energy excess by hypertrophy and is more efficient in storing fat. On the contrary, abdominal subcutaneous fat undergoes a hypertrophic response to energy excess and is less efficient in storing fat with a higher lipid turnover.[7]

Computed tomography (CT) and MRI can accurately measure subcutaneous and VAT compartments. Although dual energy X-ray absorptiometry (DEXA) cannot directly differentiate between subcutaneous and visceral adiposity, abdominal fat mass estimated by DEXA correlates with visceral adiposity as assessed by CT and MRI. Apart from being able to differentiate subcutaneous and visceral fat depots, fluorodeoxyglucose (FDG)- positron emission tomography (PET) provides additional information regarding the regional differences in metabolic status of adipose tissue including identification of brown adipose tissue.[9] However, although important from a research perspective, imaging-based assessment of adiposity is unlikely to find a place in routine clinical practice. Clinical measures of central obesity such as waist circumference and waist–hip ratio have been shown to be better predictors of metabolic and cardiovascular outcomes as compared with BMI.[10] Apart from being better, although imperfect, surrogates of visceral obesity than BMI, these clinical measures of central obesity also consider abdominal SAT. Indeed, the National Cholesterol Education Program-Adult Treatment Panel III, International Diabetes Federation, and European Group for the Study of Insulin Resistance definitions of metabolic syndrome incorporate waist circumference instead of BMI. Given the intricate relationship between metabolic syndrome risk factors and NAFLD, whether the incorporation of waist circumference as a measure of central obesity in addition to BMI will help us to better define, characterize, and prognosticate patients with lean NAFLD remains unknown and is an unmet area of research.

EPIDEMIOLOGY

Prevalence of Nonalcoholic Fatty Liver Disease in Lean Individuals

In the past, NAFLD in lean individuals was considered a unique condition in the Asian population, mainly because most initial studies came from Asia.[2] This was probably due to different fat distribution in Asians and the corresponding impact on the interpretation of normal BMI and waist circumference, as described above. However, subsequent studies clearly showed that lean individuals in North America, South America, and Europe could also have NAFLD.

Three recent systematic reviews and meta-analyses provided detailed description of the prevalence of NAFLD in lean individuals from different countries and regions.[11–13] All 3 studies defined lean as BMI less than 23 kg/m^2 in Asians and less than 25 kg/m^2 in non-Asians. Overall, the global prevalence of NAFLD among lean individuals was estimated at 9.7% to 12.1%, which was lower than the often-quoted prevalence of 25% to 30% in the total population. The estimates in the individual studies were affected by study settings (true population studies, healthy volunteers from the community or other settings, hospital patients), assessments (decreasing sensitivities from MRI, controlled attenuation parameter, abdominal ultrasonography, steatosis scores to elevated aminotransferase), and study period (increasing prevalence of NAFLD over time).[14] With these caveats in mind, the pooled prevalence of NAFLD in lean individuals is around 11.7% in East Asia, 10.0% in South Asia and 15.5% in Europe (**Table 1**).[11] At the country level, the reported prevalence of NAFLD in lean individuals was the highest in Mexico (37.0%) and Italy (26.1%), compared with around 10% in most other countries (**Figs. 1–3**).

Racial difference in NAFLD epidemiology has been most extensively studied in the United States.[15] The prevalence is the highest in Hispanics, followed by non-Hispanic Whites, Asians, and the lowest in Blacks. Compared with other racial groups, more Asian Americans with NAFLD are lean, and they are less likely to have cirrhosis.[16] The prevalence of NAFLD in lean individuals increases with age, although the impact of age and sex in this population is less than the effect of the other metabolic risk factors.[17]

Among patients with NAFLD globally, around 14.1% are lean.[13] The percentage mirrors the prevalence of obesity in different countries. In general, countries with higher mean population BMI and a higher prevalence of obesity have a smaller proportion of NAFLD patients being lean with some differences between rural and urban settings. At the country level, 73.7% of NAFLD patients in rural India and 10.6% in urban India were lean, compared with 49.9% in South Korea, 19.0% to 22.1% in Japan, 16.4% in Taiwan, 7.8% to 17.8% in China, and 17.3% in the United States.[13,18]

Incidence of Nonalcoholic Fatty Liver Disease in Lean Individuals

Incidence data of NAFLD are limited by the unreliability of abdominal ultrasonography in detecting changes in hepatic steatosis over time. In the systematic review and meta-analysis by Ye and colleagues, the pooled incidence of NAFLD in lean individuals was 23 per 1000 person-years during 10,424 person-years of follow-up.[11] One study from Hong Kong used proton-magnetic resonance spectroscopy to measure changes liver fat fraction in randomly selected subjects from the general population.[19]

Table 1
Country-level and region-level prevalence of nonobese nonalcoholic fatty liver disease in the general population[11–13]

	Prevalence (%)
East Asia	8–16
Mainland China	4–18
South Korea	7–18
Japan	11–17
Taiwan	7–22
Hong Kong	13–17
South Asia	6–17
India	5–31
Pakistan	3–6
Bangladesh	10–14
Sri Lanka	9–11
Malaysia	3–5
Middle East	-
Iran	13–22
North America	-
United States	7–11
Mexico	29–46
Europe	5–40
The Netherlands	9
Italy	23–29
Spain	6–13
Romania	6–9
United Kingdom	0

Among 565 subjects who did not have NAFLD at baseline, 78 subjects (13.8%) developed NAFLD at a median interval of 47 months, yielding an annual incidence of 3.4%. Four hundred and six subjects in this study were lean (BMI <23 kg/m^2) at baseline, and 36 subjects (8.9%) developed incident NAFLD, among whom 29 continued to have BMI <23 kg/m^2 and none had BMI increased to 25 kg/m^2 or greater. An increase in waist circumference and plasma triglycerides were independent factors associated with incident NAFLD in lean individuals.

Nonalcoholic Steatohepatitis and Liver Fibrosis

Liver biopsy is required for the diagnosis of nonalcoholic steatohepatitis (NASH). However, liver biopsy is an invasive procedure reserved for patients with features or risk factors of advanced liver disease. Therefore, studies using liver biopsy are limited by selection bias and likely overestimate the prevalence of NASH and liver fibrosis. The systematic review by Ye and colleagues identified 8 studies involving 1441 nonobese or lean patients with biopsy-proven NAFLD (11). The prevalence of NASH was 10.8% to 67.2% in nonobese patients and 17.3% to 80.8% in obese patients. Grade 2 to 3 lobular inflammation was observed in 6.5% to 51.8%, and stage 2 to 4 fibrosis was observed in 17.5% to 42.2%. One of the largest lean Caucasian liver biopsy cohorts included 1339 patients from Italy, UK, Spain, and Australia, among whom 14.4%

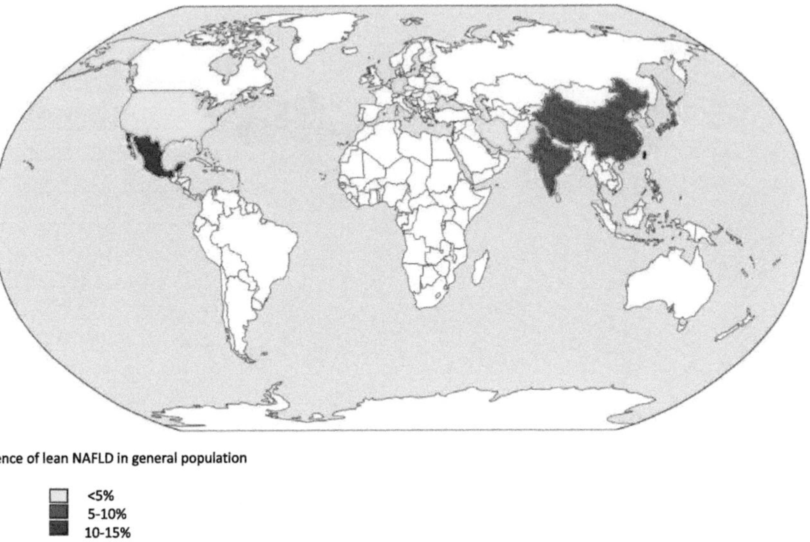

Fig. 1. Prevalence of lean NAFLD in general population.[11]

were lean.[20] Although lean patients had less severe histology overall, 54.1% had NASH and 10.2% had stage 3 to 4 fibrosis.

In contrast, population-based studies using noninvasive tests more faithfully reflect the epidemiology of lean NAFLD. In a population study of community NAFLD patients in Hong Kong, 2.6% and 5.1% of those with BMI less than 25 and 25 kg/m^2 or greater had liver stiffness by vibration-controlled transient elastography (VCTE) of 9.6 kPa or greater suggestive of advanced liver fibrosis.[17] VCTE was also used in the National Health and Nutrition Examination Surveys 2017 to 2018.[21] Using the FibroScan-aspartate aminotransferase (FAST) score cutoff of 0.67,[22] the prevalence of NASH plus stage 2 to 4 fibrosis was estimated at 1.2% in all 4218 adults with valid

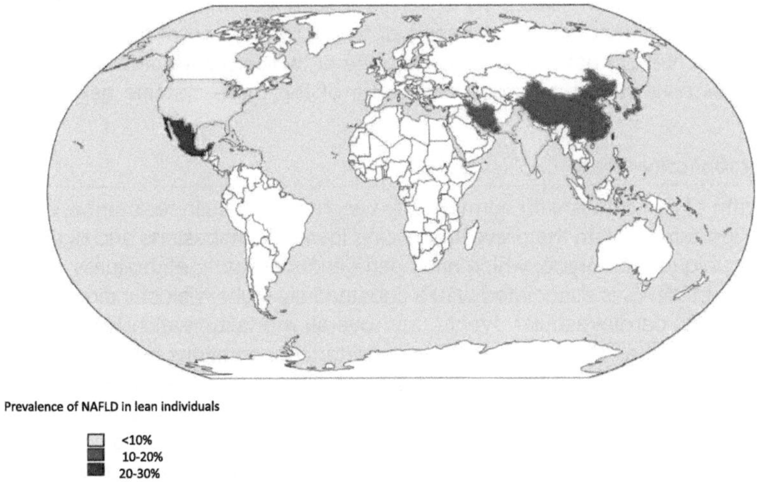

Fig. 2. Prevalence of NAFLD in lean individuals.[11]

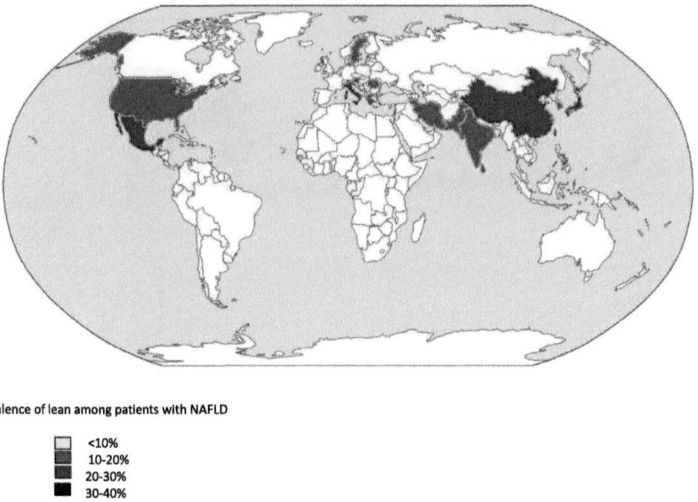

Fig. 3. Prevalence of lean individuals among patients with NAFLD.[11]

elastography measurements: 1.7% in men and 0.8% in women; and 2.2% in Hispanics, 1.0% in Asian Americans, 0.9% in non-Hispanic Whites, and 0.4% in Blacks.

PATHOGENESIS

In most patients, insulin resistance is central to the pathophysiology of NAFLD, which involves a complex interplay of multiple additional factors including sedentary lifestyle, dietary excesses, genetic risk factors, adiposopathy with altered adipokine levels, gut dysbiosis, lipotoxicity, oxidative stress, mitochondrial dysfunction, and activation of inflammatory and fibrogenic pathways.[1] Although patients with lean NAFLD have less insulin resistance compared with overweight and obese patients, a wealth of evidence suggests that these patients have higher insulin resistance compared with their healthy counterparts without NAFLD.[13] As such insulin resistance also seems to be a major player in the pathogenesis of lean NAFLD. In this context, it should be pointed out that not all patients with NAFLD have insulin resistance, and this highlights the importance of the multifactorial pathogenesis of NAFLD.[23] Instead of discussing the granular details of NAFLD pathophysiology in general, which have been extensively covered in other reviews, we will focus on some of the more specific aspects of lean NAFLD.

Lean but Metabolically Obese

Around one-fifth of individuals with normal body weight have insulin resistance, dyslipidemia, or hypertension with the prevalence being lower in Caucasians and higher in Asians.[24] This unique phenotype, which has been described as "metabolically obese normal weight" (MONW), is associated with a substantially higher risk of incident type 2 diabetes mellitus, cardiovascular events, and overall mortality, which is similar to that of overweight or obese individuals.[25] Two important observations from MONW individuals may be particularly relevant to our understanding of lean NAFLD. First, there may be an individual fat threshold independent of BMI, which when surpassed results in metabolic dysfunction in that particular individual.[26] Second, in spite of a normal total body fat mass, an aberrant body fat compartmentalization with increased VAT also predisposes to the MONW phenotype.[27]

As alluded to in the previous section, VAT is associated with NAFLD independent of BMI.[8,28,29] Further, in a longitudinal study of 2017 individuals followed up for around 4 years, an increase in VAT was associated with an increased risk of incident NAFLD while an increase in SAT was associated with NAFLD regression.[30] From a metabolic standpoint, VAT is intrinsically more insulin resistant and is associated with increased lipolysis as a consequence of suppressed insulin-mediated inhibition of lipoprotein lipase. Increased free fatty acids thus produced from VAT are able to reach the liver in high concentrations as VAT is drained by the portal venous system. Further, VAT is more susceptible to inflammation and cell death and is associated with dysregulated adipokine secretion with decrease in insulin-sensitizing adiponectin and increase in proinflammatory tumor necrosis factor alpha (TNF-α) and interleukin 6(IL-6).[3] Indeed, there is no difference in the level of adiponectin between lean and nonlean individuals with NAFLD reflecting the prevailing adiposopathy even in the lean patients.[31]

Sarcopenia and Myosteatosis

Muscles are the primary organ system involved in the uptake of circulatory glucose in response to insulin, and it is not surprising that a decrease in muscle mass is associated with perturbations in metabolic homeostasis. Sarcopenia has been associated with NAFLD, NASH, and fibrosis independent of metabolic comorbidities and BMI.[32–34] Moreover, muscle mass in lean individuals with NAFLD is lower than that in their obese counterparts.[35] In a Japanese NAFLD cohort, sarcopenic obesity defined by the authors as decreased appendicular skeletal mass index with increased fat mass percent as assessed by DEXA, was independently associated with NAFLD in individuals with BMI less than 25 kg/m^2.[36]

Abnormal muscle composition with fatty infiltration of muscles or myosteatosis has garnered much attention in recent years. Myosteatosis is not only associated with NAFLD but it also correlates with the severity spectrum ranging from simple steatosis, NASH without significant fibrosis, and NASH with significant fibrosis.[37,38] Further, myosteatosis is present in a substantial proportion of patients with NAFLD who do not have sarcopenia and it has been suggested that myosteatosis may be more important than sarcopenia in governing the risk of NAFLD.[39,40]

There is an intrinsic relationship among sarcopenia, myosteatosis, insulin resistance, and metabolic dysfunction. Sarcopenia promotes insulin resistance and worsens glycemic control due to the reduced muscle mass available for insulin-mediated glucose uptake. Further, sarcopenia is associated with poor exercise capacity, which translates to decreased caloric expenditure and further worsens insulin resistance and the metabolic milieu. Insulin resistance promotes peripheral lipolysis resulting in increased free fatty acids that suppress the growth hormone-insulin like growth factor axis, thereby impairing muscle regeneration. Increased circulating free fatty acids exacerbate myosteatosis, which in turn promotes insulin resistance via the mitogen activated protein (MAP)-kinase pathway and worsens the overall inflammatory state. Increased gluconeogenesis because of insulin resistance and the low-grade inflammatory milieu of NAFLD with increased TNF-α and IL-6 promotes proteolysis while myosteatosis decreases protein synthesis in muscles.[40]Altered myokine secretion including decreased irisin and increased myostatin also promote hepatic steatosis. Myostatin also has fibrogenic effects partly due to the activation of hepatic stellate cells. In a recent Japanese study, myostatin (a myokine) and leptin (an adipokine) were found to be associated with hepatic steatosis in nonobese patients.[41] This highlights the importance of the synergy of derangements in skeletal muscle tissue (sarcopenia and myosteatosis) and adipose tissue (increased VAT with adiposopathy) in the pathogenesis of lean NAFLD.

Genetic Predisposition

Several genetic polymorphisms have been described which predispose to NAFLD, NASH, and fibrosis. Among the commonly described genes, there seems to be no difference in the prevalence of *PNPLA3* and *TM6SF2* polymorphisms between lean and nonlean patients although the data available for comparison is scant and heterogeneous.[13] Polymorphisms of *CETP* (rs12447924 and rs12597002), *SREBP-2* (rs133291), *PEMT* (rs7946 C > T), and *IFNL4* (rs368234815 TT) have been associated with NAFLD in lean and nonobese individuals.[42] More studies are needed to get a granular understanding of the contribution of these genetic polymorphisms viz a viz other risk factors such as metabolic dysfunction, the interplay between the different genes, and the differences in genetic predisposition between lean and nonlean patients.

Gut Dysbiosis and Differential Metabolic Adaptation in Lean Nonalcoholic Fatty Liver Disease

Lean patients with NAFLD have a distinct gut-microbial signature compared with their obese counterparts with an enrichment of *Erysipelotrichaceae*, *Ruminococcus*, *Romboutsia*, and Veillonellaceae and an impoverishment of *Ruminiclostridium*, *Streptococcus*, *Lachnospiraceae*, *Desulfovibrionaceae*, Ruminococcaceae, and *Eubacterium.* Compared with healthy lean individuals, gut microbiota of lean NAFLD patients are enriched with Dorea with decreased abundance of *Marvinbryantia* and *Christensellenaceae.*[43–46] Some evidence suggest that the distinct gut microbiota profile of patients with lean NAFLD predisposes them to visceral obesity although their good metabolic adaptation including increased bile acids and fibroblast growth factor 19 (FGF-19) keeps the total body fat mass intact.[47]

Lifestyle Factors

Limited data suggest that despite having a normal body weight, lean patients with NAFLD do not have a completely healthy lifestyle. Compared with lean individuals without NAFLD, they consume more added sugars particularly soft drinks, fructose, cholesterol, and less polyunsaturated fatty acids.[48,49] Indeed, increased carbohydrate energy ratio and less than moderate level of physical activity were found to be predictors of NAFLD in nonobese individuals independent of BMI and total energy intake in a Korean study.[50]

CLINICAL FEATURES AND OUTCOMES

Metabolic Risk Factors

In a recent meta-analysis of 53 studies on lean NAFLD, data on metabolic risk factors viz a viz obese NAFLD were extractable from 7 studies including 9321obese and 4832 lean patients with NAFLD, respectively. Compared with those with lean NAFLD, patients with NAFLD of the classic phenotype had a significantly higher odds of abdominal obesity [OR: 12.09 (8.4–17.40)], hypertension [OR: 1.8 (1.5–2.2)], type 2 diabetes mellitus [OR: 1.7 (1.3–2.2)], impaired fasting glucose [OR:1.3 (1.2–1.5)], low high density lipprotein (HDL) [OR: 1.2 (1.1–1.4)], and metabolic syndrome [OR: 3 (2.2–4.2)].[13] The relative paucity of metabolic comorbidities in patients with lean NAFLD is relevant to the proposed change in the nomenclature of NAFLD to metabolic-dysfunction associated fatty liver disease (MAFLD). Indeed, 51% of the lean patients in an Indian cohort of NAFLD did not fulfill the MAFLD criteria.[51] However, this does not mean that patients with lean NAFLD are metabolically healthy. In fact, compared with healthy, lean individuals without NAFLD, patients with lean NAFLD have a significantly higher BMI and higher risk of metabolic syndrome and its components including central obesity, type 2 diabetes mellitus, impaired fasting glucose, hypertension, and low HDL.[13] Patients with lean NAFLD thus have an intermediate metabolic phenotype between lean, healthy individuals without NAFLD and nonlean patients with NAFLD.

Severity of Liver Disease

In an Indian cohort of 1040 patients with NAFLD, no difference was detected in controlled attenuation parameter, FIB-4 score, liver stiffness measurement (LSM), FAST score or the proportion of patients in whom advanced fibrosis was ruled-out or ruled-in using FIB-4 or LSM among lean and nonlean patients.[52] A community-based study from Hong Kong reported no difference in intrahepatic triglycerides among nonobese and obese patients with NAFLD although cytokeratin-18 and LSM was significantly lower in nonobese patients. However, there was no difference in the proportion of patients with advanced fibrosis (LSM of $\geq$ 9.6 kPa) between the 2 phenotypes of NAFLD (17).

Meta-analyses of histologic data suggests that patients with lean NAFLD have lower NAFLD activity score (NAS), NASH, and fibrosis scores compared with patients with nonlean NAFLD.[53] Close scrutiny of **Table 2**, which lists the various studies that have looked at the histologic severity of lean NAFLD viz a viz nonlean NAFLD, reveals several caveats most notably the heterogeneity in the results.[20,35,52,54–63] Further, some of the studies have clubbed lean and overweight patients into nonobese. Age is another confounding factor that needs to be considered while assessing liver disease severity in these patients. On the one hand, there is a correlation between age and BMI while, on the other hand, age is an important risk factor for fibrosis and poor outcomes.[64]

Clinical Outcomes

Data on long-term outcomes in lean patients with NAFLD is limited. In a 19-year follow-up of a Japanese cohort of 223 patients with biopsy proven NAFLD, no difference was observed in overall mortality or liver-related events including HCC among obese and nonobese patients on multivariate analysis. Not surprisingly, older age, type 2 diabetes mellitus, and advanced fibrosis on baseline biopsy were significantly associated with both liver-related events and overall mortality.[65] Similar long-term prognosis with respect to liver-related events and no difference in survival in lean and nonlean patients with NAFLD has also been reported in a recent multicentric study of 1339 biopsy-proven Caucasian patients with NAFLD with almost 10,500 person-years of follow-up. This study also corroborated that lean NAFLD may progress to advanced liver disease independent of longitudinal progression to obesity.[20] Intriguingly, in a Scandinavian cohort of 646 patients with biopsy-proven NAFLD, lean patients had a significantly higher risk of developing advanced liver disease including cirrhosis and HCC.[66] Analysis of the NHANES III data also suggests that patients with nonobese NAFLD have a substantially higher cumulative all-cause mortality (51.7%) during 15-year follow-up compared with obese NAFLD (27.2%).[67]

ASSESSMENT

The aims of assessment in a patient suspected to have NAFLD include confirming the diagnosis, determining the severity of liver disease, and assessing the concomitant metabolic conditions and cardiovascular risk.[68] The diagnosis of NAFLD is based

Table 2
Histologic severity of lean and nonobese nonalcoholic fatty liver disease

Study and Region	Number of Patients	Number of Lean or Nonobese Patients	Age (Years)	Steatosis Score	NASH	NAFLD Activity Score	Fibrosis Score	Significant or Advanced Fibrosis
Akyuz et al,[54] Turkey	483	Lean: 37 (7.6%)	Lean vs nonlean: 41.2 ± 11.6 vs: 45.5 ± 10.2, $P < .05$	Lean vs nonlean: 2 (1–3) vs 2 (1–3), P : ns	-	Lean: 4.6 ± 3.7 Nonlean: 5 ± 1.4 P : ns	Lean: 0.3 ± 0.74 Nonlean: 1 ± 1.4 P <0.01	-
Kumar et al,[56] India	110	Lean: 18 (16.4%)	-	-	Lean vs nonlean: 28% vs 48.9%, P : ns	-	-	Significant fibrosis in lean vs nonlean: 5.6% vs 28.2%, P : ns
Fracanzani et al,[57] Italy	669	Lean: 143 (21.4%)	Lean vs nonlean: 46 ± 13 vs 49 ± 12, $P = .04$	Grade 3 steatosis in lean vs nonlean: 18% vs 30%, $P = .01$	Lean: 17% Nonlean: 40% $P < .001$	Lean: 2.7 ± 1.6 Nonlean: 3.9 ± 1.7, $P < .01$	Lean: 0.7 ± 0.95 Nonlean: 1.4 ± 1.1 $P < .01$	Significant fibrosis in lean vs nonlean: 17% vs 42%, $P < .01$
Margariti et al,[60] Greece	56	Lean: 8 (14.3%)	-	Grade 3 steatosis in lean vs nonlean: 25% vs 42%, P : ns	Lean: 50% Nonlean: 68.8% P : ns	Lean: 3.1 ± 1.9 Nonlean: 4 ± 1.9 P : ns	Lean: 1.5 ± 1.7 Nonlean: 1.5 ± 1.2 P : ns	-
Sookoian et al,[61] Argentina	336	Lean: 25 (7.4%)	Lean vs nonlean: 52.3 ± 10.6 vs 52.9 ± 11.7, P : ns	Lean vs nonlean: 1.8 ± 0.84 vs 2.2 ± 0.8, P : ns	-	Lean vs nonlean: 3.37 ± 1.9 vs 3.7 ± 1.4, P : ns	Lean vs nonlean: 0.6 ± 0.9 vs 0.87 ± 1.22, P : ns	-
Younes et al,[20] multicentric Caucasians	1339	Lean: 195 (14.6%)	Lean v nonlean: 45 (36–55) vs 49 (38–58), $P = .03$	Grade 3 steatosis in lean vs nonlean: 10.4% vs 23.8%, $P < .001$	Lean vs nonlean: 54.1% vs 71.2% $P < .001$	-	-	Advanced fibrosis in lean vs nonlean: 10.2% vs 25%, $P < .001$

Denkmayr et al,[63] Austria	466	Lean: 74 (15.8%)	Lean: 48.7 ± 14.8 Overweight: 49.6 ± 13.8 Obese:50.4 ± 12.3 P : ns	Grade 3 steatosis in lean vs nonlean: 2.7% vs 5.1%, P : ns	Lean vs nonlean: 18.9% vs 11.7%, P : ns	-	-	Advanced fibrosis in lean vs nonlean: 21.6% vs 9.9%, P : ns
De et al,[52] India	149	Lean: 19 (12.8%)	Lean vs nonlean: 38.5 ± 12.04 vs 41.4 ± 11.1, P : ns	Grade 3 steatosis in lean vs nonlean: 15.8% vs 33%, P : ns	Lean vs nonlean: 21% vs 15.4% P : ns	Lean vs nonlean: 3.3 ± 1.2 vs 3.3 ± 1.2, P : ns	-	Significant fibrosis in lean vs nonlean: 10.5% vs 24.6%, P : ns
Alam et al,[55] Bangladesh	220	Nonobese: 56 (25.4%)	Nonobese vs obese: 41.7 ± 10.9 vs 40.5 ± 9.6, P : ns	Nonobese vs obese: 1.8 ± 0.8 vs 1.8 ± 0.7, P : ns	Nonobese vs obese: 53.6% vs 47%, P : ns	Nonobese vs obese: 4.4 ± 1.4 vs 4.4 ± 1.1, P : ns	Nonobese vs obese: 1.2 ± 0.8 vs 1.1 ± 0.8, P : ns	Significant fibrosis in nonobese vs obese: 19.6% vs 18.9% P : ns
Honda et al,[58] Japan	540	Nonobese: 134 (24.8%)	Nonobese vs obese: 48.5 ± 13.9 vs 56.6 ± 13.6, $P < .001$	Nonobese vs obese: 1.4 ± 0.6 vs 1.7 ± 0.7, $P < .001$	-	Nonobese vs obese: 3.5 ± 1.6 vs 4.2 ± 1.5, $P < .001$	Nonobese vs obese: 1.6 ± 1.1 vs 1.7 ± 1.0, p: ns	-
Leung et al,[59] Hong Kong	307	Nonobese: 72 (23.5%)	Nonobese vs obese: 54 ± 11 vs 51 ± 12, P : ns	Nonobese vs obese: 1.7 ± 0.8 vs 2 ± 0.8, P : ns	Nonobese vs obese: 43.5% vs 51.95%, P : ns	Nonobese vs obese: 3.3 ± 1.3 vs 3.8 ± 1.2, P : ns	Nonobese vs obese: 1.3 ± 1.5 vs 1.7 ± 1.4, $P < .01$	Advanced fibrosis in nonobese vs obese: 26.1% vs 27.7%, P : ns
Tan et al,[62] multicentric Asia	1812	Nonobese: 392 (21.6%)	Nonobese vs obese: 49.6 ± 12.5 vs 47.3 ± 12.9, $P = .02$	-	Nonobese vs obese: 50.5% vs 56.5% $P = .03$	-	-	Advanced fibrosis in nonobese vs obese: 14% vs 18.7%, $P = .03$)

on the detection of hepatic steatosis (usually by abdominal ultrasonography) and the exclusion of other liver diseases. In lean patients, it is important to exclude secondary causes of hepatic steatosis (eg, excessive alcohol consumption, endocrine disorders, medications, hepatitis C virus infection, Wilson disease, and lipodystrophy), especially when there is severe hepatic steatosis or active necroinflammation despite relatively mild metabolic burden.

In 2020, a group of hepatologists proposed to rename NAFLD as MAFLD.[69] Under the new definition, a patient would have MAFLD if she has fatty liver plus overweight or obesity, type 2 diabetes, or 2 other metabolic risk factors, whereas MAFLD can coexist with other liver diseases.[70] In other words, patients who are lean and metabolically healthy are not considered to have MAFLD even when fatty liver is present.[71]

Because only a minority of lean patients would have advanced liver disease, noninvasive tests should be performed first.[72] Simple fibrosis scores such as the NAFLD fibrosis score and the Fibrosis-4 index perform similarly in the lean and obese populations.[73] They also have consistent performance in patients with different racial background.[74] Although these simple fibrosis scores only have modest accuracy, they have high negative predictive values in excluding advanced fibrosis, especially in settings with a low prevalence of advanced liver disease.[75] Patients with persistently normal fibrosis scores also have extremely low risk of developing cirrhosis, hepatic decompensation, and HCC.[76] In specialist settings, specific fibrosis biomarkers such as PRO-C3 and enhanced liver fibrosis score, VCTE, ultrasound elastography, and magnetic resonance elastography are often performed as the second step to confirm the presence of significant or advanced fibrosis. VCTE is a point-of-care test and is commonly used in Europe, Asia, and North America.[77] Its use is limited by a lower success rate in obese patients but the development of the XL probe allows successful measurements in most patients.[78] The M probe can be used reliably in lean patients with a high accuracy.

In head-to-head comparisons, magnetic resonance elastography has a higher success rate and marginally higher accuracy for fibrosis staging than VCTE.[79] Recently, the MACK-3, NIS4, and FAST scores have also been developed to identify patients with NASH and stage 2 to 4 fibrosis. This is because most histology-based phase 2 and 3 clinical trials are targeting patients with NASH with significant liver fibrosis, and it is thought that clinicians will use similar algorithms to select patients for treatment when a drug is approved. Nonetheless, these newer investigations have not been specifically evaluated in the lean population.

TREATMENT

Healthy lifestyle in terms of diet and physical activity is the cornerstone for the management of obesity-related disorders. A 5% to 7% reduction in body weight can lead to resolution in hepatic steatosis and steatohepatitis, and a 10% reduction can improve fibrosis in most patients, although there is considerable individual variation in response.[80,81] Few studies have examined the safety and efficacy of weight reduction in patients with NAFLD who are lean. In one randomized controlled trial from Hong Kong, 154 patients with NAFLD were randomized to a 12-month lifestyle intervention program or usual care, among whom 78 had BMI of more than 25 kg/m^2 at baseline.[82] In both the nonobese (67% vs 18%) and obese (61% vs 21%) subgroups, patients in the intervention arm were more likely to achieve remission of NAFLD. The rate of remission also increased with the degree of weight reduction in both groups, although the nonobese subgroup did not need to lose as much weight to achieve the same

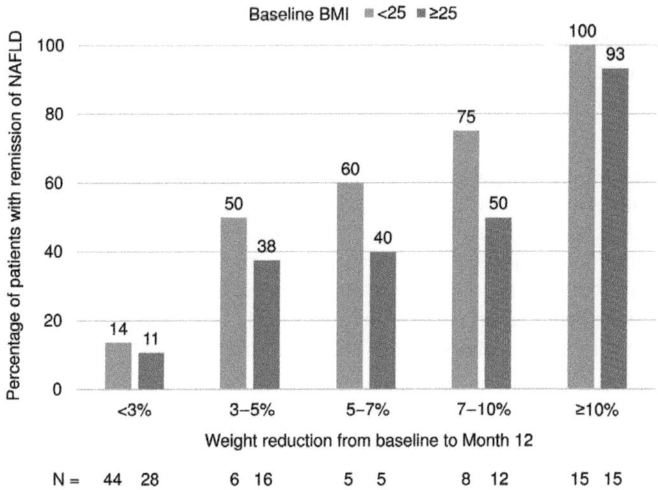

Fig. 4. Weight reduction and resolution of NAFLD in nonobese individuals. In a randomized controlled trial comparing a lifestyle intervention program with usual care in community subjects with NAFLD, a dose–response relationship between the degree of weight reduction and remission of NAFLD at 12 months (liver fat fraction <5% by proton-magnetic resonance spectroscopy) was seen in patients with baseline BMI <25 and $\geq$ 25 kg/m^2. However, the response rate was higher in nonobese patients, suggesting that they did not need to lose as much weight to achieve NAFLD remission. (The figure was reproduced with permission from the article by Wong and colleagues[82]).

degree of response (**Fig. 4**). This suggests that lifestyle intervention is also effective in nonobese patients.

However, it is important to determine if low body weight is the result of sarcopenia and nutritional deficiencies in advanced liver disease. In patients receiving liver transplantation for NASH, lean BMI paradoxically increased the risk of graft loss and overall mortality.[83] Sarcopenia is also an independent factor associated with a 2-fold increase in mortality in patients with cirrhosis.[84] Although data are limited, it would be prudent to liaise with dietitians and provide physical training to preserve muscle mass in patients with advanced liver disease.

There is currently no approved drug treatment for NASH, although several agents have reached phase 2 to 3 development.[85] Understandably, no study specifically examined the safety and efficacy of NASH drugs in lean patients, and it would be an important research topic for future real-world studies. That being said, based on the mechanisms of action, several existing drugs deserve some discussion.

Pioglitazone is a peroxisome proliferator-activated receptor (PPAR)-gamma agonist with effect on insulin resistance, steatosis and steatohepatitis.[86] Although weight gain is a known side effect, it is in part through the expansion of subcutaneous white adipose tissue, which stores fat and reduces fat deposition in the liver.[87] Recently, the pan-PPAR agonist lanifibranor was shown to both resolve NASH and improve fibrosis in the phase 2b NASH Trial to Validate IVA337 Efficacy (NATIVE) trial, and modest weight gain was again observed.[88] As weight gain is less of a problem in lean patients, the role of these treatments deserves further evaluation.

Newer antidiabetic drugs such as glucagon-like peptide-1 receptor agonists (GLP-1RA) and sodium-glucose cotransporter-2 inhibitors not only improve glycemic control but also reduce body weight and cardiovascular events.[86,89] In particular, the

GLP-1RA semaglutide at a subcutaneous dose of 0.4 mg daily led to NASH resolution in 59% of patients.[90] However, because these agents lead to weight reduction, their safety and efficacy in lean patients should be scrutinized.

SUMMARY

Accumulating evidence suggest that lean NAFLD is present in not only Asia but across different regions. Studies in the past 2 decades have shed light on the pathogenesis, risk factors, clinical characteristics, and management of lean NAFLD. Although lean patients with NAFLD in general have less severe metabolic profile and liver disease, some may nonetheless harbor NASH and advanced fibrosis, and the use of noninvasive tests for risk stratification cannot be overstated. Healthy lifestyle remains valuable in this special patient population. Future studies should define the best pharmacologic treatment of lean NASH.

CLINICS CARE POINTS

- Regular physical exercise is strongly recommended in lean patients with NAFLD to improve the insulin sensivity and hepatic steatosis.
- As per the usual concept, since lean patients with NAFLD have normal body weight, further weight reduction by lifestyle interventions may not be required in them.
- Evidence is however emerging for lesser degree of weight reduction in these patients to achieve the histological improvement.
- Indications for using pharmacotherapy in lean patients with NAFLD remain the same as for non-lean patients.

DISCLOSURE

V. Wong has served as a consultant or advisory committee member for AbbVie, Boehringer Ingelheim, Echosens, Gilead Sciences, Intercept, Inventiva, Merck, Novo Nordisk, Pfizer, ProSciento, Sagimet Biosciences, and TARGET PharmaSolutions; and a speaker for Abbott, AbbVie, Echosens, Gilead Sciences, and Novo Nordisk. He has received a research grant from Gilead Sciences, United States and is a cofounder of Illuminatio Medical Technology Limited. A. Duseja and A. De have no disclosures.

REFERENCES

1. Powell EE, Wong VW, Rinella M. Non-alcoholic fatty liver disease. Lancet 2021; 397(10290):2212–24.
2. Kim D, Kim WR. Nonobese fatty liver disease. Clin Gastroenterol Hepatol 2017; 15(4):474–85.
3. Sakers A, De Siqueira MK, Seale P, et al. Adipose-tissue plasticity in health and disease. Cell 2022;185(3):419–46.
4. Long MT, Noureddin M, Lim JK. AGA clinical practice update: diagnosis and management of nonalcoholic fatty liver disease in lean individuals: expert review. Gastroenterology 2022;163(3):764–74, e1.
5. Consultation WE. Appropriate body-mass index for Asian populations and its implications for policy and intervention strategies. Lancet (London, England) 2004; 363(9403):157–63.

6. Rothman KJ. BMI-related errors in the measurement of obesity. Int J Obes 2008; 32(Suppl 3):S56–9.
7. Neeland IJ, Ross R, Després JP, et al. Visceral and ectopic fat, atherosclerosis, and cardiometabolic disease: a position statement. Lancet Diabetes Endocrinol 2019;7(9):715–25.
8. Park BJ, Kim YJ, Kim DH, et al. Visceral adipose tissue area is an independent risk factor for hepatic steatosis. J Gastroenterol Hepatol 2008;23(6):900–7.
9. Wang H, Chen YE, Eitzman DT. Imaging body fat: techniques and cardiometabolic implications. Arterioscler Thromb Vasc Biol 2014;34(10):2217–23.
10. Ross R, Neeland IJ, Yamashita S, et al. Waist circumference as a vital sign in clinical practice: a consensus statement from the IAS and ICCR working group on visceral obesity. Nat Rev Endocrinol 2020;16(3):177–89.
11. Ye Q, Zou B, Yeo YH, et al. Global prevalence, incidence, and outcomes of non-obese or lean non-alcoholic fatty liver disease: a systematic review and meta-analysis. Lancet Gastroenterol Hepatol 2020;5(8):739–52.
12. Lu FB, Zheng KI, Rios RS, et al. Global epidemiology of lean non-alcoholic fatty liver disease: a systematic review and meta-analysis. J Gastroenterol Hepatol 2020;35(12):2041–50.
13. Young S, Tariq R, Provenza J, et al. Prevalence and profile of nonalcoholic fatty liver disease in lean adults: systematic review and meta-analysis. Hepatol Commun 2020;4(7):953–72.
14. Lin H, Zhang X, Li G, et al. Epidemiology and clinical outcomes of metabolic (Dysfunction)-associated fatty liver disease. J Clin Transl Hepatol 2021;9(6): 972–82.
15. Harrison SA, Gawrieh S, Roberts K, et al. Prospective evaluation of the prevalence of non-alcoholic fatty liver disease and steatohepatitis in a large middle-aged US cohort. J Hepatol 2021;75(2):284–91.
16. Weinberg EM, Trinh HN, Firpi RJ, et al. Lean Americans with nonalcoholic fatty liver disease have lower rates of cirrhosis and comorbid diseases. Clin Gastroenterol Hepatol 2021;19(5):996–1008 e6.
17. Wei JL, Leung JC, Loong TC, et al. Prevalence and severity of nonalcoholic fatty liver disease in non-obese patients: a population study using proton-magnetic resonance spectroscopy. Am J Gastroenterol 2015;110(9):1306–14, quiz 15.
18. Duseja A, Singh SP, Mehta M, et al. Clinicopathological profile and outcome of a large cohort of patients with nonalcoholic fatty liver disease from South Asia: interim results of the Indian consortium on nonalcoholic fatty liver disease. Metab Syndr Relat Disord 2022;20(3):166–73.
19. Wong VW, Wong GL, Yeung DK, et al. Incidence of non-alcoholic fatty liver disease in Hong Kong: a population study with paired proton-magnetic resonance spectroscopy. J Hepatol 2015;62(1):182–9.
20. Younes R, Govaere O, Petta S, et al. Caucasian lean subjects with non-alcoholic fatty liver disease share long-term prognosis of non-lean: time for reappraisal of BMI-driven approach? Gut 2022;71(2):382–90.
21. Vilar-Gomez E, Vuppalanchi R, Mladenovic A, et al. Prevalence of High-risk Nonalcoholic Steatohepatitis (NASH) in the United States: results from NHANES 2017-2018. Clin Gastroenterol Hepatol 2021;S1542-3565(21):01353–7. Online ahead of print.
22. Newsome PN, Sasso M, Deeks JJ, et al. FibroScan-AST (FAST) score for the non-invasive identification of patients with non-alcoholic steatohepatitis with significant activity and fibrosis: a prospective derivation and global validation study. Lancet Gastroenterol Hepatol 2020;5(4):362–73.

23. Singh SP, Misra B, Kar SK, et al. Nonalcoholic fatty liver disease (NAFLD) without insulin resistance: is it different? Clin Res Hepatol Gastroenterol 2015;39(4): 482–8.
24. Wang B, Zhuang R, Luo X, et al. Prevalence of metabolically healthy obese and metabolically obese but normal weight in adults worldwide: a meta-analysis. Horm Metab Res 2015;47(11):839–45.
25. Kramer CK, Zinman B, Retnakaran R. Are metabolically healthy overweight and obesity benign conditions?: a systematic review and meta-analysis. Ann Intern Med 2013;159(11):758–69.
26. Taylor R, Holman RR. Normal weight individuals who develop type 2 diabetes: the personal fat threshold. Clin Sci (Lond) 2015;128(7):405–10.
27. Albhaisi S, Chowdhury A, Sanyal AJ. Non-alcoholic fatty liver disease in lean individuals. JHEP Rep 2019;1(4):329–41.
28. Chung GE, Kim D, Kwark MS, et al. Visceral adipose tissue area as an independent risk factor for elevated liver enzyme in nonalcoholic fatty liver disease. Medicine (Baltim) 2015;94(9):e573.
29. Yu SJ, Kim W, Kim D, et al. Visceral obesity predicts significant fibrosis in patients with nonalcoholic fatty liver disease. Medicine (Baltim) 2015;94(48):e2159.
30. Kim D, Chung GE, Kwak MS, et al. Body fat distribution and risk of incident and regressed nonalcoholic fatty liver disease. Clin Gastroenterol Hepatol 2016;14(1): 132–8, e4.
31. Feldman A, Eder SK, Felder TK, et al. Clinical and metabolic characterization of lean caucasian subjects with non-alcoholic fatty liver. Am J Gastroenterol 2017; 112(1):102–10.
32. Yu R, Shi Q, Liu L, et al. Relationship of sarcopenia with steatohepatitis and advanced liver fibrosis in non-alcoholic fatty liver disease: a meta-analysis. BMC Gastroenterol 2018;18(1):51.
33. Cai C, Song X, Chen Y, et al. Relationship between relative skeletal muscle mass and nonalcoholic fatty liver disease: a systematic review and meta-analysis. Hepatol Int 2020;14(1):115–26.
34. Lee YH, Kim SU, Song K, et al. Sarcopenia is associated with significant liver fibrosis independently of obesity and insulin resistance in nonalcoholic fatty liver disease: nationwide surveys (KNHANES 2008-2011). Hepatology 2016;63(3): 776–86.
35. Tobari M, Hashimoto E, Taniai M, et al. Characteristics of non-alcoholic steatohepatitis among lean patients in Japan: not uncommon and not always benign. J Gastroenterol Hepatol 2019;34(8):1404–10.
36. Kashiwagi K, Takayama M, Fukuhara K, et al. A significant association of non-obese non-alcoholic fatty liver disease with sarcopenic obesity. Clin Nutr ESPEN 2020;38:86–93.
37. Nachit M, De Rudder M, Thissen JP, et al. Myosteatosis rather than sarcopenia associates with non-alcoholic steatohepatitis in non-alcoholic fatty liver disease preclinical models. J Cachexia Sarcopenia Muscle 2021;12(1):144–58.
38. Nachit M, Kwanten WJ, Thissen JP, et al. Muscle fat content is strongly associated with NASH: a longitudinal study in patients with morbid obesity. J Hepatol 2021;75(2):292–301.
39. Linge J, Ekstedt M, Dahlqvist Leinhard O. Adverse muscle composition is linked to poor functional performance and metabolic comorbidities in NAFLD. JHEP Rep 2021;3(1):100197.

40. Zambon Azevedo V, Silaghi CA, Maurel T, et al. Impact of sarcopenia on the severity of the liver damage in patients with non-alcoholic fatty liver disease. Front Nutr 2021;8:774030.
41. Shida T, Oshida N, Suzuki H, et al. Clinical and anthropometric characteristics of non-obese non-alcoholic fatty liver disease subjects in Japan. Hepatol Res 2020; 50(9):1032–46.
42. Kuchay MS, Martínez-Montoro JI, Choudhary NS, et al. Non-Alcoholic fatty liver disease in lean and non-obese individuals: current and future challenges. Biomedicines 2021;9(10):1346.
43. Wang B, Jiang X, Cao M, et al. Altered fecal microbiota correlates with liver biochemistry in nonobese patients with non-alcoholic fatty liver disease. Sci Rep 2016;6:32002.
44. Duarte SMB, Stefano JT, Miele L, et al. Gut microbiome composition in lean patients with NASH is associated with liver damage independent of caloric intake: a prospective pilot study. Nutr Metab Cardiovasc Dis 2018;28(4):369–84.
45. Yun Y, Kim HN, Lee EJ, et al. Fecal and blood microbiota profiles and presence of nonalcoholic fatty liver disease in obese versus lean subjects. PLoS One 2019; 14(3):e0213692.
46. Lee G, You HJ, Bajaj JS, et al. Distinct signatures of gut microbiome and metabolites associated with significant fibrosis in non-obese NAFLD. Nat Commun 2020;11(1):4982.
47. Chen F, Esmaili S, Rogers GB, et al. Lean NAFLD: a distinct entity shaped by differential metabolic adaptation. Hepatology 2020;71(4):1213–27.
48. Assy N, Nasser G, Kamayse I, et al. Soft drink consumption linked with fatty liver in the absence of traditional risk factors. Can J Gastroenterol 2008;22(10):811–6.
49. Yasutake K, Nakamuta M, Shima Y, et al. Nutritional investigation of non-obese patients with non-alcoholic fatty liver disease: the significance of dietary cholesterol. Scand J Gastroenterol 2009;44(4):471–7.
50. Kwak JH, Jun DW, Lee SM, et al. Lifestyle predictors of obese and non-obese patients with nonalcoholic fatty liver disease: a cross-sectional study. Clin Nutr 2018; 37(5):1550–7.
51. De A, Ahmad N, Mehta M, et al. NAFLD vs. MAFLD - it is not the name but the disease that decides the outcome in fatty liver. J Hepatol 2022;76(2):475–7.
52. De A, Mehta M, Singh P, et al. Lean Indian patients with non-alcoholic fatty liver disease (NAFLD) have less metabolic risk factors but similar liver disease severity as non-lean patients with NAFLD. J Clin Exp Hepatol 2022;12:S63.
53. Sookoian S, Pirola CJ. Systematic review with meta-analysis: the significance of histological disease severity in lean patients with nonalcoholic fatty liver disease. Aliment Pharmacol Ther 2018;47(1):16–25.
54. Akyuz U, Yesil A, Yilmaz Y. Characterization of lean patients with nonalcoholic fatty liver disease: potential role of high hemoglobin levels. Scand J Gastroenterol 2015;50(3):341–6.
55. Alam S, Gupta UD, Alam M, et al. Clinical, anthropometric, biochemical, and histological characteristics of nonobese nonalcoholic fatty liver disease patients of Bangladesh. Indian J Gastroenterol 2014;33(5):452–7.
56. Kumar R, Rastogi A, Sharma MK, et al. Clinicopathological characteristics and metabolic profiles of non-alcoholic fatty liver disease in Indian patients with normal body mass index: do they differ from obese or overweight non-alcoholic fatty liver disease? Indian J Endocrinol Metab 2013;17(4):665–71.

57. Fracanzani AL, Petta S, Lombardi R, et al. Liver and cardiovascular damage in patients with lean nonalcoholic fatty liver disease, and association with visceral obesity. Clin Gastroenterol Hepatol 2017;15(10):1604–16011.e1.
58. Honda Y, Yoneda M, Kessoku T, et al. Characteristics of non-obese non-alcoholic fatty liver disease: effect of genetic and environmental factors. Hepatol Res 2016; 46(10):1011–8.
59. Leung JC, Loong TC, Wei JL, et al. Histological severity and clinical outcomes of nonalcoholic fatty liver disease in nonobese patients. Hepatology 2017;65(1): 54–64.
60. Margariti A, Deutsch M, Manolakopoulos S, et al. The severity of histologic liver lesions is independent of body mass index in patients with nonalcoholic fatty liver disease. J Clin Gastroenterol 2013;47(3):280–6.
61. Sookoian S, Pirola CJ. Systematic review with meta-analysis: risk factors for non-alcoholic fatty liver disease suggest a shared altered metabolic and cardiovascular profile between lean and obese patients. Aliment Pharmacol Ther 2017;46(2): 85–95.
62. Tan EX, Lee JW, Jumat NH, et al. Non-obese non-alcoholic fatty liver disease (NAFLD) in Asia: an international registry study. Metabolism 2022;126:154911.
63. Denkmayr L, Feldman A, Stechemesser L, et al. Lean patients with non-alcoholic fatty liver disease have a severe histological phenotype similar to obese patients. J Clin Med 2018;7(12):562.
64. Meeuwsen S, Horgan GW, Elia M. The relationship between BMI and percent body fat, measured by bioelectrical impedance, in a large adult sample is curvilinear and influenced by age and sex. Clin Nutr 2010;29(5):560–6.
65. Hirose S, Matsumoto K, Tatemichi M, et al. Nineteen-year prognosis in Japanese patients with biopsy-proven nonalcoholic fatty liver disease: lean versus overweight patients. PLoS One 2020;15(11):e0241770.
66. Hagstrom H, Nasr P, Ekstedt M, et al. Risk for development of severe liver disease in lean patients with nonalcoholic fatty liver disease: a long-term follow-up study. Hepatol Commun 2018;2(1):48–57.
67. Zou B, Yeo YH, Nguyen VH, et al. Prevalence, characteristics and mortality outcomes of obese, nonobese and lean NAFLD in the United States, 1999-2016. J Intern Med 2020;288(1):139–51.
68. Wong VW, Chan WK, Chitturi S, et al. Asia-pacific working party on non-alcoholic fatty liver disease guidelines 2017-Part 1: definition, risk factors and assessment. J Gastroenterol Hepatol 2018;33(1):70–85.
69. Eslam M, Newsome PN, Sarin SK, et al. A new definition for metabolic dysfunction-associated fatty liver disease: an international expert consensus statement. J Hepatol 2020;73(1):202–9.
70. Wong VW, Wong GL, Woo J, et al. Impact of the new definition of metabolic associated fatty liver disease on the epidemiology of the disease. Clin Gastroenterol Hepatol 2021;19(10):2161–21671 e5.
71. Francque S, Wong VW. NAFLD in lean individuals: not a benign disease. Gut 2022;71(2):234–6.
72. Wong VW, Adams LA, de Ledinghen V, et al. Noninvasive biomarkers in NAFLD and NASH - current progress and future promise. Nat Rev Gastroenterol Hepatol 2018;15(8):461–78.
73. Fu C, Wai JW, Nik Mustapha NR, et al. Performance of simple fibrosis scores in nonobese patients with nonalcoholic fatty liver disease. Clin Gastroenterol Hepatol 2020;18(12):2843–2845 e2.

74. Wong VW, Tak WY, Goh GBB, et al. Performance of noninvasive tests of fibrosis among Asians, hispanic, and non-hispanic whites in the STELLAR trials. Clin Gastroenterol Hepatol 2022;S1542-3565(22):00069–76. Online ahead of print.
75. Mahady SE, Macaskill P, Craig JC, et al. Diagnostic accuracy of noninvasive fibrosis scores in a population of individuals with a low prevalence of fibrosis. Clin Gastroenterol Hepatol 2017;15(9):1453–14560 e1.
76. Hagstrom H, Talback M, Andreasson A, et al. Repeated FIB-4 measurements can help identify individuals at risk of severe liver disease. J Hepatol 2020;73(5): 1023–9.
77. Zhang X, Wong GL, Wong VW. Application of transient elastography in nonalcoholic fatty liver disease. Clin Mol Hepatol 2020;26(2):128–41.
78. Wong VW, Irles M, Wong GL, et al. Unified interpretation of liver stiffness measurement by M and XL probes in non-alcoholic fatty liver disease. Gut 2019; 68(11):2057–64.
79. Park CC, Nguyen P, Hernandez C, et al. Magnetic resonance elastography vs transient elastography in detection of fibrosis and noninvasive measurement of steatosis in patients with biopsy-proven nonalcoholic fatty liver disease. Gastroenterology 2017;152(3):598–607 e2.
80. Wong VW, Chan RS, Wong GL, et al. Community-based lifestyle modification programme for non-alcoholic fatty liver disease: a randomized controlled trial. J Hepatol 2013;59(3):536–42.
81. Vilar-Gomez E, Martinez-Perez Y, Calzadilla-Bertot L, et al. Weight loss through lifestyle modification significantly reduces features of nonalcoholic steatohepatitis. Gastroenterology 2015;149(2):367–78, e5; quiz e14-5.
82. Wong VW, Wong GL, Chan RS, et al. Beneficial effects of lifestyle intervention in non-obese patients with non-alcoholic fatty liver disease. J Hepatol 2018;69(6): 1349–56.
83. Satapathy SK, Jiang Y, Agbim U, et al. Posttransplant outcome of lean compared with obese nonalcoholic steatohepatitis in the United States: the obesity paradox. Liver Transpl 2020;26(1):68–79.
84. Tantai X, Liu Y, Yeo YH, et al. Effect of sarcopenia on survival in patients with cirrhosis: a meta-analysis. J Hepatol 2022;76(3):588–99.
85. Wong VW, Singal AK. Emerging medical therapies for non-alcoholic fatty liver disease and for alcoholic hepatitis. Transl Gastroenterol Hepatol 2019;4:53.
86. Mantovani A, Byrne CD, Targher G. Efficacy of peroxisome proliferator-activated receptor agonists, glucagon-like peptide-1 receptor agonists, or sodium-glucose cotransporter-2 inhibitors for treatment of non-alcoholic fatty liver disease: a systematic review. Lancet Gastroenterol Hepatol 2022;7(4):367–78.
87. Gastaldelli A, Sabatini S, Carli F, et al. PPAR-gamma-induced changes in visceral fat and adiponectin levels are associated with improvement of steatohepatitis in patients with NASH. Liver Int 2021;41(11):2659–70.
88. Francque SM, Bedossa P, Ratziu V, et al. A randomized, controlled trial of the pan-PPAR agonist lanifibranor in NASH. N Engl J Med 2021;385(17):1547–58.
89. Hsiang JC, Wong VW. SGLT2 inhibitors in liver patients. Clin Gastroenterol Hepatol 2020;18(10):2168–21672 e2.
90. Newsome PN, Buchholtz K, Cusi K, et al. A placebo-controlled trial of subcutaneous semaglutide in nonalcoholic steatohepatitis. N Engl J Med 2021;384(12): 1113–24.

Special Population

Pediatric Nonalcoholic Fatty Liver Disease

Eric Dybbro, MD[a,1], Miriam B. Vos, MD, MSPH[b,2], Rohit Kohli, MBBS, MS[a,*]

KEYWORDS

• Nonalcoholic steatohepatitis • Obesity • Children • Lifestyle modifications

KEY POINTS

- Pediatric nonalcoholic fatty liver disease (NAFLD) represents the most common liver disease with children and associated with significant morbidity and even with increased mortality versus age-matched controls.
- Therapeutic options are limited in pediatric patients, and the current mainstay of therapy, lifestyle modifications, has proven to have a limited efficacy due to patient adherence in the current clinical setting.
- More studies remain to elucidate improved therapeutic options and improve programs aimed at the prevention of development of NAFLD in the pediatric population.

DEFINITION

Pediatric nonalcoholic fatty liver disease (NAFLD) represents a spectrum of chronic liver disease that can range from isolated steatosis Nonalcoholic Fatty Liver (NAFL), Nonalcoholic Steatohepatitis (NASH) with the presence of hepatocellular inflammation and injury with or without fibrosis, and even cirrhosis.[1] NAFLD is defined as the accumulation of 5% or greater macrovesicular and microvesicular fat in hepatocytes in a patient in whom other causes of liver disease has been excluded. In the pediatric population, it is important to exclude other liver diseases that can present with steatosis as part of the diagnostic process. These include Wilson's disease, mitochondrial and peroxisomal disorders, lysosomal acid lipase deficiency, lipodystrophies, and more.[2–5]

EPIDEMIOLOGY

NAFLD is closely linked to obesity and thus, in parallel to the global obesity pandemic, the estimated worldwide pooled prevalence of NAFLD has increased during the past

[a] Division of Gastroenterology, Hepatology, and Nutrition, Children's Hospital Los Angeles, Los Angeles, CA, USA; [b] Division of Gastroenterology, Hepatology, and Nutrition, Emory School of Medicine, Children's Healthcare of Atlanta, Atlanta, GA, USA
[1] Present address: 400 North 2nd Avenue #472, Phoenix, AZ 85003.
[2] Present address: 1860 Haygood Drive, Atlanta, GA 30322.
* Corresponding author. 4650 Sunset Boulevard, Los Angeles, CA 90703.
E-mail address: rokohli@chla.usc.edu
Twitter: @liver4kids (R.K.)

Clin Liver Dis 27 (2023) 471–482
https://doi.org/10.1016/j.cld.2023.01.012
liver.theclinics.com
1089-3261/23/

decades with current USA-specific prevalence studies estimate it affecting up to 30% of the adult population.[6,7] Although initially considered an adult disease, it was very quickly recognized to also affect the pediatric population.[8]

Risk factors for the development of NAFLD in the pediatric population include increased body mass index (BMI), low birth weight, rapid weight gain from birth to 5 years, parental hepatic steatosis, central adiposity, and insulin resistance.[9] Given the increase in pediatric obesity rates, it is not surprising that the estimated prevalence of pediatric NAFLD has been increasing during the past several decades, both in the United States and globally.[10,11] However, epidemiological studies of the prevalence of NAFLD in pediatrics has been hampered by methodologic issues with screening methods, necessitating indirect measurements of prevalence to estimate disease burden. Although increased awareness has prompted improved screening algorithms in pediatrics, it is likely that many patients remain undiagnosed.[12] Population prevalence in the United States based on posthumous pathological examination revealed the prevalence of fatty liver disease to in up 13% of all children, with the rate increasing to 38% among obese children.[13] Given these estimates, NAFLD in children is increasingly being recognized as affecting a significant portion of the pediatric population and now represents *the most common form of pediatric chronic liver disease*.[14]

PATHOGENESIS/GENETICS

Although the pathogenesis of NAFLD remains to be fully elucidated, current evidence suggests a genetic underpinning followed by environmental hits. The prevalence of pediatric NAFLD differs by sex and race/ethnicity despite adjustment for NAFLD risk factors, with higher rates of hepatic steatosis observed among children of Hispanic origin followed by Asian and Caucasian and with relative protection in the Black population.[15,16] These race and ethnic patterns seem to be driven by inheritance of NAFLD polymorphisms. Sex seems to play a role with multiple studies suggesting increased prevalence in male children.[16,17]

[18]There is increasing recognition of the role of genetic contributions to explain the noted heterogeneity of disease. This was first suggested in studies demonstrated familial clustering of NAFLD, indicative of a more complex interplay between genetics and environmental inputs.[19] The role of genetic modulation of risk factors may be especially important in the pathogenesis of pediatric disease given the presentation at an early age.

Genome-wide association studies have identified an Single nucleotide polymorphism (SNP) in *adiponutrin/patatin-like phospholipase domain containing 3* as strong determinants in the development of steatosis and steatohepatitis in adults.[20] In children, this polymorphism was similarly noted to increase the risk of NAFLD development and correlate with steatosis severity, hepatocellular ballooning, lobular inflammation, and perivenular fibrosis.[21,22] Several other polymorphisms have been identified determinates of pediatric hepatic steatosis, and population prevalence of these also contribute to dramatic ethnic variation of disease.[23] More studies specific to pediatrics is required to further characterize genetic differences in disease progression.

COMORBIDITIES

Insulin resistance, Prediabetes, and Type 2 Diabetes

Abnormal glucose metabolism has been shown to be common in adult patients with NAFLD, and comorbid type 2 diabetes has been established as a risk factor for progressive NAFLD, NASH, cirrhosis, and liver-related mortality.[24] In pediatrics, a large multicenter study of pediatric patients with NAFLD found that nearly 30% of the patients had prediabetes or type 2 diabetes, a rate higher than would be expected in obese patients without NAFLD.[25] Concerningly, those patients with type 2 diabetes had higher rates of NASH indicating, similar to adult studies, comorbid type 2 diabetes may confer high risk of advanced liver disease in pediatrics.[26] However, the relationship between insulin resistance and NAFLD remains to be fully understood. In a study of obese children and adolescents, genetically influenced NAFLD was not associated with increased Homeostatic Model Assessement of Insulin Resitance (HOMA -IR), suggesting that the association previously described between NAFLD and insulin resistance is due to shared pathogenic pathways, rather than driven by the NAFLD polymorphisms.[27]

Obstructive sleep apnea

Obstructive sleep apnea (OSA) has been demonstrated to be associated with NAFLD in adult and animal studies and has been linked to driving the progression of NASH, although the exact mechanism remains unknown.[28] In pediatrics-focused studies, the presence of OSA was shown to be associated with NASH and advanced fibrosis on biopsy with direct correlation of severity of OSA to advanced histological features, regardless of insulin resistance/obesity parameters.[28,29] The role of OSA management and its ability to modulate NAFLD in pediatrics are yet to be fully elucidated; however, the management of pediatric OSA may have long-term benefits not-respecting NAFLD and, thus, should be identified and referred for consideration of management.[30]

SCREENING

NAFLD in pediatrics is often asymptomatic and historically was identified incidentally. Given the growing burden of disease, as well as increased awareness of need to identify patients with NAFLD, guidelines on screening and identification among pediatric patients have been recommended by several specialty groups. Current guidelines proposed by the North American Society of Pediatric Gastroenterology, Hepatology, and Nutrition (NASPGHAN) suggest screening with the measurement of serum alanine aminotransferase (ALT) starting between ages 9 and 11 for all obese children or overweight children with additional risk factors for NAFLD.[31] The use of ALT has the benefit of being an inexpensive and widely available test, though it has important limitations. The NASPGHAN guidelines suggest utilizing an ALT cutoff of greater than 2 times the upper limit of normal (for greater than 3 months) to initiate further workup for NAFLD and other causes of alcoholic steatosis.

The American Academy of Pediatrics has backed the NASPGHAN guidelines and promoted their application in outpatient general pediatrics. Review of well child visits from 2009 to 2018 using review of electronic health records in a large integrated health care network demonstrated NAFLD screening occurred in 54% of children with obesity and 24% of overweight children. Of those children with abnormal screens, only 12% were referred for further evaluation.[12] This indicates that a significant number of patients may remain undiagnosed, demonstrating the continued need to streamline and ensure the application screening guidelines in clinical practice.

It should be noted that the use of ALT for screening purposes has important limitations. Importantly, exact thresholds have not been established due to wide variability in ALT cutoffs and used reference standards across validation studies. Pooled results of various studies suggest an ALT threshold of ~40 IU/L demonstrating a sensitivity of 50% and specificity of 90%, with the ability to increase specificity although at the expense of sensitivity as cutoffs set higher.[32] In addition, serum ALT levels in pediatric patients with NAFLD have been shown to correlate with steatosis and insulin resistance versus NASH and fibrosis, histological findings seen even in patients with normal ALT levels.[33,34] Much research has been dedicated to the identification of novel biomarkers but until then clinicians must be aware of the important caveats in ALT measurement.

DIAGNOSIS

NAFLD remains a diagnosis of exclusion requiring the presence of hepatic steatosis and the exclusion of other causes including genetic/metabolic disorders, autoimmune, infections, and medication-induced steatosis. When these alternative causes are adequately ruled out, the diagnosis of NAFLD is established; however, definite diagnosis, and staging of the fibrosis, continues to require a liver biopsy. Pediatric liver biopsy procedures, historically performed by pediatric gastroenterologists, are frequently now under the purview of interventional radiology and demonstrate excellent safety parameters.[35] Although many clinicians may forgo the liver biopsy in favor of "presumptive diagnosis" to avoid an invasive procedure, the liver biopsy continues to have a role in its ability to accurately stage NASH activity and fibrosis as well as identify other chronic liver disease.

In adults, the characteristic histopathological findings in NAFLD are well characterized and include macrovesicular steatosis, perisinusoidal or pericellular fibrosis, lobular inflammation, lipid granulomas, Mallory hyaline, and megamitochondria, which has allowed for the development and clinical use of a grading score.[36,37] Pathological examination of pediatric patients with NAFLD has demonstrated distinct patterns of pathologic findings as well as important differences contrasted to adult pathological findings, again highlighting the heterogeneity of disease.[23] The exact clinical significance of these differences remains unknown.

Predictive Scores

Given the population prevalence of NAFLD, and the need for invasive liver biopsy procedure for prognostication, much effort has been expended to develop noninvasive mechanism for the identification of children with NAFLD and a way to determine those with advanced disease. Several such noninvasive fibrosis scoring systems have been developed in adult patients including AST/ALT ratio, NAFLD fibrosis score, AST/platelet ratio, and the FIB4-score[38]; however, extrapolation to pediatric patients have demonstrated poor performance in the pediatric population.[39,40]

Two specific scoring systems have been derived for the pediatric population, the Pediatric NAFLD Fibrosis Score and the Pediatric NAFLD Fibrosis Index, both developed to predict the presence and staging of fibrosis in children without requiring a liver biopsy.[41,42] However, when tested in other cohorts, they performed inadequately, raised into question their generalizability in larger population groups.[40,43]

Imaging

Ultrasound (US) imaging is commonly used in the evaluation of hepatic steatosis given its relative ease of obtaining and lower cost compared with other imaging modalities. Unfortunately, the use of US to identify hepatic steatosis has not shown adequate performance metrics, especially in obese children.[44] Indeed, in a head-to-head cohort comparison, the performance of US did not demonstrate improvement over serum ALT measurement.[45] Importantly, US has proved to be unable to distinguish inflammation and/or progression of fibrosis in pediatric NAFLD, limiting its application in NAFLD evaluation.[46]

A new US-based modality that has shown promise in NAFLD is the use of controlled attenuation parameter (CAP), which aims to assess presence and extent of hepatic steatosis by calculating the attenuation of the shear-wave propagation. This technology has been shown to have good performance in adult patients.[47,48] In a single-center study comparing the correlation between CAP measurements and histological grades demonstrated the ability of CAP to distinguish between no steatosis and steatosis as well as between grades of steatosis in pediatric patients with variety of liver disease.[49] Limited studies have shown that it may have similar accuracy in pediatric NAFLD; however, further studies are warranted due to report of decreased accuracy noted in obese children.[48,49]

Transient elastography represents another US-based modality that screens for advanced fibrosis by measuring sheer wave speed and hepatic stiffness. This has shown to be accurate in predicting fibrosis in adult patients.[50] Meta-analysis of pediatric studies demonstrated specificity of 95% and sensitivity of 90% for the prediction of >F2 fibrosis, although of note, considerable heterogeneity was noted among included studies.[51] As in CAP, use in patients with obesity may similarly affect accuracy.

Use of MRI, particularly the use of MRI-estimated liver proton density fat fraction has shown promise in accurately determining steatosis in adult patients and demonstrated improved accuracy over US-based modalities.[52] Application to pediatrics resulted in similar high accuracy in the pediatric population and was able to classify and predict steatosis grade.[53,54] Use of this technology, however, continues to be limited by availability and high cost as well as possible need for sedation in younger children.[55]

NATURAL HISTORY OF PEDIATRIC NONALCOHOLIC FATTY LIVER DISEASE

Longitudinal studies in adult patients with NAFLD demonstrate increased mortality when comparted with matched controls.[56] Cross-sectional studies have demonstrated that pediatric patietns with NAFLD are at risk of development of advanced fibrosis, cirrhosis, and even the development of hepatocellular carcinoma.[57,58] A single-center longitudinal cohort study of 66 pediatric patients with NAFLD over median follow-up time of 6.4 years demonstrated that pediatric NAFLD diagnosis was associated with significant decrease in observed survival free of liver transplantation as compared with expected survival of matched general population.[59] Available UNOS data demonstrate significant morbidity and even mortality associated with transplantation for NASH cirrhosis, with a significant number of patients requiring retransplantation.[60]

In addition, given the association with metabolic syndrome, patients with NAFLD continue to be at risk for the development of other comorbidities, and indeed, a single center cohort of patients with NAFLD followed over time demonstrated continued obesity and increased prevalence of diabetes at the end of follow-up period.[61] NAFLD has also been associated with increased cardiovascular risk profile, with pathogenic changes in lipid profiles and atherosclerotic changes being noted in pediatric patients.[62]

[59]Overall, there is insufficient 10 and 20+ year outcome data in children with NAFLD, which remains a major gap in our understanding of the disease. In the United States, data collection for such outcomes is hampered by the split medical system and lack of carryover of pediatric medical records into adult health-care systems.

THERAPEUTIC MODALITIES

The management of NAFLD involves direct treatment of liver disease as well as the associated metabolic syndrome comorbidities with the goal of therapy to improve long-term outcomes. This is especially important in pediatrics given the early age of presentation.

Lifestyle Modifications

First-line treatment of all obese children with NAFLD is lifestyle modification in the form of dietary restriction and exercise. Efficacy of weight loss in pediatrics has been demonstrated in a study in which study participants who lost approximately 20% of their body weight showed a significant reduction of serum ALT and hepatic steatosis.[63] In a rigorous, randomized controlled trial, reduction of dietary sugars added to foods to less than 3% of calories for 8 weeks in a cohort of adolescent males was shown to significantly decrease serum ALT as well as hepatic steatosis (−6%) as measured via MRI.[64] Exercise, to the tune of more than 60 min/session and more than 3 times week, has been shown to be effective in reducing hepatic steatosis.[65]

Although effective in study protocols, lifestyle modifications have shown more limited efficacy in clinical practice due to patient participation and long-term adherence. Indeed, even study programs have found long-term maintenance of weight loss to be limited.[66] Studies examining effects of obesity counseling in primary care setting have shown that the number of patients able to achieve a meaningful reduction of BMI to be limited to only around one-third, and that success was correlated with increased amount of clinical follow-up that may not be feasible in outpatient pediatric clinics.[67]

Pharmacological therapies

Given the limitations of lifestyle modifications, much attention has been directed to identifying effective pharmacological therapies. One of the largest studies in pediatrics, the Treatment of NAFLD in Children (TONIC) trial, investigated the use of Vitamin E in patients with NASH and demonstrated the reduction of NAFLD activity score and significant resolution of NASH in 58% of patients, although primary endpoint of sustained decrease in serum ALT was not reached, nor was reduction in fibrosis.[68] Widespread adoption of Vitamin E therapy is limited by some reports concerning for higher mortality during longer term usage, although repeat studies have failed to replicate the increase in mortality.[69,70] Due to these concerns, AASLD guidelines reserve Vitamin E therapy only for patients with biopsy-proven NASH after counseling on possible risks while, at this time, NASPGHAN guidelines do not recommend use.[1,31]

The use of insulin sensitizers has been suggested as role in the treatment of NAFLD given the role of insulin resistance in the pathogenesis of NAFLD. Metformin remains the most studied in the pediatric population; however, trial studies have not proven durable benefit on serum ALT or hepatic histology.[68,71] Pioglitazone, a peroxisome proliferator-activated receptor γ agonist, has shown promise in the treatment of adult NAFLD; however, adverse effects on weight gain, bone health, and increased risk of bladder cancer limit its usage in pediatric population.[1,72] A rapidly evolving category of medications that may have benefit for pediatric NAFLD in the future is the GLP1s, both because of the weight loss potential and insulin-sensitizing effect. GLP1s.[73]

Supplementation with the use of poly-unsaturated fats has resulted in mixed evidence to support its ability to reduce ALT level and long-term outcomes in pediatric NAFLD, although smaller Randomized Clinical Trial (RCT) studies have suggested supplementation with docosahexaenoic acid as able to decrease liver fat content via US measurement in children with NAFLD.[74–76] At present, it is unclear the clinical significance of these findings and thus continue to not have routine recommendations for their use in pediatrics.

Bariatric Surgery

Use of bariatric surgery has been established as effective in adult studies but its practice is more limited in the pediatric population. Use in obese adolescent populations has shown that bariatric surgery can result in durable weight loss and reduce NASH histological score in addition to improvement in insulin resistance, hypertension, and dyslipidemia.[77,78] Currently, NASPGHAN guidelines do not recommend bariatric surgery as a specific therapy for NAFLD; however, the guidelines do suggest consideration of its use in obese adolescents with noncirrhotic NASH and other obesity-related serious comorbidities.[31] The American Society for Metabolic and Bariatric Surgery Pediatric Committee 2018 guidelines stress the safety and efficacy of bariatric surgery in obese adolescent patients and stress its role in those patients with NASH highlighting the opportunity to intervene early and prevent long-term damage.[79] Currently, bariatric surgery in adolescents remains a relative uncommon procedure, despite national obesity and NAFLD rates.[80] It remains to be seen how much of a role bariatric surgery will play in pediatric NAFLD, especially given the possibilities of the relatively noninvasive and novel endoscopic-bariatric technologies.

PREVENTION IS THE KEY

Given limited therapeutic options, it is reasonable to also consider the prevention of NAFLD development. This is especially true in the pediatric population where, given the age of onset, the development of NAFLD results in many years of expected disease duration during which complications would be expected to develop. Given the ability of lifestyle modifications to prevent NAFLD as well as aid in obesity comorbidities, it has emerged as cornerstone of preventative efforts. Weight loss management in the medical home has been proven to be more effective in setting of multidisciplinary team approach, and several studies have suggested models to construct the medical home.[81–83] Research into obesity prevention has indicated prevention efforts structured as multilevel approach involving patients and their families but also communities and school systems.[84] Given the scope of childhood obesity, there exists ongoing research to ascertain an efficacious but also cost-effective manner to initiate programs on a population level. Pediatric NAFLD may be a condition to focus on for prevention starting at an early age, given the familial pattern and strong genetic predictors.

SUMMARY

- Pediatric NAFLD represents the most common liver disease with children and is associated with significant morbidity and even mortality versus age-matched controls.
- Therapeutic options are limited in pediatric patients, and the mainstay of therapy, lifestyle modifications, has proven to have limited efficacy due to patient adherence in the current clinical setting.
- More research remains to elucidate improved therapeutic options and improve programs aimed at the prevention of development of NAFLD in the pediatric population.

CLINICS CARE POINTS

- NAFLD is the most common chronic liver disease in children, although true, the prevalence is likely underrepresented due to limitations of current screening modalities.
- In youth, the diagnosis of NAFLD requires excluding other causes of hepatic steatosis.
- The diagnosis of NAFLD in pediatrics carries important long-term morbidity, and even mortality risks, and often is accompanied by other metabolic disease-related comorbidities.

- Current therapeutic options available in pediatric population remain focused on lifestyle modification. Although efficacious in research settings, current clinical approaches have demonstrated limited efficacy due to patient adherence.

DISCLOSURE

The authors have nothing to disclose. E. Dybbro: Nothing to disclose. R. Kohli: Epigen-research grant, Sanofi, Mirum, Albireo, Intercept–consulting.

REFERENCES

1. Chalasani N, Younossi Z, Lavine JE, et al. The diagnosis and management of nonalcoholic fatty liver disease: practice guidance from the American Association for the Study of Liver Diseases. J Hepatol 2018;67:328–57.
2. Alqahtani SA, Chami R, Abuquteish D, et al. Hepatic ultrastructural features distinguish paediatric Wilson disease from NAFLD and autoimmune hepatitis. Liver Int 2022;42:2482–91.
3. Wang C, Pai AK, Putra J. Paediatric non-alcoholic fatty liver disease: an approach to pathological evaluation. J Clin Pathol 2022;75:443–51.
4. Patni N, Garg A. Lipodystrophy for the diabetologist-what to look for. Curr Diab Rep 2022;22:461–70.
5. Eslam M, Sanyal AJ, George J, et al. MAFLD: a consensus-driven proposed nomenclature for metabolic associated fatty liver disease. Gastroenterology 2020;158:1999–2014.e1.
6. Mitra S, De A, Chowdhury A. Epidemiology of non-alcoholic and alcoholic fatty liver diseases. Transl Gastroenterol Hepatol 2020;5:16.
7. Masarone M, Federico A, Abenavoli L, et al. Non alcoholic fatty liver: epidemiology and natural history. Rev Recent Clin Trials 2014;9:126–33.
8. Moran JR, Ghishan FK, Halter SA, et al. Steatohepatitis in obese children: a cause of chronic liver dysfunction. Am J Gastroenterol 1983;78:374–7.
9. Schwimmer JB, Deutsch R, Rauch JB, et al. Obesity, insulin resistance, and other clinicopathological correlates of pediatric nonalcoholic fatty liver disease. J Pediatr 2003;143:500–5.
10. Welsh JA, Karpen S, Vos MB. Increasing prevalence of nonalcoholic fatty liver disease among United States adolescents, 1988-1994 to 2007-2010. J Pediatr 2013;162:496–500.e1.
11. Zhang X, et al. Increasing prevalence of NAFLD/NASH among children, adolescents and young adults from 1990 to 2017: a population-based observational study. BMJ Open 2021;11:e042843.
12. Sahota A.K., Shapiro W.L., Newton K.P., et al., Incidence of nonalcoholic fatty liver disease in children: 2009-2018, Pediatrics, 146(6):e20200771, 2020.
13. Schwimmer JB, Deutsch R, Kahen T, et al. Prevalence of fatty liver in children and adolescents. Pediatrics 2006;118:1388–93.
14. Mann J, Valenti L, Scorletti E, et al. Nonalcoholic fatty liver disease in children. Semin Liver Dis 2018;38:001–13.
15. Browning J.D., Szczepaniak L.S., Dobbins R., et al., Prevalence of hepatic steatosis in an urban population in the United States: impact of ethnicity, Hepatology, 40, 2004, 1387–1395.
16. Schwimmer JB, McGreal N, Deutsch R, et al. Influence of gender, race, and ethnicity on suspected fatty liver in obese adolescents. Pediatrics 2005;115:e561–5.

17. Wiegand S, Keller K-M, Röbl M, et al. Obese boys at increased risk for nonalcoholic liver disease: evaluation of 16 390 overweight or obese children and adolescents. Int J Obes 2010;34:1468–74.
18. Tilg H, Moschen AR. Evolution of inflammation in nonalcoholic fatty liver disease: the multiple parallel hits hypothesis. Hepatology 2010;52:1836–46.
19. Schwimmer JB, Celedon MA, Lavine JE, et al. Heritability of nonalcoholic fatty liver disease. Gastroenterology 2009;136:1585–92.
20. Romeo S, Kozlitina J, Xing C, et al. Genetic variation in PNPLA3 confers susceptibility to nonalcoholic fatty liver disease. Nat Genet 2008;40:1461–5.
21. Valenti L, Alisi A, Galmozzi E, et al. I148M patatin-like phospholipase domain-containing 3 gene variant and severity of pediatric nonalcoholic fatty liver disease. Hepatology 2010;52:1274–80.
22. Mansoor S, Maheshwari A, Di Guglielmo M, et al. The PNPLA3 rs738409 Variant but not MBOAT7 rs641738 is a risk factor for nonalcoholic fatty liver disease in obese U.S. Children of hispanic ethnicity. Pediatr Gastroenterol Hepatol Nutr 2021;24:455–69.
23. Schwimmer JB, Behling C, Newbury R, et al. Histopathology of pediatric nonalcoholic fatty liver disease. Hepatology 2005;42:641–9.
24. Younossi ZM, Gramlich T, Matteoni CA, et al. Nonalcoholic fatty liver disease in patients with type 2 diabetes. Clin Gastroenterol Hepatol 2004;2:262–5.
25. Newton KP, Hou J, Crimmins NA, et al. Prevalence of prediabetes and type 2 diabetes in children with nonalcoholic fatty liver disease. JAMA Pediatr 2016;170: e161971.
26. Newfield RS, Graves CL, Newbury RO, et al. Non-alcoholic fatty liver disease in pediatric type 2 diabetes: metabolic and histologic characteristics in 38 subjects. Pediatr Diabetes Pedi 2018;12798. https://doi.org/10.1111/pedi.12798.
27. Morandi A, Di Sessa A, Zusi C, et al. Nonalcoholic fatty liver disease and estimated insulin resistance in obese youth: a mendelian randomization analysis. J Clin Endocrinol Metab 2020;105:e4046–54.
28. Mesarwi OA, Loomba R, Malhotra A. Obstructive sleep apnea, hypoxia, and nonalcoholic fatty liver disease. Am J Respir Crit Care Med 2019;199:830–41.
29. Ahmed MH. Obstructive sleep apnea syndrome and fatty liver: association or causal link? World J Gastroenterol 2010;16:4243.
30. Thomas S, Patel S, Gummalla P, et al. Cannot hit snooze on OSA: sequelae of pediatric obstructive sleep apnea. Children 2022;9:261.
31. Vos MB, Abrams SA, Barlow SE, et al. NASPGHAN Clinical practice guideline for the diagnosis and treatment of nonalcoholic fatty liver disease in children: recommendations from the expert committee on NAFLD (ECON) and the north american society of pediatric gastroenterology, hepatology and nutrition (NASPGHAN). J Pediatr Gastroenterol Nutr 2017;64:319–34.
32. Koot BGP, Nobili V. Screening for non-alcoholic fatty liver disease in children: do guidelines provide enough guidance? Obes Rev 2017;18:1050–60.
33. Maximos M, Bril F, Portillo Sanchez P, et al. The role of liver fat and insulin resistance as determinants of plasma aminotransferase elevation in nonalcoholic fatty liver disease. Hepatology 2015;61:153–60.
34. Molleston JP, Schwimmer JB, Yates KP, et al. Histological abnormalities in children with nonalcoholic fatty liver disease and normal or mildly elevated alanine aminotransferase levels. J Pediatr 2014;164:707–13.e3.
35. Potter C, Hogan MJ, Henry-Kendjorsky K, et al. Safety of pediatric percutaneous liver biopsy performed by interventional radiologists. J Pediatr Gastroenterol Nutr 2011;53:202–6.

36. Brunt EM, Janney CG, di Bisceglie AM, et al. Nonalcoholic steatohepatitis: a proposal for grading and staging the histological lesions. Am J Gastroenterol 1999; 94:2467–74.
37. Kleiner DE, Brunt EM, Van Natta M, et al. Design and validation of a histological scoring system for nonalcoholic fatty liver disease. Hepatology 2005;41:1313–21.
38. Alkhouri N, McCullough AJ. Noninvasive diagnosis of NASH and liver fibrosis within the spectrum of NAFLD. Gastroenterol Hepatol 2012;8:661–8.
39. Mansoor S, Yerian L, Kohli R, et al. The evaluation of hepatic fibrosis scores in children with nonalcoholic fatty liver disease. Dig Dis Sci 2015;60:1440–7.
40. Yang HR. Noninvasive Parameters and hepatic fibrosis scores in children with nonalcoholic fatty liver disease. World J Gastroenterol 2012;18:1525.
41. Alkhouri N, Mansoor S, Giammaria P, et al. The development of the pediatric NAFLD fibrosis score (PNFS) to predict the presence of advanced fibrosis in children with nonalcoholic fatty liver disease. PLoS One 2014;9:e104558.
42. Nobili V, Alisi A, Vania A, et al. The pediatric NAFLD fibrosis index: a predictor of liver fibrosis in children with non-alcoholic fatty liver disease. BMC Med 2009; 7:21.
43. Jackson J.A., Konomi J.V., Mendoza M.V., et al., Performance of fibrosis prediction scores in paediatric non-alcoholic fatty liver disease, J Paediatr Child Health, 54, 2018, 172–176.
44. Bohte AE, Koot BGP, van der Baan-Slootweg OH, et al. US cannot be used to predict the presence or severity of hepatic steatosis in severely obese adolescents. Radiology 2012;262:327–34.
45. Draijer LG, Feddouli S, Bohte AE, et al. Comparison of diagnostic accuracy of screening tests ALT and ultrasound for pediatric non-alcoholic fatty liver disease. Eur J Pediatr 2019;178:863–70.
46. Shannon A, Alkhouri N, Carter-Kent C, et al. Ultrasonographic quantitative estimation of hepatic steatosis in children with NAFLD. J Pediatr Gastroenterol Nutr 2011;53:190–5.
47. Karlas T, Petroff D, Garnov N, et al. Non-invasive assessment of hepatic steatosis in patients with NAFLD using controlled attenuation parameter and 1H-MR spectroscopy. PLoS One 2014;9:e91987.
48. Chan W-K, Nik Mustapha NR, Mahadeva S. Controlled attenuation parameter for the detection and quantification of hepatic steatosis in nonalcoholic fatty liver disease. J Gastroenterol Hepatol 2014;29:1470–6.
49. Desai NK, Harney S, Raza R, et al. Comparison of controlled attenuation parameter and liver biopsy to assess hepatic steatosis in pediatric patients. J Pediatr 2016;173:160–4.e1.
50. Friedrich–Rust M, Ong MF, Martens S, et al. Performance of transient elastography for the staging of liver fibrosis: a meta-analysis. Gastroenterology 2008;134: 960–74.e8.
51. Hwang J-Y, Yoon HM, Kim JR, et al. Diagnostic performance of transient elastography for liver fibrosis in children: a systematic review and meta-analysis. Am J Roentgenol 2018;211:W257–66.
52. Imajo K, Kessoku T, Honda Y, et al. Magnetic resonance imaging more accurately classifies steatosis and fibrosis in patients with nonalcoholic fatty liver disease than transient elastography. Gastroenterology 2016;150:626–37.e7.
53. Schwimmer JB, Middleton MS, Behling C, et al. Magnetic resonance imaging and liver histology as biomarkers of hepatic steatosis in children with nonalcoholic fatty liver disease. Hepatology 2015;61:1887–95.

54. Middleton M.S., Van Natta M.L., Heba E.R., et al., Diagnostic accuracy of magnetic resonance imaging hepatic proton density fat fraction in pediatric nonalcoholic fatty liver disease, Hepatology, 67, 2018, 858–872.
55. Serai SD, Panganiban J, Dhyani M, et al. Imaging modalities in pediatric NAFLD. Clin Liver Dis 2021;17:200–8.
56. Ekstedt M, Franzén LE, Mathiesen UL, et al. Long-term follow-up of patients with NAFLD and elevated liver enzymes. Hepatology 2006;44:865–73.
57. Molleston JP, White F, Teckman J, et al. Obese children with steatohepatitis can develop cirrhosis in childhood. Am J Gastroenterol 2002;97:2460–2.
58. Nobili V, Alisi A, Grimaldi C, et al. Non-alcoholic fatty liver disease and hepatocellular carcinoma in a 7-year-old obese boy: coincidence or comorbidity? Pediatr Obes 2014;9:e99–102.
59. Feldstein AE, Charatcharoenwitthaya P, Treeprasertsuk S, et al. The natural history of non-alcoholic fatty liver disease in children: a follow-up study for up to 20 years. Gut 2009;58:1538–44.
60. Alkhouri N, Hanouneh IA, Zein NN, et al. Liver transplantation for nonalcoholic steatohepatitis in young patients. Transpl Int 2016;29:418–24.
61. Cioffi C, Welsh JA, Cleeton RL, et al. Natural history of NAFLD diagnosed in childhood: a single-center study. Children 2017;4:34.
62. Baskar S, Jhaveri S, Alkhouri N. Cardiovascular risk in pediatric nonalcoholic fatty liver disease: recent advances. Clin Lipidol 2015;10:351–62.
63. Nobili V, Manco M, Devito R, et al. Effect of vitamin E on aminotransferase levels and insulin resistance in children with non-alcoholic fatty liver disease. Aliment Pharmacol Ther 2006;24:1553–61.
64. Schwimmer JB, Ugalde-Nicalo P, Welsh J, et al. Effect of a low free sugar diet vs usual diet on nonalcoholic fatty liver disease in adolescent boys. JAMA 2019; 321:256.
65. Medrano M., Cadenas-Sanchez C., Álvarez-Bueno C., et al., Evidence-based exercise recommendations to reduce hepatic fat content in youth- a systematic review and meta-analysis, *Prog Cardiovasc Dis*, 61, 2018, 222–231.
66. Grønbæk H, Lange A, Birkebæk NH, et al. Effect of a 10-week weight loss camp on fatty liver disease and insulin sensitivity in obese Danish children. J Pediatr Gastroenterol Nutr 2012;54:223–8.
67. Kumar S., King E.C., Christison A.L., et al., Health outcomes of youth in clinical pediatric weight management programs in POWER, *J Pediatr*, 208, 2019, 57–65.e4.
68. Lavine JE, Schwimmer JB, Van Natta ML. Effect of Vitamin E or metformin for treatment of nonalcoholic fatty liver disease in children and adolescents. JAMA 2011;305:1659.
69. Miller ER, Pastor-Barriuso R, Dalal D, et al. Meta-Analysis: high-dosage vitamin E supplementation may increase all-cause mortality. Ann Intern Med 2005;142:37.
70. Gerss J, Köpcke W. The questionable association of vitamin E supplementation and mortality–inconsistent results of different meta-analytic approaches. Cell Mol Biol (Noisy-le-grand) 2009;55(Suppl):OL1111–20.
71. Nobili V, Manco M, Ciampalini P, et al. Metformin use in children with nonalcoholic fatty liver disease: an open-label, 24-month, observational pilot study. Clin Ther 2008;30:1168–76.
72. Lewis JD, Ferrara A, Peng T, et al. Risk of bladder cancer among diabetic patients treated with pioglitazone. Diabetes Care 2011;34:916–22.
73. Attia S.L., Softic S., Mouzaki M., Evolving role for pharmacotherapy in NAFLD/NASH, *Clin Transl Sci*, 14 (1), 2021, 11–19.

74. Nobili V, Alisi A, Della Corte C, et al. Docosahexaenoic acid for the treatment of fatty liver: randomised controlled trial in children. Nutr Metab Cardiovasc Dis 2013;23:1066–70.
75. Nobili V, Bedogni G, Alisi A, et al. Docosahexaenoic acid supplementation decreases liver fat content in children with non-alcoholic fatty liver disease: double-blind randomised controlled clinical trial. Arch Dis Child 2011;96:350–3.
76. Zöhrer E, Alisi A, Jahnel J, et al. Efficacy of docosahexaenoic acid–choline–vitamin E in paediatric NASH: a randomized controlled clinical trial. Appl Physiol Nutr Metabol 2017;42:948–54.
77. Inge TH, Courcoulas AP, Jenkins TM, et al. Weight loss and health status 3 years after bariatric surgery in adolescents. N Engl J Med 2016;374:113–23.
78. Manco M, Mosca A, De Peppo F, et al. The benefit of sleeve gastrectomy in obese adolescents on nonalcoholic steatohepatitis and hepatic fibrosis. J Pediatr 2017;180:31–7.e2.
79. Pratt J.S.A., Browne A., Browne N.T., et al., ASMBS pediatric metabolic and bariatric surgery guidelines, Surg Obes Relat Dis, 14, 2018, 882–901.
80. Tsai WS, Inge TH, Burd RS. Bariatric surgery in adolescents. Arch Pediatr Adolesc Med 2007;161:217.
81. Nobili V, Alisi A, Raponi M. Pediatric non-alcoholic fatty liver disease: preventive andtherapeutic value of lifestyle intervention. World J Gastroenterol 2009;15: 6017.
82. Whitlock EP, O'Connor EA, Williams SB, et al. Effectiveness of weight management interventions in children: a targeted systematic review for the USPSTF. Pediatrics 2010;125:e396–418.
83. Quattrin T, Roemmich JN, Paluch R, et al. Treatment outcomes of overweight children and parents in the medical Home. Pediatrics 2014;134:290–7.
84. Romanelli R, Cecchi N, Carbone MG, et al. Pediatric obesity: prevention is better than care. Ital J Pediatr 2020;46:103.

Economic Burden and Patient-Reported Outcomes of Nonalcoholic Fatty Liver Disease

Maria Stepanova, PhD[a,b,c], Linda Henry, PhD[a,b,c],
Zobair M. Younossi, MD, MPH[a,b,*]

KEYWORDS

• Health care costs • Advanced liver disease • Comorbidities • QALYs/ DALYs
• Physical functioning • Mental health • Health utilities • Work productivity

KEY POINTS

- Nonalcoholic fatty liver disease (NAFLD) is a chronic liver disease with a rapidly expanding prevalence that makes it a major global health concern.
- The costs of NAFLD/nonalcoholic steatohepatitis (NASH) are substantial and increasing.
- NASH with advanced liver disease is the costliest state, especially in those with renal impairment, cardiovascular disease, and/or type 2 diabetes mellitus.
- Patients with NAFLD may experience a range of symptoms that impact their health-related quality of life and other aspects of daily functioning and overall well-being.
- The impairment of quality of life is the most profound in NAFLD patients with more advanced liver disease, to include NASH and cirrhosis, and in patients with non-hepatic comorbidities.

HEALTH-RELATED QUALITY OF LIFE AND OTHER PATIENT-REPORTED OUTCOMES IN NONALCOHOLIC FATTY LIVER DISEASE

General Aspects of Health-Related Quality of Life and Other Patient-Reported Outcomes

Health-related quality of life (HRQL) is a multidimensional construct that can comprehensively evaluate patient's health status including but not limited to: physical, emotional, mental, and social well-being.[1] Although the terms HRQL and patient-reported outcomes (PROs) have often been used interchangeably, PRO is a more

[a] Department of Medicine, Center for Liver Diseases, Inova Fairfax Medical Campus, Falls Church, VA, USA; [b] Betty and Guy Beatty Center for Integrated Research, Inova Health System, Falls Church, VA, USA; [c] Center for Outcomes Research in Liver Diseases, Washington, DC, USA
* Corresponding author. Betty and Guy Beatty Center for Integrated Research, Claude Moore Health Education and Research Building, 3300 Gallows Road, Falls Church, VA 22042.
E-mail address: Zobair.Younossi@inova.org

Clin Liver Dis 27 (2023) 483–513
https://doi.org/10.1016/j.cld.2023.01.007
liver.theclinics.com
1089-3261/23/

inclusive term that includes not only HRQL but also other outcomes reported by and important to patients such as perceived fatigue, limitations in work productivity and daily activities, diet, stigma of the disease, cognitive functioning, and other aspects of overall well-being.[2]

In general, tools or instruments for the evaluation of HRQL and other PROs are divided into generic and disease-specific. Although disease-specific instruments are designed to address aspects of patients' well-being most commonly affected by the disease and, therefore, tend to be more sensitive to the disease severity and more responsive to disease progression and efficacious treatments, generic instruments can also be useful because they would allow comparing PRO scores across different clinical populations.[3] Health utility score is another type of PRO assessment that is based on a patient's preference for a state of health. These scores are essential for economic analyses to quality-adjust outcomes such as quality-adjusted years of life (QALYs) to compare different interventions. There are several algorithms to calculate health utility scores directly (standard gamble, time-trade-off); however, it is usually more practical that they are estimated using questionnaires such as health utility index (HUI) or calculated from either specifically designed multiattribute PRO instruments (EQ-5D) or approximated from general purpose PRO instruments (SF-6D from SF-36).[4]

Health-Related Quality of Life in Nonalcoholic Fatty Liver Disease

Until recently, there was a paucity of research addressing the HRQL burden of NAFLD and NASH. One of the main reasons was that, at the early stages of the disease, patients with NAFLD tend to be mostly asymptomatic or describe only mild vague symptoms of fatigue or right upper quadrant pain.[5] In fact, a review published in 2015 identified only four studies that measured HRQL in patients with NAFLD.[6] Since then, however, there has been substantial progress in both awareness of NAFLD and its total burden and also the development of potential treatments for NAFLD and NASH for which clinical trials are needed to appreciate the HRQL of those patients. Indeed, a more recent review published in 2018 found as many as 14 studies[7] and the interest in the topic has been growing ever since (**Table 1**).

Although the disease-specific chronic liver disease questionnaire (CLDQ) instrument has been developed in 1999,[8] some of the early studies of HRQL in NAFLD have been conducted primarily using generic instruments such as SF-36. As such, one of the first studies suggested that patients with NAFLD may have a substantially impaired HRQL as measured by physical component summary (PSC) and mental component summary (MCS) scores of SF-36: in the study sample ($N = 67$), mean patients' scores were 35 and 43, respectively, which was substantially lower than the general population norms (50 for both scores) or similarly assessed scores of patients with other etiologies of chronic liver disease; that study, however, included 73% NAFLD patients with cirrhosis.[9] In a larger study of adults with NAFLD who were enrolled in the Non-Alcoholic Steatohepatitis Clinical Research Network (NASH-CRN; $N = 713$), patients with NAFLD had worse PCS (mean 45.2) and MCS (mean 47.6) when compared with the US population norm scores and especially with individuals without any chronic illnesses.[10] In that study, patients with a diagnosis of NASH had even lower PCS scores and so did patients with cirrhosis; at the same time, there was no additional impairment in MCS in patients with more advanced liver disease. Similar findings were reported in another study where a significant reduction in all SF-36 domains including PCS and MCS was observed among participants with NASH ($N = 79$) when compared with normative data.[11] More recently, baseline HRQL data collected from NASH participants of clinical trials were consistent with

Table 1
Summary of studies of patient-reported outcomes in nonalcoholic fatty liver disease or nonalcoholic steatohepatitis

Study	Study Sample	Reference Group	PRO Instrument(s)	Main Findings
Afendy et al,[9] 2009	*N* = 67 (73% cirrhosis)	General population norm; other chronic liver diseases; cirrhosis	SF-36	Patients with NAFLD scored significantly lower compared with all other liver disease patients on physical functioning scores; lower than general population norms in physical and mental summary scores
David et al,[10] 2009	*N* = 713 (61% NASH, 28% bridging fibrosis)	General population norm; cirrhosis	SF-36	Patients with NAFLD had worse physical and mental health when compared with the US population norm with and without chronic illnesses; patients with NASH and cirrhosis had even lower physical health-related scores
Chawla et al,[11] 2016	*N* = 79 (100% NASH, no cirrhosis)	General population norm	SF-36	Patients with NASH reported worse scores in physical health-related domains compared with the general population
Younossi et al,[12] 2019	*N* = 1667 clinical trial enrollees (100% NASH, 48% bridging fibrosis and 52% cirrhosis)	General population norm; cirrhosis	SF-36, CLDQ, WPAI, EQ-5D	Physical and select mental health-related scores lower than general population norm in both bridging fibrosis and cirrhosis NASH groups; patients with cirrhosis have lower disease-specific scores (by CLDQ) and select generic physical health-related scores (SF-36) than bridging fibrosis; utility scores lower than in general population and additionally lower in cirrhosis

(*continued on next page*)

Table 1
(continued)

Study	Study Sample	Reference Group	PRO Instrument(s)	Main Findings
Younossi et al,[13] 2022	*N* = 125 clinical trial enrollees (100% NASH, no cirrhosis)	General population norm	SF-36	Physical and mental health scores were not significantly different from the general population norms; SF-6D utility scores lower than the general population norm; reduction in hepatic fat linked to improvement in PROs
Dan et al,[14] 2007	*N* = 106 (14% cirrhosis)	Chronic hepatitis B, chronic hepatitis C	CLDQ	Patients with NAFLD had lower HRQL scores than patients with chronic viral hepatitis B (five out of six CLDQ domains) or hepatitis C (two domains)
Younossi et al,[15] 2019	*N* = 1338 clinical trial enrollees (45% bridging fibrosis, 55% cirrhosis)	Chronic hepatitis C	SF-36, CLDQ, WPAI	Patients with NASH had significantly lower HRQL scores related to physical health (Physical Functioning, Bodily Pain, General Health, Vitality, Physical Summary of SF-36, Fatigue of CLDQ) than matched patients with hepatitis C but better mental health scores and work productivity
Golabi et al,[16] 2016	*N* = 3333 NHAHES participants (NAFLD diagnosed by FLI)	NHANES participants without liver disease or with chronic hepatitis C	HRQOL-4	Three out of four scores were lower in NAFLD than controls without liver disease; the impairment was less pronounced in NAFLD than in hepatitis C

Younossi et al,[17] 2020	*N* = 4250 enrollees of the Global Liver Registry from 18 countries (8% cirrhosis)	Enrollees of the Global Liver Registry with chronic hepatitis B and chronic hepatitis C	FACIT-F, CLDQ, WPAI	Compared with patients with viral hepatitis, PRO scores of patients with NAFLD were significantly impaired in all domains of FACIT-F and CLDQ
Younossi et al,[18] 2021	*N* = 5691 enrollees of Global Liver Registry from 18 countries (15% cirrhosis)	General population norm	FACIT-F, CLDQ, WPAI	CLDQ-NASH and FACIT-F PRO scores were lower in patients with NAFLD than in general population norms
Younossi et al,[19] 2017	*N* = 104 (15% cirrhosis)	Socio-demographic and clinical groups	CLDQ-NASH	Patients with metabolic syndrome had lower PRO scores; development and pilot validation of CLDQ-NASH instrument
Younossi et al,[20] 2019	*N* = 1667 (100% NASH, 48% bridging fibrosis and 52% cirrhosis)	Socio-demographic and clinical groups	CLDQ-NASH	NASH patients with cirrhosis, obesity, type 2 diabetes, and comorbidities had lower PRO scores; independent validation of CLDQ-NASH instrument
Huang et al,[21] 2021	*N* = 5181 (4% NASH, <1% cirrhosis)	Socio-demographic and clinical groups	CLDQ	Patients with cirrhosis and comorbidities had lower PRO scores
Younossi et al,[22] 2021	*N* = 1218 enrollees of clinical trials (100% NASH, no cirrhosis)	General population norm	CLDQ-NASH, EQ-5D	The EQ-5D utility and VAS scores were significantly lower than age- and sex-matched general population norms; no difference in scores between fibrosis stages in the absence of cirrhosis; reduction in NAS or resolution of NASH linked to improvement in PROs

(*continued on next page*)

Table 1
(continued)

Study	Study Sample	Reference Group	PRO Instrument(s)	Main Findings
Newton et al,[28] 2008	$N = 36$	Matched controls without liver disease and with PBC	CLDQ, FIS	Fatigue was markedly higher in patients with NAFLD than in controls
Sayiner et al,[31] 2016	$N = 89$ (34% cirrhosis)	General population norm; cirrhosis	SF-36	Patients with NAFLD had significantly lower PRO and health utility scores than the general population; patients with cirrhosis had an additional impairment in all PRO scores
Rustgi et al,[33] 2022	Literature search, multiple sources	General population norm	SF-6D, HUI2	Utility scores of NAFLD patients with no fibrosis (stage 0) were only marginally lower than the general population norm; starting from the stage of compensated cirrhosis, utilities were significantly lower than the general population norm
McSweeney et al,[35] 2020	Literature search, multiple sources; NASH cirrhosis only	General population norm, NASH without cirrhosis	SF-36, CLDQ-NASH, FIS	Patients with NASH-cirrhosis had lower HRQL scores than patients with non-cirrhotic NASH and the general population with respect to physical health/functioning, emotional health and worry, and mental health
Huben et al,[36] 2019	$N = 304$ (69% NASH, 15% cirrhosis)	NASH	CLDQ	Patients with NASH had significantly lower scores in all domains of CLDQ in comparison to non-NASH NAFLD

Younossi et al,[37] 2020	N = 1669 clinical trial enrollees (100% NASH, 48% bridging fibrosis, 52% cirrhosis)	Pruritus	SF-36, CLDQ-NASH, EQ-5D, WPAI	NASH patients with pruritus had a substantial impairment in all PRO scores in comparison to NASH patients without pruritus
Younossi et al,[38] 2021	N = 2154 (48% bridging fibrosis, 52% cirrhosis)	Histology- and NIT-based groups	SF-36, CLDQ-NASH, EQ-5D, WPAI	NASH patients with hepatocyte ballooning, higher ELF, greater % hepatic collagen, or greater liver stiffness had significant PRO impairment; improvement in fibrosis NITs (liver stiffness by transient elastography, serum-based ELF, FIB-4, APRI) was linked to improvement in select PRO scores
Tapper & Lai,[39] 2016	N = 151 (21% bridging fibrosis or cirrhosis)	Weight change groups	CLDQ	a decrease in BMI was associated with improved PRO scores
Younossi et al,[40] 2018	N = 72 (100% NASH, 65% bridging fibrosis, no cirrhosis)	Histology-based groups	SF-36, CLDQ, WPAI	patients who experienced a $\geq$2 point decrease in NAS, $\geq$1-stage reduction in fibrosis or at least 50% relative reduction in collagen showed significant improvements in their PROs, whereas those with an increase in % collagen experienced a significant PRO worsening
Armstrong et al,[41] 2016	N = 26 (100% NASH, 46% bridging fibrosis or cirrhosis)	Treatment with liraglutide	SF-36	48-wk treatment with liraglutide was associated with a significant improvement in physical summary score of SF-36 compared with placebo

(*continued on next page*)

Table 1
(continued)

Study	Study Sample	Reference Group	PRO Instrument(s)	Main Findings
Sanyal et al,[42] 2010	$N = 247$ (no diabetes, 100% NASH, no cirrhosis)	Treatment with pioglitazone or vitamin E	SF-36	No difference in posttreatment PRO scores between patients treated with pioglitazone, vitamin E, or placebo
Karaivazoglou et al,[43] 2019	Literature review	General population, non-NAFLD clinical groups	multiple	Pediatric NAFLD is associated with neuropsychiatric symptoms and poor quality of life; the level of impairment does not correlate with liver disease severity

Abbreviations: APRI, AST-to-platelet index; CLDQ, chronic liver disease questionnaire; ELF, enhanced liver fibrosis; EQ-5D, EuroQol-5 dimension; FIB-4, fibrosis-4; FIS, fatigue impact scale; FLI, fatty liver index; HRQL, health-related quality of life; NAFLD, nonalcoholic fatty liver disease; NASH, nonalcoholic steatohepatitis; NHAHES, National Health and Nutrition Examination Survey; NIT, non-invasive test; PBC, primary biliary cholangitis; PRO, patient-reported outcome; SF-36, short form-36; VAS, visual analog scale; WPAI, work productivity and activity impairment.

prior smaller studies showing that patients with NAFLD and NASH have impaired HRQL, primarily its physical health-related aspect, which tends to get worse with more advanced disease.[12,13]

In a study that used CLDQ to assess HRQL in patients with different etiologies of liver disease, patients with NAFLD (N = 106) had lower HRQL scores than patients with chronic viral hepatitis B (five out of six CLDQ domains) or hepatitis C (two domains).[14] Another study compared SF-36 scores of patients with NASH and advanced fibrosis (N = 1338) to the scores of matched patients with chronic hepatitis C, and concluded that patients with NASH and advanced fibrosis have more impairment of their physical health-related scores than patients with hepatitis C with advanced fibrosis.[15]

Although most studies assessed HRQL in relatively small single-center cohorts of patients with NAFLD and NASH, there was a report regarding HRQL in NAFLD which used population data collected from National Health And Nutrition Examination Survey (NHANES), a representative US population sample.[16] In that study, in the absence of a biopsy- or imaging-based diagnosis of NAFLD, the Fatty Liver Index (FLI) was used to select the sample of patients (N = 3333). Patients with NAFLD were found to have some impairment in their HRQL as measured by HRQOL-4 (an instrument that assesses four HRQL domains via healthy days measures) in comparison to non-NAFLD controls but that impairment was smaller in magnitude in comparison to that of patients with chronic hepatitis C. More recently, a large multinational study (Global Liver Registry and Global NAFLD/NASH Registry) found that patients with an established diagnosis of NAFLD had lower HRQL scores than patients with chronic hepatitis B or C or the general population norms as measured by a generic Functional Assessment of Chronic Illness Therapy (FACIT) instrument.[17,18]

In the context of assessment of HRQL in NAFLD, it is important to note that in 2017, a disease-specific PRO instrument (CLDQ-NAFLD/NASH) was developed.[19] Having been developed in a similar fashion to the original CLDQ with extra items but an identical domain structure and comparably good psychometric properties, CLDQ-NAFLD/NASH has been validated[20] and is currently being used in clinical trials and other studies of HRQL in patients with NAFLD and NASH.[21,22] Although other PRO instruments such as NASH-Check have been developed, it has not undergone full validation.[23]

Other Patient-Reported Outcomes in Nonalcoholic Fatty Liver Disease: Fatigue, Health Utilities, and Work Productivity

In addition to the most commonly studied HRQL, some other PROs reflect essential aspects of patients' overall well-being. In the context of NAFLD, one such special PRO is fatigue which is known to accompany multiple chronic diseases and conditions where systemic inflammation is present.[24] In fact, the liver is believed to be central in the pathogenesis of fatigue because it uniquely regulates much of the storage, release, and production of substrate for energy generation.[25] Although commonly related to impaired physical functioning, fatigue is a multifaceted condition that may consist of peripheral (physical health-related) and central components[26]; in fact, both dimensions of fatigue have been shown to be present in those with chronic liver disease.[25–27]

In patients with NAFLD, fatigue is usually studied among other HRQL domains as it is routinely returned by most commonly used PRO instruments (Vitality by SF-36, Fatigue by CLDQ or CLDQ-NAFLD/NASH, and Fatigue Scale by FACIT-F). As such, increased fatigue in patients with NAFLD has been reported in the studies reviewed above. However, fatigue is sometimes evaluated using specifically designed instruments. In one study of patients with NAFLD (N = 156), fatigue was markedly higher in patients with NAFLD than in age-, sex- and BMI-matched controls as measured by Fatigue Impact Scale (FIS).[28]

Self-reported work productivity impairment (WPI) in patients with NAFLD has been studied using the Work Productivity and Activity Impairment – Specific Health Problem (WPAI-SHP) instrument in which employed patients are asked to evaluate their impairment in productivity while working (presenteeism) and loss of work hours (absenteeism) owing to their disease. In one study which included patients with advanced fibrosis or compensated cirrhosis (CC) (N = 1667), the mean WPI was 0.12 and not different between the two groups.[12] In another study that enrolled patients without cirrhosis (N = 1218), it was 0.16 and not different between patients with and without bridging fibrosis.[22] In both studies, between 20% and 33% of the total WPI was owing to absenteeism and the remainder was presenteeism. In the multinational Global Liver Registry (N = 1065), the mean WPI varied substantially between countries and regions of the world, with some regions reporting mean WPI as high as 0.38 or 0.53 and an average in the registry of 0.22;[18] in that study, the share of absenteeism in WPI was 24%. In this context, although not studied extensively in NAFLD yet, for patients with chronic hepatitis C it has been shown that even moderately impaired work productivity resulted in at least hundreds of millions of dollars or euros in annual societal losses[29,30]; with a substantially higher prevalence, the impact of WPI owing to NAFLD is expected to be even greater.

Health utilities in NAFLD have been evaluated as primary outcomes or included as supplementary material for health economic studies. In a study that included patients with NAFLD seen in an outpatient clinic, SF-6D utility scores (derived from the SF-36 generic PRO instrument) were found to be as low as 0.66 in non-cirrhotic NAFLD and 0.55 in cirrhotic NAFLD[31] both of which were substantially lower than the general population norm of 0.78.[32] Another study found that EQ-5D-based utility scores of NASH patients with cirrhosis were lower than the general population norms or the scores of non-cirrhotic patients.[12] Similar findings regarding impaired health utility scores in comparison to the general population norms were reported from studies of NAFLD patients without cirrhosis (using SF-6D and EQ-5D).[13,22] Finally, a study that assessed the cost-effectiveness and potential value of pharmaceutical treatments estimated health utility scores of patients with NAFLD by fibrosis stage using approximations from other HRQL metrics and/or other chronic liver disease populations where applicable.[33] In that study, the authors projected that NAFLD patients with no fibrosis (stage 0) would have a health utility score of 0.85 (which is only marginally lower than the general population norm of 0.87 for EQ-5D[34]) but which would gradually decrease to 0.80 in patients with CC and then deteriorate to as low as 0.60 in the event of decompensation.

Health-Related Quality of Life in the Presence of Risk Factors and Disease Progression

Although NAFLD is not an asymptomatic disease by itself, patients' HRQL and other PROs can be affected by several additional risk factors. As reviewed above, most studies have found a greater impairment in PROs in patients with cirrhosis in comparison to non-cirrhotic NAFLD/NASH patients;[10,12,18,35] however, there was little to no significant association of HRQL with fibrosis stage in the absence of cirrhosis.[22]

Other factors that have been consistently shown to affect PROs in patients with NAFLD included older age (primarily for physical health-related domains), female sex, and the presence of psychiatric comorbidities such as depression and other non-hepatic comorbidities.[9,12,18] The impact of type 2 diabetes has been shown in some studies[10–12,36] but not in others.[18,31] Considering disease-specific factors, in one study, NASH patients with pruritus were found to have a substantial impairment in all aspects of their HRQL in comparison to NASH patients without pruritus.[37] The association of some PRO scores with NAFLD Activity Score (NAS) and, in particular, its hepatocyte ballooning component has also been reported.[38] With reference to other liver disease-related tests, a large study has shown the association of NASH patients' PRO scores with % collagen and with commonly used noninvasive tests (NITs) for fibrosis; as a result, patients with high ELF scores (≥11.3, which is a commonly used threshold for ruling in cirrhosis) had significant PRO impairment and so did patients with % hepatic collagen ≥11.2% or liver stiffness by transient elastography ≥23.4 kPa.[12,38]

Although there is a paucity of prospectively collected data regarding the dynamics in NAFLD or NASH patients' HRQL over time, some interventional studies have identified clinical predictors of HRQL changes in patients with NAFLD. In one study, a decrease in BMI was associated with improved quality of life so that those who achieved at least a 5% reduction in weight had a mean 0.45-point improvement in the total CLDQ score (range 1 to 7) compared with less than 0.01 in those who did not[39]; this adds to other known clinical benefits of weight loss for patients with NAFLD. More recently, in the era of clinical trials for NASH, prospective association of histologic and other liver function parameters with PROs has been studied more extensively using both generic (SF-36) and disease-specific (CLDQ and CLDQ-NAFLD/NASH) instruments. In a phase 2 study of selonsertib, patients who experienced a ≥2 point decrease in NAS, ≥1-stage reduction in fibrosis or at least 50% relative reduction in collagen showed significant improvements in their PROs, whereas those with a >17% increase in their collagen experienced a significant decrease in their PROs.[40] Other clinical trials linked improvement in PROs to the reduction in NAS or resolution of NASH (phase 3 obeticholic acid),[22] reduction in hepatic fat (phase 2 resmetirom),[13] and improvement in select fibrosis NITs (liver stiffness by transient elastography, serum-based ELF, FIB-4, APRI) (phase 3 selonsertib).[38] One other phase 2 study has shown that 48-week treatment with liraglutide was associated with a significant improvement in PCS of SF-36 compared with placebo but the pathologic mechanism of the improvement was not studied.[41] Taken together, these reports consistently show that improvement of liver function is strongly associated with better quality of life in patients with NAFLD and NASH. On the other hand, treatment with pioglitazone or vitamin E was not associated with PRO improvement in comparison to placebo in a randomized clinical trial despite improvement in some histologic parameters and liver function tests in patients who received the active treatment.[42]

Out of subgroups of special interest, there is pediatric NAFLD which is a growing concern in the developed world. There is limited data regarding HRQL in the pediatric NAFLD population. One recent review concluded that pediatric NAFLD is frequently accompanied by neuropsychiatric symptoms and poor quality of life, and the level of impairment does not seem to correlate with the degree of hepatic damage.[43] Further research is needed to cover this knowledge gap.

ECONOMIC BURDEN OF NONALCOHOLIC FATTY LIVER DISEASE

In addition to the significant negative impact of NAFLD on PROs, studies have shown that NAFLD also is associated with increased health care utilization and costs[44] (**Table 2**). One of the first studies quantifying the health care utilization of those with NAFLD was conducted in the United States using data from the US Health and Human Services Department. These data were for all persons aged 65 years and older as well

Table 2
Economic studies for nonalcoholic fatty liver disease and nonalcoholic steatohepatitis

Study	Country	Years of Study	Sample	Economic Outcome Measured	Main Findings
Younossi et al,[44] 2015	United States—Medicare	2005 to 2010	Retrospective study of 29,528 Medicare beneficiaries who sought outpatient care for principal or secondary diagnosis of NAFLD	Outpatient Health care Utilization Among those with NAFLD	Both total of outpatient visits and the prevalence of diabetes, hyperlipidemia, and hypertension increased significantly over the study. The mean yearly inflation-adjusted charges increased from \$2624–\$3308 in 2005 to \$3608–\$5132 in 2010 (in 2010 USD). The main predictors of the increase were having cardiovascular disease, diabetes, hypertension, and the number of outpatient visits.
Sayiner et al,[45] 2017	United States—Medicare	2005 to 2010	Retrospective study 976 Medicare inpatients and 4742 Medicare outpatients with NAFLD were included.	Inpatient and Outpatient Health care costs for patients with NAFLD and for patients with NAFLD-related cirrhosis- compensated and decompensated.	Median total hospital charge for Patients with NAFLD was reported as \$36,289 [IQR: \$18,359-\$71,225] in 2010 Total charges for NAFLD patients without cirrhosis were significantly lower than

NAFLD patients with cirrhosis ($33,863 vs $61,151). Charges for the NAFLD patients with DCC were significantly higher than for patients with CC ($66,554 vs $34,860) Inpatient mortality (258%, *P*<.001), presence of CC (90%, *P*<.001), and presence of CVD (51%, *P*<.001) were associated with increased inpatient total charges For outpatients, the median total charge was $9011. NAFLD patients with cirrhosis had higher charges than non-cirrhotic NAFLD patients ($12,049 vs $8830. Patients with DCC had approximately $5000 higher charges than patients with CC ($15,187 vs $10,379) CVD, hypertension, and obesity were all associated with increased outpatient charges

(*continued on next page*)

Table 2
(continued)

Study	Country	Years of Study	Sample	Economic Outcome Measured	Main Findings
Gordon et al,[46] 2020	United States–Medicare	2007 to 2015	Longitudinal-Retrospective study—255,681 total patients—72.5% did not progress; 1.3% progressed to CC; 25.8% progressed to DCC, 0.2% underwent a liver transplant, and 0.2% developed HCC	Health care costs consisted of costs associated with inpatient medical services, outpatient visits, physician visits, and pharmacy fills-Had 2 periods of study prehospitalization (pre-index) and post-hospitalization (post-index)	Patients with NAFLD/NASH had the lowest total annual costs of $19,908, whereas those who had DCC had costs exceeding $74,000 with costs for liver transplantation totaling greater than $129,276. Those with CC, DCC, LT, or HCC incurred costs that were 1.2, 3.2, 5.0, and 3.3 times higher, respectively, compared with patients with NAFLD/NASH who did not experience disease progression. Those with renal impairment had 1.6 times higher costs, whereas those with CVD had 1.4 times higher costs. The majority of costs were experienced in the post-index period of time for those who had disease progression

Romero-Gomez, et al,[47] 2020	Spain	2006 to 2017	A longitudinal, retrospective cohort study using data from the Spanish National Health System's Hospital Discharge Records Database 8205 patients;72.9% did not progress; 1.7% progressed to CC, 24.7% progressed to DCC, 1.4% to liver transplant; 0.7% developed HCC.	Pre- and post-index health care resource utilization and costs per patient per mo (PPPM) were calculated. Costs included outpatient, inpatient, and pharmacy expenditures and were adjusted to 2017 euros. Measures of health care resource utilization included the number of readmissions per patient and average LOS per admission	From the prehospitalization time (pre-index) to the post-hospitalization time (post-index) the all-cause PPPM costs increased between 44% and 46% mostly driven by inpatient health care costs. The NAFLD/NASH nonprogressors post-index costs were €4230 compared with € 11,356 for liver transplantation, €7053 for DCC, and €7213 for HCC. Having renal impairment, CVD, and/or being a tobacco user past or present were all associated with increased costs.
Petta et al,[48] 2020	Italy	2011 to 2017	Retrospective study of 9729 patients hospitalized with NAFLD/NASH—3% had advanced liver disease	Costs included inpatient stays, health services requiring hospital assistance, outpatient services, and the pharmacy fills and were annualized to costs in 2017 Compared costs pre-index	The cumulative mean all-cause costs increased exponentially over 7 y in NAFLD/NASH patients overall. The percentage of increase in the cumulative costs was 1361% (range 838% to

(continued on next page)

Table 2
(*continued*)

Study	Country	Years of Study	Sample	Economic Outcome Measured	Main Findings
				date (6 mo before hospitalization) and post-index date (post hospitalization).	1364%) for patients with advanced liver disease mainly driven by inpatient costs. Steepest increase of costs occurred in the y before and after the index date and the steepest slope was noted for those who had a liver transplant.
Canbay et al,[49] 2018	Germany	2011 to 2016	Retrospective longitudinal cohort study using the German health care claims data 215,655 adult patients diagnosed with NAFLD and/or NASH were categorized as NAFLD, NAFLD nonprogressors, compensated cirrhosis, decompensated cirrhosis, liver transplant, or HCC. Within each stage, annual all-cause HRU and costs were measured during the pre- and post-index periods	All-cause HRU data covered outpatient visits, inpatient hospitalizations, and emergency department visits. All-cause health care cost data included costs of inpatient care, outpatient care, outpatient pharmacotherapy, devices and aids, and total costs	Mean annual costs were significantly higher among patients with advanced liver disease: compensated cirrhosis, €10,291; decompensated cirrhosis, €22,561; liver transplant, €34,089; HCC, €35,910. Nonprogressors costs were €3,818,

Hagström et al,[50] 2020	Sweden	1971 to 2009	Retrospective study using data from national registers (thru Dec 2014) of 646 patients with biopsy-proven NAFLD in Sweden. Each patient was matched for age, sex, and county of residence with 10 persons from the general population (controls).	All costs are based on 2016 prices and the estimated unit costs from Swedish sources were converted to US dollars using an exchange rate of $1 = 9 Swedish krona. Total costs included hospitalization, outpatient visits, and prescribed drugs attributed to liver disease.	Follow-up of 19.9 y. Incremental cost of $635 per y for inpatients with NAFLD. Mean increase of $255 in outpatient visits for patients with NAFLD. Total costs incurred by patients with stage 3 to 4 fibrosis were higher than patients with fibrosis stage 0 to 2 (mean annual costs, $4397 vs $629). Cumulative costs were higher for all stages of fibrosis compared with controls.
O'Hara et al,[51] 2020	France, Germany, Italy, Spain, UK, USA	2018	NASH patients (N=3,754) recruited by 337 physicians in 6 countries.	Mean total annual per patient direct medical, direct non-medical, and indirect costs (in euros of 2018). The costs were estimated using national unit price data and extrapolated to the population level to calculate the economic burden.	The mean total annual per patient cost of NASH was €2,763, €4,917, and €5,509 for direct medical, direct non-medical, and indirect costs, respectively. The national per-patient cost was highest in the USA and lowest in France, and the costs increased with fibrosis and decompensation driven by hospitalization and comorbidities while indirect costs were driven by work loss.

(*continued on next page*)

Table 2
(*continued*)

Study	Country	Years of Study	Sample	Economic Outcome Measured	Main Findings
Younossi et al,[52] 2016	United States, Germany, France, Italy, and the United Kingdom	2016	Markov Modeling constructed using a series of interlinked Markov chains with 4 individual health states for those with NAFLD with an embedded disease-specific Markov structure to allow for patients with NAFLD to transition to a different liver disease health states	Total Cost and Burden of NAFLD by Country both direct medical costs and societal costs (QALYs)	In the United States, they determined that 64 million people had NAFLD at a cost of $1613 per person and an overall cost of 103 billion USD. For the studied European countries, 52 million persons were considered to have NAFLD at a cost of €354 to €1163 per person or a total cost of €52 million. The highest cost regardless of the country was found in those aged 45 to 65 y.
Younossi et al,[53] 2020	United States—those with T2DM and NAFLD	2017—projected costs over 20 y	Markov Modeling—10 health states with 1-y cycles.	Costs included inpatient, outpatient, liver transplant, and diabetes care.	Over the 20-y the total cost of NASH with T2DM would be $1.67 trillion with $504.2 billion (75.5%) related to diabetes management and $163.7 billion (24.5%) related to NASH care. For all patients with NAFLD and T2DM, the total cost per-person-

					per-y is $7,700, with costs attributable to diabetes comprising $6900 (89.4%) of total cost and NAFLD-attributable costs comprising $819 (10.6%). Highest costs in 65+ group
Younossi et al,[54] 2019	United States–NASH and Advanced Fibrosis NASH	2017–lifetime costs	Markov Model 11 health stages over the lifetime horizon with each model cycle of 1 y. Separate model for advanced fibrosis and NASH, the model state started at F3.	Costs were inclusive of inpatient, outpatient, professional services, emergency department, and drug costs in addition to discounting all future costs at an annual rate of 3%	The estimated lifetime costs for those with NASH in 2017 dollars was $222.6 billion, whereas the cost for those with advanced NASH population was $95.4 billion at $139,724 per patient. The highest costs would occur for those aged 18 to 39 y at $72,000 Without any change in treatment or the rising rates of obesity and T2DM, from 2017 to 2060, there will be 10.8 million new cases of NASH at a cost of $359 billion
Tampi et al,[57] 2020	Hong Kong—NASH and Advanced Fibrosis NASH	2017—lifetime costs	Markov Model 11 health stages over the lifetime horizon with each model cycle of 1 y.	Costs were inclusive of inpatient, outpatient, professional services, emergency department, and drug costs in addition to discounting all future	Total costs for both prevalence and incidence of NASH were 1.32 billion USD with an average per person cost of $257. The costs of NASH in 2017

(continued on next page)

Table 2
(*continued*)

Study	Country	Years of Study	Sample	Economic Outcome Measured	Main Findings
				costs at an annual rate of 3%	to 2018 accounted for 0.41% of Hong Kong's total health expenditures which is most likely underestimated as the costs in the study excluded costs of comorbidities and societal costs.
Phisalprapa et al,[58] 2021	Thailand representing low–middle-income countries	NASH with fibrosis state F2 and greater	Markov Model 11health stages over the lifetime horizon with each model cycle of 1 y.	Health care utilization costs were composed of outpatient medication care and laboratory testing with the assumption that patients with NAFLD visit an outpatient clinic four times a y. Costs of more advanced disease were based on costs obtained for patients with HCV but minus the cost of viral load testing and hepatitis C medications.	First-y costs would be $886,664,483, the fifth-y costs would be $886,376,246, and the total lifetime cost for NASH with significant fibrosis is projected at $15.2 billion or $5174 per case in 2019 accounting for approximately 3% of Thailand's GDP. Adults over 60 y of age had the highest costs ($9492 per case) compared with the 18

				They estimated costs over the estimated costs of NASH with significant fibrosis at the first-y, fifth y and over a lifetime	to 39 age cohort ($4393 per case) But, the lifetime cost of the population aged 18 to 39 would account for 42% of the total amount compared with 21% for patients aged over 60
Schattenberg et al,[59] 2021	France, Germany, Italy, Spain, and the United Kingdom	NASH population diagnosed in 2018	Cost of Illness Analysis (only diagnosed patients incur costs)	Costs included health system primary and secondary (inpatient) health care, diagnostic tests, pharmaceuticals, and medical research. Well-being was defined using productivity costs which were estimated via a human capital approach and included reduced workforce participation, lost productive time caused by absenteeism and presenteeism, forgone income because of premature mortality or morbidities as well as the search, hiring, and training costs required if the employee was to be replaced.	In 2018, the estimated economic costs were: €8319 to 13,845 M for France, €10,824 to 30,878 M for Germany, €5388 to 14,150 M for Italy, €4525 to 7942 M for Spain and €7773 to 14,404 M for the UK. Average per person health system costs are estimated to range between €699 and 771 for France, €795 to 852 for Germany, €1915 to 2242 for Italy, €1919 and 2568 for Spain and €890 and 918 for the United Kingdom. The majority of health system costs were incurred in the inpatient health care setting followed by diagnostic tests, primary health care, and pharmaceuticals.

(*continued on next page*)

Table 2
(*continued*)

Study	Country	Years of Study	Sample	Economic Outcome Measured	Main Findings
					The disability-adjusted life y (DALYs) ranged as well by country and were driven primarily by a higher rate of mortality among patients with NASH
Younossi et al,[60] 2019	Simulation for the economic impact of NASH if NASH treatment were available	NASH	Markov Model—estimated differences in outcomes between Standard of Care (SOC) and 2 hypothetical NASH treatments (A and B) using 10,000 50-year-old biopsy-proven NASH patients over lifetime horizon. Treatment A encompassed successful treatment followed by a maintenance regimen stopping disease progression. Treatment B, patients remained at risk of disease progression after successful treatment.	Treatment success was defined as regression to fibrosis and treatment failure was progression to stages beyond cirrhosis	Using an annual probability of treatment (ATP) ranging from 10% to 70% of treatment, they determined that treatment A averted 353 to 782 liver transplants and 1277 to 2381 liver-related deaths and treatment B averted 129 to 437 liver transplants and 386 to 1043 liver-related deaths compared with lifestyle intervention.

as those with certain disabilities who receive government-sponsored health care, more commonly known as Medicare. Among the Medicare patients who had NAFLD, investigators reported that between 2005 and 2010, the prevalence of diabetes, hyperlipidemia, and hypertension increased significantly which occurred alongside a significant increase in the number of outpatient visits per year. As a result, both total service charge per year and total payment per year increased significantly whereby the mean yearly inflation-adjusted charges increased from $2624 to $3308 in 2005 to $3608 to $5132 in 2010 (in 2010 USD). The main predictors of the increase were cardiovascular disease, diabetes, hypertension, and the number of outpatient visits.

In a follow-up study of both outpatient and inpatient Medicare resource use, the enormous impact of NAFLD was reiterated and the median total hospital charge for patients with NAFLD was reported as $36,289 (interquartile range [IQR] $18,359 to $71,225) in 2010.[45] Investigators also found that those without cirrhosis had significantly lower inpatient charges than those with cirrhosis ($33,863 vs $61,151) but among those with cirrhosis, those with DCC had the highest costs compared with those with CC ($66,554 vs $34,860). However, dying in the hospital had the most significant impact on inpatient charges (an increase in charges of 258%). This study also reviewed charges among outpatients the median total charge was $9011 and again NAFLD patients with cirrhosis had higher charges than non-cirrhotic NAFLD patients ($12,049 vs $8830), whereas those with DCC had approximately $5000 higher charges than patients with CC ($15,187 vs $10,379). The presence of cardiovascular diseases (CVDs), hypertension, and obesity were all associated with increased outpatient charges.[45]

Another study using a like approach with the Medicare population determined costs over 8 years from 2007 to 2015.[46] Among their total sample of 255,681patients with NAFLD/NASH, 185,407 (72.5%) did not have any disease progression, whereas 3454 (1.3%) progressed to CC, 65,926 (25.8%) progressed to decompensated cirrhosis (DCC), 473 (0.2%) underwent a liver transplant, and 421 (0.2%) developed hepatocellular carcinoma (HCC). Health care costs consisted of costs associated with inpatient medical services, outpatient visits, physician visits, and the pharmacy fills incurred during each pre-index and post-index period. Patients with NAFLD/NASH had the lowest total annual costs of $19,908, whereas those who had DCC had costs exceeding $74,000 with costs for liver transplantation totaling greater than $129,276. In fact, after the investigators controlled for patient characteristics and comorbid health conditions, those with CC, DCC, LT, or HCC incurred costs that were 1.2, 3.2, 5.0, and 3.3 times higher, respectively, compared with patients with NAFLD/NASH who did not experience disease progression. In addition, comorbid CVD, renal impairment, diabetes, dysrhythmia, hypertension, obesity, and current or past tobacco use were also associated with higher health care costs compared with NAFLD/NASH patients without these conditions. Those with renal impairment had 1.6 times higher costs, whereas those with CVD had 1.4 times higher costs. The majority of costs were experienced in the post-index period of time for those who had disease progression.[46]

A study using a similar economic methodology was conducted in Spain and validates prior studies whereby advanced liver disease is the major driver of the economic burden of NAFLD/NASH.[47] In this retrospective study, researchers examined the impact of liver disease severity, comorbidities, and demographics on health care resource utilization and costs in Spain from 2006 to 2017. Pre- and post-index health care resource utilization and costs per patient per month (PPPM) were calculated. Costs included outpatient, inpatient, and pharmacy expenditures and were adjusted to 2017 euros. Measures of health care resource utilization included the number of readmissions per patient and average LOS per admission. There were 8205 patients in the study of which 5984 (72.9%) did not have disease progression, 139 (1.7%) progressed to CC, 2028 (24.7%) to DCC, 115 (1.4%) to liver transplant, and 61 (0.7%) to HCC. As in other studies, the most common comorbidities were hypertension and type 2 diabetes where the prevalence of comorbidities was higher in patients with advanced liver diseases compared with those in the NAFLD/NASH nonprogressor group. From the prehospitalization time (pre-index) to the post-hospitalization time (post-index) the all-cause PPPM costs increased between 44% and 46% mostly driven by inpatient health care costs. The more severe the liver disease, the higher the costs. For example, the NAFLD/NASH nonprogressor post-index costs were €4230 compared with € 11,356 for liver transplantation, €7053 for DCC and €7213 for HCC. As in other studies among the comorbidities, having renal impairment, CVD, and/or being a tobacco user past or present were all associated with increased costs.[47]

A study conducted in Italy investigated the costs (comorbidities and health care resource utilization) associated with advanced liver disease in those with NASH for the years 2011 to 2017 who had been hospitalized.[48] Investigators compared costs pre-index date (6 months before hospitalization) and post-index date (post hospitalization). Costs included inpatient stays, health services requiring hospital assistance, outpatient services, and pharmacy fills and were annualized to costs in 2017. Patients were followed from index-date until the date of disease progression, end of coverage, death, or the end of the study. Among the 9729 patients hospitalized with NAFLD/NASH, 3% had advanced liver disease (1.3% had CC, 3.1% DCC, 0.8% HCC, 0.1% LT, and patients could be in more than one group). Comorbidity burden was high across the study group but those with advanced liver disease had higher rates than those without advanced liver disease and more frequently had all three comorbidities of T2DM, renal impairment and CVD. Results showed that the cumulative mean all-cause costs increased exponentially over 7 years in NAFLD/NASH patients overall where the percentage of increase in the cumulative costs was 1361% for NAFLD/NASH and ranged from 838% to 1364% for patients with advanced liver disease mainly driven by inpatient costs. The steepest increase in costs occurred in the year before and after the index date and the steepest slope was noted for those who had a liver transplant. Researchers concluded that better screening and management of those at risk for NAFLD/NASH is needed to reduce the risk of disease progression and subsequent health care resource utilization and costs.[48]

Similar findings were reported for Germany and Sweden.[49,50] In Germany, researchers found that patients who had CC and progressed had cost about 130% higher than those that did not progress and costs increased as disease severity increased.[49] Investigators from Sweden compared costs among patients with NASH fibrosis and determined that those with a fibrosis stage of 3 or 4 had costs that were seven times higher than those with fibrosis stage 0 to 2.[50]

In the Global Assessment of the Impact of NASH (GAIN) study which is a prevalence-based burden of illness study across Europe and the USA, for 2018, the mean total annual per patient cost of NASH was €2,763, €4,917, and €5,509 for direct medical, direct non-medical, and indirect costs, respectively. The authors found that the national per-patient cost was highest in the USA and lowest in France, and the costs increased with fibrosis and decompensation driven by hospitalization and comorbidities while indirect costs were driven by work loss.[51]

In addition to these retrospective studies, modeling studies using decision analysis-Markov Models have been undertaken to gain a further appreciation of the economics of NAFLD among different groups and in the future. In 2016, using Markov modeling, investigators looked at the economic burden of NAFLD for five countries: the United States, Germany, France, Italy, and the United Kingdom. In the United States, they determined that 64 million people had NAFLD at a cost $1613 per person and an overall cost of 103 billion USD.[52] For the studied European countries, 52 million persons were considered to have NAFLD at a cost of €354 to €1163 per person or a total cost of €52 million. The highest cost regardless of the country was found in those aged 45 to 65 years.

A similar study was carried out to estimate costs of among those with NAFLD and type 2 diabetes mellitus (T2DM) in the United States for the year 2017.[53] From their analysis, they determined that there were 18.2 million people in the United States living with T2DM and NAFLD and of which 6.4 million were estimated to have NASH. Over the 20-year horizon of their study, they predicted that the costs would be $55.8 billion along with 65,000 transplants, 1.37 million cardiovascular-related deaths, and 812,000 liver-related deaths.[53]

Again, using a similar approach, the investigators studied the economics of NASH and advanced NASH in the United States using a Markov model for all stages of NASH and a Markov model specifically designed to identify the economics of NASH with advanced fibrosis (fibrosis stage > 3).[54] The costs were inclusive of inpatient, outpatient, professional services, emergency department, and drug costs in addition to discounting all future costs at an annual rate of 3%. Results suggested that there were 6.65 million adults living with NASH in the United States in 2017 along with 232,000 incident cases. The estimated lifetime costs for those with NASH in 2017 dollars were $222.6 billion, whereas the cost for those with advanced NASH population was $95.4 billion at $139,724 per patient. Interestingly, they determined that the highest costs would incur in those aged 18 to 39 years at $72,000 suggesting that NAFLD may be impacting those of younger age as a result of the increasing global rate of obesity and T2DM and increasing the long-term economic impact of this disease.[55,56] In fact, the researchers did determine that without any change in treatment or the rising rates of obesity and T2DM, from 2017 to 2060, there will be 10.8 million new cases of NASH at a cost of $359 billion.[54]

A comparative study on the cost of NASH was also conducted in Hong Kong.[57] Results showed that the total costs for both the prevalence and incidence of NASH were 1.32 billion USD with an average per person cost of $257. Owing to the low number of organ donors, Hong Kong is expected to have a higher mortality rate due to a low number of liver transplants which were found to most likely occur in the younger group of 30 to 39 years old. In fact, the investigators estimated that over 20-year span of the study there would only be 124 liver transplants but 1596 liver-related deaths with the highest rate occurring in those aged 50 to 59 years old. However, there were 28,018 cardiovascular deaths projected with the highest rate in the 70 to 79 years age group. In addition, investigators found that the costs of NASH from 2017 to 2018 accounted for 0.41% of Hong Kong's total health expenditures which is most likely underestimated as the costs in the study excluded costs of comorbidities and societal costs.

To represent the potential economic impact among low–middle-income countries, a group of researchers investigated the health care utilization cost of NASH with fibrosis (fibrosis stage ≥2) in Thailand in the outpatient setting.[58] Health care utilization costs were composed of outpatient medication care and laboratory testing with the assumption that patients with NAFLD visit an outpatient clinic four times a year. Costs of more advanced disease were based on costs obtained for patients with HCV but minus the cost of viral load testing and hepatitis C medications. They estimated costs of NASH with significant fibrosis at the first year, fifth year, and over a lifetime and found that in the first-year costs would be $886,664,483, the fifth-year costs would be $886,376,246, and the total lifetime cost for NASH with significant fibrosis was projected to be $15.2 billion or $5174 per case in 2019 accounting for approximately 3%

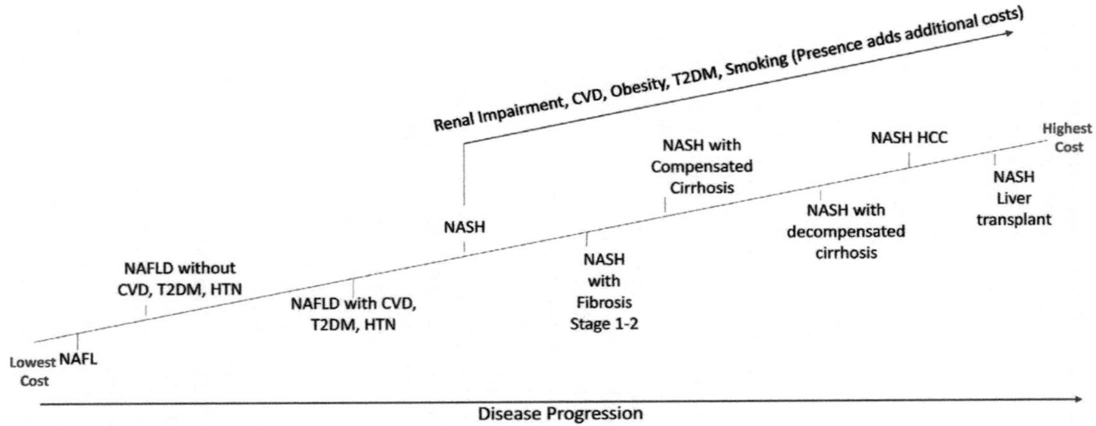

Fig. 1. Economic burden of NAFLD/NASH.

of Thailand's GDP. Although they found that adults over 60 years of age had the costs ($9492 per case) compared with the 18 to 39 age cohort ($4393 per case), the lifetime cost of the population aged 18 to 39 would account for 42% of the total amount compared with 21% for patients aged over 60.[58]

A cost of illness study for 2018 was conducted for France, Germany, Italy, Spain, and the United Kingdom.[59] Unlike other economic studies, a cost of illness relies on the population that has been diagnosed and does not include the costs of comorbidities. However, in this study, investigators did account for the costs associated with well-being. Costs included health system primary and secondary (inpatient) health care, diagnostic tests, pharmaceuticals, and medical research Well-being was defined using productivity costs that were estimated via a human capital approach and included reduced workforce participation, lost productive time caused by absenteeism and presenteeism, forgone income because of premature mortality or morbidities as well as the search, hiring and training costs required if the employee was to be replaced. Per the model, if 100% of the prevalent NASH population was diagnosed in 2018, the estimated total economic costs would have totaled: €8319 to 13,845 M for France, €10,824 to 30,878 M for Germany, €5388 to 14,150 M for Italy, €4525 to 7942 M for Spain and €7773 to 14,404 M for the UK. Average per person health system costs were estimated to range between €699 to 771 for France, €795 to 852 for Germany, €1915 to 2242 for Italy, €1919 and 2568 for Spain, and €890 and 918 for the United Kingdom. The majority of health system costs were incurred in the inpatient health care setting followed by diagnostic tests, primary health care, and pharmaceuticals. The disability-adjusted life years (DALYs) ranged as well by country and were driven primarily by a higher rate of mortality among patients with NASH.[59]

Presently, there are no medication-based treatments approved for NASH such that treatment interventions are centered around a weight loss of 5% to 10% of one's body weight through a healthy diet (eg, Mediterranean Diet) and engaging in physical activity. With this viewpoint in mind, investigators set out to determine the economic impact of NASH if treatment was available by using Markov models to estimate the differences in outcomes between the use of lifestyle modification and 2 hypothetical NASH treatments (A and B).[60] Treatment success was defined as regression to fibrosis and treatment failure was progression to stages beyond cirrhosis. Using an annual probability of treatment (ATP) ranging from 10% to 70% of treatment, they determined that treatment A averted 353 to 782 liver transplants and 1277 to 2381 liver-related deaths, and treatment B averted 129 to 437 liver transplants and 386 to 1043 liver-related deaths compared with lifestyle intervention. They concluded that treatment of NASH that leads to regression of fibrosis can have a positive impact on clinical outcomes; however, further analysis once medications are approved will need to be done on the true economic impact.[60]

In summary, around the world the economic burden of NAFLD and NASH may be substantial, especially in those with more advanced diseases. Modeling studies suggest that these costs are going to continue to increase over time if the disease trajectory of NAFLD and NASH is not supplanted with early diagnosis and intervention. The presence of comorbidities especially renal impairment, T2DM, CVD, obesity, and using or having used tobacco products all significantly increase the costs associated with NASH (**Fig. 1**). Therefore, from the economic burden perspective, early identification of patients at risk for both the development of NAFLD and advanced liver disease for those with NAFLD is necessary. In this context, as our understanding of this complex liver disease continues to evolve, efforts to raise awareness must be maintained to assist clinicians and the public in reversing the course of this liver disease. Further economic work should continue to explore how best to incorporate QALYs and/or

DALYs into the studies. Cost-effectiveness research will also be required when treatments for NASH become available.

SUMMARY

Nonalcoholic fatty liver disease and its progressive form NASH pose a substantial and rapidly growing economic burden on the societies worldwide. For patients, NAFLD is not an asymptomatic disease as even those without advanced fibrosis or cirrhosis experience impairment in their HRQL and work productivity. The increasing health care costs and decreasing quality of life associated with NAFLD make it a formidable disease of significant public health importance in need of an urgent address at the national level.

CONFLICTS OF INTEREST

There are no conflicts of interest to disclose for any of the authors.

FUNDING

None.

REFERENCES

1. Wilson IB, Cleary PD. Linking clinical variables with health-related quality of life. JAMA 1995;1995:59–65.
2. Centers for Medicare and Medicaid Services. Patient-reported outcome measures. 2022. Available at: https://mmshub.cms.gov/sites/default/files/Patient-Reported-Outcome-Measures.pdf. Accessed June 14, 2022.
3. Patrick DL, Deyo RA. Generic and disease-specific measures in assessing health status and quality of life. Med Care 1989;27:S217–32.
4. Tarride JE, Burke N, Bischof M, et al. A review of health utilities across conditions common in paediatric and adult populations. Health Qual Life Outcomes 2010; 8:12.
5. Ahmed M. Non-alcoholic fatty liver disease in 2015. World J Hepatol 2015;7(11): 1450–9.
6. Younossi ZM, Henry L. Economic and quality-of-life implications of non-alcoholic fatty liver disease. Pharmacoeconomics 2015;33(12):1245–53.
7. Assimakopoulos K, Karaivazoglou K, Tsermpini EE, et al. Quality of life in patients with nonalcoholic fatty liver disease: a systematic review. J Psychosom Res 2018; 112:73–80.
8. Younossi ZM, Guyatt G, Kiwi M, et al. Development of a disease specific questionnaire to measure health related quality of life in patients with chronic liver disease. Gut 1999;45(2):295–300.
9. Afendy A, Kallman JB, Stepanova M, et al. Predictors of health-related quality of life in patients with chronic liver disease. Aliment Pharmacol Ther 2009;30(5): 469–76.
10. David K, Kowdley KV, Unalp A, et al. Quality of life in adults with nonalcoholic fatty liver disease: baseline data from the nonalcoholic steatohepatitis clinical research network. Hepatology 2009;49(6):1904–12.
11. Chawla KS, Talwalkar JA, Keach JC, et al. Reliability and validity of the chronic liver disease questionnaire (CLDQ) in adults with non-alcoholic steatohepatitis (NASH). BMJ Open Gastroenterol 2016;3(1):e000069.

12. Younossi ZM, Stepanova M, Anstee QM, et al. Reduced patient-reported outcome scores associate with level of fibrosis in patients with nonalcoholic steatohepatitis. Clin Gastroenterol Hepatol 2019;17(12):2552–60.e10.
13. Younossi ZM, Stepanova M, Taub RA, et al. Hepatic fat reduction due to resmetirom in patients with nonalcoholic steatohepatitis is associated with improvement of quality of life. Clin Gastroenterol Hepatol 2022;20(6):1354–61.e7.
14. Dan AA, Kallman JB, Wheeler A, et al. Health-related quality of life in patients with non-alcoholic fatty liver disease. Aliment Pharmacol Ther 2007;26(6):815–20.
15. Younossi ZM, Stepanova M, Lawitz EJ, et al. Patients with nonalcoholic steatohepatitis experience severe impairment of health-related quality of life. Am J Gastroenterol 2019;114(10):1636–41.
16. Golabi P, Otgonsuren M, Cable R, et al. Non-alcoholic fatty liver disease (NAFLD) is associated with impairment of health related quality of life (HRQOL). Health Qual Life Outcomes 2016;14:18.
17. Younossi ZM, Yilmaz Y, Yu ML, et al. The clinical and patient reported outcomes (PROs) profile of patients with non-alcoholic fatty liver disease (NAFLD) from real-world practices varies across the world. J Hepatol 2020;73:S111.
18. Younossi ZM, Yilmaz Y, Yu ML, et al. Clinical and patient-reported outcomes from patients with nonalcoholic fatty liver disease across the world: data from the global non-alcoholic steatohepatitis (NASH)/non-alcoholic fatty liver disease (NAFLD) registry. Clin Gastroenterol Hepatol 2021;20(10):2296–306.e6.
19. Younossi ZM, Stepanova M, Henry L, et al. A disease-specific quality of life instrument for non-alcoholic fatty liver disease and non-alcoholic steatohepatitis: CLDQ-NAFLD. Liver Int 2017;37(8):1209–18.
20. Younossi ZM, Stepanova M, Younossi I, et al. Validation of chronic liver disease questionnaire for nonalcoholic steatohepatitis in patients with biopsy-proven nonalcoholic steatohepatitis. Clin Gastroenterol Hepatol 2019;17(10):2093–100.e3.
21. Huang R, Fan JG, Shi JP, et al. Health-related quality of life in Chinese population with non-alcoholic fatty liver disease: a national multicenter survey. Health Qual Life Outcomes 2021;19(1):140.
22. Younossi ZM, Stepanova M, Nader F, et al. Obeticholic acid impact on quality of life in patients with nonalcoholic steatohepatitis: REGENERATE 18-month interim analysis. Clin Gastroenterol Hepatol 2021;20(9):2050–8.e12.
23. Doward LC, Balp MM, Twiss J, et al. Development of a patient-reported outcome measure for non-alcoholic steatohepatitis (NASH-CHECK): results of a qualitative study. Patient 2021;14(5):533–43.
24. Karshikoff B, Sundelin T, Lasselin J. Role of inflammation in human fatigue: relevance of multidimensional assessments and potential neuronal mechanisms. Front Immunol 2017;8:21.
25. Gerber LH, Weinstein AA, Mehta R, et al. Importance of fatigue and its measurement in chronic liver disease. World J Gastroenterol 2019;25(28):3669–83.
26. Weinstein AA, Diao G, Baghi H, et al. Demonstration of two types of fatigue in subjects with chronic liver disease using factor analysis. Qual Life Res 2017;26(7):1777–84.
27. Swain MG. Fatigue in liver disease: pathophysiology and clinical management. Can J Gastroenterol 2006;20(3):181–8.
28. Newton JL, Jones DE, Henderson E, et al. Fatigue in non-alcoholic fatty liver disease (NAFLD) is significant and associates with inactivity and excessive daytime sleepiness but not with liver disease severity or insulin resistance. Gut 2008;57(6):807–13.

29. Younossi Z, Brown A, Buti M, et al. Impact of eradicating hepatitis C virus on the work productivity of chronic hepatitis C (CH-C) patients: an economic model from five European countries. J Viral Hepat 2016;23(3):217–26.
30. Younossi ZM, Jiang Y, Smith NJ, et al. Ledipasvir/sofosbuvir regimens for chronic hepatitis C infection: insights from a work productivity economic model from the United States. Hepatology 2015;61(5):1471–8.
31. Sayiner M, Stepanova M, Pham H, et al. Assessment of health utilities and quality of life in patients with non-alcoholic fatty liver disease. BMJ Open Gastroenterol 2016;3(1):e000106.
32. Fryback DG, Dunham NC, Palta M, et al. US norms for six generic health-related quality-of-life indexes from the National Health Measurement study. Med Care 2007;45(12):1162–70.
33. Rustgi VK, Duff SB, Elsaid MI. Cost-effectiveness and potential value of pharmaceutical treatment of nonalcoholic fatty liver disease. J Med Econ 2022;25(1):347–55.
34. Janssen B, Szende A. Population norms for the EQ-5D. In: Szende A, Janssen B, Cabases J, editors. Self-reported population health: an international perspective based on EQ-5D. Dordrecht (the Netherlands): Springer; 2014. p. 19–30.
35. McSweeney L, Breckons M, Fattakhova G, et al. Health-related quality of life and patient-reported outcome measures in NASH-related cirrhosis. JHEP Rep 2020;2(3):100099.
36. Huber Y, Boyle M, Hallsworth K, et al. Health-related quality of life in nonalcoholic fatty liver disease associates with hepatic inflammation. Clin Gastroenterol Hepatol 2019;17(10):2085–92.e1.
37. Younossi ZM, Wong VW, Anstee QM, et al. Fatigue and pruritus in patients with advanced fibrosis due to nonalcoholic steatohepatitis: the impact on patient-reported outcomes. Hepatol Commun 2020;4(11):1637–50.
38. Younossi ZM, Anstee QM, Wai-Sun Wong V, et al. The association of histologic and noninvasive tests with adverse clinical and patient-reported outcomes in patients with advanced fibrosis due to nonalcoholic steatohepatitis. Gastroenterology 2021;160(5):1608–19.e13.
39. Tapper EB, Lai M. Weight loss results in significant improvements in quality of life for patients with nonalcoholic fatty liver disease: a prospective cohort study. Hepatology 2016;63(4):1184–9.
40. Younossi ZM, Stepanova M, Lawitz E, et al. Improvement of hepatic fibrosis and patient-reported outcomes in non-alcoholic steatohepatitis treated with selonsertib. Liver Int 2018;38(10):1849–59.
41. Armstrong MJ, Gaunt P, Aithal GP, et al. Liraglutide safety and efficacy in patients with non-alcoholic steatohepatitis (LEAN): a multicentre, double-blind, randomised, placebo-controlled phase 2 study. Lancet 2016;387(10019):679–90.
42. Sanyal AJ, Chalasani N, Kowdley KV, et al. Pioglitazone, vitamin E, or placebo for nonalcoholic steatohepatitis. N Engl J Med 2010;362(18):1675–85.
43. Karaivazoglou K, Kalogeropoulou M, Assimakopoulos S, et al. Psychosocial issues in pediatric nonalcoholic fatty liver disease. Psychosomatics 2019;60(1):10–7.
44. Younossi ZM, Zheng L, Stepanova M, et al. Trends in outpatient resource utilizations and outcomes for Medicare beneficiaries with nonalcoholic fatty liver disease. J Clin Gastroenterol 2015;49:222–7.
45. Sayiner M, Otgonsuren M, Cable R, et al. Variables associated with inpatient and outpatient resource utilization among Medicare beneficiaries with nonalcoholic

fatty liver disease with or without cirrhosis. J Clin Gastroenterol 2017;51(3): 254–60.
46. Gordon SC, Fraysse J, Li S, et al. Disease severity is associated with higher healthcare utilization in nonalcoholic steatohepatitis Medicare patients. Am J Gastroenterol 2020;115(4):562–74.
47. Romero-Gomez M, Kachru N, Zamorano MA, et al. Disease severity predicts higher healthcare costs among hospitalized nonalcoholic fatty liver disease/ nonalcoholic steatohepatitis (NAFLD/NASH) patients in Spain. Medicine (Baltimore) 2020;99(50):e23506.
48. Petta S, Ting J, Saragoni S, et al. Healthcare resource utilization and costs of nonalcoholic steatohepatitis patients with advanced liver disease in Italy. Nutr Metab Cardiovasc Dis 2020;30(6):1014–22.
49. Canbay A, Meise D, Haas JS. Substantial comorbidities and rising economic burden in real-world non-alcoholic fatty liver disease (NAFLD)/non-alcoholic steatohepatitis (NASH) patients with compensated cirrhosis (CC): a large German claims database study. J Hepatol 2018;68:S32.
50. Hagström H, Nasr P, Ekstedt M, et al. Healthcare costs of patients with biopsy-confirmed nonalcoholic fatty liver disease are nearly twice those of matched controls. Clin Gastroenterol Hepatol 2020;18(7):1592–9.e8.
51. O'Hara J, Finnegan A, Dhillon H, et al. Cost of non-alcoholic steatohepatitis in Europe and the USA: The GAIN study. JHEP Rep 2020;2(5):100142.
52. Younossi ZM, Blissett D, Blissett R, et al. The economic and clinical burden of nonalcoholic fatty liver disease in the United States and Europe. Hepatology 2016;64(5):1577–86.
53. Younossi ZM, Tampi RP, Racila A, et al. Economic and clinical burden of nonalcoholic steatohepatitis in patients with type 2 diabetes in the U.S. Diabetes Care 2020;43(2):283–9.
54. Younossi ZM, Tampi R, Priyadarshini M, et al. Burden of illness and economic model for patients with nonalcoholic steatohepatitis in the United States. Hepatology 2019;69(2):564–72.
55. World Health Organization (WHO). Diabetes. Obtained from the world wide web at: https://www.who.int/news-room/fact-sheets/detail/diabetes. Accessed July 7, 2022.
56. World Health Organization (WHO). Obesity and overweight. Obtained from the world wide web at: https://www.who.int/news-room/fact-sheets/detail/obesity-and-overweight. Accessed July 7, 2022.
57. Tampi RP, Wong VW, Wong GL, et al. Modelling the economic and clinical burden of non-alcoholic steatohepatitis in East Asia: data from Hong Kong. Hepatol Res 2020;50(9):1024–31.
58. Phisalprapa P, Prasitwarachot R, Kositamongkol C, et al. Economic burden of non-alcoholic steatohepatitis with significant fibrosis in Thailand. BMC Gastroenterol 2021;21(1):135.
59. Schattenberg JM, Lazarus JV, Newsome PN, et al. Disease burden and economic impact of diagnosed non-alcoholic steatohepatitis in five European countries in 2018: a cost-of-illness analysis. Liver Int 2021;41(6):1227–42.
60. Younossi ZM, Tampi RP, Nader F, et al. Hypothetical treatment of patients with non-alcoholic steatohepatitis: potential impact on important clinical outcomes. Liver Int 2019;1:1–11.

Physicians' Use of Digital Health Interventions in the Management of Nonalcoholic Fatty Liver Disease

Jeffrey V. Lazarus, PhD[a,b,c,*], Marcela Villota-Rivas, MGH[a], Carolina Jiménez-González, MSc[d], Alvaro Santos-Laso, PhD[d], Paula Iruzubieta, MD, PhD[d], María Teresa Arias-Loste, MD, PhD[d], Lisa Rice-Duek, MBA[e], Simon Leigh, PhD[f,g], Christopher J. Kopka, JD[h], Juan Turnes, MD[i], José Luis Calleja, MD, PhD[j], Javier Crespo, MD, PhD[d]

KEYWORDS

- Digital health interventions • Hepatology • Liver disease
- Nonalcoholic fatty liver disease (NAFLD) • Nonalcoholic steatohepatitis (NASH)
- Spain

Continued

INTRODUCTION

Approximately 41 million deaths annually are attributable to noncommunicable diseases (NCDs), accounting for 71% of all global deaths, with liver cancer being responsible for an estimated 830,000 of these.[1,2] The NCD nonalcoholic fatty liver disease (NAFLD) is the leading cause of chronic liver disease globally,[3] affecting an estimated 25% to 48% of the global adult population.[4] NAFLD progresses to the more severe nonalcoholic steatohepatitis (NASH) in approximately 20% of cases.[5] NASH is a

[a] Barcelona Institute for Global Health (ISGlobal), Hospital Clínic, University of Barcelona, Barcelona, Spain; [b] Faculty of Medicine and Health Sciences, University of Barcelona, Barcelona, Spain; [c] CUNY Graduate School of Public Health and Health Policy (CUNY SPH), New York, NY, USA; [d] Gastroenterology and Hepatology Department, Marqués de Valdecilla University Hospital, Clinical and Translational Digestive Research Group, IDIVAL, Avenida Valdecilla s/n, 39008, Santander, Spain; [e] Health Information Management Systems Society (HIMSS), Berlin, Germany; [f] Organization for the Review of Care and Health Applications, Daresbury, UK; [g] Institute of Digital Healthcare, University of Warwick, Coventry, UK; [h] Independent Researcher, Salida, CO, USA; [i] Department of Gastroenterology and Hepatology, Complejo Hospitalario Universitario Pontevedra & IIS Galicia Sur, Spain; [j] Department of Gastroenterology and Hepatology, Hospital Universitario Puerta de Hierro de Majadahonda, Universidad Autónoma de Madrid, Madrid, Spain

* Corresponding author. Barcelona Institute for Global Health (ISGlobal), Hospital Clínic, University of Barcelona, Calle del Rossellón 171, ENT-2, Barcelona ES-08036, Spain.
E-mail address: Jeffrey.Lazarus@isglobal.org

Clin Liver Dis 27 (2023) 515–533
https://doi.org/10.1016/j.cld.2023.01.021 liver.theclinics.com

Continued

KEY POINTS

- Awareness about the utilization of digital health interventions (DHIs) in the management of chronic liver disease, including nonalcoholic fatty liver disease (NAFLD), is quite poor around the world. We used Spain as a case example to survey physicians about their knowledge, beliefs, attitudes, practices, and access with regard to DHIs for patient care, and in particular for liver disease, including their potential implementation in the field of fatty liver disease.
- Most surveyed physicians across Spain reported understanding what DHIs are but only a minority had received education/training on their use.
- Most respondents reported that they had never recommended DHIs to patients but did have an interest in receiving training on choosing and recommending appropriate DHIs for their patients.
- The main identified facilitating factors that would motivate physicians to recommend DHIs were having enough time and having evidence of their utility for the patient.
- Physicians mainly recommended organizational and patient care management procedure DHIs versus those more directly tied to patient health outcomes to patients with NAFLD and nonalcoholic steatohepatitis.

leading cause of progression to cirrhosis and liver cancer,[6,7] with liver cancer being the second leading cause of years of life lost among all cancers.[8]

NAFLD often results from having an unbalanced diet and sedentary lifestyle, is considered the hepatic complication of metabolic syndrome (MetS), and is strongly associated with other NCDs such as obesity, cardiovascular disease (CVD), and type 2 diabetes mellitus (T2DM).[3,9] Lifestyle modification with weight reduction is the only established treatment for NAFLD.[10] Nonetheless, consistent lifestyle adjustments and sustained weight loss over time can be challenging in this population[11]; the intensive coaching needed to promote adherence to weight management programs[10] may be expensive and unsustainable.

Globally, with about 5 billion Internet[12] and more than 6.5 billion smartphone users,[13] digital health intervention (DHI) opportunities are expanding rapidly. DHIs are defined as health services delivered electronically through formal or informal care (eg, telemedicine, electronic medical record [EMR], ePrescribing, telemonitoring, health applications, digital therapeutics, digital health peer groups) accessed by the care provider and receiver via digital devices (eg, telemonitoring devices, computer/tablet, mobile phone, wearable).[14] People are increasingly turning to DHIs, especially since the COVID-19 pandemic, with a study showing a 343% increase in internet searches for DHIs immediately following the first lockdown in the United Kingdom (UK).[15] The scientific evidence of the effectiveness of DHIs in health management is also expanding. A recent randomized controlled trial (RCT) systematic review and meta-analysis found that DHIs have a positive effect on physical activity outcomes in people with NCDs immediately after the intervention, with this effect lasting long-term in individuals with minimal human contact and supervision.[16] This expansion in DHI uptake and their proven health benefits is shifting health care toward personalized, patient-centric medicine that expands beyond hospitals and clinics and into homes and daily life.[17] DHIs thus provide a tremendous opportunity to address the challenges of having no pharmaceutical treatment specifically for NAFLD.

Worldwide, researchers have investigated DHI use in managing conditions such as MetS, obesity, CVD, and T2DM, with recent findings proving their efficacy in this regard.[18–20] A UK study looked at people's perspectives and use of DHIs and found that although only 38% of respondents had used such technology, 65% were open to it.[21] Two additional UK studies researched barriers and facilitators to effective DHI uptake by health care providers and found that a lack of awareness about and trust in DHIs were barriers, whereas factors such as evidence of efficacy, health care system stamps of approval, and peer-to-peer recommendations were facilitators.[22,23] In Spain, researchers have assessed people's knowledge, perspectives, ability to use, and use of DHIs, with findings showing that, overall, participants were receptive to them[24] and thought that they had a positive impact on their health[25] but that their promotion was lacking.[24,26] In addition, a study on determining factors for the intention to use DHIs by health care providers in Andalusia found that institutional support, perceived usefulness, and ease of use were influential factors.[27]

At present, only one study from the UK, involving 21 physicians, carried out a needs assessment regarding DHIs for NAFLD,[28] and an RCT from Singapore (n = 55) concluded that DHIs can be effective in improving anthropometric measures and liver enzymes in patients with NAFLD.[29] Compared with the broader DHI evidence base in other areas, there is a dearth of research around the adoption of DHIs targeting health-related behaviors by health professionals in liver disease management. In this context, and considering that the prevalence of NAFLD and NASH in Spain was reported to be 22.9% and 3.9% in 2016 and forecasted to increase to 27.6% and 5.9% by 2030, respectively,[30] and that the country is poorly prepared to address these conditions,[31–33] a better understanding of issues related to DHI use for liver disease management in the country is important. Thus, this study surveyed physicians in Spain to investigate their knowledge, beliefs, attitudes, practices, and access with regard to DHIs for patient care and in particular for liver disease, including NAFLD and NASH.

METHODS

An 18-item survey in Spanish, designed using the Research Electronic Data Capture online platform, was shared with all members of the Spanish Association for the Study of the Liver (*Asociación Española para el Estudio del Hígado* [*AEEH*]) and the Spanish Society of Digestive Diseases (*Sociedad Española de Patología Digestiva* [*SEPD*]) from February to March 2022. Members were contacted via both a medical association newsletter and through Twitter. Collected data included respondent demographics: membership status with regard to *AEEH* and *SEPD*, position/job held, university work experience, specialty, place, location, and area of practice, percentage of time spent providing liver health care weekly, number of beds in hospital of practice (if applicable), country of birth, age, gender, and number of years practicing. Further survey items inquired about participants' knowledge (eg, "I understand what DHIs are"), beliefs (eg, "I think that DHIs can have benefits in"), attitudes (eg, "I would recommend at least one form of DHI in general liver disease patient care management"), practices (eg, "Have you recommended DHIs to your patients in your clinical practice?"), and access (eg, "Which of the following DHIs are available at and provided by your workplace?") with regard to DHIs for patient care and in particular for liver diseases, including NAFLD and NASH, patient care management (refer to Supplementary File 1 for an English version of the survey). Respondents included physicians and other health care providers such as nurses. As the purpose of this study was to analyze physician data, only their responses were included in the analyses. Anonymized data were analyzed descriptively. Quantitative variables were expressed as means and standard deviations and qualitative variables as absolute values and proportions.

Qualitative variables were compared with the chi-square test or Fisher exact test, as appropriate.

RESULTS

A total of 295 physicians from all 17 autonomous communities and the autonomous city of Melilla, Spain, participated (**Fig. 1**). The demographic data of participants are summarized in **Table 1**. The average participant age was 44.4 years. Most participants were women (55.8%), had been practicing for more than 15 years (52.3%), were consulting physicians (67.1%), did not hold a university position (63.3%), worked in secondary care (95.9%), worked in the public sector (76.3%), were gastroenterologists (59.7%), and worked in more than 500 bed hospitals (50.2%). Less than half (41.1%) of participants spent 40% or more of their time per week providing liver health care.

Most participants reported understanding what DHIs are (91.2%). Only a minority (24.5%) had received education/training on the use of DHIs, with 84.7% of these receiving said education/training via work and 29.2% via self-directed learning. A comparative analysis based on age found that participants older than 40 years were more likely to have received DHI education/training (29.2% vs 17.9%, $P = 0.0255$) (**Fig. 2**). An additional comparative analysis of the questions "'I have received education/training on the use of DHIs" and "Have you recommended DHIs to your patients in your clinical practice" demonstrated that respondents were more likely to recommend DHIs if they had received said education/training ($P = <0.0001$) (**Fig. 3**). Most physicians (93.6%) reported that they thought that it would be useful to receive focused training on how to choose and recommend appropriate DHIs for their patients, without significant differences between those who had already received DHI education/training and those who had not (**Fig. 4**).

As for beliefs, more respondents reported thinking that DHIs can have benefits in areas such as improving general patient care management (65.8%) and administrative processes (65.4%) and less so in areas such as improving patient engagement and

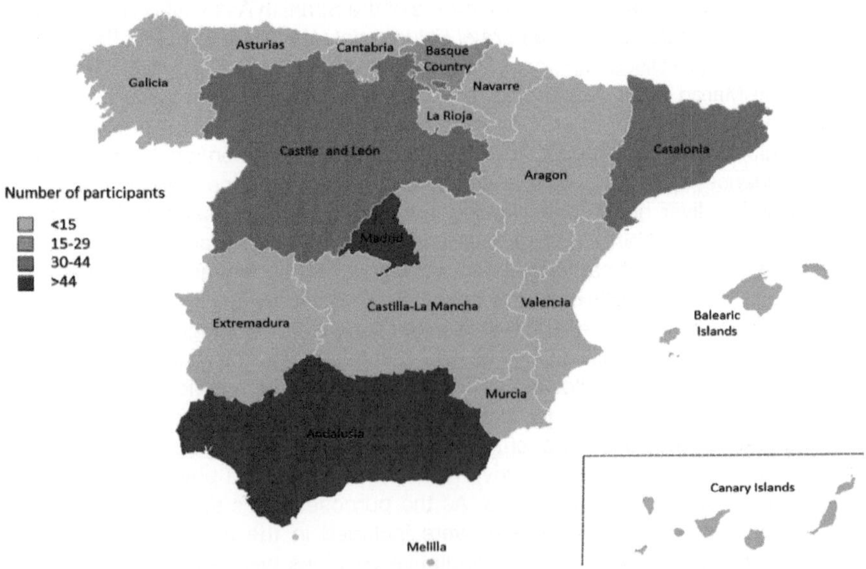

Fig. 1. Number of survey participants per autonomous community/city (n=295).

Table 1
Participant demographic data

Survey Item	Number (%) n = 295
[a]I am a member of	
AEEH	48 (16.3)
SEPD	97 (32.9)
Both	92 (31.2)
Neither	58 (19.7)
[b]Gender	
Male	128 (43.5)
Female	164 (55.8)
Nonbinary	2 (0.7)
Age	
Average—all	44.4 ± 11.2
Average age—male	46.7 ± 12.0
Average age—female	42.4 ± 10.1
Average age—nonbinary	57.5 ± 6.7
Participants ≤40	124 (42.0)
Participants >40	171 (58.0)
[b]Country of origin	
Spain	260 (88.4)
Other	34 (11.6)
[a]Number of years practicing	
0–5	59 (20.0)
6–10	36 (12.2)
11–15	46 (15.6)
16–20	45 (15.3)
21–25	38 (12.9)
>25	71 (24.1)
Position/job	
Department head	31 (10.5)
Head of unit	34 (11.5)
Consulting physician	198 (67.1)
Resident physician	27 (9.2)
Researcher	5 (1.7)
[b]University experience	
Permanent professor	15 (5.1)
Associate professor	62 (21.1)
Assistant professor	31 (10.5)
I do not have a university position	186 (63.3)
[c]Place of practice	
Primary care	8 (7.7)
Secondary care	283 (95.9)
Research center	4 (1.4)

(*continued on next page*)

Table 1
(*continued*)

Survey Item	Number (%) n = 295
Area of work	
Public sector	225 (76.3)
Private sector	18 (6.1)
Both	52 (17.6)
Specialty	
Hepatology	89 (30.2)
Gastroenterology	176 (59.7)
Internal medicine	6 (2.0)
Other	24 (8.1)
Number of beds in the hospital where you work	
<200	39 (13.2)
200–500	95 (32.2)
>500	148 (50.2)
I do not work in a hospital	13 (4.4)
[a,b]Percentage of time spent providing liver health care per week (%)	
0–9	46 (15.6)
10–19	42 (14.3)
20–29	48 (16.3)
30–39	37 (12.6)
40–49	20 (6.8)
50–59	29 (9.9)
60–69	19 (6.5)
70–79	21 (7.1)
80–89	11 (3.7)
90–100	21 (7.1)

Abbreviations: AEEH, Asociación Española para el Estudio del Hígado (Spanish Association for the Study of the Liver); *SEPD, Sociedad Española de Patología Digestiva* (Spanish Society of Digestive Diseases).

[a] Percentages may add up to just greater than or less than 100 due to rounding.
[b] n = 294 due to lack of response to survey item.
[c] Total number is more than 295, as respondent was asked to choose all answers that applied.

self-management of health (51.9%) and diagnosis efficiency (39.0%) (**Fig. 5**). In terms of access, most participants reported that they had workplace availability and provision of technologies such as ePrescribing and treatment compliance (78.6%), peer-to-peer professional consultation (67.1%), and administrative procedures (61.0%), whereas only 37.6% had such access to telemedicine/remote health, 10.2% to clinic-to-patient monitoring (at home), and 8.4% to symptom checkers (**Fig. 6**).

Most respondents reported that they had never recommended DHIs to their patients in their clinical practice (56.3%). When asked which facilitating factors would motivate them to recommend DHIs specifically for liver care management, 58.6% reported that they would recommend them if they had enough time during the consult, 50.8% if they had evidence of the utility of using DHIs for the patient, and 49.2% if the patient demonstrated evidence of digital literacy (**Fig. 7**A). Among those participants who

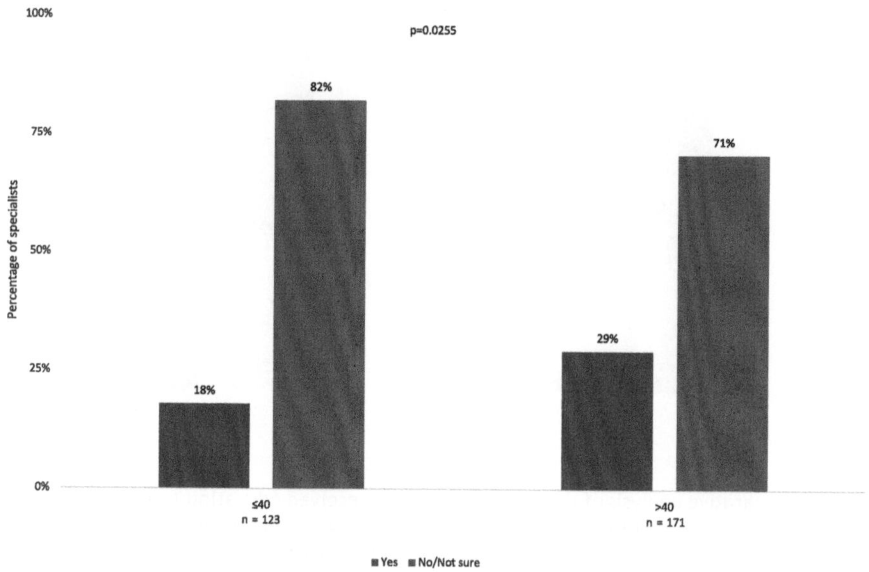

Fig. 2. Comparative analysis of the question: "I have received education/training on the use of digital health interventions" by age.

had not recommended DHIs, again, most reported that they would if they had enough time during the consult with the patient to discuss and recommend them (58.4%) and 51.2% if they had evidence of the utility of using DHIs for the patient (**Fig. 7**B). When asked which health care providers at their workplace recommend DHIs for patient care management, participants reported that it was primarily specialists (endocrinologists, cardiologists and gastroenterologist—69.2%) and primary care physicians (60.3%) and less so allied health professionals such nurses (26.1%) and dietitians

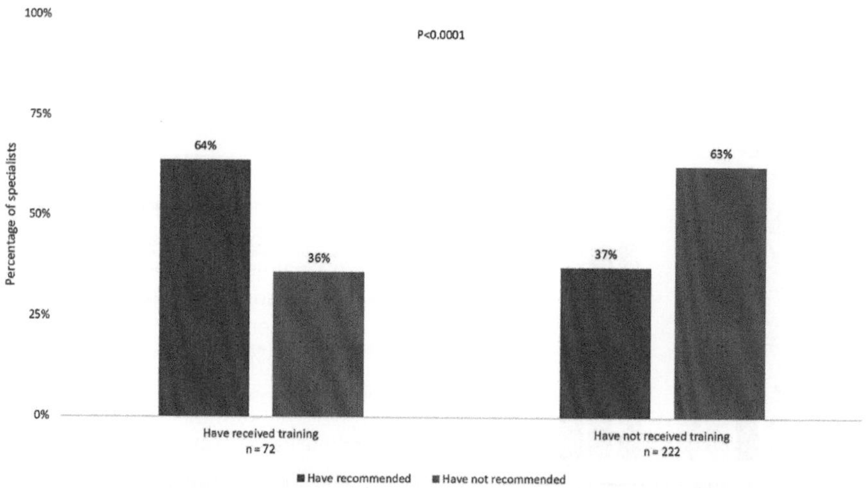

Fig. 3. Comparative analysis of the questions: "I have received education/training on the use of digital health interventions (DHIs)" and "Have you recommended DHIs to your patients in your clinical practice?"

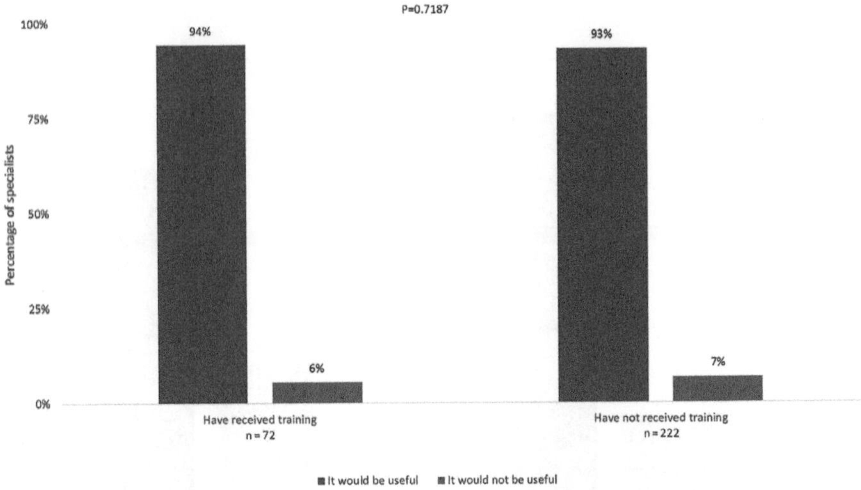

Fig. 4. Comparative analysis of the questions: "I have received education/training on the use of digital health interventions (DHIs)" and "I think it would be useful to receive focused training on how to choose and recommend appropriate DHIs for my patients."

(16.9%). As for the manner of recommending DHIs to their patients, most respondents did so via in-person consultations.

As for the types of DHIs that physicians recommended to patients with NAFLD and NASH, most reported recommending ePrescribing and EMR access at 76.9% and 54.5%, respectively, whereas 41.3% reported recommending health applications (**Fig. 8**). In terms of the types of DHIs that respondents recommended to patients for general liver disease patient care management, 58.8% and 57.9% of respondents chose weight management (nutrition) and weight management (exercise), respectively (**Fig. 9**). Regarding which aspects respondents would appreciate in a digital health

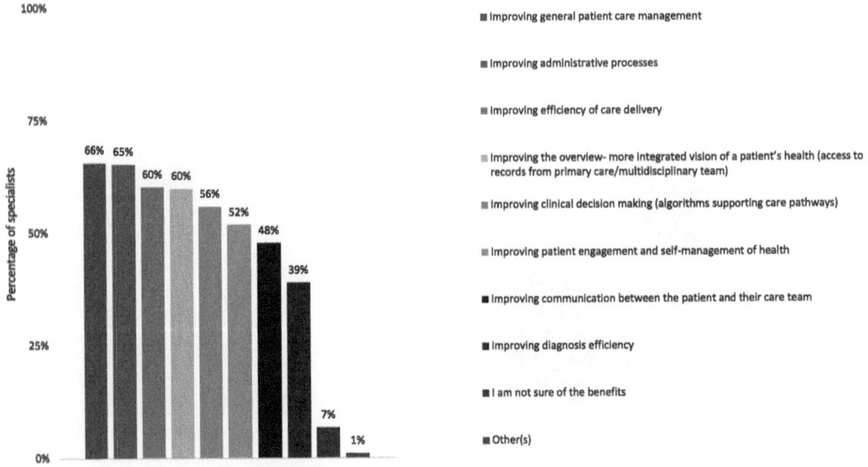

'Other(s)' responses included: 'Safety [benefits] for both patients and physicians (n=1)'; and others that referred to risks: 'Risk of turning the physician into an administrator and of purchasing medical data for big data (n=1)'; and '[Risk of] increasing the bureaucracy of the system' (n=1).

Fig. 5. Percentage of participants' answers to the question: "I think that digital health interventions can have benefits in the following (choose all that apply)" (n=295).

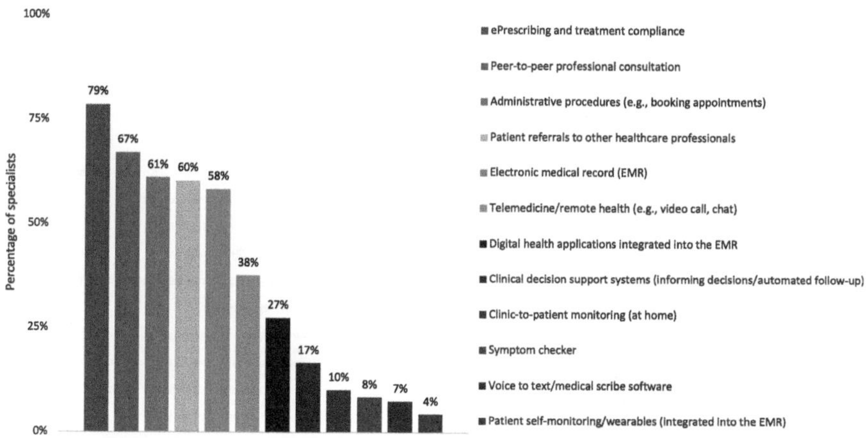

Fig. 6. Percentage of participants' answers to the question: "Which of the following digital health interventions are available at and provided by your workplace? (choose all that apply)" (n=295).

application for NAFLD and NASH, most clinicians (63.7%) chose "access to current protocols and referral flowchart" (**Fig. 10**A). However, among clinicians who reported working in a hospital with more than 500 beds, there was a greater appreciation for a "disease risk stratification calculator" (**Fig. 10**B).

DISCUSSION

This study is the first to investigate DHIs in Spain with respect to NAFLD management. We chose Spain as an example of a country with a sizable prevalence of NAFLD, a lack of NAFLD preparedness, and potentially low provider awareness about DHI. The findings may be relevant in other countries with similar characteristics. Based on data from surveyed physicians, we found that there are 2 main categories of DHIs that are available and provided in clinical workplaces that support NAFLD management: those focused on organizational and patient care management procedures (ie, administrative procedures such as booking appointments, peer-to-peer professional consultation, ePrescribing and treatment compliance, patient referrals to other health care professionals, EMR, telemedicine/remote health, clinical decision support systems, and voice to text/medical scribe software) and those that are more overtly and directly tied to patient health outcomes (ie, digital health applications and patient self-monitoring/wearables being integrated into the EMR, clinic-to-patient monitoring [at home], and symptom checkers).

Participants reported that they have greater clinical workplace access to DHIs focused on organizational and patient care management procedures, which could be explained by the fact that these types of DHIs have been in use for longer and are better established. EMR, ePrescribing, and telemedicine technologies, for instance, date back to the 1960s.[34–36] Nonetheless, even though digital innovations and transformation are perceived as an opportunity to improve the quality of and access to care in a cost-effective way, health care providers have historically been hesitant to adopt this technology and thus, digitalization in health care has progressed slowly.[37]

The study's results demonstrated a lower clinical workplace access in Spain of DHIs directly focused on health outcomes, such as digital health applications and patient

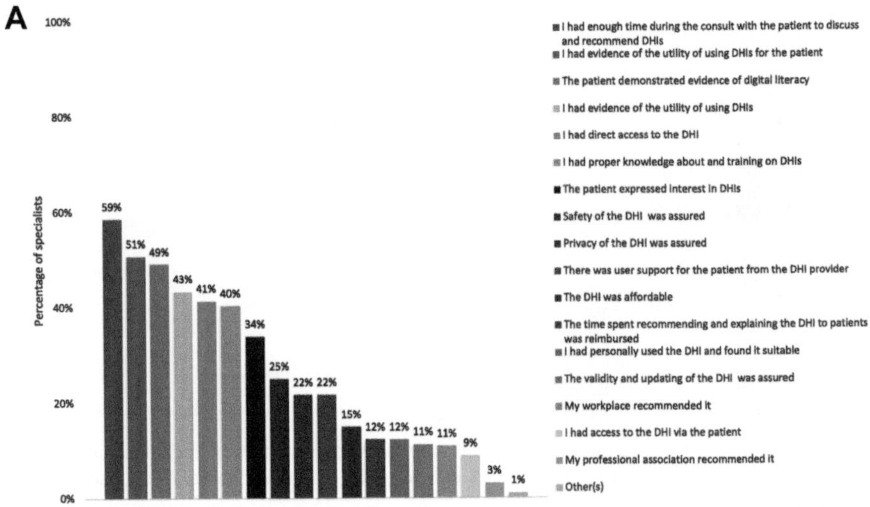

'Other(s)' responses included: 'I think [DHIs] will mean a loss of the patient's co-responsibility in the process of diagnosis and cure' (n=1); '[There was] scientific evidence of its usefulness and safety' (n=1); and 'Not applicable' (n=1).

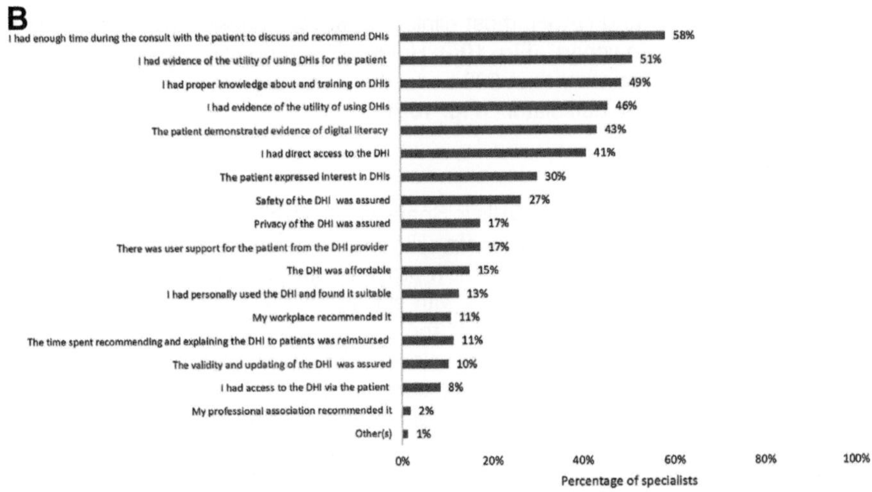

'Other(s)' responses included '[I would be willing to recommend DHIs for general liver patient care management if there was] scientific evidence of its usefulness and safety' (n=1); and 'Not applicable' (n=1).

Fig. 7. (*A*) Percentage of participants' answers to the question: "I would be willing to recommend digital health interventions (DHIs) for general liver patient care management if (choose all that apply)" (n=295). (*B*) Percentage of participants' answers to the question: "I would be willing to recommend digital health interventions (DHIs) for general liver patient care management if" among participants who had never recommended DHIs (n=166).

self-monitoring/wearables being integrated into the EMR. The COVID-19 outbreak, though, has generated an urgent demand to modify health care delivery. By way of example, prevention measures, such as physical distancing, have resulted in a strong worldwide increase in the uptake of DHIs such as telemedicine.[37] The pandemic effect also revealed a surge in the use of mobile applications for COVID-19 contact tracing, diagnosis, and treatment.[37] Health care continues to be the midst of a digital transformation, accelerated by the effects of the pandemic.

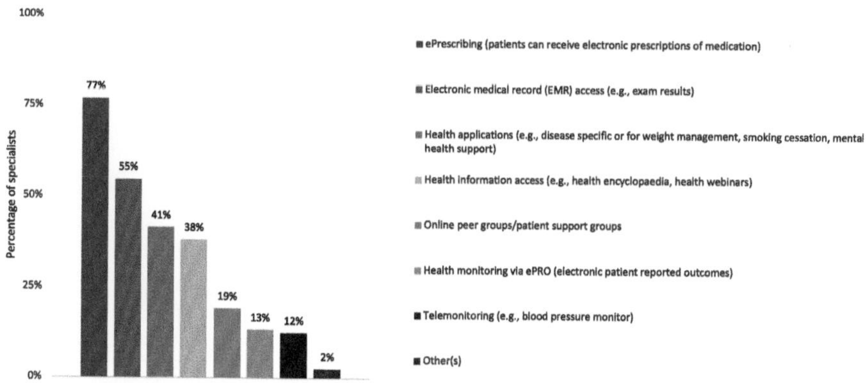

'Other(s)' responses included: 'I do not attend to this type of patients' (n=3).

Fig. 8. Percentage of participants' answers to the question: "What type of DHIs do you recommend for nonalcoholic fatty liver disease/nonalcoholic steatohepatitis patient care management? (choose all that apply)" (n=121).

This ongoing digitalization of health care is likely to affect not just operational procedures in clinical settings but also health care provider perceptions and practices regarding DHIs and patient experiences via this technology. In line with the results about DHI availability in the workplace, more physicians reported thinking that DHIs can have benefits in organizational areas such as improving administrative processes and general patient care management. In contrast, physicians were less likely to report believing that DHIs would have benefits in areas directly affecting patient health outcomes, such as diagnosis efficiency and improving patient engagement and self-management of health. Furthermore, most respondents reported that they had never recommended DHIs in their clinical practice to their patients. When asked about facilitating factors that would motivate them to recommend DHIs specifically for liver care management, including NAFLD, most physicians reported that they would recommend them if they had evidence of the utility of using DHIs for the patient. Two UK

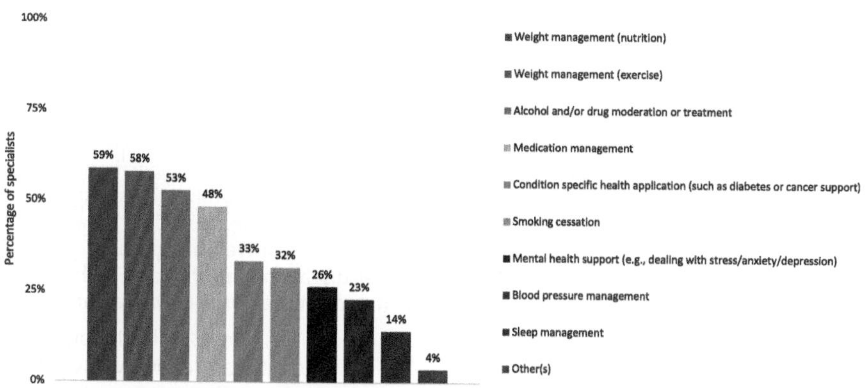

'Other(s)' responses included: 'Edpuzzle platform with tips on how to improve your disease' (n=1); 'Searching for dietary recommendations in the Spanish gastroenterology societies' (n=1); 'None' (n=1); and 'I do not attend to this type of patients' (n=1).

Fig. 9. Percentage of participants' answers to the question: "What type of digital health application (mobile or web-based) do you recommend for general liver disease patient care management? (choose all that apply)" (n=114).

A

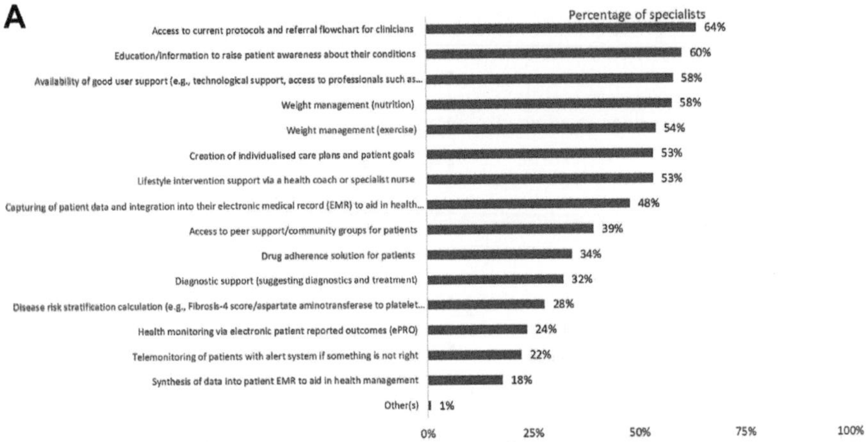

'Other(s)' responses included: 'The vital prognosis of these patients depends on the cardiovascular risk... cardiologists, endocrinologists are not mentioned' (n=1); and 'None' (n=1).

B

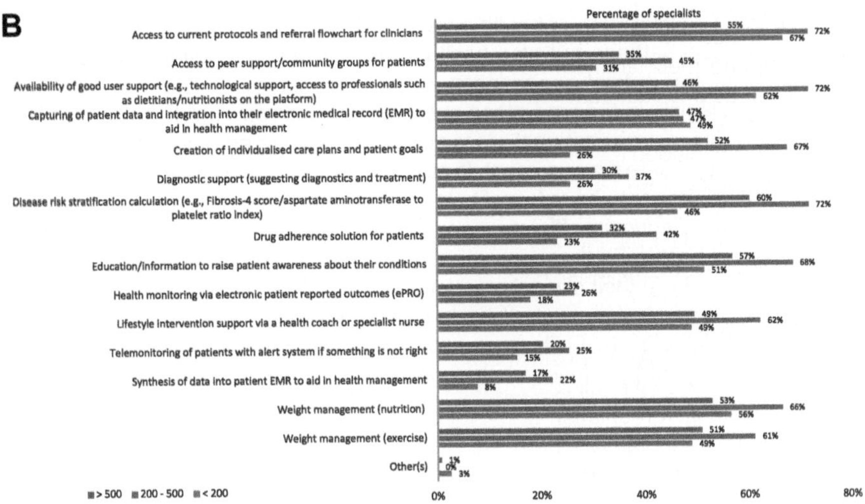

'Other(s)' responses included: 'The vital prognosis of these patients depends on the cardiovascular risk... cardiologists, endocrinologists are not mentioned' (n=1); and 'None' (n=1). Total n per hospital bed size group: >500, n=148; 200-500, n=95; and <200, n=39.

Fig. 10. (*A*) Percentage of participants' answers to the question: "What aspects would you appreciate in a digital health application (mobile or web-based) tailored specifically for the management of nonalcoholic fatty liver disease/nonalcoholic steatohepatitis? (choose all that apply)" (n=292). (*B*) Percentage of participants' answers to the question: "What aspects would you appreciate in a digital health application (mobile or web-based) tailored specifically for the management of nonalcoholic fatty liver disease/nonalcoholic steatohepatitis? (choose all that apply)" analyzed by the number of beds in the hospital where participants reported working (n=282).

studies, which investigated barriers and facilitators to effective DHI uptake by health care providers, found that a lack of awareness of and trust in DHIs were barriers and that factors such as evidence of efficacy, health care system stamps of approval, and peer-to-peer recommendations were facilitators.[22,23] Another study on determining factors for the intention to use DHIs by health providers in Andalusia found that institutional support in terms of technology availability and development and perceived usefulness were influential factors.[27] The adaption and, in some cases, outright suspension of regulations during the COVID-19 pandemic enabled an increase in DHI uptake by the health care system.[37] Assuming that the regulatory environment continues to enable DHI uptake, physicians will be increasingly exposed to this technology. Further assuming that DHIs demonstrate continued, positive impacts on health care management, physicians' beliefs and practices may continue to evolve.

In addition to firsthand evidence of the utility of using DHIs for patient care management, scientific evidence is a key driver in changing perceptions and practices in health care. To this end, DHIs have recently been shown to improve the health care management of patients with NAFLD and conditions related to NAFLD and NASH, such as MetS, obesity, CVD, and T2DM. An RCT from Singapore, albeit with a small sample size of 55 and a short follow-up time of 6 months, demonstrated that DHIs can be effective in improving anthropometric measures and liver enzymes in patients with NAFLD,[29] which is a promising start to the evidence base in this field. In terms of Mets, an RCT systematic review and meta-analysis found that DHIs have a positive effect on physical activity outcomes immediately after the intervention, with this effect lasting long-term in individuals with minimal human contact and supervision.[16] As for obesity, a systematic review of RCTs concluded that self-monitoring via DHIs is consistently associated with weight loss in behavioral treatment.[18] In terms of CVD, a systematic review and meta-analysis of RCTs showed that DHIs may improve behavioral factors such as physical activity, diet, and medication adherence and are even more potent when used to treat multiple behavioral outcomes.[19] As for T2DM, a systematic meta-review concluded that DHIs might be clinically effective in improving disease control overall and that they may significantly improve hemoglobin A_{1c} concentrations.[20]

According to the World Health Organization, all of the previously mentioned DHI evaluation methods, from the more simple observing and documenting of daily occurrences, that is, firsthand experience, to the more thorough methods, such as RCTs, are valid and warrant their discrete uses.[38] Gathering data on DHI utility does not necessarily need to be a lengthy and complicated process but it does need to be robust and validated. A recent study demonstrated that digital health technology companies have a low level of clinical robustness in their manufacturing process and that their claims can lack regulation and transparency.[39] Verified databases of approved DHIs that have been validated for clinical use, both at an institutional level, within a hospital or a specific department for instance, or nation-wide, as is the case for the National Health System in the UK,[40] are ways to facilitate DHI uptake by physicians. Physicians can then feel assured of the positive impact of DHIs on patient outcomes while accounting for usability and patients' safety and privacy. About a quarter of respondents thought that safety and privacy were important in recommending DHIs for general patient liver care management. Safety and privacy have previously been identified as major components in DHI uptake by health care providers, with a systematic review on DHI adoption by health care professionals finding that these were crucial adoption factors.[41] Available DHIs in the field of liver care management could potentially be reviewed by hepatology and gastroenterology professional bodies taking into account the social determinants of health, with results communicated to members via social media or publications, giving reassurance and building trust as to their clinical validity, safety, privacy, and inclusivity.

Increased exposure to DHIs and their impact alone will not lead to a successful digital transformation of health care management. As demonstrated in the findings, even though most participants reported understanding what DHIs are, only a minority had received education/training on their use, with a comparative analysis showing that older participants were more likely to have received said education/training. An additional comparative analysis of the questions "I have received education/training on the use of DHIs" and "Have you recommended DHIs to your patients in your clinical practice" showed that respondents were more likely to recommend DHIs if they had received said education/training (P = <0.0001). Most physicians also reported that they thought that it would be useful to receive focused training on how to choose and recommend appropriate DHIs for their patients, without significant differences between those who had already received DHI education/training and those who had not. Education and training have been found to be important factors in DHI uptake by health care providers previously, with a systematic review on DHI adoption by health care professionals finding that familiarity with the technology was a major adoption component.[41] As the findings also showed that most physicians who had been educated/trained on DHIs had received said education/training via their clinical workplace, the focus should be on adding exposure to DHI education/training earlier in the career path (eg, medical school) and continuing the momentum throughout their career (eg, on-the-job training about DHIs).

Three additional factors are important in DHI uptake: physician time, staff delegation, and patients' digital literacy. Most physicians reported that they would recommend DHIs if they had sufficient time during the consult with the patient. In clinical workplaces that support NAFLD management, physicians are already pressed for time during a consultation, and adding another task could overburden them and engender resistance to new technologies. The findings of this study also demonstrated that the physician's perception of a patients' digital literacy was a major consideration for recommending DHIs in general liver patient care management. The previously mentioned systematic review on DHI adoption by health care professionals similarly found that time and digital literacy were major uptake components.[41] In addition, survey respondents perceived that, within health care teams, physicians were most likely to recommend DHIs via in-person consultations. Delegation and task-shifting to an allied health professional, such as a nurse[42] or dietitian, may increase DHI uptake. These allied health professionals will likely require a combination of experience in patient education, available time, the ability to assess digital literacy, and the opportunity to provide proper patient education and support on the DHI to the patient and, in some cases, those caregivers closely involved in the patients' health care management.

To fully leverage the potential benefits of DHIs for liver health, all of the previously discussed factors should be considered and addressed by health systems. As demonstrated by our findings, most Spanish physicians in clinical workplaces that support NAFLD management are not making use of this technology in patient care management. For NAFLD and NASH care for instance, when physicians are recommending DHIs, they tend to be more focused on organizational and patient care management aspects (eg, ePrescribing and EMR access) and less so on patient outcomes (eg, health applications and monitoring via electronic patient-reported outcomes, online peer/patient support groups, and telemonitoring). When asked about which aspects physicians would appreciate in a digital health application for NAFLD and NASH, even though the most highly ranked option reflected organizational and patient care management aspects ("access to current protocols and referral flowchart"), a promising finding is that physicians would also appreciate DHI features centered around patient outcomes (eg, patient education, nutrition- and exercise-based weight management, creation of individualized care plans, lifestyle intervention support via a health care provider). Another encouraging result is that when participants were asked about the type of digital health applications that they recommend for general liver disease patient care management, nutrition- and exercise-based weight management were the top ranked responses, both of which are the cornerstone of NAFLD and NASH treatment.[10]

One of the main limitations of this study is that although there were 295 participants from across Spain and 89.9% were liver specialists, this figure represents approximately 25% of all liver specialists in the country. Nevertheless, this study is the first to look into utilization of DHIs in clinical settings associated with liver disease management in Spain. Given that, to date, there are very few studies of this type in the world, this study contributes to building a more robust evidence base around DHI utilization for liver care in Spain and beyond. Future studies could build on this survey to reach a higher proportion of physicians focused on liver care in Spain and in other countries around the world. Previous research, both outside and inside Spain, has looked at people's knowledge, perspectives, abilities with, and use of DHIs, with findings demonstrating that participants were open to their uptake[21,24] and thought that they had a positive impact on their health[25] but that their promotion was lacking.[24,26] Future research could survey patients with liver disease, specifically, to see about their knowledge, beliefs, attitudes, practices, and access with regard to DHIs for their health care management. Performing the suggested research for liver care management, from both a care provider and receiver perspective, could provide the evidence to help in optimizing utilization of a technology that has the potential to transform the way in which health care is approached and lead to improved patient outcomes.

SUMMARY

Although a high level of familiarity with DHIs among physicians in Spain was found, most reported that they do not recommend these tools in patient care management and when they do, most recommend DHIs focused on organizational aspects, such as ePrescribing and EMR access, and less on those that directly affect patient health outcomes, such as health applications and telemonitoring. Addressing concerns, including an absence of time, evidence of DHI utility, education, training, and access, may contribute to increased utilization of these technologies overall and more importantly to directly improve the health of patients. DHIs have the potential to help in caring for people with or at risk of noncommunicable liver diseases, including NAFLD and NASH, which represent an enormous and growing burden on the health care system.

CLINICS CARE POINTS

- Although familiarity with DHIs among surveyed physicians in Spain in clinical workplaces that support NAFLD management is high, only a minority have been educated/trained on their use, which results in a lower likelihood that they will recommend them for patient care.
- Most physicians are interested in receiving focused training on how to choose and recommend appropriate DHIs for their patients, regardless of whether or not they have already received DHI education/training.
- The 3 main facilitating factors that would motivate physicians to recommend DHIs, specifically for liver care management, are having enough time in the clinical workplace during the consult to do so, having evidence of the utility of using DHIs for the patient, and that the patient demonstrates evidence of digital literacy.
- Physicians' clinical workplace access to DHIs focused on organizational and patient care management procedures (eg, EMR) is higher than those more directly tied to patient health outcomes (eg, digital health applications and patient self-monitoring/wearables

being integrated into the EMR), with this finding being mirrored in terms of their perceptions of the areas in which DHIs can have benefits.

- This trend was also mirrored in terms of the types of DHIs that physicians recommended to patients with NAFLD and NASH, with most recommending DHIs such as ePrescribing and EMR access and less recommending DHIs such as health applications and telemonitoring.
- Even though when asked about which aspects they would appreciate in a digital health application for fatty liver disease, the most highly ranked option reflected organizational and patient care management aspects ("access to current protocols and referral flowchart"), a promising finding is that physicians also reported a high interest in DHI features centered around patient outcomes (eg, patient education, nutrition- and exercise-based weight management, creation of individualized care plans, lifestyle intervention support via a health care provider).
- When asked about the type of digital health applications that they recommend for general liver disease patient care management, nutrition- and exercise-based weight management were the top ranked responses by physicians, both of which are the cornerstone of NAFLD and NASH treatment.
- A clinicians' ability to delegate DHI management, administration, and patient engagement to allied health professionals may facilitate uptake in clinical environments.

DISCLOSURE

Unrestricted funding from Gilead Sciences was provided to IDIVAL, Cantabria, Spain, to carry out this study. J.V. Lazarus acknowledges grants and speaker fees from AbbVie, Gilead Sciences, and MSD and speaker fees from Genfit, Intercept, Janssen, Novo Nordisk, and ViiV, outside of the submitted work. J.L. Calleja reports grants to his institution from Gilead Sciences and personal fees from AbbVie, Gilead Sciences, MSD, and Intercept, outside of the submitted work. J. Crespo reports consulting and personal fees from Gilead Sciences, AbbVie, MSD, Shionogi, Intercept Pharmaceuticals, Janssen Pharmaceuticals Inc, Celgene, and Alexion, outside of the submitted work. M. Villota-Rivas, C. Jiménez-González, A. Santos-Laso, P. Iruzubieta, M.T. Arias-Loste, L. Rice-Duek, S. Leigh, C.J. Kopka, and J.T. Vázquez have nothing to disclose.

ACKNOWLEDGMENTS

J.V. Lazarus and M. Villota-Rivas acknowledge institutional support to ISGlobal from the Spanish Ministry of Science and Innovation and the State Research Agency through the "Centro de Excelencia Severo Ochoa 2019-2023" Program (CEX2018-000806-S) and from the "Generalitat de Catalunya" through the CERCA Program. A. Santos-Laso acknowledges support from the Institute of Health Carlos III (Spanish Ministry of Science and Innovation), Spain, through the "Sara Borrell" award (CD21/00039).

SUPPLEMENTARY DATA

Supplementary data related to this article can be found online at https://doi.org/10.1016/j.cld.2023.01.021.

REFERENCES

1. World Health Organization. Noncommunicable diseases. Available at: https://www.who.int/news-room/fact-sheets/detail/noncommunicable-diseases. Accessed July 1, 2022.

2. World Health Organization. Cancer. Available at: https://www.who.int/news-room/fact-sheets/detail/cancer. Accessed July 1, 2022.
3. Younossi ZM, Henry L. Fatty liver through the ages: nonalcoholic steatohepatitis. Endocr Pract 2022;28(2):204–13.
4. Ekstedt M, Nasr P, Kechagias S. Natural history of NAFLD/NASH. Curr Hepatol Rep 2017;16:391–7.
5. Estes C, Razavi H, Loomba R, et al. Modeling the epidemic of nonalcoholic fatty liver disease demonstrates an exponential increase in burden of disease. Hepatology 2018;67(1):123–33.
6. Ruth Araújo A, Rosso N, Bedogni G, et al. Global epidemiology of non-alcoholic fatty liver disease/non-alcoholic steatohepatitis: what we need in the future Fondazione Italiana Fegato-Onlus, Trieste, Italy. Liver Int 2018;38:47.
7. Kanwal F, Kramer JR, Mapakshi S, et al. Risk of hepatocellular cancer in patients with non-alcoholic fatty liver disease. Gastroenterology 2018;155(6):1828–37.
8. Fitzmaurice C, Abate D, Abbasi N, et al. Global, regional, and national cancer incidence, mortality, years of life lost, years lived with disability, and disability-adjusted life-years for 29 cancer groups, 1990 to 2017: a systematic analysis for the global burden of disease study. JAMA Oncol 2019;5(12):1749–68.
9. Younossi Z, Tacke F, Arrese M, et al. Global perspectives on nonalcoholic fatty liver disease and nonalcoholic steatohepatitis. Hepatology 2019;69(6):2672–82.
10. Romero-Gómez M, Zelber-Sagi S, Trenell M. Treatment of NAFLD with diet, physical activity and exercise. J Hepatol 2017;67:829–46.
11. Hallsworth K, Adams LA. Lifestyle modification in NAFLD/NASH: facts and figures. JHEP Reports 2019;1(6):468–79.
12. Internet Statista. Users in the world 2022. Available at: https://www.statista.com/statistics/617136/digital-population-worldwide/. Accessed July 1, 2022.
13. Statista. Smartphones - statistics & facts. Available at: https://www.statista.com/topics/840/smartphones/#dossierKeyfigures. Accessed July 1, 2022.
14. Soobiah C, Cooper M, Kishimoto V, et al. Identifying optimal frameworks to implement or evaluate digital health interventions: a scoping review protocol. BMJ Open 2020;10(8):e037643.
15. Leigh S, Daly R, Stevens S, et al. Web-based internet searches for digital health products in the United Kingdom before and during the COVID-19 pandemic: a time-series analysis using app libraries from the Organisation for the Review of Care and Health Applications (ORCHA). BMJ Open 2021;11(10):e053891.
16. Stavric V, Kayes NM, Rashid U, et al. The effectiveness of self-guided digital interventions to improve physical activity and exercise outcomes for people with chronic conditions: a systematic review and meta-analysis. Front Rehabil Sci 2022;0:120. https://doi.org/10.3389/FRESC.2022.925620.
17. Wu T, Simonetto DA, Halamka JD, et al. The digital transformation of hepatology: the patient is logged in. Hepatology 2022;75(3):724–39.
18. Patel ML, Wakayama LN, Bennett GG. Self-monitoring via digital health in weight loss interventions: a systematic review among adults with overweight or obesity. Obesity 2021;29(3):478–99.
19. Akinosun AS, Polson R, Diaz-Skeete Y, et al. Digital technology interventions for risk factor modification in patients with cardiovascular disease: systematic review and meta-analysis. JMIR Mhealth and Uhealth 2021;9(3):e21061. Available at: https://mhealth.jmir.org/2021/3/e21061.
20. Eberle C, Stichling S. Clinical improvements by telemedicine interventions managing type 1 and type 2 diabetes: systematic meta-review. J Med Internet Res 2021;23(2):e23244. Available at: https://www.jmir.org/2021/2/e23244.

21. Digital ORCHA. Health in the UK: national attitudes and behaviour research. 2021. Available at: https://orchahealth.com/wp-content/uploads/2021/07/2107_ICS_Research_Report_2021_National_final.pdf. Accessed July 1, 2022.
22. Leigh S, Ashall-Payne L, Andrews T. Barriers and facilitators to the adoption of mobile health among health care professionals from the United Kingdom: discrete choice experiment. JMIR Mhealth and Uhealth 2020;8(7):e17704. Available at: https://mhealth.jmir.org/2020/7/e17704.
23. Leigh S, Ashall-Payne L. The role of health-care providers in mHealth adoption. Lancet Digit Heal 2019;1(2):e58–9.
24. Sotillos-González B, Buiza-Camacho B, Herrera-Usagre M, et al. Visión ciudadana sobre la prescripción de aplicaciones móviles de salud y el uso de tecnologías de la información y la comunicación en el entorno sanitario en Andalucía. J Healthc Qual Res 2018;33(4):225–33.
25. Observatorio Nacional de las Telecomunicaciones y de la SI. Los ciudadanos ante la e-Sanidad: opiniones y expectativas de los ciudadanos sobre el uso y aplicación de las TIC en el ámbito sanitario. 2016. Available at: https://www.ontsi.es//sites/ontsi/files/los_ciudadanos_ante_la_e-sanidad.pdf. Accessed July 1, 2022.
26. Oñate CG, Peyró CF. Mobile applications for the elderly: a study of their current strategy. Aula Abierta 2018;47(1):107–12.
27. Determinantes de la intención de uso de la telemedicina en una organización sanitaria - dialnet. Available at: https://dialnet.unirioja.es/servlet/articulo?codigo=6905102. Accessed July 1, 2022.
28. Hallsworth K, McPherson S, Anstee QM, et al. Digital intervention with lifestyle coach support to target dietary and physical activity behaviors of adults with nonalcoholic fatty liver disease: systematic development process of VITALISE using intervention mapping. J Med Internet Res 2021;23(1):e20491. Available at: https://www.jmir.org/2021/1/e20491.
29. Lim SL, Johal J, Ong KW, et al. Lifestyle intervention enabled by mobile technology on weight loss in patients with nonalcoholic fatty liver disease: randomized controlled trial. JMIR Mhealth and Uhealth 2020;8(4):e14802. Available at: https://mhealth.jmir.org/2020/4/e14802.
30. Estes C, Anstee QM, Arias-Loste MT, et al. Modeling NAFLD disease burden in China, France, Germany, Italy, Japan, Spain, United Kingdom, and United States for the period 2016–2030. J Hepatol 2018;69(4):896–904.
31. Lazarus JV, Ekstedt M, Marchesini G, et al. A cross-sectional study of the public health response to non-alcoholic fatty liver disease in Europe. J Hepatol 2020;72(1):14–24.
32. Lazarus JV, Palayew A, Carrieri P, et al. European 'NAFLD Preparedness Index' — is Europe ready to meet the challenge of fatty liver disease? JHEP Reports 2021;3(2):100234.
33. Lazarus JV, Mark HE, Villota-Rivas M, et al. The global NAFLD policy review and preparedness index: are countries ready to address this silent public health challenge? JHEP 2022;76(4):771–80.
34. Evans RS. Electronic health records: then, now, and in the future. Yearb Med Inform 2016;25(S 01):S48–61.
35. Salmon JW, Jiang RE-. Prescribing: history, issues, and potentials. Online J Public Health Inform 2012;4(3). https://doi.org/10.5210/OJPHI.V4I3.4304.
36. Board on health care services; institute of medicine. The role of telehealth in an evolving health care environment: workshop summary. The evolution of telehealth: where have we been and where are we going? - the role of telehealth in

an evolving health C. 2012. Available at: https://www.ncbi.nlm.nih.gov/books/NBK207141/. Accessed July 1, 2022.
37. Glauner P, Plugmann P, Lerzynski G. In: Glauner P, Plugmann P, Lerzynski G, editors. Digitalization in healthcare. Implementing innovation and artificial intelligence. Springer; 2021. https://doi.org/10.1007/978-3-030-65896-0.
38. Johns. Monitoring and Evaluating Digital Health Interventions A practical guide to conducting research and assessment Global mHealth Initiative Monitoring and evaluating digital health interventions: a practical guide to conducting research and assessment. 2016. Available at: http://apps.who.int/bookorders. Accessed July 1, 2022.
39. Day S, Shah V, Kaganoff S, et al. Assessing the clinical robustness of digital health startups: cross-sectional observational analysis. J Med Internet Res 2022;24(6):e37677. Available at: https://www.jmir.org/2022/6/e37677.
40. NHS Apps Library - NHS Digital. Available at: https://digital.nhs.uk/services/nhs-apps-library. Accessed July 1, 2022.
41. Gagnon MP, Ngangue P, Payne-Gagnon J, et al. m-Health adoption by healthcare professionals: a systematic review. J Am Med Informatics Assoc 2016;23(1):212–20.
42. Ferguson C, Hickman L, Wright R, et al. Preparing nurses to be prescribers of digital therapeutics 2018;54(4–5):345–9.

Research Priorities for Precision Medicine in NAFLD

Paula Iruzubieta, PhD, MD[a], Ramon Bataller, PhD, MD[b], María Teresa Arias-Loste, PhD, MD[a], Marco Arrese, MD[c], José Luis Calleja, PhD, MD[d], Graciela Castro-Narro, MD, MSc[e], Kenneth Cusi, PhD, MD[f], John F. Dillon, MD[g], María Luz Martínez-Chantar, PhD[h], Miguel Mateo, MD[i], Antonio Pérez, PhD, MD[j], Mary E. Rinella, PhD, MD[k], Manuel Romero-Gómez, PhD, MD[l], Jörn M. Schattenberg, PhD, MD[m], Shira Zelber-Sagi, RD, PhD[n,o], Javier Crespo, PhD, MD[a,*], Jeffrey V. Lazarus, PhD[p,q,r,*]

KEYWORDS

• NAFLD • Non-invasvie tests (NITs) • Precision medicine • Multidisciplinary care
• Disease phenotyping

Continued

[a] Gastroenterology and Hepatology Department, Clinical and Translational Research in Digestive Diseases, Valdecilla Research Institute (IDIVAL), Marqués de Valdecilla University Hospital, Avenida Valdecilla 25, 39008, Santander, Spain; [b] Division of Gastroenterology, Hepatology and Nutrition, Center for Liver Diseases, University of Pittsburgh Medical Center, PA, USA; [c] Department of Gastroenterology, School of Medicine, Pontificia Universidad Católica de Chile, Avenida Libertador Bernardo O'Higgins 340, 8331150, Santiago, Chile; [d] Department of Gastroenterology and Hepatology, Puerta de Hierro University Hospital, Puerta de Hierro Health Research Institute (IDIPHIM), CIBERehd, Universidad Autonoma de Madrid, Calle Joaquín Rodrigo 1, 28222, Majadahonda, Spain; [e] Department of Gastroenterology, Instituto Nacional de Ciencias Médicas y Nutrición Salvador Zubirán, Department of Hepatology and Transplant, Hospital Médica Sur, Asociación Latinoamericana para el Estudio del Hígado (ALEH), Mexico City, Mexico; [f] Division of Endocrinology, Diabetes & Metabolism, Department of Medicine, University of Florida, Gainesville, FL, USA; [g] Division of Molecular and Clinical Medicine, University of Dundee, Ninewells Hospital and Medical School, Dundee, UK; [h] Liver Disease Laboratory, Center for Cooperative Research in Biosciences (CIC BioGUNE), Basque Research and Technology Alliance (BRTA), Centro de Investigación Biomedica en Red de Enfermedades Hepáticas y Digestivas (CIBERehd), Derio, Bizkaia, Spain; [i] Pharmacy Organisation and Inspection, Government of Cantabria, Santander, Spain; [j] Endocrinology and Nutrition Department, Santa Creu I Sant Pau Hospital, Universitat Autónoma de Barcelona, IIB-Sant Pau and Centro de Investigación Biomedica en Red de Diabetes y Enfermedades Metabólicas Asociadas (CIBERDEM), Barcelona, Spain; [k] Department of Medicine, University of Chicago, Chicago, IL, USA; [l] UCM Digestive Diseases and CIBERehd, Virgen Del Rocío University Hospital, Institute of Biomedicine of Seville, University of Seville, Seville, Spain; [m] Metabolic Liver Research Program, I. Department of Medicine, University Medical Centre Mainz, Mainz, Germany; [n] University of Haifa, School of Public Health, Mount Carmel, Haifa, Israel; [o] Department of Gastroenterology, Tel- Aviv Medical Centre, Tel- Aviv, Israel; [p] Barcelona Institute for Global Health (ISGlobal), Hospital Clínic, University of Barcelona, Calle del Rossellón 171, ENT-2, Barcelona ES-08036, Spain; [q] Faculty of Medicine and Health Sciences, University of Barcelona, Barcelona, Spain; [r] CUNY Graduate School of Public Health and Health Policy (CUNY SPH), New York, NY, USA

* Corresponding authors. Clinical and Translational Research in Digestive Diseases, Valdecilla Research Institute (IDIVAL), Marqués de Valdecilla University Hospital, Avenida Valdecilla 25, 39008, Santander, Spain (J.C.); Barcelona Institute for Global Health (ISGlobal), Hospital Clínic, University of Barcelona, Calle del Rossellón 171, ENT-2, Barcelona ES-08036, Spain (J.V.L.).
E-mail addresses: javiercrespo1991@gmail.com (J.C.); jeffrey.lazarus@isglobal.org (J.V.L.)

Clin Liver Dis 27 (2023) 535–551
https://doi.org/10.1016/j.cld.2023.01.016
1089-3261/23/

Continued

KEY POINTS

- Despite its enormous burden and impact, NAFLD has received little public health attention globally, with weak and fragmented responses.
- Population-based screening is not considered cost-effective, but several studies and expert guidelines suggest that individuals with diabetes and other metabolic risk factors, such as obesity, should be considered for case-finding strategies.
- NAFLD's heterogeneity represents a major challenge in developing highly effective therapies. The identification of NAFLD phenotypes could favor precision medicine in this liver disease.
- The development of patient-centered models of care, including the use of telemedicine, is key to personalized and precision medicine in NAFLD.
- To advance the field of fatty liver disease, we developed a set of strategic research priorities addressing public health and clinical issues, including screening and diagnosis strategies, clinical trial design, multidisciplinary approaches, and novel therapies.

INTRODUCTION

NAFLD and its inflammatory condition NASH, which is more likely to progress to fibrosis and advanced liver disease, are the histologic manifestation of a heterogeneous disease closely associated with insulin resistance and obesity.[1] NAFLD is a complex and heterogeneous condition that involves multiple signaling pathways that regulate disease development and progression. Despite extensive efforts to find effective treatments, there is no approved drug therapy for NAFLD. Progress in NAFLD prevention and treatment requires a better understanding of its pathophysiology and clinical subtypes, identification of risk factors, the definition of phenotypes, and development of personalized and precision medicine. This review summarizes the presentations and discussions by a panel of experts during the *International Precision Medicine Forum: NAFLD Updated*, held in May 2022. Research priorities in NAFLD care include social and economic implications, interindividual variations, clinical trial design, multidisciplinary models of care, and patient management approaches.

A PUBLIC HEALTH PROBLEM

Disease Burden and Economic Impact of NAFLD

NAFLD is the most prevalent chronic liver disease (CLD) globally, affecting roughly one in three adults and 10% of children and adolescents.[2,3] Its prevalence is expected to increase, mainly due to its close association with obesity and type 2 diabetes mellitus (T2DM).[4,5] NAFLD costs about US $103 billion in the United States and €35 billion in Europe annually, in direct medical costs alone.[6] Despite its enormous burden and impact, NAFLD has received little public health attention globally, with weak and fragmented responses.[7,8] A NAFLD policy review of 102 countries found that a comprehensive public health response was lacking overall and that it was rarely mentioned in the strategies for related conditions like obesity and T2DM.[9] Research priorities should thus include more robust national prevalence studies, including in the pediatric population, a better understanding of the health system and overall costs for addressing NAFLD, and further investigation into the policies in place at the global, national, and subnational levels, including for common comorbidities like obesity and T2DM.[10]

Tackling NAFLD will also entail revising its terminology. The American Association for the Study of Liver Diseases and the European Association for the Study of the Liver, along with the Asian Pacific Association for the Study of the Liver, the *Asociación Latinoamericana para el Estudio del Hígado,* and other societies are leading a global multi-stakeholder process to revise the nomenclature, taking into account stigma and ensuring that it advances disease and treatment understanding.[11]

The Recognition of Hidden Chronic Liver Disease as a Silent Condition

CLD, including NAFLD, develops slowly and can remain undiagnosed for years until clinical manifestations become apparent or a diagnosis is made incidentally.[12] There is evidence suggesting that even early stages of CLD are associated with decreased overall survival. Therefore, early diagnosis may delay or prevent complications and decrease liver fibrosis-associated morbidity and mortality.[13] Estimating the prevalence of significant liver fibrosis and cirrhosis in the general population and in subjects at risk of CLD is possible. Although methodological differences exist in published studies, conservative estimates suggest that significant liver fibrosis and cirrhosis are present in 5% to 7% and 0.5% to 0.8% of the general population, respectively.[13] These figures are much higher among individuals with metabolic risk factors such as abdominal obesity and T2DM,[14] with an estimated prevalence of advanced fibrosis in patients with NAFLD and T2DM of 17%.[4]

Although there are no data supporting screening for liver fibrosis in the general population, several studies and expert guidelines suggest that individuals with T2DM and multiple metabolic risk factors should be considered for case-finding strategies, as they have an increased prevalence of advanced liver fibrosis.[15,16] However, although appropriate screening tools are not sufficiently defined, there is agreement that noninvasive tests (NITs) for liver fibrosis, either via blood or elastography, can confidently exclude advanced liver fibrosis in low-prevalence populations.[16] Future studies should investigate whether universal screening with NITs is cost-effective, in terms of treatment and health outcomes.

Research Priorities in One of the Countries with the Highest Prevalence of NAFLD: Mexico

The prevalence of obesity and T2DM in Mexico is the first and sixth highest globally, respectively, and CLD represents the sixth most common cause of death.[17] NAFLD is currently the main cause of cirrhosis in this country, overtaking the hepatitis C virus (HCV) and alcohol consumption.[18] A recent study using a screening score (MAFLD-S) that considers the following NAFLD predictors: age and gender and the presence of diabetes, hypertension, and dyslipidemia, found an estimated prevalence of NAFLD of 49.7%.[19] The high prevalence of obesity and metabolic syndrome (MetS) in the context of high genetic susceptibility, with a prevalence of 77% of the G risk allele in PNPLA3 (patatin-like phospholipase domain-containing protein 3) in Mexicans, are major contributors to the high prevalence of NAFLD in the country,[20] as is the growing trend of ultra-processed food consumption in the last three decades, which has contributed to the high rate of obesity.[21] Research in Mexico should address factors such as the lack of awareness about NAFLD among health care providers, fragmentation of the health system in terms of providing multidisciplinary care, and developing effective strategies for NAFLD prevention and treatment, given the size of the country and its diverse population.[22]

RESEARCH TO IMPROVE THE DIAGNOSIS OF NAFLD

Screening for NAFLD

The case for early detection of NAFLD builds on the opportunity to provide interventions or lifestyle advice that will positively affect liver health.[23] Population-based screening is not considered cost-effective. Today, the major challenge is to identify the small subgroup of patients that show an advanced disease stage and have an unfavorable outcome. Strategies based on case finding in response to risk factors such as T2DM, obesity, features of MetS, or routinely performed abnormal liver function tests are being evaluated.[24] These risk stratification strategies build on a combination of clinical risk factors and surrogate scores that use indirect blood-based tests of hepatic fibrosis. Both the European and North American liver societies recommend a two-tier approach to risk stratification in those suspected or incidentally found to have hepatic steatosis on imaging, using sequential NITs.[16,25] The FIB-4 score that was initially developed to identify patients with cirrhosis in an HIV (human immunodeficiency virus) and HCV-coinfected population is most widely found in referral and screening pathways. The FIB-4 has an acceptable specificity, allowing us to rule out many patients with NAFLD that do not show advanced fibrosis. Based on its low sensitivity, sequential combinations with mostly imaging biomarkers, for example, transient elastography allowing for liver stiffness measurements (LSM), are used. Inaccuracies seem to be acceptable based on the slow, progressive course of the disease and highlight the need for repeated assessment when risk factors are maintained. The approval of new pharmacologic treatment options for NASH will certainly stimulate early detection in at-risk populations.

NAFLD Phenotyping

There are multiple factors that interact to influence the development and clinical course of NAFLD.[26] Importantly, morbimortality in patients with NAFLD involves extrahepatic organs, as it is considered a mediator of systemic diseases including cardiovascular disease.[27] This further contributes to NAFLD's heterogeneity, representing a major challenge in discovering highly effective therapies. Recognizing NAFLD as a systemic metabolic dysfunction should facilitate patient stratification and identification of disease subtypes.[28] Although NAFLD is usually associated with excess body weight, it may also affect normal-weight individuals, a condition termed lean-NAFLD. Recent data suggest that lean-NAFLD shows cardiovascular and cancer-related mortality comparable to obese NAFLD individuals and a similar increased risk of all-cause mortality.[29,30] However, lean-NAFLD has unique pathogenic underpinnings.[31] Thus, identifying and addressing factors influencing lean NAFLD is crucial to improve patient outcomes and developing precise treatment strategies.[32]

The existence of patient phenotyping has been highlighted in several recent studies based on omics techniques.[33–35] One study stratified patients with NAFLD according to their risk of developing hepatocellular carcinoma (HCC) using a polygenic risk score of hepatic fat content,[33] which predicted HCC independently of classical risk factors and the presence of advanced fibrosis, suggesting that liver fat accumulation directly favors hepatic carcinogenesis. In fact, different pathogenic mechanisms have been reported between NAFLD patients with insulin resistance and different genetic profiles, which may have implications for diagnosis and treatment.[36] Another study identified two NAFLD metabolic phenotypes, M-subtype, and non-M-subtype, based on the serum metabolic profile of methionine adenosyltransferase 1a knockout mice, which have low hepatic S-adenosylmethionine (SAMe) and high stearoyl-CoA dehydrogenase 1 levels. This study suggests that NAFLD patients with an M-subtype profile will likely benefit from SAMe or Aramchol treatment.[34] However, this approach results in several unclassified patients. The potential integration of multi-omics data as well as clinical parameters may thus improve research into this novel subtyping approach of patients with NAFLD, paving the way for precision medicine.

CHALLENGES IN NAFLD CLINICAL TRIALS

Despite two decades of investigation into a therapeutic solution for NAFLD, there are no approved drugs. NAFLD clinical trials are challenging to perform, with multiple promising agents failing in phase IIb and III trials.[37–39] There are multiple wide-ranging reasons for this. Here, we discuss some of the main current challenges.

Endpoints in NAFLD

Full US Food and Drug Administration (FDA) approval requires that a drug improves how a patient feels, functions, or survives. NAFLD, even at advanced stages, is mostly asymptomatic with a slow progression rate. As a consequence, surrogate endpoints, such as improving liver histologic stage, which is known to predict clinical outcomes, are needed for conditional approval, with the expectation that longer follow-up studies will show improvement in clinical outcomes.[40] Two endpoints are currently accepted in trials including noncirrhotic NASH.[41,42] These include either the complete resolution of NASH, without worsening of fibrosis, or an improvement of greater than 1 stage in fibrosis, without worsening of NASH. Changes in histologic parameters of fibrosis and NASH as surrogates for clinical outcomes are widely used endpoints in most clinical trials. However, the high variability in the interpretation of histologic findings by expert pathologists and the issue of sampling error led to a reluctance from the FDA and the European Medicines Agency to rely on histology-based endpoints alone.[43]

There are growing data from large databases (eg, Non-invasive Biomarkers of Metabolic Liver Disease [NIMBLE] and Liver Investigation: Testing Marker Utility in Steatohepatitis [LITMUS] consortia) and from clinical trials on the benefits and limitations of various noninvasive serum and imaging biomarkers, compared with histologic parameters.[44–46] Importantly, emerging data suggest that serum biomarkers are able to predict adverse clinical outcomes.[47,48] Once sufficient data are accrued, it is likely that nonhistological endpoints will gain acceptance by regulatory authorities, so both patient selection and treatment response will be assessed noninvasively.

Modifiers of NAFLD and the Placebo Effect

NAFLD represents a syndrome with a wide spectrum of physiologic adaptations and diseases. Although there are commonalities in the pre-disposing factors, there is no single clear etiologic factor, suggesting that there are multiple contributing causes and therefore metabolic pathways involved.[49] Manipulation of single pathways is likely to lead to compensation by other pathways ameliorating any drug effect. Moreover, disease modifiers, such as alcohol intake, genetic factors, and microbial dysbiosis accentuate differences in disease progression across individuals. These factors may influence specific cellular and molecular drivers of disease development and progression.[50] Differences in such drivers of the disease may explain the highly variable interindividual response rates in clinical trials.

Another important challenge in NASH drug development is the "placebo" response, which, depending on the endpoint, can be as high as 40%.[51] Modest differences, compared with placebo, have accentuated the variable and often high interobserver variability in the histologic interpretation of liver biopsy. A meta-analysis of control arms in NASH randomized controlled trials (RCTs) found that 25% of patients given a placebo had an improvement in their NAFLD activity score (NAS) by $\geq$ 2 points.[51] Further analysis showed improvements in placebo arms larger than previously anticipated therapeutic effect sizes, including a resolution of NASH without worsening of fibrosis in 9% to 21% of participants and a significant reduction in liver fat.[52] The cause of this seems to be multi-factorial. Being South American, changes in body mass index, a higher baseline NAS, frequent medical visits, and the Hawthorne effect have been suggested as contributing factors. Innovative trial designs in NAFLD should take into account the placebo effect and disease modifiers.

MULTIDISCIPLINARY APPROACHES

Dietary Treatment for NAFLD

Lifestyle intervention (LSI), with modifications in diet and physical activity, has become the first line of therapy in patients with NAFLD,[53] with dietary adjustments having been shown to be effective.[54] The Mediterranean diet has been associated with an improvement in NAFLD, mortality, and risk of T2DM and cardiovascular events in follow-up.[55] However, modifications in the composition of specific macro- or micronutrients in the diet are not the only central point. A new approach, called 'nutritional geometry', considers the importance of integrating nutrition, science, and the environment to understand how food components interact to regulate the properties of diets affecting health and disease.[56] Age, sex, T2DM, and genes impact the effect of the diet on weight loss and NASH resolution. Stratifying patients according to the geometry of nutrition could improve the rate of response.[57] In fact, patients bearing the genotype GG in PNPLA3 and fat mass and obesity-associated TT showed a more pronounced response to the Mediterranean diet, promoting a better improvement of liver stiffness. In responders, we should keep all of these modifications and in nonresponders, we should consider their inclusion in clinical trials to obtain drug therapy with an antifibrotic effect.

Recently, a patient guideline for all patients at risk of or living with NAFLD was developed by clinicians, scientists, and patient representatives.[58] Its goals are to support patients in taking an active role in their own health care, develop a better understanding of what the doctor is discussing with them, and enable them to monitor their condition. Patients are also encouraged to ask the treating multidisciplinary team questions regarding personalized information on LSI. The guideline also summarizes a significant amount of scientific literature concerning lifestyle, translated into simple patient recommendations regarding weight reduction, dietary composition, physical activity, alcohol consumption, and smoking.

Influence of Alcohol on NAFLD

MetS and excessive alcohol use are the two main causes of acquired fatty liver disease worldwide. Although in academic medicine we tend to separate these two etiologies (ie, NAFLD and alcohol-related liver disease), in the real world many patients have both components and they synergize to cause a more advanced stage of the disease. There are many reports indicating that daily alcohol intake exacerbates the clinical course of NAFLD, increasing liver damage, the presence of steatosis in imaging, the development of advanced fibrosis, and the development of HCC.[59,60] These studies suggest that having a body mass index >30 kg/m^2 and drinking three or more alcoholic beverages per day have a strong synergistic effect. A controversial issue is whether low to moderate alcohol consumption could be protective against liver damage in patients with MetS. Some epidemiologic studies suggest that having one drink per day, especially wine, could be protective.[61] However, studies analyzing individual data indicate that even small amounts of alcohol could exacerbate liver injury in patients with obesity and diabetes.[62] As a result, most clinical practice guidelines recommend to patients with NAFLD abstain from alcohol.[63,64]

The difficulty in obtaining reliable information about the quantity of alcohol consumption hampers preventive interventions. Many patients underreport alcohol use for several reasons, including social stigma.[65] Simple biochemical tests such as an aspartate transaminase/alanine aminotransferase ratio greater than 1 in the absence of cirrhosis or high gamma-glutamyl-transpeptidase, suggest concomitant alcohol use. Alcohol metabolites are more specific and are being increasingly used in clinical practice.[66] Although blood alcohol detects recent alcohol intake, the presence of urine metabolites (ethyl-glucuronide and ethyl sulfate) can detect 1 to 3 days of alcohol intake. These metabolites can also be detected in hair and a recent study using this approach revealed that up to 25% of patients with presumed NAFLD have significant alcohol intake.[67] More recently, phosphatidyl-ethanol (PEth), a minor metabolite of ethanol that is stored in membranes of red blood cells and can be measured in whole blood samples, has emerged as a reliable biomarker of alcohol use. Blood PEth can detect alcohol use in the last 1 to 3 weeks, is quantitative, and is highly informative in patients being listed for liver transplantation.[68] However, the validity of this biomarker in patients with NAFLD is unknown and should be assessed in prospective clinical trials.

Diagnosis and Management of NAFLD in Endocrinology Clinical Settings

Endocrinologists are in an ideal position to identify persons at risk or to prevent the development of adverse outcomes of NAFLD. Screening for NAFLD is justified based on recent studies, indicating a high prevalence of liver fibrosis in individuals with T2DM or components of MetS and the association of liver fibrosis with the future risk of developing liver-related complications and overall higher mortality.[4,69] A guideline recently published by the American Association of Clinical Endocrinology provides endocrinologists and primary care clinicians with practical recommendations for the diagnosis and management of NAFLD.[70] The presence of T2DM and/or features of MetS should warrant further investigation for NAFLD and liver fibrosis. To identify patients with NAFLD at high risk of progression, the use of NITs for liver fibrosis is essential, especially the FIB-4 index, which offers an easy, inexpensive, and well-validated method of noninvasive diagnosis of advanced fibrosis in patients with NAFLD.

The ideal therapy for patients with NAFLD and T2DM or MetS would effectively improve liver injury and fibrosis and promote cardiometabolic health. Primary targets can be addressed concurrently and not necessarily sequentially, and the most appropriate strategy is the staggered use of the different therapeutic measures but giving priority to those that act on the causal factors (unhealthy diet, sedentarism, obesity) and/or improve a greater number of pathophysiological elements and components of MetS or, at least, have no negative effects on other metabolic parameters or cardiovascular comorbidities.[71,72] When choosing initial glucose-lowering medications, in addition to the hypoglycemic effect, those that have evidence of hepatic and cardiovascular benefit must be selected, such as pioglitazone and glucagon-like peptide-1 receptor agonists. Moreover, new drugs for T2DM in development to become FDA-approved, like tirzepatide, could radically change the treatment of NASH.[73] Therefore, raising the awareness of all health care providers, especially endocrinologists and primary care physicians, about the need for early diagnosis and treatment of NAFLD is critical.

NOVEL APPROACHES IN NAFLD MANAGEMENT

Metabolic Endoscopic Techniques

A study showed that a total body weight loss (TBWL) of 10% guaranteed NASH resolution in 90% of participants, fibrosis regression in 80%, and steatosis disappearance in 100%. Only 10% of participants reached enough body weight reduction,[74] though, suggesting that LSI might be insufficient for adequate and sustained weight loss. Therapies such as bariatric surgery (BS) and metabolic endoscopic techniques (METs) can be useful alternatives. BS produces a significant long-term weight loss and has been shown to ameliorate NAFLD.[75] However, BS is associated with acute and chronic postoperative complications, and is costly. The advantages of METs include their reversibility, short procedure time, technical ease, and lower adverse event rates.[76,77] METs may provide an effective treatment approach to obesity and associated comorbidities, including NAFLD. Intragastric balloons, a type of MET, have shown a TBWL of 11% at 12 months in obese subjects[78] and NASH resolution in 50% of patients with NAFLD.[79] However, only 50% of subjects will maintain the weight loss for >1 year.[80] Endoscopic sleeve gastroplasty (ESG), another type of MET, has gained recognition for being an effective weight loss procedure with an adequate safety profile. This technique involves an endoscopic suturing device to reduce gastric volume. A meta-analysis of studies with ESG showed a TBWL of 15% to 16% at 6 to 12 months.[81] A NASH RCT with ESG is currently underway, showing significant improvement in NAS score at 18 months in interim results (NCT03426111). Likewise, its efficacy is being evaluated in comparison with the surgical sleeve (NCT04060368).[82] Future research in METs should focus on defining its role in NAFLD treatment and its place in the NAFLD management algorithm.

Fecal Microbiota Transplantation

The gut microbiota is a modifiable organism in both health and disease and there is mounting evidence that it plays an important role in NAFLD. However, there are conflicting findings on the main microorganisms that mediate this effect.[83–85] Gut microbiome dysbiosis may contribute to NAFLD development by dysregulating the gut barrier, leading to the transfer of microbial metabolites and microbes into the liver, and affecting metabolic regulation of glucose and lipids in the host.[86] Most human microbiome studies are cross-sectional and analyze microbiota composition using 16S rRNA gene sequencing (identification bacteria at the species level); thus, how the gut microbiome influences liver disease susceptibility and the impact of strategies targeting it, like via fecal microbiota transplantation (FMT), for NASH treatment are largely unknown. FMT aims to re-balance the gut microbiome taken from the stool of healthy subjects. Recent clinical trials, with a short follow-up period (6 months) and a small sample size, found that allogenic FMT can reduce intestinal permeability and expression of hepatic genes involved in inflammation and lipid metabolism. FMT is emerging as a potential therapeutic option against NASH that deserves further investigation.[87,88] However, with the integration of multi-omics technologies, these untargeted therapies will likely be replaced by personalized and precision medicine approaches including bacteriophages that modulate specific bacterial enzymes and metabolic pathways.[89,90] Currently, we are still searching for the "ideal gut microbiota" for donation, a consortium of microbes that could improve NAFLD, although finding this formula will be very complex, given the variability of the composition of the microbiome depending on ethnicity, geography, and diet.[91] Furthermore, rather than the species of microbes, we may have to target their functions, such as metabolism. We need large RCTs in patients with NAFLD to evaluate the efficacy of microbiota-centered therapeutics and address the role of microbes and microbial factors on NAFLD progression and consider the complex interactions with confounding effects.

NAFLD Therapy Based on Hepatocyte Targeting

The fact that different cell types are implicated in the development of NAFLD (eg, hepatocytes and stellate and Kupffer cells) hampers the search for a therapeutic solution. In this context, the use of iRNA through therapeutic oligonucleotides has emerged as a promising new strategy to silence genes involved in the disease.[92] Targeting hepatocytes via delivery of oligonucleotides, such as antisense oligonucleotides or siRNA, have shown great efficacy in various liver diseases,[93,94] including NASH.[95,96] The key features of these molecules include: (a) specific delivery to the hepatocyte, avoiding undesirable side effects; (b) their stability with a half-life of about 1 month; (c) their subcutaneous administration; (d) their chemical synthesis; and (e) the possibility of personalized therapy based on the patient's profile of deregulated genes. These novel approaches will certainly open new avenues targeting not only the hepatocyte, but also other cell types involved in NAFLD. Identification of dysregulated genes will allow for patient-tailored predictions and testing of drug combinations, ultimately leading to personalized medicine in NAFLD.

Telemedicine and Digital Health Interventions in NAFLD

Telemedicine must combine synchronous services, such as video consultation, and asynchronous services, such as telemonitoring and mobile applications (mHealth).[97] Telemedicine is poised to accelerate personalized/precision medicine. Strong evidence exists for the use of telemedicine in improving screening rates for viral hepatitis and for the treatment of HCV in both community and prison settings,[98,99] as well as in other diseases such as hypertension and T2DM.[100,101] However, the usefulness of telemedicine in NAFLD is not well established. There is only one United Kingdom study that carried out a needs assessment with regards to digital health interventions for NAFLD[102] and an RCT from Singapore that concluded that mHealth can be effective in improving anthropometric measures and liver enzymes in patients with NAFLD.[103] Electronic medical records and mHealth can be used by primary care physicians to risk stratify patients with suspected NAFLD and guide referral and/or follow-up. Given that adherence to LSI is critical for NAFLD treatment, telemedicine might prove to play an important role in this sense. mHealth aimed at patients to induce changes in lifestyle regarding diet and physical activity needs to be better studied, including the maintenance of these changes over a prolonged period of time. Telemedicine-based interventions in NAFLD also require further investigation to determine their impact on screening, clinical outcomes, and prevention targets.

SUMMARY

As described in **Box 1** research priorities were identified to advance the agenda and better address fatty liver disease. The main priorities were divided into five sections: public health, diagnosis of NAFLD, NAFLD clinical trials, multidisciplinary approaches, and novel approaches in NAFLD management. Priorities range from improvements in

Box 1
NAFLD/NASH research priorities

Public Health

- The prevalence of NAFLD and NASH in all countries, including in key affected populations, must be better estimated.
- Establish fatty liver disease national registries to evaluate real-world disease burden, long-term disease progression, and clinical outcomes, to enable proper adjustment of health care services for the increasing liver disease burden.
- Socioeconomic costs must be reported at the national and, where relevant, sub-national levels.
- Policies that need to be in place to address fatty liver disease must be regularly studied, including in the context of the 2030 United Nations Sustainable Development Goals.
- Health inequities in NAFLD must be identified to address the "root-cause" at a societal level.

Diagnosis of NAFLD

- Define the population subgroup(s) and appropriate noninvasive tests (NITs) for liver fibrosis screening and staging.
- Determine the factors that may contribute to the development and progression of fatty liver disease in lean individuals.
- Holistically characterize patients with NAFLD to identify subphenotypes.

NAFLD clinical trials

- Conditional approval pathways building on NITs need to be defined for clinical trials by regulators.
- Barriers to clinical trial access to all patients affected, including minorities, marginalized populations, and those in low-resource countries, should be studied.

Multidisciplinary approaches

- Define which health care providers should be involved in NAFLD management and when.
- Calculate the costs of better integrating the management of NAFLD with different scenarios, such as co-location and telemedicine.
- Develop and evaluate integrated care models for patients with NAFLD.
- Investigate the use of short- and long-term alcohol biomarkers in patients with NAFLD, to improve patient stratification for adequate management.

Novel approaches in NAFLD management

- Continually assess combination therapies, as well as personalized approaches.
- Assess the determining factors of outcomes of metabolic endoscopic techniques and define their position within the NAFLD and obesity management algorithm.
- Evaluate the efficacy of microbiota-centered therapeutics and the role of microbes and microbial factors on NAFLD progression.
- Determine the best characteristics of telemedicine for screening, clinical outcomes, and prevention targets in NAFLD and analyze the cost-effectiveness of various telemedicine strategies.
- Evaluate the effectiveness of novel long-term, web-based, comprehensive behavioral lifestyle intervention programs for the treatment of NAFLD, among children, adolescents, and adults.
- Assess the contribution of additional technological tools, such as artificial intelligence.

clinical practice, identification of main molecular drivers, and development of personalized approaches to health policy issues. The next steps include further developing, with stakeholders from around the world, fatty liver disease research and action priorities, including a change in the nomenclature and definitions to better account for metabolic factors and concomitant alcohol intake. The global NAFLD community should continue to collaborate[104] to increase awareness of this prevalent disease, influence health authorities and policymakers, work with regulatory agencies in designing clinical trials, promote programs for early detection, and develop effective personalized therapies to improve the quality of life and prolong survival in patients with advanced liver disease.

CLINICS CARE POINTS

- Early diagnosis of NAFLD may delay or prevent complications and decrease liver fibrosis associated morbidity and mortality. Therefore, defining the population subgroups and appropriate non-invasive tests for liver fibrosis screening and staging is required.
- There are multiple signaling pathways and factors that regulate the development and progression of NAFLD. Identification of NAFLD subphenotypes is crucial to improve patient outcomes and develop precise treatment strategies.
- Lifestyle intervention is the first line of therapy in NAFLD patients. Importantly, age, sex, type 2 diabetes mellitus, and genes impact the effect of the diet on weight loss and NASH resolution; thus, a personalized diet could improve the rate of response.

- Metabolic endoscopic techniques, fecal microbiota transplantation, and therapeutic oligonucleotides may provide an effective treatment approach to NAFLD. Further research, focused on defining their role in NAFLD treatment, is needed.
- Telemedicine-based interventions in NAFLD might prove to play an important role in early diagnosis, management,and referral of patients with NAFLD.
- Progress in NAFLD prevention and treatment requires a better understanding of health system and costs for addressing NAFLD and further investigation into its pathophysiology, clinical subtypes, and precision medicine.

DISCLOSURE

J.L. Calleja reports consultancy and speaker fees from Echosens, Advanz Ph, and MSD, outside of the submitted work. K. Cusi is a consultant for Altimmune, Akero, Arrowhead, AstraZeneca, 89Bio, BMS, Coherus, Intercept, Lilly, Madrigal, Merck, Novo Nordisk, Quest, Sagimet, Sonic Incytes, Terns, Thera Technologies, and MSD, outside of the submitted work. J.F. Dillon has received research grants and lecture honoraria from MSD, AbbVie, and Gilead, outside of the submitted work. M.L. Martínez-Chantar advises for Mitotherapeutix LCC, outside of the submitted work. J.M. Schattenberg reports consultancy for Apollo Endosurgery, Albireo Pharma Inc, Bayer, BMS, Boehringer Ingelheim, Echosens, Gilead Sciences, GSK, Intercept Pharmaceuticals, Ipsen, Inventiva Pharma, Madrigal, MSD, Nordic Bioscience, Novartis, Novo Nordisk, Pfizer, Roche, Sanofi, and Siemens Healthcare GmbH and research Funding from Gilead Sciences, Boehringer Ingelheim, Nordic Bioscience, and Siemens Healthcare GmbH, outside of the submitted work. J. Crespo reports consulting and personal fees from Gilead Sciences, AbbVie, MSD, Shionogi, Intercept Pharmaceuticals, Janssen Pharmaceuticals Inc, Celgene, and Alexion, outside of the submitted work. J.V. Lazarus acknowledges grants and speaker fees from AbbVie, Gilead Sciences, and MSD and speaker fees from Genfit, Intercept, Janssen, Novo Nordisk, and ViiV, outside of the submitted work. P. Iruzubieta, R. Bataller, M.T. Arias-Loste, M. Arrese, G. Castro-Narro, M. Mateo, A. Pérez, M.E. Rinella, M. Romero-Gómez, and S. Zelber-Sagi have nothing to disclose.

ACKNOWLEDGMENTS

The authors acknowledge the Valdecilla Biomedical Research Institute (Santander, Spain) for supporting the International Precision Medicine Forum: NAFLD Updated. J.V. Lazarus acknowledges institutional support to ISGlobal from the Spanish Ministry of Science and Innovation and the State Research Agency through the “Centro de Excelencia Severo Ochoa 2019-2023” Program (CEX2018-000806-S) and from the “Generalitat de Catalunya” through the CERCA Program. Funding from the Spanish Instituto de Salud Carlos III Grant (FIS - PI18/01304 to J. Crespo) and from the Chilean Agencia Nacional de Investigación y Desarrollo (ANID) through the Fondo Nacional de Desarrollo Científico y Tecnológico (FONDECYT 1191145 to M. Arrese) is also acknowledged.

REFERENCES

1. Byrne CD, Targher G. NAFLD: a multisystem disease. J Hepatol 2015;62(1): S47–64.
2. Younossi ZM, Henry L. Fatty liver through the ages: nonalcoholic steatohepatitis. Endocr Pract 2022;28(2):204–13.

3. Riazi K, Azhari H, Charette JH, et al. The prevalence and incidence of NAFLD worldwide: a systematic review and meta-analysis. Lancet Gastroenterol Hepatol 2022;7(9):851–61.
4. Younossi ZM, Golabi P, de Avila L, et al. The global epidemiology of NAFLD and NASH in patients with type 2 diabetes: a systematic review and meta-analysis. J Hepatol 2019;71(4):793–801.
5. Machado M, Marques-Vidal P, Cortez-Pinto H. Hepatic histology in obese patients undergoing bariatric surgery. J Hepatol 2006;45(4):600–6.
6. Younossi ZM, Blissett D, Blissett R, et al. The economic and clinical burden of nonalcoholic fatty liver disease in the United States and Europe. Hepatology 2016;64(5):1577–86.
7. Lazarus JV, Mark HE, Anstee QM, et al. Advancing the global public health agenda for NAFLD: a consensus statement. Nat Rev Gastroenterol Hepatol 2022;19(1):60–78.
8. Lazarus JV, Anstee QM, Hagström H, et al. Defining comprehensive models of care for NAFLD. Nat Rev Gastroenterol Hepatol 2021;18(10):717–29.
9. Lazarus JV, Mark HE, Villota-Rivas M, et al. The global NAFLD policy review and preparedness index: are countries ready to address this silent public health challenge? J Hepatol 2022;76(4):771–80.
10. Díaz LA, Fuentes-López E, Ayares G, et al. The establishment of public health policies and the burden of non-alcoholic fatty liver disease in the Americas. Lancet Gastroenterol Hepatol 2022;7(6):552–9.
11. Reaching consensus on NAFLD nomenclature | AASLD. Available at: https://www.aasld.org/news/reaching-consensus-nafld-nomenclature. Accessed July 21, 2022.
12. Marcellin P, Kutala BK. Liver diseases: a major, neglected global public health problem requiring urgent actions and large-scale screening. Liver Int 2018; 38(Suppl 1):2–6.
13. Ginès P, Castera L, Lammert F, et al. Population screening for liver fibrosis: toward early diagnosis and intervention for chronic liver diseases. Hepatology 2022;75(1):219–28.
14. Caballería L, Pera G, Arteaga I, et al. High prevalence of liver fibrosis among European adults with unknown liver disease: a population-based study. Clin Gastroenterol Hepatol 2018;16(7):1138–45, e5.
15. Llop E, Iruzubieta P, Perelló C, et al. High liver stiffness values by transient elastography related to metabolic syndrome and harmful alcohol use in a large Spanish cohort. United Eur Gastroenterol J 2021;9(8):892–902.
16. Berzigotti A, Tsochatzis E, Boursier J, et al. EASL Clinical Practice Guidelines on non-invasive tests for evaluation of liver disease severity and prognosis - 2021 update. J Hepatol 2021;75(3):659–89.
17. Inegi. ESTADÍSTICA DE DEFUNCIONES REGISTRADAS DE ENERO A JUNIO DE 2021 (PRELIMINAR). Available at: https://www.paho.org/hq/dmdocuments/2016/2016-cha-epidemiological-calendar.pdf. Accessed July 17, 2022.
18. Gonzalez-Chagolla A, Olivas-Martinez A, Ruiz-Manriquez J, et al. Cirrhosis etiology trends in developing countries: transition from infectious to metabolic conditions. Report from a multicentric cohort in central Mexico. Lancet Reg Health-Americas 2022;7:100151.
19. Ruiz-Manriquez J, Olivas-Martinez A, Chávez-García LC, et al. Prevalence of metabolic-associated fatty liver disease in Mexico and development of a screening tool: the MAFLD-S score. Gastro Hep Adv 2022;1(3):352–8.

20. Martínez LA, Larrieta E, Calva JJ, et al. The expression of PNPLA3 polymorphism could be the key for severe liver disease in NAFLD in hispanic population. Ann Hepatol 2017;16(6):909–15.
21. Marrón-Ponce JA, Tolentino-Mayo L, Hernández -FM, et al. Trends in ultra-processed food purchases from 1984 to 2016 in Mexican households. Nutrients 2018;11(1). https://doi.org/10.3390/NU11010045.
22. Arab JP, Díaz LA, Dirchwolf M, et al. NAFLD: challenges and opportunities to address the public health problem in Latin America. Ann Hepatol 2021;24:100359.
23. Armandi A, Schattenberg JM. Beyond the paradigm of weight loss in non-alcoholic fatty liver disease: from pathophysiology to novel dietary approaches. Nutrients 2021;13(6):1977.
24. Dillon JF, Miller MH, Robinson EM, et al. Intelligent liver function testing (iLFT): a trial of automated diagnosis and staging of liver disease in primary care. J Hepatol 2019;71(4):699–706.
25. Kanwal F, Shubrook JH, Adams LA, et al. Clinical care pathway for the risk stratification and management of patients with nonalcoholic fatty liver disease. Gastroenterology 2021;161(5):1657–69.
26. Hardy T, Oakley F, Anstee QM, et al. Nonalcoholic fatty liver disease: pathogenesis and disease spectrum. Annu Rev Pathol Mech Dis 2016;11:451–96.
27. Dulai PS, Singh S, Patel J, et al. Increased risk of mortality by fibrosis stage in nonalcoholic fatty liver disease: systematic review and meta-analysis. Hepatology 2017;65(5):1557–65.
28. Eslam M, Sanyal AJ, George J. An international consensus panel. MAFLD: a consensus-driven proposed nomenclature for metabolic associated fatty liver disease. Gastroenterology 2020;158(7):1999–2014.
29. Ahmed OT, Gidener T, Mara KC, et al. Natural history of nonalcoholic fatty liver disease with normal body mass index: a population-based study. Clin Gastroenterol Hepatol 2022;20(6):1374–81, e6.
30. Younes R, Govaere O, Petta S, et al. Caucasian lean subjects with non-alcoholic fatty liver disease share long-term prognosis of non-lean: time for reappraisal of BMI-driven approach? Gut 2022;71(2):382–90.
31. Younes R, Bugianesi E. NASH in lean individuals. Semin Liver Dis 2019;39(1):86–95. https://doi.org/10.1055/s-0038-1677517.
32. Long MT, Noureddin M, Lim JK. AGA clinical practice update: diagnosis and management of nonalcoholic fatty liver disease in lean individuals: expert review. Gastroenterology 2022. https://doi.org/10.1053/J.GASTRO.2022.06.023.
33. Bianco C, Jamialahmadi O, Pelusi S, et al. Non-invasive stratification of hepatocellular carcinoma risk in non-alcoholic fatty liver using polygenic risk scores. J Hepatol 2021;74(4):775–82.
34. Alonso C, Fernández-Ramos D, Varela-Rey M, et al. Metabolomic identification of subtypes of nonalcoholic steatohepatitis. Gastroenterology 2017;152(6):1449–61, e7.
35. Martínez-Arranz I, Bruzzone C, Noureddin M, et al. Metabolic subtypes of patients with NAFLD exhibit distinctive cardiovascular risk profiles. Hepatology 2022. https://doi.org/10.1002/HEP.32427.
36. Luukkonen PK, Qadri S, Ahlholm N, et al. Distinct contributions of metabolic dysfunction and genetic risk factors in the pathogenesis of non-alcoholic fatty liver disease. J Hepatol 2022;76(3):526–35.

37. Harrison SA, Wong VWS, Okanoue T, et al. Selonsertib for patients with bridging fibrosis or compensated cirrhosis due to NASH: results from randomized phase III STELLAR trials. J Hepatol 2020;73(1):26–39.
38. Harrison SA, Goodman Z, Jabbar A, et al. A randomized, placebo-controlled trial of emricasan in patients with NASH and F1-F3 fibrosis. J Hepatol 2020; 72(5):816–27.
39. Harrison SA, Abdelmalek MF, Caldwell S, et al. Simtuzumab is ineffective for patients with bridging fibrosis or compensated cirrhosis caused by nonalcoholic steatohepatitis. Gastroenterology 2018;155(4):1140–53.
40. Allen AM, Therneau TM, Ahmed OT, et al. Clinical course of non-alcoholic fatty liver disease and the implications for clinical trial design. J Hepatol 2022. https://doi.org/10.1016/J.JHEP.2022.07.004.
41. EMA. Reflection paper on regulatory requirements for the development of medicinal products for chronic non-infectious liver diseases (PBC, PSC, NASH). 2018. Available at: www.ema.europa.eu/contact. Accessed July 17, 2022.
42. Noncirrhotic nonalcoholic steatohepatitis with liver fibrosis: developing drugs for treatment guidance for industry DRAFT GUIDANCE. Available at: https://www.fda.gov/Drugs/GuidanceComplianceRegulatoryInformation/Guidances/default.htm. Accessed July 17, 2022.
43. Loomba R, Ratziu V, Harrison SA, et al. Expert panel review to compare FDA and EMA guidance on drug development and endpoints in nonalcoholic steatohepatitis. Gastroenterology 2022;162(3):680–8.
44. Sanyal AJ, Shankar SS, Calle RA, et al. Non-invasive biomarkers of nonalcoholic steatohepatitis: the FNIH NIMBLE project. Nat Med 2022;28(3):430–2.
45. Johnson K, Leary PJ, Govaere O, et al. Increased serum miR-193a-5p during non-alcoholic fatty liver disease progression: diagnostic and mechanistic relevance. JHEP reports Innov Hepatol 2021;4(2). https://doi.org/10.1016/J.JHEPR.2021.100409.
46. Rinella ME, Dufour JF, Anstee QM, et al. Non-invasive evaluation of response to obeticholic acid in patients with NASH: results from the REGENERATE study. J Hepatol 2022;76(3):536–48.
47. Boursier J, Hagström H, Ekstedt M, et al. Non-invasive tests accurately stratify patients with NAFLD based on their risk of liver-related events. J Hepatol 2022;76(5):1013–20.
48. Vieira Barbosa J, Milligan S, Frick A, et al. Fibrosis-4 index can independently predict major adverse cardiovascular events in nonalcoholic fatty liver disease. Am J Gastroenterol 2022;117(3):453–61.
49. Armandi A, Schattenberg JM. NAFLD between genes and environment: what drives fibrogenesis? Gut 2021;70(5):815–6.
50. Tilg H, Adolph TE, Moschen AR. Multiple parallel hits hypothesis in nonalcoholic fatty liver disease: revisited after a decade. Hepatology 2021;73(2):833.
51. Han MAT, Altayar O, Hamdeh S, et al. Rates of and factors associated with placebo response in trials of pharmacotherapies for nonalcoholic steatohepatitis: systematic review and meta-analysis. Clin Gastroenterol Hepatol 2019;17(4):616–29. Available at: https://pubmed.ncbi.nlm.nih.gov/29913275/. Accessed February 9, 2021.
52. Noureddin N, Han MAT, Alkhouri N, et al. Accounting for the placebo effect and optimizing outcomes in clinical trials of nonalcoholic steatohepatitis (NASH). Curr Hepatol Reports 2020;19(1):63–9.
53. Romero-Gómez M, Zelber-Sagi S, Trenell M. Treatment of NAFLD with diet, physical activity and exercise. J Hepatol 2017;67(4):829–46.

54. Hassani Zadeh S, Mansoori A, Hosseinzadeh M. Relationship between dietary patterns and non-alcoholic fatty liver disease: a systematic review and meta-analysis. J Gastroenterol Hepatol 2021;36(6):1470–8.
55. Abenavoli L, Boccuto L, Federico A, et al. Diet and non-alcoholic fatty liver disease: the mediterranean way. Int J Environ Res Public Health 2019;16(17):3011.
56. Berná G, Romero-Gomez M. The role of nutrition in non-alcoholic fatty liver disease: pathophysiology and management. Liver Int 2020;40(S1):102–8.
57. Simpson SJ, Raubenheimer D, Cogger VC, et al. The nutritional geometry of liver disease including non-alcoholic fatty liver disease. J Hepatol 2018;68(2):316–25.
58. Francque SM, Marchesini G, Kautz A, et al. Non-alcoholic fatty liver disease: a patient guideline. JHEP Reports Innov Hepatol 2021;3(5):100322.
59. Loomba R, Bettencourt R, Barrett-Connor E. Synergistic association between alcohol intake and body mass index with serum alanine and aspartate aminotransferase levels in older adults: the Rancho Bernardo Study. Aliment Pharmacol Ther 2009;30(11–12):1137–49.
60. Ascha MS, Hanouneh IA, Lopez R, et al. The incidence and risk factors of hepatocellular carcinoma in patients with nonalcoholic steatohepatitis. Hepatology 2010;51(6):1972–8.
61. Moriya A, Iwasaki Y, Ohguchi S, et al. Roles of alcohol consumption in fatty liver: a longitudinal study. J Hepatol 2015;62(4):921–7.
62. Blomdahl J, Nasr P, Ekstedt M, et al. Moderate alcohol consumption is associated with advanced fibrosis in non-alcoholic fatty liver disease and shows a synergistic effect with type 2 diabetes mellitus. Metabolism 2021;115:154439.
63. European Association for the Study of the Liver (EASL). Electronic address: easloffice@easloffice.eu, European association for the study of diabetes (EASD), European association for the study of obesity (EASO). EASL–EASD–EASO clinical practice guidelines for the management of non-alcoholic fatty liver disease. J Hepatol 2016;64(6):1388–402.
64. Aller R, Fernández-Rodríguez C, lo Iacono O, et al. Consensus document. Management of non-alcoholic fatty liver disease (NAFLD). Clinical practice guideline. Gastroenterol Hepatol 2018;41(5):328–49.
65. Carol M, Pérez-Guasch M, Solà E, et al. Stigmatization is common in patients with non-alcoholic fatty liver disease and correlates with quality of life. PLoS One 2022;17(4):e0265153.
66. Cabezas J, Lucey MR, Bataller R. Biomarkers for monitoring alcohol use. Clin Liver Dis 2016;8(3):59–63.
67. Staufer K, Huber-Schönauer U, Strebinger G, et al. Ethyl glucuronide in hair detects a high rate of harmful alcohol consumption in presumed non-alcoholic fatty liver disease. J Hepatol 2022. https://doi.org/10.1016/J.JHEP.2022.04.040.
68. Selim R, Zhou Y, Rupp LB, et al. Availability of PEth testing is associated with reduced eligibility for liver transplant among patients with alcohol-related liver disease. Clin Transplant 2022;36(5):e14595.
69. Taylor RS, Taylor RJ, Bayliss S, et al. Association between fibrosis stage and outcomes of patients with nonalcoholic fatty liver disease: a systematic review and meta-analysis. Gastroenterology 2020;158(6):1611–25, e12.
70. Cusi K, Isaacs S, Barb D, et al. American association of clinical Endocrinology clinical practice guideline for the diagnosis and management of nonalcoholic fatty liver disease in primary care and Endocrinology clinical settings: Co-sponsored by the American association for the study of liver diseases (AASLD). Endocr Pract 2022;28(5):528–62.

71. Stefan N, Cusi K. A global view of the interplay between non-alcoholic fatty liver disease and diabetes. Lancet Diabetes Endocrinol 2022;10(4):284–96.
72. Liao HW, Saver JL, Wu YL, et al. Pioglitazone and cardiovascular outcomes in patients with insulin resistance, pre-diabetes and type 2 diabetes: a systematic review and meta-analysis. BMJ Open 2017;7(1):e013927.
73. Jastreboff AM, Aronne LJ, Ahmad NN, et al. Tirzepatide once weekly for the treatment of obesity. N Engl J Med 2022;387(3). https://doi.org/10.1056/NEJMOA2206038.
74. Vilar-Gomez E, Martinez-Perez Y, Calzadilla-Bertot L, et al. Weight loss through lifestyle modification significantly reduces features of nonalcoholic steatohepatitis. Gastroenterology 2015;149(2):367–78, e5.
75. Lassailly G, Caiazzo R, Ntandja-Wandji LC, et al. Bariatric surgery provides long-term resolution of nonalcoholic steatohepatitis and regression of fibrosis. Gastroenterology 2020;159(4):1290–301, e5.
76. Hill C, Khashab MA, Kalloo AN, et al. Endoluminal weight loss and metabolic therapies: current and future techniques. Ann N Y Acad Sci 2018;1411(1):36–52.
77. Lopez-Nava G, Asokkumar R, Bautista-Castaño I, et al. Endoscopic sleeve gastroplasty, laparoscopic sleeve gastrectomy, and laparoscopic greater curve plication: do they differ at 2 years? Endoscopy 2021;53(3):235–43.
78. Abu Dayyeh BK, Kumar N, Edmundowicz SA, et al. ASGE Bariatric Endoscopy Task Force systematic review and meta-analysis assessing the ASGE PIVI thresholds for adopting endoscopic bariatric therapies. Gastrointest Endosc 2015;82(3):425–38, e5.
79. Bazerbachi F, Vargas EJ, Rizk M, et al. Intragastric balloon placement induces significant metabolic and histologic improvement in patients with nonalcoholic steatohepatitis. Clin Gastroenterol Hepatol 2021;19(1):146–54, e4.
80. Courcoulas A, Abu Dayyeh BK, Eaton L, et al. Intragastric balloon as an adjunct to lifestyle intervention: a randomized controlled trial. Int J Obes 2017;41(3):427–33.
81. Singh S, Hourneaux de Moura DT, Khan A, et al. Safety and efficacy of endoscopic sleeve gastroplasty worldwide for treatment of obesity: a systematic review and meta-analysis. Surg Obes Relat Dis 2020;16(2):340–51.
82. Lavín-Alconero L, Fernández-Lanas T, Iruzubieta-Coz P, et al. Efficacy and safety of endoscopic sleeve gastroplasty versus laparoscopic sleeve gastrectomy in obese subjects with Non-Alcoholic SteatoHepatitis (NASH): study protocol for a randomized controlled trial (TESLA-NASH study). Trials 2021;22(1):1–11.
83. Henao-Mejia J, Elinav E, Jin C, et al. Inflammasome-mediated dysbiosis regulates progression of NAFLD and obesity. Nature 2012;482(7384):179–85.
84. Zhou D, Pan Q, Shen F, et al. Total fecal microbiota transplantation alleviates high-fat diet-induced steatohepatitis in mice via beneficial regulation of gut microbiota. Sci Rep 2017;7(1):1529.
85. Le Roy T, Llopis M, Lepage P, et al. Intestinal microbiota determines development of non-alcoholic fatty liver disease in mice. Gut 2013;62(12):1787–94.
86. Iruzubieta P, Medina JM, Fernández-López R, et al. A role for gut microbiome fermentative pathways in fatty liver disease progression. J Clin Med 2020;9(5):1369.
87. Craven L, Rahman A, Nair Parvathy S, et al. Allogenic fecal microbiota transplantation in patients with nonalcoholic fatty liver disease improves abnormal

small intestinal permeability: a randomized control trial. Am J Gastroenterol 2020;115(7):1055–65.
88. Witjes JJ, Smits LP, Pekmez CT, et al. Donor fecal microbiota transplantation alters gut microbiota and metabolites in obese individuals with steatohepatitis. Hepatol Commun 2020;4(11):1578–90.
89. Bajaj JS, Ng SC, Schnabl B. Promises of microbiome-based therapies. J Hepatol 2022;76(6):1379–91.
90. Duan Y, Llorente C, Lang S, et al. Bacteriophage targeting of gut bacterium attenuates alcoholic liver disease. Nature 2019;575(7783):505–11. Available at: https://pubmed.ncbi.nlm.nih.gov/31723265/. Accessed December 20, 2019.
91. Erdmann J. How gut bacteria could boost cancer treatments. Nature 2022; 607(7919):436–9.
92. Alkhouri N, Gawrieh S. A perspective on RNA interference-based therapeutics for metabolic liver diseases. Expert Opin Investig Drugs 2021;30(3):237–44.
93. Wooddell CI, Blomenkamp K, Peterson RM, et al. Development of an RNAi therapeutic for alpha-1-antitrypsin liver disease. JCI Insight 2020;5(12). https://doi.org/10.1172/JCI.INSIGHT.135348.
94. Balwani M, Sardh E, Ventura P, et al. Phase 3 trial of RNAi therapeutic givosiran for acute intermittent porphyria. N Engl J Med 2020;382(24):2289–301.
95. Lindén D, Ahnmark A, Pingitore P, et al. Pnpla3 silencing with antisense oligonucleotides ameliorates nonalcoholic steatohepatitis and fibrosis in Pnpla3 I148M knock-in mice. Mol Metab 2019;22:49–61.
96. Cansby E, Nuñez-Durán E, Magnusson E, et al. Targeted delivery of Stk25 antisense oligonucleotides to hepatocytes protects mice against nonalcoholic fatty liver disease. Cell Mol Gastroenterol Hepatol 2019;7(3):597–618.
97. Telehealth Basics - ATA. Available at: https://www.americantelemed.org/resource/why-telemedicine/. Accessed July 22, 2022.
98. MacLean CD, Berger C, Cangiano ML, et al. Impact of electronic reminder systems on hepatitis C screening in primary care. J Viral Hepat 2018;25(8):939–44.
99. Cuadrado A, Cobo C, Mateo M, et al. Telemedicine efficiently improves access to hepatitis C management to achieve HCV elimination in the penitentiary setting. Int J Drug Policy 2021;88:103031.
100. Yin BD, Tu DH, Yang N, et al. The application effect of internet technology on managing patients with hypertension in a medical center: a prospective case-control study. Medicine (Baltim) 2021;100(50):E28027.
101. Faruque LI, Wiebe N, Ehteshami-Afshar A, et al. Effect of telemedicine on glycated hemoglobin in diabetes: a systematic review and meta-analysis of randomized trials. CMAJ (Can Med Assoc J) 2017;189(9):E341–64.
102. Hallsworth K, McPherson S, Anstee QM, et al. Digital intervention with lifestyle coach support to target dietary and physical activity behaviors of adults with nonalcoholic fatty liver disease: systematic development process of VITALISE using intervention mapping. J Med Internet Res 2021;23(1):e20491.
103. Lim SL, Johal J, Ong KW, et al. Lifestyle intervention enabled by mobile technology on weight loss in patients with nonalcoholic fatty liver disease: randomized controlled trial. JMIR mHealth uHealth 2020;8(4):e14802.
104. Schattenberg J.M., Allen A.M., Jarvis H., et al., A multistakeholder approach to innovations in NAFLD care, Commun Med (Lond), 3 (1), 1.

Printed and bound by CPI Group (UK) Ltd, Croydon, CR0 4YY
03/10/2024
01040466-0007